Management
of Common
Musculoskeletal
Disorders

Randolph M. Kessler, B.S., R.P.T.

Instructor, Division of Physical Therapy
Department of Rehabilitation Medicine
University of Washington School of Medicine
Seattle, Washington

Darlene Hertling, B.S., R.P.T.

Lecturer, Division of Physical Therapy
Department of Rehabilitation Medicine
University of Washington School of Medicine
Seattle, Washington

with three contributors

Illustrations by Elizabeth Kessler

Management of Common Musculoskeletal Disorders

Physical Therapy Principles and Methods

HARPER & ROW, PUBLISHERS

PHILADELPHIA

Cambridge
New York
Hagerstown
San Francisco

1817

London
Mexico City
São Paulo
Sydney

Acquisitions Editor: Lisa A. Biello
Sponsoring Editor: Sanford Robinson
Manuscript Editor: Janet Baker
Indexer: Norman Duren
Art Director: Maria S. Karkucinski
Designer: Ronald Dorfman
Production Assistant: Barney Fernandes
Compositor: Bi-Comp, Incorporated

The authors and publisher have exerted every effort to ensure that drug selection and dosage set forth in this text are in accord with current recommendations and practice at the time of publication. However, in view of ongoing research, changes in government regulations, and the constant flow of information relating to drug therapy and drug reactions, the reader is urged to check the package insert for each drug for any change in indications and dosage and for added warnings and precautions. This is particularly important when the recommended agent is a new or infrequently employed drug.

7   9   11   12   10   8

Library of Congress Cataloging in Publication Data

Kessler, Randolph M.
  Management of common musculoskeletal disorders.

  Includes bibliographies and index.
  1. Physical therapy. 2. Musculoskeletal system—
Diseases—Patients—Rehabilitation. I. Hertling,
Darlene. II. Title. [DNLM: 1. Muscular diseases—
Therapy. 2. Bone diseases—Therapy. 3. Physical
therapy. WE 140 K42p]
RM700.K43   616.7′062   82-6072
ISBN 0-06-141429-8

To
Max, Tess, Tera
Gunter, Sonja, and Dieter

Contributors

DANIEL JONES, B.S., R.P.T.
Practicing Physical Therapist
Portland, Oregon

MAUREEN K. LYNCH, B.S., R.P.T.
Physical Therapist
Seattle, Washington

C. GERALD WARREN, M.P.H., R.P.T.
Associate Professor and Coordinator of Research
Department of Rehabilitation Medicine
University of Washington
Seattle, Washington

Preface

Management of Common Musculoskeletal Disorders: Physical Therapy Principles and Methods was written to fill a void in the rapidly expanding area of musculoskeletal medicine. The trend toward increased physical activity in a population living close to the limits of life expectancy has significantly increased the number of patients suffering musculoskeletal pain or dysfunction: more individuals are troubled with athletic injuries during their active years, and more are living long enough to experience one or more "degenerative" musculoskeletal ailments.

Patients presenting with musculoskeletal disorders which are not severely disabling and for which surgical intervention is not warranted have been among the most ignored and are perhaps the most mismanaged in modern medicine. Such patients have generated little interest among our highly trained specialists, the orthopaedist tending to be more concerned with surgically correctable problems, the rehabilitation team with permanent disabilities, and the family practitioner with "medical" disorders.

There are certainly excellent books available that deal with managing surgical orthopaedic disorders, with rehabilitating the severely disabled, and with specific areas of musculoskeletal medicine. However, few, if any, cover pertinent background material, principles of examination, concepts of management, and techniques of treatment as they relate to nonsurgical musculoskeletal medicine. *Management of Common Musculoskeletal Disorders* is a first and, we feel, very important step in developing a multifaceted approach to the musculoskeletal system.

This book was written for the student in the advanced stages of training and for the practicing clinician. Originally it was directed toward physical therapists, but we soon recognized that its cross-sectional appeal should be much broader. Patients with musculoskeletal disorders are likely to consult any one of a wide variety of practitioners, and we trust that orthopaedists, physiatrists, rheumatologists, family practitioners, orthopaedic assistants, physical therapy assistants, athletic trainers, orthopaedic nurses, and chiropractors will also find it useful.

The book is comprised of three sections: Basic Concepts, Selected Techniques, and Clinical Applications. Part One, dealing with background material, is not meant to be a comprehensive discussion of the musculoskeletal system, which is well covered in other texts. Our purpose is to expand the traditional taxonomies of joint structure and function so as to provide a conceptual model of the musculoskeletal system that can serve as a basis for the discussions of evaluation and treatment procedures which follow. The reader is led from the notion of a joint as the junction of two bones to a concept of the synovial joint as the basic unit of the musculoskeletal system. This approach is developed by considering the functional and structural joint components in detail, under both normal and pathological conditions. Included is a discussion of pain of deep somatic origin, a topic not extensively covered in current literature. Various phenomena associated with the perception of pain arising from the musculoskeletal tissues are discussed from a neurophysiological standpoint and related to various pain theories, including the currently popular "gate control" model. The key chapter in this first section, from a clinical standpoint, is the last one, on evaluation. A comprehensive system of patient evaluation is a crucial component of the clinician's overall approach to management. Ways to elicit subjective and objective data are presented, along with guides to the interpretation of findings. The whole section on background material is included to provide a scientific rationale for some of the physical therapy modalities and procedures used in the management of patients with common musculoskeletal disorders. This approach is much needed in an area of medicine in which treatment programs often incorporate remedies which are not well supported by experimental or empirical evidence of their efficacy.

Part Two, which concerns techniques, is not intended to include all the procedures that might be used in the management of patients with common musculoskeletal disorders. Rather, it introduces those techniques that are not traditionally included in most professional training programs. The most important of these are the specific joint mobilization techniques which, while not widely accepted by the medical profession, have been used for many years by a few medical practitioners and other types of health-care personnel. Because over the past century considerable misunderstanding and confusion have been associated with the use of joint mobilization techniques, a chapter dealing with the history of their use and misuse is included. (A considerable portion of the chapter on Arthrology in the section on Basic Concepts is devoted to providing a rationale and indications for the use of these techniques.) We consider this a major contribution of this book. A satisfactory rationale for using these techniques has not previously been presented in the literature, and this fact has contributed considerably to the confusion and misunderstanding just mentioned.

Part Three encompasses the clinical applications of the preceding material as it relates to selected conditions affecting the extremities, with reference to some common spinal disorders. Each of the regional chapters in this section is organized to include functional anatomy and biomechanics, specific regional evaluation, and common lesions and their management.

We believe that the distinguishing strong point of this work is the integration of well established principles of human structure, mechanics, physiology, and pathology, from numerous sources, to form a rational basis for the clinician's approach to managing patients with common musculoskeletal disorders. Growing consumerism and increasing governmental regulation of the health-care industry are placing heavier demands upon accountability. These demands must be met by increased emphasis on experimental and clinical research. An organized and scientifically based rationale for commonly used therapeutic procedures is essential in providing direction and guidance to research efforts. The material contained in this book, having evolved through descriptive research, provides just such a framework for further clinical and experimental investigations.

Randolph M. Kessler, B.S., R.P.T.
Darlene Hertling, B.S., R.P.T.

Acknowledgments

We are gratefully indebted to our expert contributors, critical colleagues, and fine typists, and to our patient publishers. We are particularly appreciative of the critical and enthusiastic support received from Dorothy Nelson, R.P.T., and Hal Egbert, R.P.T., who provided much of the original impetus which led to this study. Special acknowledgment and thanks must go to Elizabeth Kessler for her invaluable contribution; her creativity and technical talents have made the artwork an outstanding feature of this book. Drs. Benjamin Moffett and Ronald Guttu receive our thanks as well, for having critically reviewed the temporomandibular segment of this study. We are indebted to JoAnn McMillan, R.P.T., and Dr. Justus Lehmann, without whose support and encouragement this book would not have been written. Jenny Cole's expertise and efficiency in preparing the original manuscript were also important factors in the completion of this book.

Contents

Management
of Common
Musculoskeletal
Disorders

Part One
BASIC CONCEPTS

1 Embryology of the Musculoskeletal System

Randolph M. Kessler

Knowledge of the development of the musculoskeletal tissues is of particular value to the clinician, whether he deals mainly with patients with developmental disabilities, long-term rehabilitation problems, or common musculoskeletal disorders, because it yields insight into the phenomenon of pain perception, segmental innervation, repair processes, and general body organization. Surely every clinician must at some time have wondered, "Why does my patient with a neck problem feel pain in the scapula?" "Why do my patients with shoulder problems not feel pain in the shoulder, but in the upper arm?" "Why do some muscles receive innervation from all of the segments that they cross, whereas some muscles crossing many segments, such as the latissimus dorsi, receive innervation from relatively few segments?" Or "What is the explanation for the 'spiraling' nature of the dermatomes, especially in the lower limb?" The answers to some of these questions are not essential for competent clinical performance. However, some concepts, such as patterns of pain referral, are of the utmost importance in patient evaluation and treatment and should be pursued in depth. The study of embryology adds to our understanding of these concepts and deserves consideration here.

AXIAL COMPONENTS

The early developing embryo is composed of three primary, or germinal, layers— ectoderm, endoderm, and mesoderm. By the fourth week of development, the neural plate lying centrally in the ectoderm begins to invaginate into the underlying mesoderm. As this occurs, the peripheral margins of the neural plate gradually become more prominent and begin to approximate one another. Eventually they meet, forming the neural tube, which pinches off from the ectoderm and ends up lying within the mesoderm (Fig. 1-1). A similar phenomenon occurs ventrally; the notochordal process migrates and pinches off to form the notochord, which lies free in the ventral mesodermal layer.

The intrusion of the notochord and neural tube results in compaction of the mesodermal cells lying lateral to them. The compaction of the paraxial mesoderm forms the somites, of which there are originally 42 to 44 pairs: 4 occipital, 8 cervical, 12 thoracic, 5 lumbar, 5 sacral, and 8 to 10 coccygeal. These roughly coincide with what are to become the craniovertebral segments. The ventromedial cells of the vertebral somites, the sclerotomes, migrate medially to surround the notochord and neural tube (Fig. 1-2). Looking longitudinally (Fig. 1-3), each sclerotome is divided by a layer of cells called the *perichordal disc*. The cranial half of one sclerotome then unites with the

3

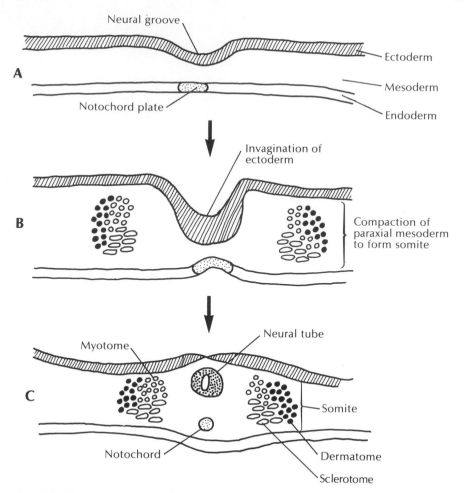

Fig. 1-1. Germinal layers of the early embryo. Invagination of the ectoderm forms the neural tube.

Fig. 1-2. Ventromedial migration of sclerotomic cells

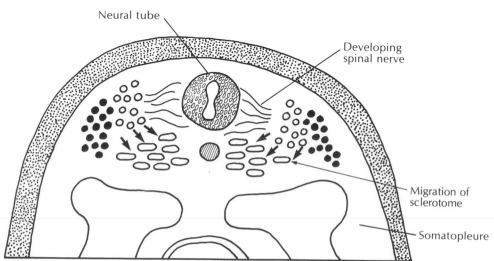

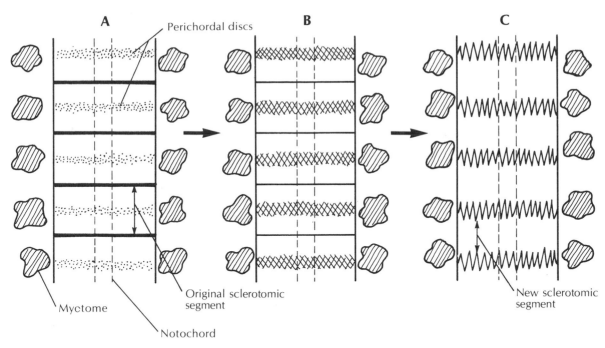

A Perichordal discs **B** **C**

Myctome

Original sclerotomic segment

Notochord

New sclerotomic segment

Fig. 1-3. Diagram illustrates the shift in relationship between a sclerotome and remaining somatic segments.

caudal half of the adjacent sclerotome, causing a shift in the relationship between sclerotomes and the remaining somites. The sclerotomes eventually chondrify, or become cartilaginous, then ossify to become the vertebrae. They also form cartilage, capsules, ligaments, and blood vessels. The perichordal disc becomes the annulus fibrosis, while the notochord becomes the original nucleus pulposis. The neural tube gradually differentiates into nerve tissue, becoming the spinal cord and sending out peripheral nerves to the adjacent mesoderm.

The more dorsomedial somite cells are the myotomes. These cells divide into the hypomere, which migrates around to form the ventrolateral trunk muscles, and the epimere, which forms the segmental muscles of the back. As this occurs, the spinal nerve divides to form the anterior primary ramus, which invades the hypomere, and the posterior primary ramus, which innervates the segmental back muscles. Because of the segmental shift in relation-

ship between the sclerotomes and myotomes, the segmental back muscles each cross at least one segment.

The remaining somatic cells are the dermatomes. These cells migrate out around the body wall, beneath the ectoderm, to form the dermal layer of skin. The dermis becomes innervated by sensory branches of the division (ramus) of the spinal nerve that innervates the muscles underlying it. The epidermal layer of skin is derived from the ectoderm.

LIMBS

The limb buds appear during the fourth week in the developing embryo. The forelimb, which appears a few days before the hindlimb, develops at the lateral body wall level with the C4–T2 segments. The hindlimb appears at an area level with the L1–S2 segments (Fig. 1-4). The early limb bud is a mass of mesenchymal cells arising from the laterally located somato-

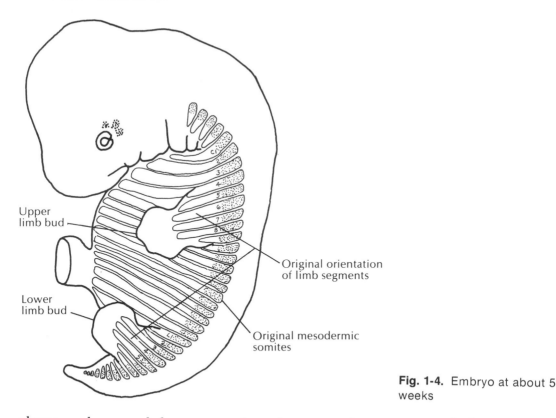

Upper
limb bud

Original orientation
of limb segments

Lower
limb bud

Original mesodermic
somites

Fig. 1-4. Embryo at about 5
weeks

pleure and covered by an ectodermal layer. The mesenchymal cells are pluripotential in that some will develop into osteoblasts, some into fibroblasts, some into myoblasts, and some into chondroblasts. The muscles of the limb buds develop *in situ* rather than from an invasion of cells from the myotome of the somite; this occurs as a result of differentiation of primitive mesenchymal cells into myoblasts, which become multinucleated muscle cells or fibers. The anterior primary divisions of the spinal nerve invade the developing limb buds to innervate the early muscle masses. Because of the intertwining of segmental nerves throughout the regional plexus and because the early muscle masses tend to divide or fuse with one another, each muscle typically receives innervation from more than one segment, and each segmental nerve tends to innervate more than one muscle. The intertwining of segments through the plexus also explains the overlapping, somewhat unpatterned skin innervation of the limbs.

The original orientation of the limb buds is such that the upper limb is positioned laterally, lying in the frontal plane at about 90° abduction, with the palm facing foreword. The lower limb is positioned similarly, with the hip externally rotated, the patella facing posteriorly, and the sole facing forward. Gradually the limbs rotate down into the fetal position. This rotation and abduction of the limb buds explains the spiraling nature of the limb segments (dermatomes, myotomes, and sclerotomes), especially in the lower limb, which undergoes more rotation. It also explains the anteversion and varus angle of the normal femoral neck in relation to the shaft of the femur, and the external torsion of the tibial shaft, which compensates for the internal torsion of the femur.

A guide to determining approximate segmental innervation of a limb is to imagine the limb in the original embryologic position. In this position, the more cranial aspects of the limb are innervated by cranial segments, the more caudal aspects by caudal segments. Thus the inner thigh, which was originally located cranially, is innervated by L2, while the outer lower leg, which was positioned caudally, is innervated by S1. Also worth noting is the fact that the scapula originates as part of the developing limb bud. As the limb develops, the scapula migrates to become "folded back" on the posterior body wall. This explains why the scapula, although it lies level with thoracic segments, is innervated primarily by cervical segments. Thus, pain of cervical origin is often referred to the scapulae, as well as to the arms. While most limb muscles split or fuse as they develop, some migrate. The latissimus is the most obvious example; it migrates so far as to attain a pelvic attachment. However, like other limb muscles it is innervated by the anterior primary divisions of mostly cervical segments, in spite of the fact that it lies over the back and extends over thoracic and lumbar segments.

The bones of the limbs also develop *in situ*. A condensation of mesenchymal cells first appears in the axial region of the limb bud. These differentiate into chondrocytes that form a "cartilage model" of the developing bone. Through the process of endochondral ossification, the cartilage model is gradually replaced by bone tissue. This occurs first in the diaphyseal regions of the long bones, extending toward both ends. Secondary centers of ossification appear at both ends, or epiphyses, and are separated from the primary area of ossification by the epiphyseal plates. The epiphyseal plate of cartilage tissue continues to develop cartilage cells that continue to undergo ossification, adding to the bone formed by the primary ossification site. In this way, the bone continues to grow in length until the epiphyseal plate closes in response to hormonal influence during the second decade of post

partum life (Fig. 1-5). The outer layer of the cartilage model remains as mesenchymal tissue that continually produces chondroblasts and osteoblasts that form bone tissue. This perichondrium—later becoming the periosteum—is responsible for the growth in width of the bones. It becomes highly innervated and highly vascularized, whereas the underlying layers of bone receive blood supply but little if any innervation.

The axial regions of the developing limb bud, which later become the joints, remain as condensations of mesenchymal tissue., In the case of synovial joints, the layers of "interzonal" mesenchyma adjacent to the developing bone ends differentiate into chondrocytes that secrete cartilage matrix, thus forming articular cartilage. The intervening middle zone undergoes cavitation to form the joint cavities, or discongruities, between joint surfaces. The surrounding layers of cells, which are continuous with the perichondrium, differentiate into fibrous capsule and synovium. The innervation of synovial joints is discussed in Chapter 2, Arthrology.

The development of the cartilage models and joint spaces and the subsequent rotation and abduction of the limb buds occurs by the seventh to eighth week of fetal life. By eight weeks, often before the mother realizes she is pregnant, the status and form of the fetal musculoskeletal system has largely been determined, and any significant teratogenic influences will have taken effect. The development of the musculo-skeletal system may be summarized as follows:

1. The musculoskeletal system is largely derived from the mesoderm.
2. The ectoderm forms the epidermal layer of skin and, through its invagination into the mesoderm, the nervous system.
3. Somites form in the paraxial mesoderm. These are (a) sclerotomes,

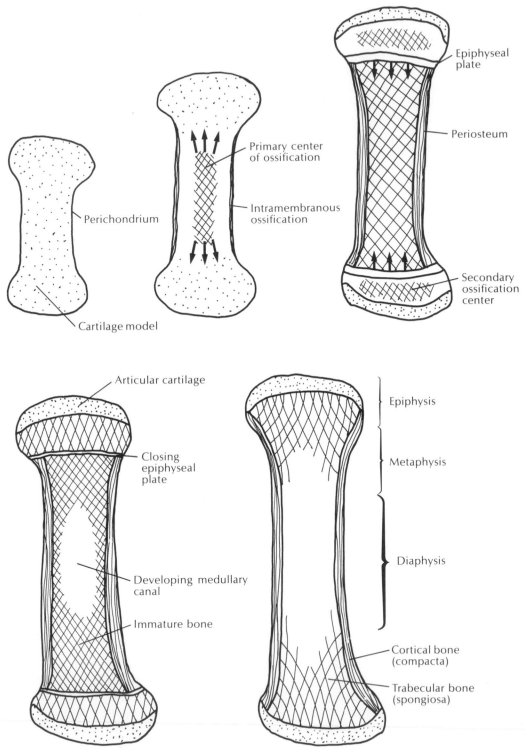

Fig. 1-5. Development of bone

which form bones, capsules, ligaments, cartilage, and blood vessels; (b) myotomes, which form muscles; and (c) dermatomes, which form the dermal layer of skin.

4. Because of the division of sclerotomes and subsequent fusion of caudal and cranial divisions of adjacent segments, a shift occurs that off-sets the relationship between axial sclerotomes and myotomes.

5. The limbs are not formed from somatic myotomes, sclerotomes, or dermatomes, but from the lateral somatic mesoderm, the somatopleure. The musculoskeletal structures of the limbs develop *in situ* from differentiation of primitive mesenchymal cells.

TERMINOLOGY

Although the limbs do not form from invasion of cells from the somatic myotomes, dermatomes, and sclerotomes, we do often refer to these segments as existing in the limbs. We speak of pain being referred to a particular sclerotome, weakness occurring within a particular myotome, or sensory changes in a dermatome. It is important to understand that these terms are useful in clinical description, but that they refer only to the source of innervation for a particular type of tissue and not the embryologic origin of the tissue, unless the terms are applied to the axial tissues. Thus when we speak of the C5 myotome we refer to those muscles in the limb receiving a significant innervation from the C5 anterior primary division or those muscles of the trunk innervated by the posterior primary division of C5. If we refer to the C5 sclerotome in the limb we mean those structures (capsules, ligaments, periosteum, etc.) receiving innervation from C5. We often say a particular joint is largely derived from a particular segment. In doing so, we imply that innervation to the structures forming the joint has its source in that spinal segment. More discussion concerning the clinical importance of segmental innervation is found in Chapter 3, Pain.

RECOMMENDED READINGS

Hollinshead H: Anatomy for Surgeons: Back and Limbs, 2nd ed, pp 207–211. New York, Harper & Row, 1969

Lewis WH: The development of the arm in man. Am J Anat 1:145, 1902

Lewis WH, Bardeen CF: The development of the limbs, body wall and back in man. Am J Anat 1:1, 1901

Warwick R, Williams P (eds): Gray's Anatomy, 35th ed, pp 81–90, 110–115, 126–132. Philadelphia, W B Saunders, 1973

2 *Arthrology*

Randolph M. Kessler

A complete study of human joints would include synchondroses, syndesmoses, symphyses, gomphoses, sutures, and synovial joints. For the sake of simplicity, and because the emphasis of clinical application is on joint mobilization techniques, this chapter will be restricted to discussion of the synovial joints, which are the most numerous and most freely movable of the various types of human joints. However, each of the above classifications of human joints includes joints capable of movement. Movement definitely takes place at most syndesmoses, such as the distal tibiofibular joint. The symphysis pubis moves, especially during pregnancy. There is some movement of the teeth in their sockets (gomphoses). In fact, even the sutures of the skull are movable, at least through the third decade of life. Some investigators have claimed that they move spontaneously, with a rhythm independent of heart rate or respiratory rate.[21] Based upon this claim, a few practitioners actually apply therapeutic mobilization to the sutures of the cranium.[21,40]

This discussion of synovial joints will emphasize the mutual influences of structure and function because the two cannot be dealt with adequately or understood when considered independently. We must expand our traditional "anatomical" concept of synovial joints to a "physiological" concept. In addition to those structures that anatomically define a joint, we must also include those structures responsible for normal movement at the joint (Fig. 2-1). With this approach we may consider the synovial joint as the basic unit of the musculoskeletal system and use it as a reference for discussing normal function and disorders of this system.

KINEMATICS

CLASSIFICATION OF JOINT SURFACES AND MOVEMENTS

The nature of movement at any joint is largely determined by the joint structure, especially the shapes of the joint surfaces. The traditional classification of synovial joints by structure includes the categories of spheroid, trochoid, condyloid, ginglymoid, ellipsoid, and planar joints.[50] It should be apparent even to someone with only a basic knowledge of human anatomy and kinesiology that this classification does not accurately define the shapes of joint surfaces or the movements that occur at each type of joint. The heads of the femur and humerus do not form true spheres or even parts of true spheres. A ginglymus, such as the humeroulnar joint, does not allow a true hinge motion on flexion and extension but rather a helical movement involving considerable rotation. The humeroradial joint, which is a trochoid joint, does not move about a single axis, or pivot, because the head of the radius is oval-shaped, having a longer diameter anteroposteriorly than mediolaterally. We can consider the interphalangeal joints, the carpometacarpal

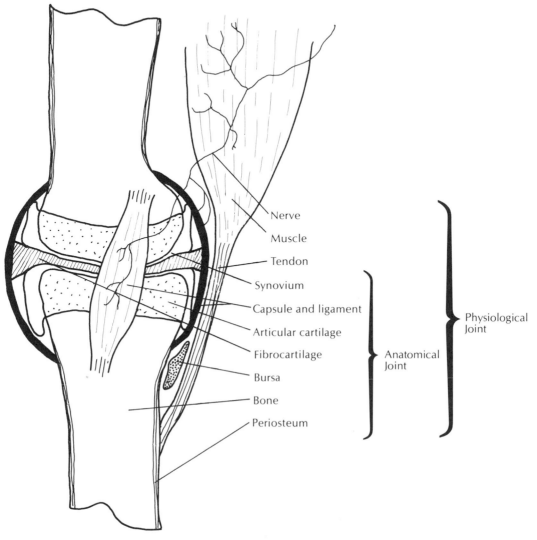

Fig. 2-1. Anatomical versus physiological concept of the synovial joint

Nerve

Muscle

Tendon

Synovium

Capsule and ligament

Articular cartilage

Fibrocartilage

Bursa

Bone

Periosteum

Anatomical Joint

Physiological Joint

joint of the thumb, the humeroulnar joint, and the calcaneocuboid joints as being sellar. However, the movements occurring at these joints vary greatly, as do the shapes of the joint surfaces. Therefore, although this classification of joint structures may serve a purpose for the anatomist, in itself it is not adequate for the clinician, such as the physical therapist, who must be concerned with the finer details of joint mechanics.

A similar problem exists with classify-

ing joint movement. The traditional classification of joint movement includes the following:[50]

Angular—Indicating an increase or decrease in the angle formed between two bones, for example, flexion–extension at the elbow

Circumduction—Movement of a bone circumscribing a cone, for example, circumduction at the hip or shoulder

Rotation—Movement occurring about the longitudinal axis of a bone, for example, internal–external rotation at the shoulder

Sliding—One bone slides over another with little or no appreciable rotation or angular movement, for example, movement between carpals

There are two problems with this classification that make it inadequate for those concerned with joint mechanics. First, it describes movement occurring between bones but ignores movement occurring between joint surfaces. We all will agree that movement takes place at joints, but often when we define movement we ignore what happens *at the joint.* An analogy would be to consider the movement of a door but to ignore the hinge. Secondly, angular movements almost never occur without some rotation, rotation nearly always occurs with some angular movement, gliding usually involves angular and rotary movement, and so on. Again, for our purposes, we need to expand our

classification to take into consideration the specifics of joint movement.

To expand our study of joint mechanics we must be able to define movements occurring between bones in such a way that they can easily be related to movements occurring between respective joint surfaces. Therefore, it is helpful to define the *mechanical axis* of any joint as a line that passes through the moving bone, touching the center of the relatively stationary joint surface and perpendicular to it (Fig. 2-2). We can now define *osteokinematic* movement—or movement occurring between two bones—according to the mechanical axis rather than according to the long axis of the moving bone as has been done in the past.[28,50] By relating osteokinematic movement to *arthrokinematic* movement—those movements occurring between joint surfaces—we will consider the movement of the mechanical axis of the moving bone relative to the stationary joint surface. In other words, we

Fig. 2-2. Osteokinetic movements may be defined by the mechanical axis. These movements are (*A*) spin and (*B*) swing.

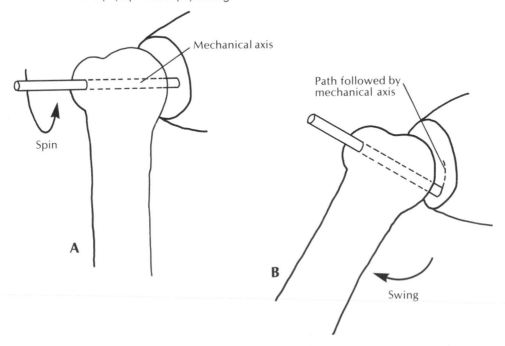

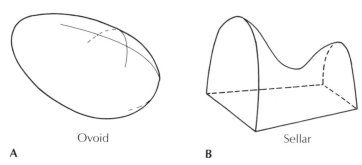

Fig. 2-3. Joint surfaces may be (*A*) ovoid or (*B*) sellar.   **A**   Ovoid   **B**   Sellar

will consider one joint surface as stationary and its opposing joint surface as moving relative to it. This relative movement will be defined according to the path traced by the line representing the mechanical axis of the joint on the stationary surface. The mechanical axis is determined at the starting point of a movement; once movement has begun, it maintains the same relationship to the moving bone, while moving relative to the stationary bone.

Joint Surfaces

Before discussing types of movement, it is necessary to define the shapes of joint surfaces since they largely determine the types of movements that may occur at the joint. No joint surface resembles a true geometric form; joint surfaces are neither spheres, ovals, or ellipses, nor are they true parts of these. We can, however, think of any joint surface as being part of an ovoid surface, that is, resembling the surface of an egg (Fig. 2-3,*A*). If we examine any cross section of an ovoid surface, we see that the radius of the joint surface changes constantly, forming a cardioid curve (Fig. 2-4). A typical example would be a sagittal section of a femoral condyle. Some joint surfaces, rather than representing part of a simple ovoid, might be considered a complex ovoid, or sellar, surface (Fig. 2-3,*B*). A sellar surface is convex in one cross-sectional plane and concave in the plane perpendicular to it, although the surfaces of each of these cross sections may be represented by a cardioid curve.

Referring again to a simple ovoid (Fig. 2-5), we call the shortest distance between any two points on the surface a *chord*, and any other line of continuous concavity toward the chord an *arc*. A three-sided figure made up of three chords is a *triangle*. A three-sided figure in which at least one side is formed by an arc is a *trigone*.

Joint Movements

Any movement in which the bone moves but the mechanical axis remains stationary is called a *spin* (see Fig. 2-2,*A*). True spin of the humerus, then, would be a movement of flexion combined with some adduction, since the glenoid cavity faces slightly forward. The bone, during true spin, would rotate about its mechanical

Fig. 2-4. A cardioid curve is representative of the cross-sectional shape of synovial joint surfaces. Because of the constantly changing radius, there is one position at which the radius of the opposing joint surface attains maximal congruency.

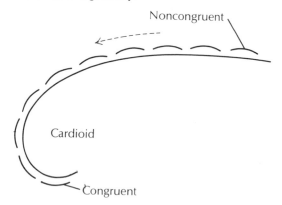

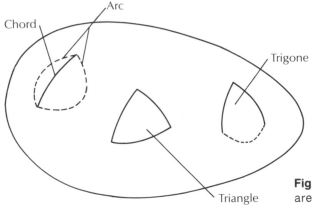

Fig. 2-5. Chords, arcs, a triangle, and a trigone are depicted on an ovoid surface.

axis. Note that when the mechanical axis of the joint and the long axis of the moving bone coincide, such as at the metacarpophalangeal and the femorotibial joints, the spin is what we traditionally call *rotation* at the joint. Where axes do not necessarily coincide, such as at the hip and shoulder, spin does not always occur when the joint "rotates." For example, spin occurs during internal and external rotation at the shoulder when the humerus is in a position of 90° of abduction; the mechanical axis (defined according to the starting position of movement) does coincide with the long axis of the humerus. However, internal and external rotations, performed with the arm to the side, do not involve spin at the joint surfaces; in this position, the mechanical axis does not coincide with the long axis of the humerus. A movement in which the mechanical axis follows the path of a chord is called a *chordate*, or *pure*, swing. If the end of the mechanical axis should trace the path of an arc during movement of the bone, we say that the bone has undergone an *arcuate*, or *impure*, swing (see Fig. 2-2,*B*).

Note that with flexion or abduction of the humerus, the movement is an impure swing. Pure swing of the humerus occurs during elevation in a plane somewhat midway between the planes of flexion and abduction (because the glenoid cavity faces about 40° forward). Also note that

internal and external rotation with the arm at the side is a movement of swing. We should be aware that an impure swing can be thought of as a pure swing with an element of spin, or rotation, about the mechanical axis. This element of rotation, which accompanies every impure swing, is called *conjunct* rotation. Habitual movements at any joint are usually impure swings. It follows that most habitual movements, or those movements that occur most frequently at any joint, involve some conjunct rotation. It is well known, for example, that the tibia rotates during flexion–extension at the knee. If you carefully watch the ulna flexing and extending on the humerus, you will see a similar rotation; the ulna pronates at the limits of extension and supinates at the extremes of flexion. The interphalangeal joints rotate considerably during flexion and extension. This is easily observed by holding the extended small fingers together, then flexing them simultaneously. The distal phalanges, especially, can be seen to supinate during flexion. Although such conjunct rotation occurs at every joint, it occurs to a much greater degree at joints with sellar surfaces than at those with simple ovoid surfaces. By now it should be evident that most of what we have traditionally considered "angular" movements are actually helical movements because of this element of conjunct rotation that accompanies them. This rotary component is an essential feature of normal joint mechanics.

ARTHROKINEMATICS

We can now examine more closely the study of what happens between joint surfaces on joint movement—arthrokinematics. When a bone swings relative to another bone, one of two types of movement may occur between joint surfaces.[28,50] If points at certain intervals on the moving surface contact points at the same intervals on the opposing surface, one surface is said to *roll* on the opposing surface (Fig. 2-6,A). This is analogous to a tire on a car contacting the road surface as the car rolls down the street— various points on the tire contact

various points on the road, the distance between contact points on the tire and road being the same. If, however, only one point on the moving joint surface contacts various points on the opposing surface, we say that *slide* is taking place (Fig. 2-6,B). This is analogous to a tire on a car that is skidding on ice. The tire is not turning, but is moving relative to the road surface—it is sliding.

Actually, in most movements at human synovial joints, both slide and roll take place simultaneously. If only roll were to take place, the moving bone would tend to dislocate before much movement could occur; if only slide were to occur, impingement of joint surfaces would prevent full movement (Fig. 2-7). Stated in another way, the moving bone must rotate about a particular center of motion (or centers of

Fig. 2-6. Arthrokinematic movements showing (A) *roll* and (B) *slide.*

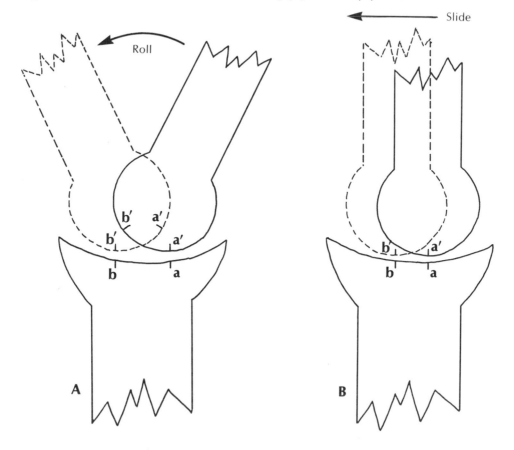

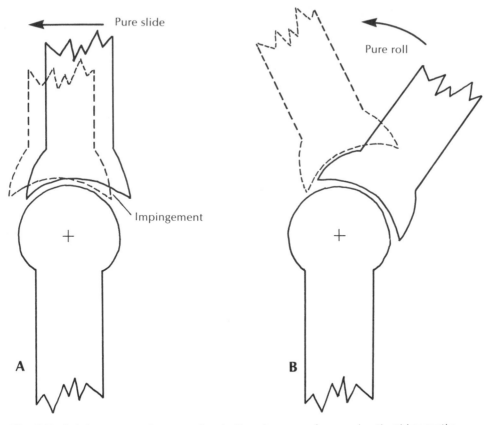

Fig. 2-7. Joint movements occurring in the absence of normal arthrokinematic movement cause (*A*) inpingement or (*B*) dislocation.

motion) in order for normal gliding to occur at the joint surfaces. If the bone should move about any other centroid of movement than what is normal for that joint, abnormal movement will occur between joint surfaces. Conversely, if normal movement does not or cannot occur between joint surfaces, the moving bone cannot move about its normal centroid of movement. This will be discussed later in the section Analysis of accessory joint motions. Clinically, a meniscus tear, which causes abnormal movement between joint surfaces, alters the normal centroid of movement at a joint.[16] This often results in abnormal stresses to the joint capsule, which are manifested as pain and muscle guarding. A tight joint capsule, which causes alteration in the normal centroid of movement, will result in abnormal

movement between joint surfaces, usually with premature cartilaginous compression before the movement is completed. Physiologically, the fact that slide and roll take place together allows for economy of articular cartilage with respect to the size of the joint surface necessary for movement. It also prevents undue wearing of isolated points on joint surfaces, which would occur if, for example, only slide took place.

The Concave-Convex Rule

Obviously, roll always occurs in the same direction as the swing of the bone. However, we can determine the direction of joint slide only by knowing the shapes of the joint surfaces. This is an important rule for anyone concerned with joint mechanics and will be referred to as the *concave-convex rule:* If a concave surface moves on a convex surface, roll and slide must occur in the same direction; if a convex surface moves on a concave surface, roll and slide occur in opposite directions (Fig. 2-8). Therefore, if the tibia extends on the stationary femur, the tibial joint surfaces must roll forward and slide forward on the femoral condyles in order for full movement to take place. However, if the femur extends on the stationary tibia, the femoral condyles must roll forward but slide backward on the tibia. If the humerus is elevated, the humeral head rolls upward but must slide inferiorly. During external rotation, with the arm at the side (a movement of swing), the head of the humerus must slide forward, whereas during internal rotation it must slide backward.

Clinically, we must apply these concepts in our approach to restoration of restricted joint motion. Traditionally, in our attempts to restore joint movement we have tended to work only on osteokinematic movements. For example, if flexion of the humerus is restricted, we use active or passive motion into flexion in an attempt to increase this movement. However, we must also consider that inferior slide of the head of the humerus on the glenoid cavity may be restricted as well. The manual therapist may use passive joint mobilization techniques to restore inferior slide in order to facilitate the restoration of upward swing of the humerus. Thus, by knowing the concave-convex rule, the therapist knows in which direction to apply joint slide mobilizations in order to increase any restricted swing of a bone.

The type of joint surface motion that occurs with a spin of a bone about its mechanical axis is actually a form of slide. However, it should be apparent that while slide occurs in one direction at one half of the joint, it occurs in the opposite direction at the other half of the joint surface.

Fig. 2-8. Relationship between arthrokinematic movements and osteokinematic movements for the "concave-convex rule"

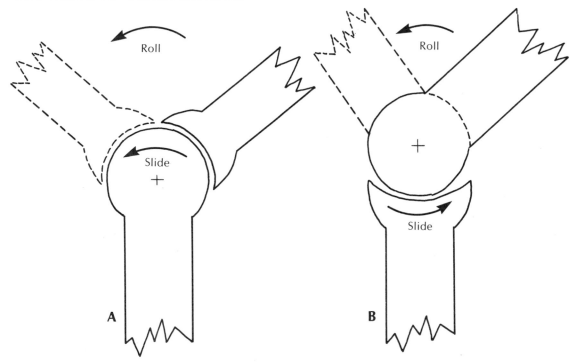

This type of slide is referred to as *spin*, as is the osteokinematic movement it accompanies.

The Close-Packed Position

Separation of joint surfaces is termed *distraction*; approximation of opposing surfaces is *compression*. While some bone movements are accompanied by a relative compression of joint surfaces, other movements involve distraction. By knowing the close-packed position at a joint, one can determine which movements involve compression and which involve distraction.

As mentioned, ovoid surfaces are irregular in that in any one cross-sectional plane the ovoid surface is of constantly changing radius, defining a cardioid curve. If we imagine an opposing joint surface moving along this curve, it is clear that in most positions the two surfaces do not fit, or are noncongruent. However, one position exists in which the joint surfaces become relatively congruent because their contacting radii are approximately the same (see Fig. 2-4). Thus, while synovial joint surfaces tend to be noncongruent, at least one position exists for each joint in which the surfaces becomes maximally congruent. This position is termed the *close-packed position* of a joint. (The close-packed position for each extremity joint is listed in the Appendix.) At any joint, movement into the close-packed position involves an impure swing and so necessarily involves a conjunct rotation. The rotary component of movement into this position causes the joint capsule and major ligaments supporting the joint to twist, which in turn causes an approximation of joint surfaces. Once the close-packed position is reached, no further movement in that direction is possible.

We can say, then, that movement toward the close-packed position involves an element of compression, whereas movement out of this position involves

distraction. MacConnaill points out that habitual movements at any joint involve movements directed into and out of the close-packed position.[28] It is likely that the resultant intermittent compression of joint surfaces has a bearing on nutrition and lubrication of articular cartilage. The squeezing out of synovial fluid with each compression phase facilitates exchange of nutrients and helps to maintain a lubricant film between surfaces (see sections Joint nutrition and Lubrication).

Interestingly, moving the upper extremity in a reciprocating pattern, such that every joint is first moved simultaneously toward its close-packed position and then directly out of the close-packed position, resembles one of the basic patterns used by Knott in her proprioceptive neuromuscular facilitation (PNF) techniques.[26] Considering the twisting and untwisting of the capsules and ligaments that occurs, and considering what is known of joint neurology with respect to joint–muscle reflexes (see the section on neurology later in this chapter), it seems likely that the faciliatory effect of the pattern may be related to joint position as well as muscle position.

The close-packed position also has important implications with respect to pathomechanics of many injuries. For instance, many upper extremity injuries occur from falling on the outstretched hand; Colles' fracture at the wrist, supracondylar elbow fractures, posterior dislocation of the elbow, and anterior dislocation of the shoulder are but a few. This is not surprising if we realize that falling on the outstretched hand, in such a way that the body rolls away from the arm on impact, throws every major upper extremity joint (except the metacarpophalangeal and acromioclavicular joints) into closepacking. As mentioned, once the closepacked position is reached, the joint becomes locked, and no further movement is possible in that direction. If further force is added, either a joint must dislocate or a bone must give, or both. The weak link tends to be determined by age; the juvenile is likely to fracture the humerus above the elbow, the adolescent or teenager may dislocate the shoulder, and the middle-aged or elderly invariably sustain a Colles' fracture. Generally speaking, most fractures and dislocations occur when a joint is in the close-packed position. Most capsular or ligamentous sprains occur when the joint is in a loose-packed position. This is simply because the tight fit of the adjoining bones in the close-packed position causes forces applied to the joint to be taken up by the bones rather than by the supporting structures; there is more "intrinsic stability" at the joint.

Joint Play

It was mentioned that in a loose-packed position, or in any position of the joint other than the close-packed position, the joint surfaces are incongruent. An obvious example is the knee joint in some position of flexion, although the menisci help to make up for the marked incongruence. It was also implied that in the loose-packed position the capsule and major supporting ligaments remain relatively lax. This must be so in order to allow a normal range of movement. It can be said, then, that in most joint positions a joint has some "play" in it because joint surfaces do not fit tightly, and because the capsule and ligaments remain somewhat lax.

This joint play is essential for normal joint function. First, the small spaces that exist because of joint incongruence are necessary to the hydrodynamic component of joint lubrication (see section on lubrication later in this chapter). Secondly, because the joint surfaces are of varying radii, movement cannot occur around a rigid axis, and so the joint capsule must allow some play in order for full movement to occur. Related to this is the fact that if normal joint distraction (one form of joint play) is lost, then joint sur-

faces will become prematurely approximated when moving toward the close-packed position, and movement in this direction will, therefore, be restricted. We cannot compare human synovial joints to a door hinge, except in a limited sense, since a door moves about a single axis at its hinge and requires little or no play. Thirdly, it was indicated that most joint movements are helical, involving movement about more than one axis simultaneously. In order for this type of movement to occur, a certain amount of joint play must exist, unless the movement is track-bound, which is usually not the case. One may, therefore, presume that loss of joint play from some pathology, such as a tight joint capsule, will lead to alteration in joint function, usually involving restriction of motion, pain, or both. Mennell uses the term *joint dysfunction* for loss of joint play.[38] This term is useful in a general discussion of joint mechanics but should be avoided clinically in favor of terms that more precisely identify the responsible pathology, since there are many possible causes of loss of joint play.

Conjunct Rotation

At this point in our discussion of joint kinematics we should elaborate on a concept introduced earlier, conjunct rotation. It was mentioned that conjunct rotation is the component of spin, or rotation, that accompanies any impure swing of a bone (see Fig. 2-9). It is easily observed when the tibia extends on the femur, the distal phalanges of the fingers flex when held together, or the ulna flexes and extends on the humerus; such movements are helical. This rotation causes the joint capsule to twist when moving toward the close-packed position. At the shoulder, where a particularly large range of movement is possible, some rotation opposite the direction of normal conjunct rotation must occur at the later stages of movement. Thus, pure abduction in the frontal plane

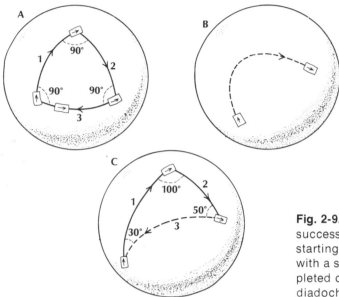

Fig. 2-9. Conjunct rotation occurring (*A*) with a succession of pure swings with return to the starting position (diadochal movement), (*B*) with a single impure swing, (*C*) with a completed cycle of pure and impure swings (also a diadochal movement).

involves an impure swing with a medial conjunct rotation at the early phase, the first 90° to 120° of movement. This is because the glenoid cavity faces somewhat forward, and the humerus on abduction swings out of the plane of the scapula. If this impure swing were left to continue, at full elevation the joint capsule would be completely twisted upon itself. This, however, is impossible, since the twisting of the joint capsule would cause a premature approximation of joint surfaces before full elevation could be attained. To prevent this premature locking of the joint on abduction, the humerus must rotate laterally on its long axis during the final phase of movement, bringing the humeral head back toward the plane of the scapula. Similarly, sagittal flexion involves a lateral conjunct rotation, but a medial longitudinal rotation during the final phase. This is best appreciated by observing it on a skeleton, noting the end position of the humerus on abduction or flexion without rotation and comparing it to elevation in the plane of the scapula, that is, about midway between flexion and abduction.

In addition to accompanying any impure swing, conjunct rotation may occur with a succession of swings, even if each of the swings is a pure swing. In a triangle drawn on a curved surface, such as an ovoid surface, the sum of the interior angles of the triangle may exceed 180° if the surface is convex, or the sum may be less than 180° if the surface is concave. During a succession of movements, in which the mechanical axis follows the path of a triangle or trigone, the amount of conjunct rotation that accompanies the completed cycle will be equal to the difference between the sum of the interior angles of the triangle or trigone and 180° (see Fig. 2-9). This type of conjunct rotation can be visualized by moving the humerus through a succession of movements: starting with the arm at the side, elbow bent, fingers facing forward, flex the humerus 90°, abduct 90° horizontally, then adduct 90°. The fingers are now directed laterally, indicating that the humerus, during this succession of movements, rotated outward 90°. The succession may only be carried out once or twice without derotating the humerus medially because of the twisting of the capsule which results from the lateral conjunct rotation.

SUMMARY OF JOINT FUNCTION

We have expanded our terminology of joint function to accommodate the more specific features of joint kinematics, including the relationships between joint structure and function, and the types of movements occurring between joint surfaces. In doing so we defined the following osteokinematic terms, or those terms defining movement between two bones:

Mechanical axis—Line drawn through the moving bone, at the starting position of a movement, that passes through the center of the opposing joint surface and is perpendicular to it

Spin—Movement of a bone about the mechanical axis

Pure swing—Movement of a bone in which an end of the mechanical axis traces the path of a chord with respect to the ovoid formed by the opposing joint surface; also called *chordate swing*

Impure swing—Movement in which the mechanical axis follows the path of an arc with respect to the opposing ovoid surface

Conjunct rotation—Element of spin that accompanies impure swing; also the rotation that may occur with a succession of swings

We also defined the following arthrokinematic terms, or those that define the types of movement occurring between joint surfaces:

Roll—Movement in which points at intervals on the moving joint surface contact points at the same intervals on the opposing surface

Slide—Movement in which a single contact point on the moving surface contacts various points on the opposing surface

Spin—Type of slide that accompanies spin of a bone; one half on the joint surface slides in one direction while the other half slides in the opposite direction, that is, the moving joint surface rotates about some point on the opposing joint surface.

Distraction—Separation of joint surfaces

Compression—Approximation of joint surfaces; always occurs when moving toward the close-packed position

The *close-packed position* was defined for a joint in which the following three conditions exist:

The joint surfaces become maximally congruent.

The joint capsule and major ligaments become twisted, causing joint surfaces to approximate.

The joint becomes locked so that no further movement is possible in that direction.

CLINICAL APPLICATION

Terminology

A rationale for the approach to management of joint dysfunction, including the use of specific joint mobilization techniques, can now be discussed based upon the above analysis of joint movement. However, some additional terms must first be presented. Unfortunately, a jargon has evolved relating to the clinical application of these concepts and is often the source of confusion since the terms are used inconsistently. Therefore, the most common and useful definitions of important terms are presented.

Accessory joint movements are simply those arthrokinematic movements that must occur in order for normal osteokinematic movement to take place. These might include slides, rolls, distractions, compressions, or conjunct rotations. Consider the osteokinematic movement of the humerus moving from the resting position with the arm at the side to the closed-packed position. We know that the joint is convex on concave. The head of the humerus must roll in the same direction in which the bone swings. It must slide opposite this direction or somewhat inferiorly and inward. Because the close-packed position is being approached, the joint surfaces are becoming approximated. It is a movement of impure swing, so a conjunct rotation, in this case a lateral rotation, must occur. If any one of these accessory movements does not or cannot occur, then this particular swing of the humerus cannot be performed painlessly or harmlessly through the full range. If full osteokinematic movement does occur, it does so at the expense of the capsule or ligaments, which must be abnormally stretched, or of the articular cartilage, which must be abnormally compressed.

Component motions, for our purposes, can be used synonymously with *accessory movements*. We speak of lateral rotation of the tibia as being a component of knee extension. Likewise, spreading of the distal tibia and fibula is a component of dorsiflexion at the ankle. The clinician must be aware of the component motions necessary for each osteokinematic movement at a joint. Many of these are listed in the Appendix.

Joint play movements are those accessory movements that can be produced passively at a joint but cannot be isolated actively. They might include distractions, compressions, slides, rolls, or spins at a joint in a particular position. We use joint play movements when applying specific mobilization techniques to restore accessory movements so that full and painless osteokinematic movement may be restored. For example, inferior glide occurs at the shoulder during active elevation. It can be performed passively, but in itself cannot be performed actively by voluntary muscle contraction; inferior glide is a joint play movement at the glenohumeral joint.

Joint mobilization is a very general term that may be applied to any active or passive attempt to increase movement at a joint. In addition to traditional methods of increasing joint movement, such as active, passive, and active-assisted range of motion techniques, joint mobilization includes specific passive mobilization techniques. These techniques are aimed at restoring those component movements that permit pain-free or harmless osteokinematic movement. They are used especially to restore those joint play movements that cannot be isolated actively. Specific passive mobilization techniques are graded (Fig. 2-10). Grades one through four are often referred to as *articulation* techniques, which are passive rhythmic oscillations. Grade five is a *manipulation* technique that is a high-velocity, low-amplitude passive thrust. These grades are relative to the pathologic amplitude of joint play movement that exists at the joint and *not* to the normal amplitude that should exist. There are two

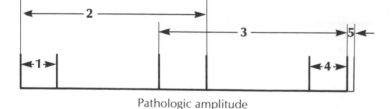

Pathologic amplitude

Fig. 2-10. Grades of joint-play movement

main criteria for the selection of the particular grade to be used: (1) the degree of pain or protective muscle spasm during passive joint play movement (irritability), and (2) the degree of restriction of joint play movement. The greater the irritability, the lower the numerical grade of movement used. Pain and spasm must be avoided. Manipulation is used primarily when a very slight, minimally painful restriction exists. A third criterion of selection might apply here, namely the skill and experience of the operator, since manipulative maneuvers should only be attempted after articulation techniques have been mastered and after much practice. The terms of joint movement are presented schematically in Figure 2-11.

Specific accessory joint motions that are limited may be restored by manual oscillations or thrusts. The primary goal of using specific joint mobilization techniques is restoration of normal, pain-free use of the joint. The emphasis is not on forcing a particular anatomical (osteokinematic) movement at a joint, as has been done in the past with traditional methods of mobilization; rather, it is on restoring normal joint mechanics in order to allow full, pain-free osteokinematic movement to occur. In this way, range of motion is restored to the joint with less risk of damaging the joint by compressing isolated portions of articular cartilage, and with less pain and muscle guarding from overstretching isolated capsuloligamentous structures, as may well occur if an osteokinematic movement is forced in the absence of necessary component movements. This is to say that specific passive mobilization, correctly applied, is a safer, more efficient, and less painful method of increasing range of motion at a joint. Mennell, in his lectures, often uses the analogy of a door having lost movement because of a faulty hinge. Efforts to restore motion by pushing hard on the door are likely to result in further damage to the hinge. The logical method to remedy the situation is to direct one's attention to the hinge—to restore normal mechanics to the hinge, thereby restoring normal movement of the door.[38]

Note that this discussion ignores the physiological concept of the joint. This is done solely for the sake of simplicity. Obviously when we consider restoring normal joint mechanics, we must consider the anatomical joint along with those structures responsible for active movement of the joint. For example, active abduction at the shoulder is often lost because of the absence of inferior glide. Relative to the anatomical joint, the joint play movement of inferior glide may be limited. However, the problem may also be physiological, in that inferior glide may not be occurring due to weakness of the supraspinatus. These are very different problems leading to similar results. The nature of the problem must be brought out by a thorough evaluation.

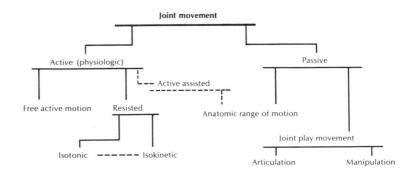

Fig. 2-11. Scheme illustrating terms related to joint movement

Analysis of Accessory Joint Motions

Clinical Assessment. We have already alluded to many of the means of determining which accessory movements are components of specific osteokinematic movements. For instance, the direction of roll is always the same as that for the swing of the bone. If a convex surface moves on a concave surface, slide will occur in the direction opposite to the roll; if concave on convex, slide occurs in the same direction as the roll. Distraction occurs when moving out of the close-packed position; compression occurs when moving into the close-packed position. These can all be determined for any joint moving in any direction. Some of the other component motions, as listed for each joint in the Appendix, must be memorized or deduced anatomically.

One way of assessing the state of a particular accessory movement (its amplitude and irritability) is clinically, by evaluating the joint play movements. These examination maneuvers are essentially the same as the specific mobilization techniques. Rather than being performed as a graded, therapeutic technique, they are used to determine the amplitude of a joint play movement, and whether or not the movement causes pain or spasm. The amplitude of movement and possible restriction must be compared to the operator's concept of "normal" for that movement, at that joint, for that body type. This requires experience in evaluating normal as well as pathologic joints. Whenever possible, the state of the pathologic joint must be compared to a healthy contralateral joint. The degree of irritability is determined by the patient's subjective response, as well as by the presence of protective muscle spasm when performing the examination movement. (Refer to regional chapters for the joint play techniques at each joint. These are performed using the same handholds as those for the therapeutic techniques included in Chapter 7. Joint Mobilization Techniques.) Proficiency in clinically evaluating joint play movements and correlating findings to knowledge of accessory movements at the joint, as well as other symptoms and signs presenting on examination, is essential to the effective application of joint mobilization techniques and management of musculoskeletal disorders.

Instant Center Analysis. The more scientific method of analyzing arthrokinematic movement has been described by Sammarco and co-workers.[45] This involves a determination of the centroid of movement, or instant center of movement, at various points throughout a joint movement. For any joint, the axis about which motion takes place changes constantly during a particular movement. This is because joint surfaces are irregular in shape. The instant centers of motion can be plotted for a movement through the use of careful radiographic studies of a joint that record the relative position of the bones at various points throughout the movement. This is done by choosing two reference points on the moving bone; in Figure 2-12 the points lie on the central axis of the bone, point A on the joint surface, point B 7 cm up on the shaft of the bone. A second radiograph taken after the bone has moved is superimposed over the original. In the new position, points A' and B' are determined along the central axis; A' is on the joint surface, B' 7 cm up on the shaft. Now lines A–A' and B–B' are constructed, and perpendicular bisectors for each of these lines are drawn. The intersection of these bisectors is the instant center of motion, or the point of zero velocity, for this particular motion of the bone. Using this instant center of motion, point C, a velocity vector can be constructed showing the direction of surface motion that occurred for the particular movement. This is done by drawing a radius from the instant center to the point

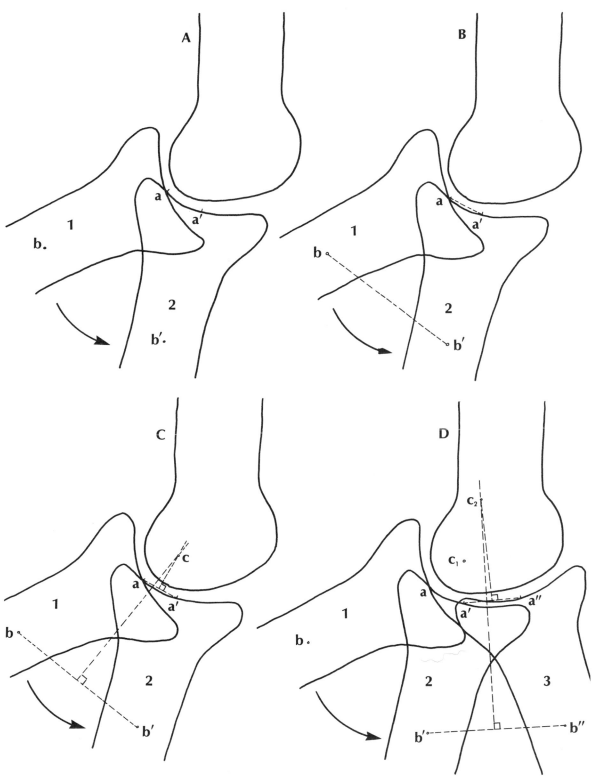

Fig. 2-12. Determination of instant centers of motion (C_1, C_2)

of contact between bones at the time for which the instant center was determined. In this case, we will call our point of contact—the point at which the center axis of the bone crosses the joint surface—point P (Fig. 2-13). A perpendicular drawn to this radius, at the joint surface, will indicate the direction of surface motion, with the arrow directed toward the movement of the bone.

Once the instant center and surface-velocity vector are determined, an interpretation can be made. An instant center lying on the joint surface at the point of contact between the bones indicates that pure roll is taking place. An instant center lying far from the joint surface point of contact indicates that pure sliding is taking place. A velocity vector pointed away from the opposing (stationary) surface indicates a distraction of the surfaces. A velocity vector aimed into the stationary surface indicates a compression of the surfaces. A velocity vector tangen-

tial to the joint surface suggests a smooth gliding motion is taking place.

The above analysis might seem somewhat complex at first, but is actually quite simple. The difficult step is obtaining reliable radiographs that can be superimposed on each other. Plotting instant centers and surface velocity vectors for a particular movement throughout the range of motion can yield some very specific information about that motion. It reveals the relative amounts of roll and slide for various points throughout the range, and how these values change during the complete motion: the closer the instant center comes to the point of contact, the more roll is taking place; the further it moves away, the more slide is occurring. Perhaps more importantly it reveals possible abnormal compression or distraction of joint surfaces throughout the range (e.g., by comparison to what the operator considers "normal"). This type of scientific analysis of arthrokinematics is not practical

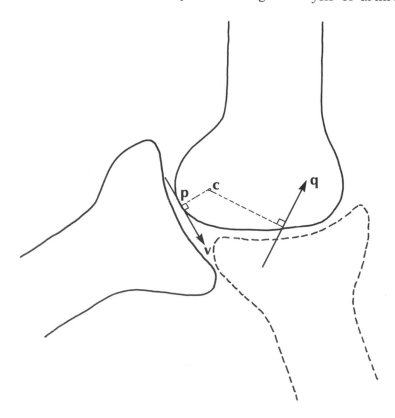

Fig. 2-13. Determination of surface velocity vectors. P is the point of contact during the arc of motion for which C applies. V is the calculated velocity vector indicating tangential surface motion. If Q were the vector for the arc of motion for which C applies, one could conclude that joint compression took place during this motion.

for routine diagnostic purposes. However, it offers clinicians an opportunity to demonstrate the value of specific therapeutic interventions in improving abnormal joint mechanics. It has been used already to show the value of certain surgeries, for example, meniscectomy at the knee, in restoring normal joint mechanics.[16]

Note that because the information is obtained from radiographs, which are two dimensional, arthrokinematic movements in only two dimensions can be studied. This analysis will not yield information concerning the amount of spin or conjunct rotation occurring.

NEUROLOGY

The neuroanatomy and, especially, the neurophysiology of joints are subjects not well covered in the current literature. Following the original works of Sherrington on neuromuscular physiology, a vast amount of information was collected concerning the role of muscle and tendon receptors in influencing posture, movement, muscle tone, and various reflex phenomena.[47] Little has been done until recently to identify specific joint receptors, and even less has been done to determine their clinical significance.[48,54] Since the subject of joint neurology is directly relevant to the management of common musculoskeletal disorders, an overview will be presented here.

INNERVATION

Joints tend to receive innervation from two sources: (1) articular nerves that are branches of adjacent peripheral nerves, and (2) branches from nerves that supply muscles controlling the joint. Each joint is usually supplied by several nerves, and their distributions tend to overlap considerably. Generally speaking, a particular aspect of a joint capsule is innervated by branches of the nerve supplying the muscle or muscles that would, when contracting, prevent overstretching of that part of the capsule. One notable exception is the anterior inferior aspect of the glenohumeral capsule, which is innervated by a branch from the axillary nerve. The nerve fibers of an articular nerve are purely afferent, with the exception of small vasomotor efferents to the blood vessels. The fiber sizes range from large myelinated fibers to small myelinated and unmyelinated fibers.

RECEPTORS

Four types of joint receptors have been identified, each serving a relatively specific role in the sensorimotor integration of joint function.[48,50,54]

Type I
Description: encapsulated ending, similar to Ruffini corpuscle
Location: numerous in the superficial joint capsule; usually found in clusters of six
Related fiber: small (6μ–9μ) myelinated (relatively slow conduction)
Action: slowly adapting, low threshold; mechanoreceptor
Function: provides information concerning the static position of the joint, is constantly firing; contributes to regulation of postural muscle tone; contributes to kinesthetic (movement) sense, senses direction and speed of movement; contributes to regulation of muscle tone during movement of the joint

Type II
Description: thickly encapsulated, similar to pacinian corpuscle
Location: sparse (relative to type I), in joint capsule (deeper layers) and fat pads
Related fiber: medium (9μ–12μ) myelinated
Action: rapidly adapting, low threshold; dynamic mechanoreceptor
Function: fires only on quick changes in movement; provides information concerning acceleration and deceleration of joint movement; acts at initiation of

movement as "booster" to help overcome inertia of body parts

Type III
Description: thinly encapsulated, similar
to Golgi end organ
Location: intrinsic and extrinsic joint ligaments
Related fiber: large $(13\mu - 17\mu)$ myelinated (fast conduction)
Action: very slowly adapting, high
threshold; dynamic mechanoreceptor
Function: monitors direction of movement; has reflex effect on muscle tone to
provide a "braking" mechanism against
movement tending to overdisplace the
joint (movement too fast or too far)

Type IV
Description: free nerve endings and
plexus
Location: fibrous capsule, intrinsic and
extrinsic ligaments, fat pads, periosteum
(*absent* in articular cartilage, intra-
articular fibrocartilage, and synovium)
Fiber: small $(92\mu - 5\mu)$ myelinated and
unmyelinated (2μ) (slow conduction).
Action: nonadapting, high threshold;
pain receptors
Function: inactive under normal conditions; active when related tissue is subject to marked deformation or other noxious mechanical or chemical stimulation

CLINICAL CONSIDERATIONS

It is apparent from the above descriptions
that stimulation of joint receptors contributes to sense of static position (type I),
sense of speed of movement (type I), sense
of change in speed of movement (type II),
sense of direction of movement (types I
and III), regulation of postural muscle
tone (type I), regulation of muscle tone at
the initiation of movement (type II), regulation of muscle tone during movement
(coordination) (type II), and regulation of
muscle tone during potentially harmful
movements (type III). Of course, skin receptors, connective tissue receptors, and
muscle receptors also contribute to many
of these same functions. Some of the clinical problems that remain unresolved, or
only partially resolved, include the following:

> How important are these joint receptors,
> relative to muscle and skin receptors, for
> example, in the regulation of muscle
> tone, posture, and movement?
> Are some of the persistent problems,
> such as chronic limp, residual incoordi-
> nation, chronic instability ("giving
> way"), and chronic muscle atrophy, en-
> countered in patients following some
> joint injuries the result of damage to
> these receptors?
> How might treatment techniques, such
> as joint mobilization, neuromuscular
> facilitation, and inhibition, be refined to
> accommodate the functions of these joint
> receptors?

One particularly interesting study demonstrates a case in which malocclusion of
dentures, causing abnormal afferent discharge from the temperomandibular joint
capsules, resulted in an almost total reflex
inhibition of the temporal muscles during
active occlusion by the patient.[25] Restoration of normal joint mechanics, by remodeling of the dentures, restored normal
muscular activity. A study by Wyke
showed rather marked postural changes
in a boy with apparent alteration of afferent impulses from the ankle capsule following injury to the lateral aspect of the
capsule.[54] The postural deficit persisted in
spite of an otherwise complete recovery,
with restoration of normal strength and
range of motion and with no residual pain.
The boy's only complaint was that of occasional "giving way" of the ankle.
Freeman advocates the use of coordination exercises on a balance board for patients with chronic ankle "instability" in
the absence of demonstrable structural instability.[20] He reports good results with
such a program, attributing such giving
way at the ankle to alteration of normal
joint afferent flow following injury to the
joint, such as from an ankle sprain. Most
physical therapists have encountered the

common phenomenon of gross quadriceps atrophy following knee injury in spite of preventive efforts to maintain muscle function. Although there is little current literature on the subject, it seems reasonable to attribute this to reflex muscle inhibition by abnormal joint receptor stimulation.[9]

As far as techniques of treatment are concerned, it is interesting to relate what we know about the function of these joint receptors, and what we know of arthrokinematics, to techniques that have already evolved. Consider the diagonal pattern commonly used in PNF techniques—moving the arm from flexion–abduction–external rotation to extension–adduction–internal rotation. Part of the explanation of this pattern speaks of moving from a position of maximum elongation and unspiraling of functionally related muscles to a position of spiraling and shortening of these same muscles.[26] We can add to this the fact that this pattern involves moving all joints simultaneously from a close-packed to a loose-packed position. In doing so, the joint capsule of each joint moves from a position of maximum shortening and spiraling to a position of lengthening and unspiraling. Studies thus far on animals have indicated that maximum afferent stimulation occurs when approaching the close-packed position of a joint; this is to be expected since it is the position of maximum tightening of the capsule and ligaments in which the receptors lie. The techniques of PNF evolved with primary consideration of the neurophysiology of muscles, using movement patterns that combine actions of functionally related muscles to bring about a mutual facilitation of each muscle in the chain. It is now suggested that these patterns also combine functionally related joint movements that add to the facilitative effect of the patterns on the muscles involved through joint receptor stimulation. It also seems probable that the joint receptors play a significant role in other techniques of facilitation, such as "quick stretch," that tend to stimulate the type II receptor.

It is important to consider the function of joint receptors when using joint mobilization or other treatment techniques involving joint movement. The effectiveness of our efforts to increase movement at a joint will naturally be compromised by any muscle contraction tending to restrict joint movement. Emphasis, then, must be made on avoiding reflex muscle contractions that would tend to prevent or restrict a desired joint movement. For this reason—and for other obvious reasons—pain must be avoided during joint mobilization, since it is well known that pain at a joint tends to elicit a reflex muscle response to restrict movement at the joint. We also know that sudden joint movement tends to stimulate firing of the type III receptors, which sets up a reflex muscle contraction to restrict further movement. Gradual initiation of movement tends to stimulate the type II receptor, which affects a small facilitative muscular response. Passive and active mobilization techniques are best performed rhythmically, without sudden changes in speed or direction of movement. A manipulation must be performed so quickly that it is completed before the reflex muscular response produced by stimulation of the type III receptor can act to interfere with the movement. Similarly, it must be performed through a very small amplitude to minimize the number of type III receptors stimulated.

With respect to the type IV pain receptors, it is worth emphasizing that articular cartilage, fibrocartilage (*e.g.*, menisci), synovium, and compact bone are essentially aneural. This is well documented in anatomical studies as well as clinically.[24,48,54] In the anatomical joint the major pain-sensitive structures are the fibrous capsule, ligaments, and periosteum. This carries some important clinical implications. It suggests that pathologic conditions that might alter joint mechanics, such that the articular cartilage undergoes undue compression stress, may go unnoticed by the patient in their initial stages. In fact, the patient may notice nothing until either joint mechanics are altered sufficiently to place an abnormal stress on the joint capsule or until the joint cartilage undergoes sufficient degeneration, causing a low-grade synovitis with resultant pressure on the capsule from effusion. This may explain why persons with "frozen shoulders" or osteoarthrosis of other joints often do not present to a physician until the disease has progressed considerably. It also suggests that clinicians must learn to routinely examine for subtle changes in joint mechanics rather than considering only gross range of motion, strength, and complaints of pain by the patient. Patients presenting with very early symptoms or signs of osteoarthrosis could enjoy complete arrest or reversal of the joint problem if properly managed, rather than resigning themselves to future joint replacement.

As will be discussed later in Chapter 3, Pain, small oscillatory articulations may, in themselves, be useful in reducing pain at the joint being moved or at other joints derived from the same segment. The added proprioceptive input may inhibit the perception of pain through modulation at the substantia gelatinosa in the dorsal horn of the spinal cord.

JOINT NUTRITION

In addition to being aneural, articular cartilage is for the most part avascular. This is also true of intra-articular fibrocartilage. Since, generally speaking, bodily tissues depend upon blood supply for nutrition, these structures would seem to be at a disadvantage. It is generally believed that the articular margins do receive some nutrients from the highly vascularized synovium and periosteum adjacent to them.[17] The menisci at the knee also receive nutrients at their peripheral capsular attachments, and it is suggested that the deep layers of articular cartilage are fed by the blood supply to the subchondral bone. However, the problem of nutrition to the more superficial, centrally located portions of the articular cartilage and to the more centrally located parts of the intra-articular fibrocartilage remains. These cartilaginous areas are primary articulating surfaces, not the more peripheral areas or deeper layers. It is generally agreed that nutrition to these regions occurs by diffusion and inhibition of synovial fluid. This is a unique situation because nutrients must cross at least two barriers in order to reach the chondrocytes embedded within the cartilage. First, they must pass from the capillary bed of the highly vascularized synovium. They must then diffuse through the superficial matrix layers of the cartilaginous surface, before reaching the cell wall of the chondrocyte. Thus, synovial fluid serves a major function as a source of nutrition for articular cartilage and intra-articular fibrocartilage.[17,31–33]

Intermittent compression and distraction of joint surfaces must occur in order for an adequate exchange of nutrients and waste products to take place. A joint that is immobilized undergoes atrophy of articular cartilage, just as a joint in which there is prolonged compression of joint surface undergoes similar atrophic changes.[3,12,13,52] The three primary mechanisms by which synovial joints undergo normal compression and distraction are the following: (1) weight bearing in lower extremity and spinal joints; (2) intermittent contraction of muscles crossing a joint; (3) twisting and untwisting of the joint capsule as the joint moves toward and away from the close-packed position during habitual movements. With respect to the last mechanism, recall that as the joint approaches the close-packed position, its joint surfaces not only become compressed but also approach a position of maximal congruency. Thus, compression normally occurs in a position in which greater areas of the opposing joint surfaces are in contact. This ensures that relatively large portions of the joint surfaces undergo adequate exchange of nutrients. From a pathologic standpoint, a joint that has lost movement, as from a tight joint capsule, does not receive a normal exchange of nutrients over the parts of the joint surfaces that no longer come into contact. This is especially true in the case of a tight joint capsule, since movements toward the close-packed position in which there is maximal joint surface contact are usually the movements that are most restricted.

Attritional changes in articular cartilage related to aging are observed in the relatively noncontacting portions of the joint surfaces.[4,35-37] Several reasons for this may be postulated. First, these are the areas of articular cartilage that undergo less deformation with use of the joint over time; as a result, the rate and degree of exchange of nutrient fluids is less in these areas. Also, with age there is a reduction of the chondroitin sulfate component of cartilaginous tissue. Since the fluid-binding capacity of articular cartilage is largely dependent upon its chondroitin sulfate content, a decrease in this constituent might interfere with normal nutrition to the tissue. Furthermore, because loss of joint range of motion occurs with advancing age the exchange of nutrients to portions of the articular cartilage is reduced.

LUBRICATION

Synovial fluid, in addition to serving as a nutritional source for articular cartilage, also acts as a lubricant to prevent undue wear of joint surfaces from fiction.[11,15,34,53] In studying lubrication of human joints, however, we cannot consider just the properties of synovial fluid and how they affect movement and friction between two surfaces. We must also take into consideration the shape and consistency of the joint surfaces as well as the types of movement that occur between joint surfaces. Many models have been proposed for human joint lubrication. Some of the earlier models tend to ignore many of the unique properties of human joints. The more recent models evolved with the sophistication of engineering principles, which are better able to deal with some of the complex factors involved in human joint lubrication. However, it is generally agreed that no one model of joint lubrication applies to all joints under all circumstances. The major mode of lubrication in a particular joint may change, depending upon such factors as loading and speed of movement.

Synovial fluid has essentially the same composition as blood plasma, except for the addition of mucin. Mucin is the mucopolysaccharide, hyaluronic acid, which is a long-chain polymer. The viscous properties of synovial fluid are attributed to hyaluronic acid. The most important property to be considered in this respect is the *thixotropic* or non-Newtonian quality of synovial fluid; the viscosity decreases with increased shear rate (increased speed of joint movement).

MODELS OF JOINT LUBRICATION

One cannot accurately draw an analogy between a machine model of lubrication and lubrication of synovial joints. One of the major reasons is that the physical properties of articular cartilage differ considerably from the physical properties of most machine components. Articular cartilage is porous and relatively spongelike in that it has the capacity to absorb and bind synovial fluid. Articular cartilage is also viscoelastic; the deformation rate is high upon initial application of the load and levels off with time. When the load is removed, the initial "reformation" rate is high and decreases over time (Fig. 2-14). Although macroscopically articular cartilage appears quite smooth and shiny, it is, in fact, relatively rough microscopically. Articular cartilage also has the tendency to adsorb large molecules, such as hyaluronic acid in synovial fluid, to its surface. The significance of this will be discussed below.

The early model of joint lubrication described a hydrodynamic, or fluid film, situation (Fig. 2-15,A).[27] In this case, synovial fluid fills in the wedges of space left by the joint surface incongruencies. Upon movement between surfaces the synovial fluid is attracted to the area of contact between the surfaces. This occurs because of (1) the pressure gradient produced by the movement and (2) the fact that relative movement tends to pull the viscous fluid in the direction of the moving surface. The result of this is the maintenance of a layer of fluids between joint surfaces during movement. Any friction occurring as a result of movement occurs within the fluid rather than between joint surfaces. This meets the requirements of a good lubrication system because it allows free movement and prevents wear to the joint surfaces. This system works well during movement; however, it would tend to fail under very slow velocity or under heavy loading. It would also fail under reciprocal motion, since it would not adapt well to changes in direction of motion, at which time the velocity of movement is zero. Since human joints often move slowly, under heavy loads, and reciprocally, by itself it seems an unsatisfactory model for human joint lubrication.

The hydrodynamic model, however, cannot be completely repudiated because the above description does not consider the viscoelasticity of joint surfaces. This model can be modified to an elastohydrodynamic system (Fig. 2-15,B). Because of the nature of articular cartilage to deform, not all of the energy of heavy loading goes to decreasing the thickness of the layer of film between the surfaces, thereby increasing friction between the surfaces. Instead, a deformation of the joint surfaces occurs, increasing the effective contact area between surfaces and thereby reducing the effective compression stress (force per unit area) to the lubrication fluid. This allows the protective layer of fluid to remain at about the same thickness. Thus, the elastohydrodynamic model describes a system that withstands loading in the presence of movement. It lacks an explanation, however, for the means of lubrication at the initiation of movement or at the period of relative zero velocity during reciprocating movements or during very heavy loading with very little movement.

We can further expand our model of joint lubrication by including the concepts

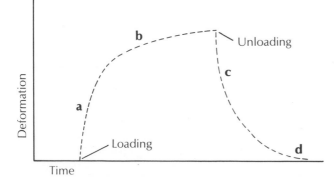

Fig. 2-14. Viscoelastic response of articular cartilage. Parts A and C of the curve are due to elastic properties, while parts B and D show viscous behavior.

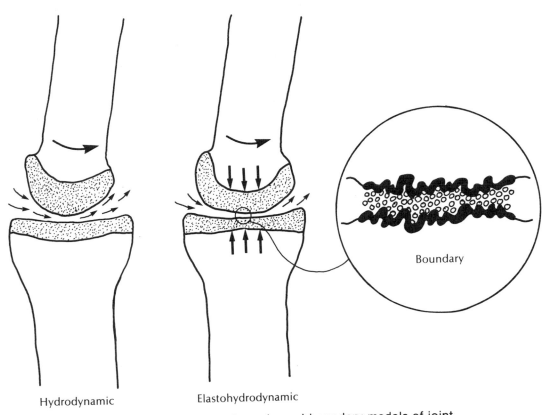

Hydrodynamic   Elastohydrodynamic   Boundary

Fig. 2-15. Hydrodynamic, elastohydrodynamic, and boundary models of joint lubrication

of boundary lubrication and weeping lubrication.[34,49,53] With any materials undergoing relative shear between two surfaces, friction is the result of the irregularities of the surfaces; the greater the irregularities, the greater the friction. Effective lubrication must reduce this friction to a minimum, thereby reducing wear of the surfaces to a minimum. In the case of boundary lubrication, the lubricant is adsorbed to the surface of the material, in effect reducing the roughness of the surfaces by filling in the irregularities. Because articular cartilage is able to adsorb long-chain molecules of hyaluronic acid, these molecules are able to fill in the irregularities as well as to coat the surface. Any friction occurring as the result of shear movement occurs between molecules of the lubricant rather than between the joint surfaces themselves. This probably serves as an adjunct to the elastohydrodynamic system, especially in cases of extreme loading sufficient to significantly decrease the thickness of the layer of fluid maintained by the elastohydrodynamic model under lighter loads. It may also play a role at the initiation of movement or periods of zero velocity, since a layer of fluid would not be present because of its dependence upon movement under an elastohydrodynamic system. The concept of weeping lubrication is actually an expansion of the elastohydrodynamic model. Because of the porosity and elastic qualities of articular cartilage, loading sufficient to cause a deformation of the articular surfaces also causes a "squeezing out" of the synovial fluid absorbed by the cartilage. The fluid that is squeezed .out further serves to maintain a protective layer of lubricant between joint surfaces.

Using this "mixed lubrication" model that combines elastohydrodynamic concepts with boundary lubrication concepts, we meet the demands of human synovial joints.[11,43] The system allows movement, change in direction of movement, loading, and variations in congruencies of joint surfaces. It takes into consideration, at least in general terms, the properties of the lubricant—synovial fluid—and the surface materials. There is still considerable controversy over the relative importance of each of the lubrication models under various conditions, but most authors agree with the general concepts presented above. Since it is still unknown how each model contributes to normal joint lubrication, very little investigation into the mutual effects of pathologic joint conditions and joint lubrication has taken place. It almost goes without saying that a breakdown in some aspect of the lubrication system is likely to cause or add to the progression of joint disease, such as degenerative joint disease. On the other hand, certain joint diseases result in changes in structure and function of joint constituents. For instance, there is a loss of joint cartilage in degenerative joint disease and changes in synovial fluid viscosity in rheumatoid arthritis. It is probable that in such cases the disease will, in turn, alter the function of the lubrication system, thus contributing to a progressive degenerative cycle.

RESOLVING PROBLEMS OF JOINT-SURFACE WEAR

It has been emphasized that synovial joint surfaces are incongruent. Because of the incongruency that exists in most positions of movement, a relatively small contact area exists between joint surfaces. It has been mentioned that the wedges of space that surround this contact area are necessary in order for a hydrodynamic lubrication system to operate effectively; without these spaces the lubricant could not be drawn, or forced, between the contacting surfaces. We may wonder if such a small area of contact might increase the likelihood of wear between joint surfaces, since loading forces from weight bearing and muscle contraction would be distributed over a small surface area, thereby increasing the compressive stress to the joint. This would, in fact, be the case if the area of contact on one or both surfaces was consistently the same throughout habitual movements. In this respect we might be concerned about a joint that is relatively tract-bound, such as the humeroulnar, patellofemoral, ankle mortise, and interphalangeal joints. In each of these joints movement tends to be restricted to one arc of movement that is determined almost entirely by the shapes of the joint surfaces. It would seem that during movement at these joints, the contacting area on one joint surface would consistently "follow a rut" on the opposing surface, increasing the likelihood of excessive wear in the rut or at the area of the surface contacting the rut. In these joints the problem of excessive wear is resolved in a number of ways. First, these joint surfaces are, relatively speaking, the most congruent in the body, so that forces are distributed over a somewhat larger area. Consider, for example, the close fit between the ulna and trochlear surface of the humerus. Secondly, the contact area on each surface is constantly changing throughout an arc of movement. A change in contact areas occurs in one sense because a combination of roll and slide takes place between joint surfaces. In another sense, the contact area changes because contact alternates from the "bottom of the valley to the sides of the slopes" on one surface and correspondingly on the opposing surface. For instance, with the knee in full extension, the articular surface of the patella makes contact with the femur at a strip extending mediolaterally across the middle of the patellar surface. In flexion, however, only the medial and lateral margins of the patella make contact with the femoral condyles while the ridge in the middle of the patellar facets lies freely in the intercondylar notch.[22] A comparable situation occurs at the elbow, ankle, and finger joints mentioned throughout their respective movements. Note that at the ankle mortise, which undergoes intermittent heavy loading in habitual use, maximal loading (stance) takes place with the joint closer to its close-packed position, dorsiflexion. This is the position of maximal congruence and, therefore, the position in which the compressive force per unit area would tend to be smallest.

But at joints such as the knee, a more complex situation exists. The knee is markedly incongruent compared to the joints discussed above; it must be in order to allow some degree of rotation to occur independently of flexion or extension or in conjunction with them. The knee must also withstand heavier loading, from weight bearing, in a wide variety of positions. Thus, the knee is often required to undergo heavy loading in positions of flexion, a position in which the surfaces are very incongruent—a small area of contact withstands relatively large compressive forces. We might be concerned that in a situation of heavy loading, relatively low velocity, and small contact area between surfaces, the lubrication system as described above would not be sufficient to prevent excessive friction (shear) and wear between joint surfaces. This might very well be the case in a joint such as the knee which must undergo such conditions during normal daily activities, such as climbing stairs, squatting, and lifting. We might also be concerned about the tendency for the femur to slip forward on the tibia under such conditions, again because of the incongruency of joint surfaces and the lack of intrinsic stability. Are the posterior cruciate and popliteus and other extrinsic stabilizers sufficient to prevent this?

The knee, then, is a joint that must allow movement of spin between the tibia and the femur and swing between the tibia and femur because of the functional demands placed upon it. In order for this to be possible, the joint surfaces must be sufficiently noncongruent. But because of this noncongruence and because of normal heavy loading in a variety of positions, the knee appears susceptible to excessive shear forces between contacting joint surfaces during movement, excessive compressive forces between contacting surfaces on static loading, and intrinsic instability when loaded in flexion. It is probable that the intra-articular menisci serve to compensate for what would otherwise be unsatisfactory engineering at the knee joint, unsatisfactory in that the joint would not withstand the normal forces applied to it without giving way or undergoing premature wearing of joint surfaces.[27] Under heavy static loading, the menisci act to increase the effective load-bearing surface area at the joint, thereby reducing the force per unit area. Being firmly attached to the joint capsule and tibia but mobile enough to conform to the shape of the articulating segments of the femoral condyles, they serve to increase the intrinsic stability of the joint by increasing the effective congruency between joint surfaces. During movement with heavy loading, they again act to increase the load-bearing surface area, but also to maintain a wedge-shaped interval surrounding the area of contact into which the lubricant fluid can be drawn.[27] Since the menisci are semicartilaginous they can also absorb synovial fluid. With increased loading, fluid can be squeezed out from the menisci as well as the articular load-bearing surface, thereby contributing to a weeping lubrication phenomenon. Also, as the menisci recede before the advancing condyles during movement, they can act to spread a layer of lubricant over the joint surfaces just prior to contact. This, incidentally, may also be a function of the rather large infrapatellar fat pad at the knee.[5] The menisci, because they are semimobile, allow the knee to act as though it were maximally congruent with respect to the requirements of lubrication and intrinsic stability, but to actually function as though it were very incongruent with respect to the types of movement that occur at the joint.

One should also take note of the considerable slide of the femoral condyles along the tibial surface during the complete range of flexion–extension. This feature also reduces the likelihood of excessive wear to the tibial surfaces by distributing the load-bearing surface over a larger area. The degree of slide could not occur normally without the extrinsic control provided by the cruciates, nor without the intrinsic stability provided by the menisci. This type of motion, in which the area of contact of a particular joint surface constantly changes with movement at the joint, is necessary to allow for the intermittent compression of articular cartilage essential to normal nutrition and lubrication. Loss of a constantly changing area of contact during use of a joint is likely to increase the probability of degeneration of articular cartilage by interfering with normal nutrition and normal lubrication, and by increasing the compressive forces over time per unit area per unit time. Unused areas of articular cartilage would not undergo necessary exchanges of nutrients; areas of cartilage in which loading occurs would eventually fail from fatigue (see section on arthrosis later in this chapter).

It is worth mentioning that fibrillation of articular cartilage in normal hip and shoulder joints occurs first in non-weight-bearing surfaces.[36] Also, a marked acceleration of degenerative changes is shown to occur in weight-bearing animal joints in which a joint is immobilized but full use of the limb is allowed.[12] These are both examples of the effects on articular cartilage of the load-bearing contact area not being distributed over a large area of the opposing surfaces. This is perhaps a partial explanation for the frequency of degenerative arthritis occurring in human hip joints; a relatively small surface area is used for weight bearing, while much of the articular cartilage receives little or no compression. As will be discussed later in the section on arthrosis, it also contributes to the explanation of how abnormal joint arthrokinematics may lead to joint pathology.

APPROACH TO MANAGEMENT OF JOINT DYSFUNCTION

We have established as our rationale for specific joint mobilization the restoration of normal joint play in order that full, pain-free motion may occur at the joint. The term *joint dysfunction* is used by Mennell to indicate loss of normal joint play.[38] There are many explanations for the causes of joint dysfunction, some of which are specific for certain joints and some of which may be applied to all joints. In the spine, entrapment of "meniscoid inclusions" is postulated by some as a cause of joint dysfunction. Frankel and co-workers have demonstrated through instant center analysis the presence of joint dysfunction at the knee from meniscus tears (confirmed later by surgery) and dysfunction in ankle joints that had been classified as unstable, postfracture, or having degenerative disease.[16,45] It has also been shown that joint dysfunction in "frozen shoulders" is often caused by adherence of the anteroinferior aspect of the joint capsule to the humeral head.[39] A loose body in a joint may be a cause of dysfunction, as may joint effusion causing some distention of the capsule. The list goes on, the point being that *there is no single cause of joint dysfunction*.

The use of specific mobilization is not indicated in all cases of dysfunction. For this reason, a thorough evaluation performed in an attempt to clarify the nature and extent of the lesion is a necessary step in the management of joint problems.

Those cases in which a physical therapist must play a major role in treatment of joint dysfunction are those dysfunctions occurring as a result of isolated or generalized capsular tightness or adhesion. These typically follow traumatic sprains to the capsule or immobilization. In some cases, they occur for no *apparent* reason, for example, "adhesive capsulitis" at the shoulder.

The traditional approach to management of patients presenting with loss of pain-free movement at a joint usually involves various modes of pain relief, active and passive measures to improve osteokinematic movement, and encouragement of normal use of the part. It should be clear that this approach is inadequate and perhaps dangerous. First, it ignores the basic problem, which is often loss of normal arthrokinematics. Secondly, it involves considerable forcing of osteokinematic movements in the absence of normal arthrokinematic movement, which may only occur at the expense of the articular cartilage. This is to say that the resiliency of the cartilage may allow a certain amount of osteokinematic movement to occur without the normal accompanying arthrokinematic movements. Frankel and co-workers describe the case of a boy who continued to use his knee in the absence of normal external rotation of the tibia on the femur during knee extension.[14] One and a half years later, at surgery, dimpling of the articular cartilage of the medial femoral condyle was observable with the naked eye, presumably due to continued abnormal compression of this portion of the articular surface from loss of normal arthrokinematic movement.

A more logical approach to the management of these patients emphasizes the restoration of joint play to allow free movement between bones. This can only be achieved by (1) evaluating to determine the nature and extent of the lesion, (2) deciding if joint mobilization is indicated based upon the evaluation, (3) choosing the appropriate techniques based upon the direction and extent of restrictions, and (4) skillfully applying techniques of specific mobilization. Efforts to relieve pain and reduce muscle guarding are, of course, important adjuncts to treatment but do not in themselves constitute a treatment program. Also, some movement should be encouraged in the cardinal planes, but only as normal kinematics are restored. To a certain extent, functional use of the part should be restricted through careful instructions to the patient until normal joint mechanics are restored. This approach minimizes the possible danger of undue stresses to the articular cartilage during attempts to restore movement. It also minimizes the possibility of discharging a patient who has relatively pain-free functional use of the joint, but who may have some residual kinematic disturbance sufficient to cause cartilage fatigue over time and perhaps osteoarthrosis in later years.

PATHOLOGIC CONSIDERATIONS

A high percentage of the chronic musculoskeletal problems seen clinically are fatigue disorders. These are disorders in which abnormal stresses imposed upon a structure over a prolonged period result in a tendency toward an increased rate of tissue breakdown. All tissues, including those with low metabolic activity such as articular cartilage, undergo a necessary process of repair to continuously replace the microdamage resulting from normal use. In bone, such microdamage would involve fracturing of bony trabeculae, whereas in other connective tissues there is disruption of individual collagen fibers. So long as the rate of microtrauma does not exceed normal limits, and the rate at which the tissue is able to repair itself is not compromised, the tissue remains "normal." The tendency to maintain an equilibrium against opposing, unbalancing factors is a homeostatic mechanism; a shift in the nature of one factor will cause a compensatory reaction by the body to correspondingly alter the other factor in order to maintain balance.

In general, we can consider the nature of the various pathologies affecting the musculoskeletal tissues according to this homeostatic model. In doing so we will consider the two factors that the body is attempting to balance as (1) the process of tissue breakdown and (2) the process of tissue production or repair. In discussing abnormal, or pathologic, situations then, we must give consideration to the causes of and homeostatic responses to a tendency toward increased tissue breakdown and a tendency toward a decreased rate of breakdown. We must also be concerned with factors that might disturb the body's ability to maintain an appropriate balance, such as those that might cause an abnormal degree of tissue production, and those that might compromise the body's ability to produce enough tissue.

INCREASED RATE OF TISSUE BREAKDOWN

Increased tissue breakdown results when the frequency or magnitude of stresses to the part increases or when the capacity of the tissue to repair itself is reduced or both. Under conditions of significantly increased stress over time, the body attempts to compensate by laying down more tissue in order to increase the capacity of the tissue to withstand the higher stress levels. The result is tissue hypertrophy. In well-vascularized tissues, this occurs in conjunction with a low-grade inflammatory process incited by the increased rate of tissue damage. A new equilibrium is reached in favor of a more massive structure, better able to withstand higher stress levels without failing. Typical examples include muscle hypertrophy in response to increased loading of a muscle over time; subchondral bony sclerosis in response to increased compressive forces over a joint; and fibrosis of a joint capsule receiving increased stresses from faulty joint movement occurring over a prolonged period of time.

Such tissue hypertrophy, especially when affecting bone and capsuloligamentous structures, causes tissue to gain in strength at the expense of extensibility; the tissue becomes better able to withstand loads without undergoing gross failure, but does not deform as readily when loaded. An increase in the ratio of collagen (mineralized collagen in the case of bone) and the remaining extracellular ground substance (mucopolysaccharide) reduces extensibility. This is thought to allow increased interfiber bond formation, with a subsequent reduced mobility, or gliding capacity, of individual elements. The added stiffness reduces the energy-attenuating capacity of the structure. Less of the energy of loading is attenuated as work, and more of the energy must be absorbed internally by the structure or attenuated by increased deformation of other structures that are in series with the hypertrophic tissues. Thus, with sclerosis of subchondral bone, the overlying articular cartilage is made to undergo greater strain per unit of load because of the reduced deformability of the subjacent bone. This is thought to be an important factor in the progressive degeneration of cartilage occurring with degenerative joint disease.[43] With fibrosis of tendon tissue, such as the extensor carpi radialis brevis origin at the elbow, the reduced extensibility of the tendon fibers results in greater strain to the tenoperiosteal junction of the tendon at the lateral humeral epicondyle. The ensuing inflammatory process is responsible for the symptoms and signs of the "tennis elbow" syndrome.

Although in such situations the hypertrophic structure is more massive and less likely to fail when loaded, the rate of microdamage may remain elevated. Although the stress to the structure tends to be reduced because of the increased cross-sectional area resulting from the hypertrophy, the internal energy within the structure may be increased because of the reduced extensibility. An increase in internal energy must be dissipated as heat or microfracturing of individual structural components. Clinically, a painful, low-grade inflammatory reaction may result from the added mechanical and thermal stimulation.

Thus, when a tissue hypertrophies in response to increased stress levels, the rate of microdamage tends to remain elevated—there is simply more tissue present to assure that the structure, as a whole, does not fail. Pain may arise from the increased internal stresses to the involved tissue or from increased strain to connected tissues.

For any tissue there is a critical point past which the rate of breakdown may exceed the rate at which the tissue is able to repair or strengthen itself. Under normal metabolic conditions, this critical point is reached soonest in tissues with limited capacity for regeneration and repair. These are tissues that are poorly vascularized and have a low metabolic turnover. The typical example of such a tissue is articular cartilage. With increased compressive stress levels to a joint, the well-vascularized bone will tend to hypertrophy, while the cartilage degenerates. Even bone, however, can be stressed at a frequency or magnitude at which it can no longer repair itself fast enough to prevent progressive breakdown. A common clinical disorder in which this occurs is the stress fractures affecting athletes or other individuals who habitually engage in high-stress-level activities.

REDUCED RATE OF TISSUE BREAKDOWN

Decreased stress levels to tissue over time will reduce the rate of breakdown. Thus, with relative inactivity the rate of microdamage is less, and the body takes the opportunity to economize by reducing the rate of tissue production. The tissue no longer needs to be as strong because of the reduction in the everyday stresses it must withstand. The typical condition in which this occurs is disuse atrophy. When a part is immobilized, the bone becomes less dense, and capsules, ligaments, and muscles atrophy. The important clinical consideration in such situations is to increase gradually the stress levels to the tissue in order to promote strengthening of the structure by stimulating increased tissue production, but without causing the weakened structures to fail. This is especially true following healing of a structure such as bone or ligament; not only must new tissue be produced, but it must also mature. Maturation involves reorientation of major structural elements along the lines of stress that the structure will normally undergo. The process of maturation takes time, and the necessary stimulus is judiciously applied loading of the part in ways that simulate the loads the part will need to withstand with normal use.

INCREASED RATE OF TISSUE PRODUCTION

The rate of tissue production increases in conjunction with any inflammatory process. The reparative phase that follows acute inflammation usually involves a proliferation of collagen tissue. This is especially true in certain virulent inflammatory processes associated with bacterial infections. Chronic, low-grade inflammation, such as that mentioned above in conjunction with increased stress levels, is also accompanied by increased collagen production. Regardless of the cause, the result is a relatively fibrosed, less extensible structure. Loss of extensibility will be especially marked if the part is immobilized during the period of increased collagen production. The new collagen will not be laid down along the appropriate lines of stress, and abnormal interfiber cross-links develop that do not accommodate normal deformation. If, on the other hand, some movement of the part occurs during the period of increased collagen production, the loss of extensibility will not be so great. Appropriate orientation of the newly laid fibers is stimulated by the stresses imposed upon the tissue by movement. Loss of extensibility in the immobilized part is due to the increased density of the structure, as well as abnormal orientation of the structured elements, whereas in the part in which some movement occurs reduced extensibility is primarily a result of the change in density.

Clinically, then, a part that is strictly immobilized during an acute inflammatory process, such as that induced by surgery, trauma, infection, or rheumatoid arthritis, is likely to lose more movement, and the loss of movement is likely to be more persistent than in the case of a part in which some movement continues in the presence of a chronic, low-grade inflammation, such as degenerative joint disease.

Restoration of normal extensibility of the tissue requires (1) removing the stimulus of increased tissue production (stress, infection, trauma, etc.); (2) gradually stretching the structure to break down abnormal interfiber cross-links; and (3) restoring normal use of the part to induce normal orientation of structural elements.

REDUCED RATE OF TISSUE PRODUCTION AND REPAIR

As mentioned above, reduced rate of tissue production and repair occurs with reduced stress levels to the tissue, but it may also occur with some change in the metabolic status of the tissue. Examples of the latter include nutritional deficiencies, reduced vascularity, and abnormal hormone levels. When the cause is related to reduced stress levels, amelioration simply involves a gradual return to normal stress conditions. However, when the cause is metabolic in nature, treatment is more complex and will vary with the type of disturbance. In these cases, stress levels must be reduced, since the body is unable to keep up with the normal rate of tissue breakdown. Continued use of the part will result in fatigue failure of the involved tissues.

Typical examples of common musculoskeletal disorders that are related to such an alteration in the metabolic status of the involved tissues include the following:

Supraspinatus tendinitis at the shoulder— The tendon begins to fatigue from reduced vascularity to an area of the tendon close to its insertion. Occasionally the body attempts to compensate for its inability to produce new tendon tissue by laying down calculous deposits. These lesions often progress to complete tendon ruptures because the rate of breakdown continues to exceed the capacity of the tissue to repair itself.

Reflex sympathetic dystrophy—Generalized hypovascularity to a part, caused by increased sympathetic activity, results in atrophy of bone, nails, muscle, and skin—in short, all musculoskeletal components.

Senile and postmenopausal osteoporosis—Bone metabolism is comprised as a result of alteration in hormone levels and other age-related influences. The bone atrophy is most marked in cancellous bone, such as that of the vertebral bodies. Radiographs often show collapsed vertebrae, resulting from progressive trabecular buckling.

Age-related tissue changes—Aging, in itself, does not seem to result in changes in the collagen content of musculoskeletal tissues. However, with advancing age, the protein-polysaccharide (glyco–amino–glycan) content of most somatic tissues is reduced. There is also an associated reduction in water content, since the protein-polysaccharide component of the tissue matrices is responsible for the fluid binding capacity of the tissues. The result is a relative fibrosis of the involved tissues, since the ratio of collagen to ground substance is increased. It is postulated that the protein-polysaccharide ground substance normally acts as a lubricating spacer between collagen fibers. As its content is reduced, the collagen fibers approximate one another and form increased numbers of interfiber cross-links (intermolecular bonds), and the fibers no longer glide easily with respect to each other. Thus, the stiffness of the structure increases. Because of the increased stiffness, the tissue as a whole looses its deformability and therefore looses its ability to attenuate the energy of loading. With loading more stress is imposed upon individual structural elements, and the rate of tissue breakdown subsequently increases. For many elderly individuals this does not pose a problem since activity levels, and therefore stress levels, decrease with advancing age.

The reduced fluid-binding capacity of the tissue, associated with protein-polysaccharide depletion, may alter the nutritional status of the tissue. This is especially important in structures, such as articular cartilage and intervertebral discs, that depend on fluid inhibition for normal exchange of nutrients. Thus, the capacity of the tissue to repair itself will also be reduced. This is a likely explanation for the degeneration of intervertebral discs and articular cartilage that occurs with advancing age.

INTERVENTION AND COMMUNICATION

From a clinical standpoint, the therapist should be prepared to estimate the nature of a pathologic process according to this scheme. This is necessary in order to plan a treatment program specific for the type of pathology present. The therapist must also be aware of the various ways he can effectively intervene so as to appropriately alter the pathologic state.

The terms used to refer to common musculoskeletal pathologies usually provide little information relating to the nature of the disorder. The same term may be applied to different conditions in which the cause and nature of the pathologic process are quite distinct. *Tendinitis* at the shoulder is an atrophic, degenerative condition resulting from reduced vascularity to an area of the rotator cuff tendons; *tendinitis* at the elbow is a hypertrophic, fibrotic condition often related to increased stress levels. Also, many terms, such as *degenerative joint disease*, refer to situations in which a number of tissues may be involved, and the nature of the changes affecting the involved tissues may differ. In the case of degenerative joint disease, for example, the subchondral bone and the joint capsule tend to hypertrophy, while the articular cartilage atrophies and degenerates.

Therapeutically, there are many physical agents and procedures that may be used in order to influence various types of pathologic processes. Perhaps the most important form of intervention is well-planned instructions to the patient regarding the performance of specific activities. In order to give appropriate instructions the clinician must gear the patient's activity level to the nature of the pathology. This requires a knowledge of the response of tissues to various loading conditions under normal and abnormal circumstances. A careful examination must be carried out, including a biomechanical assessment. It also requires that the clinician be aware of the types of stresses imposed upon a part by various activities. The patient must understand what he is told, and he must be able and willing to carry out the instructions.

ARTHROSIS

When considering a diseased joint we usually think in terms of the physiological changes that have occurred at the joint. There is much information concerning the histologic and biochemical changes in periarticular tissues, changes in hemodynamics, and synovial fluid changes that accompany some of the more common joint diseases.[2,7,29,30–32,35] Although it is recognized that mechanical changes also occur, these are usually not dealt with until advanced structural changes have resulted. The treatment then is usually surgical. The earlier, conservative treatment in joint disease typically involves measures to counter the physiological changes taking place. This seems the logical approach in arthropathies in which the etiology is apparently some physiological change and in which the primary joint changes are physiological. Thus, in rheumatoid arthritis, gout, and spondylitis, the primary treatments are those aimed at control of inflammation and metabolic disturbances. The mechanical changes in joint function are generally agreed to be secondary and often left to improve (or degenerate) along with the primary physiological changes.

Although our knowledge of normal joint mechanics is becoming more sophisticated, little has been written concerning the mechanical changes that occur with, or possibly lead to, joint disease. It is well accepted, however, that joint disease may result from some mechanical disturbance. These cases are usually referred to as *secondary osteoarthritis*, in which some past joint trauma can be cited as a precipitating factor. This is distinguished by many researchers from *primary osteoarthritis*, in which several joints may be involved with no known causative factor. However, the pathologies of primary and secondary osteoarthritis are essentially identical, and since they are for the most part noninflammatory, they are best referred to as *osteoarthroses*. As the probable etiologies of osteoarthroses are investigated, the more it appears that the classifications of primary and secondary are often arbitrary. Although it has been postulated by some that primary osteoarthrosis has a physiological or metabolic etiology, it appears that in many cases it is due to mechanical changes, the onset of which are much more subtle than those causing secondary osteoarthrosis.[18,19,46]

It is generally agreed that changes in the articular cartilage trigger a cycle leading to the progression of degenerative joint disease. Cartilage damage may occur following a single traumatic incident causing a tension or compression strain sufficient to interfere with the structural integrity of the cartilage. This is relatively rare and usually accompanies a fracture of the adjacent bone. More common is cartilage wearing from fatigue, or the cumulative effects of abnormal stresses, none of which is sufficient in itself to cause structural damage.[18,51] Cartilage may be susceptible to fatigue in part because it is aneural; any other musculoskeletal tissue is relatively immune to fatigue because protective reflex inhibition occurs with abnormal stress. This inhibitory response requires, of course, intact innervation. Cartilage is also susceptible to damage because it is avascular. It lacks the normal inflammation and repair response that would replace damaged parts of the tissue. In fact, when cartilage is lacerated without involvement of the vascularized subchondral bone, there is a brief proliferation of chondrocytes, but no repair of the defect ensues. If the lesion is sufficient to penetrate the subchondral bone, it immediately fills with blood, and a clot is formed. This clot is invaded with new blood vessels that apparently bring in undifferentiated mesenchymal cells. These cells proceed to fill the defect with fibrocartilage (not hyaline cartilage).[10,23]

Hyaline cartilage in part makes up for the fact that it is aneural and avascular by its considerable ability to deform when loaded in compression. Much of the substance of articular cartilage is a mucopolysaccharide ground substance, a chief component of which is chondroitin sulfate. Chondroitin sulfate is highly hydrophilic with the ability to bind large quantities of water. Cartilage is about 70% to 80% water and depends upon this water content for its resiliency—its ability to withstand compression stresses without structural damage. The energy of compressive loading is dissipated as cartilage undergoes strain, or deformation. This strain results in tension stresses that are absorbed by the collagen fibers embedded within the ground substance (Fig. 2-16). Thus, the extracellular cartilage matrix normally withstands compression stresses, through the mucopolysaccharide gel, and tension stresses, through the collagen fibers. Interspersed throughout this matrix are the chondrocytes, or cartilage cells, that are responsible for production of the matrix components. It must be added that a considerable proportion of compressive forces is attenuated by the cancellous sub-

Fig. 2-16. (*A*) Compressive loading of articular cartilage results in (*B*) tensile stresses to the collagenous elements and compressive stresses to the mucopolysaccharide-water complex. (*C*) The total response is viscoelastic in nature. The viscous creep with sustained loading is largely the result of a time-dependent squeezing out of fluid.

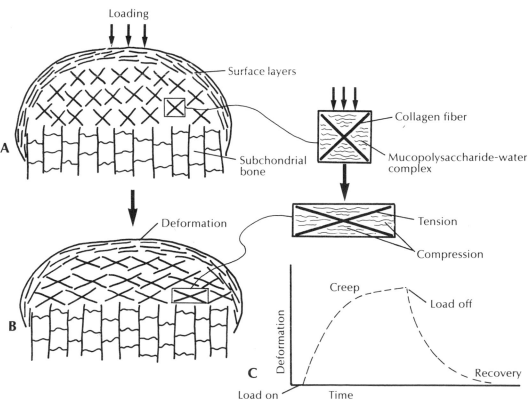

chondral bone that, although stiffer than the articular cartilage, is thicker and has more volume for energy attenuation.[43]

Although cartilage was once thought to be inert metabolically, studies now indicate that turnover of cartilage does occur.[32] Chondrocytes apparently secrete some matrix material continuously to replace that lost by normal attrition. It has also been shown that in response to mild or moderate osteoarthrosis in which cartilage degradation has increased, proliferation and metabolic activity of chondrocytes also increase. At least for a while the chondrocytes are able to keep pace with the disease. For some reason as yet unknown, this process shuts down in later stages of the disease. It is also poorly understood why lacerations of cartilage do not undergo repair, whereas some repair does take place in the earlier stages of osteoarthrosis.

The Degenerative Cycle

The initial changes that occur in the cartilage when abnormal stresses leading to acute damage or chronic fatigue are applied are (1) fibrillation, or fracturing of collagen fibers, and (2) depletion of ground substance, primarily a loss of chondroitin sulfate.[7,29,30,35-37,51] There remains some

dispute over which change takes place first; however, it seems to be agreed that once initiated, a vicious cycle of degeneration will follow. This cycle is countered up to a point by the proliferation of chondrocytes and the increased secretion of cartilage matrix by the chondrocytes. A cycle, such as depicted in Figure 2-17 is likely to develop. Loss of chondroitin sulfate leaves the collagen fibers more susceptible to fracture; fracturing of these fibers causes a "softening" of the surface layers of the cartilage; the cartilage becomes less able to withstand stresses in this region, with the resultant death of local chondrocytes; the death of chondrocytes is thought to allow the release of proteolytic enzymes that have a further degradatory effect on chondroitin sulfate. The adjacent areas of cartilage, peripheral and deep to this damaged area, must now absorb increased stresses, so the process of cartilage degeneration tends to spread. Added to this mechanical factor in spreading is the chemical factor due to destructive enzyme release.[44]

Because of the absence of pain receptors in articular cartilage, considerable degeneration may take place before symptoms bring the problem to the attention of the patient. Pain or stiffness may not occur until synovial effusion causes sufficient

Fig. 2-17. Cycle of degenerative changes in a joint

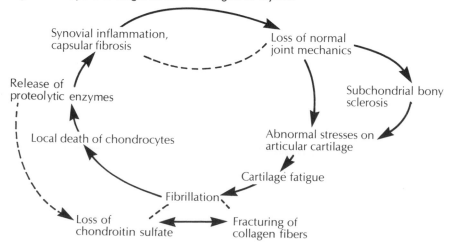

pressure to the joint capsule to fire pain- or pressure-sensitive receptors. The effusion is a result of synovial irritation caused by the release of proteolytic enzymes and other cartilaginous debris. Further irritation may result from abnormal stresses to the joint capsule from altered joint mechanics. In the case of low-grade, chronic inflammation of the synovial lining, the patient may be aware of only transient symptoms. Such a low-grade inflammation, if chronic, will result in capsular fibrosis, or thickening, which will further alter joint mechanics. Fibrosis of the joint capsule may be thought of as a relative increase in the collagen-mucopolysaccharide ratio. The result is that which occurs with any scarring process—reduced extensibility from loss of elasticity, gradual contracture, and adherence to adjacent tissues. The loss of capsular mobility often goes unnoticed by the patient until it causes sufficient limitation of motion to interfere with daily activities. In joints such as the shoulder, which in the inactive person may be used only through a small range of motion to perform daily activities, a rather marked limitation of movement may occur before the patient realizes that a problem exists. Such a lack of mobility of the joint capsule will, of course, contribute significantly to the cycle of degeneration depicted in Figure 2-17 because of the resultant alteration of normal joint mechanics. Other reactive joint tissue changes will also occur if the process is allowed to continue, including osteophyte formation, subchondral sclerosis, subchondral cyst formation, and eburnation of exposed bone. It should be realized that subchondral bone changes are likely to lead to an alteration in the forces that must be absorbed by the articular cartilage since normally subchondral bone takes up much of the force of compressive loading.[53] In fact, some researchers feel that subchondral bone changes, such as sclerotic changes due too altered blood flow, are often the first changes to take place in the degenerative cycle.[7]

Changes in composition and structure of the articular surface, owing to fibrillation and chondroitin sulfate depletion, are also likely to compromise the lubrication system of the joint. Large irregularities would gradually make boundary lubrication less effective; loss of cartilage resiliency from chondroitin sulfate loss would interfere with weeping lubrication. These potential changes in lubrication efficiency would also seem to contribute further to the progression of degeneration.

CAPSULAR TIGHTNESS

As indicated in the section on clinical application, specific joint mobilization techniques are primarily used in cases of capsuloligamentous tightness or adherence. There are, of course, cases in which an isolated portion of a joint capsule or supporting ligament is injured and heals in a state of relative shortening or becomes adhered to adjacent tissues during the healing process. Such pathologies are usually of traumatic origin, with a well-defined mechanism of injury and subsequent course. More often, however, the therapist is confronted with cases in which the entire joint capsule is "tight," as suggested by the presence of a capsular pattern of restriction at the joint. Conditions that cause a capsular pattern of restriction at a joint can be classified into two general categories: (1) conditions in which there is considerable joint effusion or synovial inflammation, and (2) conditions in which there is a relative capsular fibrosis. It is important to make this distinction since the implications for management will vary according to the cause of the restriction.

Joint Effusion

Joint effusion causes a capsular pattern of restriction because of the distension of the joint capsule by the excessive intra-articular synovial fluid. Portions of the capsule that are normally lax in order to allow a certain range of movement become taut because of capsular distention. The joint tends to assume a position in which the joint cavity—the space enclosed by the joint capsule—is of maximum volume. The continuous pressure applied to the capsule by the joint fluid may effect abnormal firing of joint receptors, which results in an alteration in function of the muscles controlling the joint.[54] The rapid wasting of the quadriceps in the presence of knee joint effusion is thought to be a result of reflex muscle inhibition from abnormal receptor firing.[9] There may also be reflex facilitation of muscle activity, observed as muscle spasm or guarding, when the joint is moved. Those conditions that cause limited movement due to articular effusion may be broadly classified as cases of inflammatory arthritis. These may, of course, include traumatic arthritis, in which some portion of the joint capsule is torn or stretched, rheumatoid arthritis, in which the synovial layer of the capsule is inflamed, infectious arthritis, gout, and others. In the acute stage of each of these conditions, the capsular restriction is primarily a result of the increased secretion of synovial fluid accompanying the acute stage of the inflammatory process or one result of reflex muscle guarding from abnormal firing of joint receptors. The cause of the restriction must be appreciated since, in such cases, we do not wish to stretch the joint capsule to restore movement, but rather to assist in the resolution of the acute inflammatory process.

Relative Capsular Fibrosis

Relative capsular fibrosis most commonly accompanies one, or some combination, of the three following situations: (1) resolution of an acute articular inflammatory process; (2) a chronic, low-grade articular inflammatory process; and (3) immobilization of a joint.[3,12,13] The term *relative capsular fibrosis* has been used, up to this point, since histologically the capsular changes do not necessarily involve an increase in collagen content. It seems, instead, that inextensibility of capsular tissue may come about from either an increase in collagen content with respect to mucopolysaccharide content, or by internal changes in the nature of the collagen tissue, such as changes in intermolecular cross-linking. The former might arise from an increased laying down of collagen, such as takes place during the repair phase of any inflammatory process.[1,8] It might also occur from a net loss of mucopolysaccharide content, with the total collagen content remaining constant. This typically occurs with prolonged immobilization of a joint.[12,41,52] One might consider the mucopolysaccharide content of connective tissue as serving as a lubricant for the collagen fibers; loss of the lubricant permits collagen fibers to approximate each other and to form abnormal interfiber cross-links. This inhibits their ability to glide against each other and thus reduces extensibility of the tissue.[1]

Clinically, it seems that conditions in which there is an actual increase in collagen content are more resistant to efforts to restore motion than are those cases of capsular restriction in which there is a net loss of mucopolysaccharide due simply to immobilization. Also, inflammatory arthritis from infection resolves with a much greater degree of fibrosis (increase in collagen) than the capsular fibrosis that accompanies low-grade, noninfectious joint inflammation such as degenerative joint disease. Thus, we might expect the rate of improvement in range of motion to be more rapid in conditions at the top of the following list, and slower when dealing with the capsular fibrosis which follows conditions near the bottom:

Simple immobilization
Traumatic arthritis

Degenerative arthrosis
Rheumatoid arthritis
Infectious arthritis

Several explanations might be offered to account for the differences in rates of improvement noted above. First, relatively destructive processes, such as infectious arthritis or rheumatoid arthritis, might be met with a more vigorous repair response and, therefore, more collagen production during the resolution of the acute inflammatory process. Secondly, the period of immobilization, either prescribed or owing to pain, is usually greater in acute inflammatory conditions, such as infectious or rheumatoid arthritis, than in relatively chronic conditions such as degenerative joint disease. The tendency, then, is for them to heal with less mobility. Thirdly, during the mobilization period, the tissues may adapt more readily to increased mobility by laying down more mucopolysaccharide ground substance than they could by remodeling collagen. The maturation of the highly collagenous "scar tissue" is a longer, more involved process, involving reabsorption of excess collagen, realignment of collagen fiber orientation, and changes in the intermolecular cross-links within the collagen tissue.[1] In this way, capsular restriction from immobilization only, in which there is no increase in collagen content, is more easily resolved than conditions that lead to an actual increase in the collagen content of the joint capsules. It should be clear from this discussion that in order to accurately set treatment goals, the therapist should understand the nature of the pathologic process and its implications.

CLINICAL CONSIDERATIONS

Considering what we now know of the pathogenesis of osteoarthrosis, the accompanying biochemical responses, the pathologic tissue changes, and the clinical manifestions, some important conclusions and correlations are worth considering in the management of patients with arthrosis.

Subtle changes in joint kinematics, persisting over a period of time, may cause abnormal stresses sufficient to result in gradual cartilage fatigue, which may, in turn, trigger a progression of changes leading to osteoarthrosis. Perhaps the most convincing evidence of this are studies by Frankel and co-workers that show changes in the normal instant centers of motion in knee joints with minimal clinical signs or symptoms.[14,16] These changes suggested premature compression of joint surfaces accompanying knee extension. On careful clinical testing, loss of longitudinal external rotation of the tibia, with respect to the normal side, was found during extension on the involved side. Subsequent surgery revealed obvious "dimpling" of the cartilaginous joint surface, in the area of the cartilage compressed at full knee extension. In these cases internal derangement of the knee, while not sufficient to cause significant symptoms or signs, was responsible for altering normal knee mechanics enough to cause early cartilaginous changes, observable with the naked eye.

Up to a point in the progression of the disease, the cartilaginous destruction is repaired by increased proliferation and metabolic activity of chondrocytes, with laying down of new cartilage. The suggestion here is that osteoarthrosis is indeed somewhat reversible if managed correctly before severe progression has taken place. It is well known that osteotomy in the case of hip osteoarthrosis will cause the femoral head to become covered with fibrocartilage, with resultant restoration of the joint space on radiograph. Studies suggest that it is partly a biologic phenomenon, perhaps from the hyperemia induced by the surgical procedure, as well as a mechanical phenomenon from the redistribution of stresses over the joint.[6]

If we accept that subtle changes in joint

kinematics can lead to osteoarthrosis, or taken one step further, if we accept that this is the etiology in many of the cases that are considered primary or secondary osteoarthrosis, then we must agree that evaluation techniques that can detect these changes are valuable. Instant center analysis is probably the best technique at our disposal for detection of altered joint kinematics. However, because of the extra number of radiographs necessary, this technique is not practical for routine evaluation. In view of this, it seems that testing of joint play movements is the most valuable technique, clinically, for detecting subtle joint changes that may be causing only minor signs or symptoms but may eventually lead to more serious joint changes in the form of osteoarthrosis. Joint play techniques are important not only in evaluation of the patient presenting with obscure musculoskeletal complaints, but also in evaluating the patient recovering from more serious trauma. Simply because a patient has regained full range of motion and strength does not guarantee that normal joint kinematics have been restored.

If osteoarthrosis may be caused by loss of normal joint mechanics, then primary treatments should be aimed at restoration of normal mechanics. This may entail surgery in cases such as meniscus tears and malalignment of bony structures. In cases of capsular tightness or capsular adhesion, treatment must consist of specific mobilization aimed at restoration of normal accessory movements at the joint. Our approach to treatment of joint problems that appear to be mechanical in nature should have a biomechanical basis. At the present time, treatment is too often "supportive" until obvious physiological changes occur. Currently, treatment tends to be directed at those physiological changes, including various modalities for pain relief and pharmaceuticals for controlling inflammation. Efforts to restore joint mechanics too often consist only of range of motion exercises and muscle strengthening, carried out without regard for the possible deleterious effects to the joint and without regard for abnormal reflex activity accompanying joint movement in the absence of normal arthrokinematics.

I believe that we, as clinicians, have yet to realize our full potential in the management of patients with mechanical joint disturbances. Knowledge of normal kinematics, ability to detect changes in joint mechanics through joint play movements, and ability to restore normal component movements to a joint are necessary in successful management of patients with joint problems that are of a mechanical etiology or in which mechanical dysfunction is a prime factor.

REFERENCES

1. Akeson WH: An experimental study of joint stiffness. J Bone Joint Surg 43A:1022– 1034, 1961
2. Akeson WH, Woo SL, Amiel D: Biomechanical and biochemical changes in periarticular connective tissues during contracture development in the immobilized rabbit knee. Connect Tissue Res 2(4):315– 323, 1974
3. Akeson WH, Amiel D, LaViolette D: The connective tissue response to immobility. Clin Orthop 51:183– 197, 1967
4. Barnett CH, Cochrane W, Palfray AJ: Age changes in articular cartilage of rabbits. Ann Rheum Dis 22:389– 400, 1963
5. Barnett CH, Davies DV, MacConnaill MA: Synovial Joints, Their Structure and Function. Springfield, IL, Charles C Thomas, 1961
6. Bentley G: Articular cartilage studies and osteoarthrosis. Ann R Coll Surg Engl 57(2):86– 100, 1975
7. Bollet AJ: Connective tissue polysaccharide metabolism and the pathogenesis of osteoarthritis. Adv Intern Med 13:33– 60, 1967
8. Clayton ML, James SM, Abdulla M: Experimental investigations of ligamentous healing. Clin Orthop 61:146, 1968

9. de Andrade JR, Grant C, Dixon A: Joint distension and reflex muscle inhibition in the knee. J Bone Joint Surg 47A:313–322, 1965

10. de Palma A, McKeever LD, Subin DK: Process of repair of articular cartilage demonstrated by histology and autoradiography with tritiated thymidine. Clin Orthop 48:229–242, 1966

11. Dowson D: Modes of lubrication in human joints. In Lubrication and Wear in Living and Artificial Joints, Vol 181. Institute of Mechanical Engineers, London, 1967

12. Ely LW, Mensor MC: Studies on the immobilization of the normal joints. Surg Gynecol Ostet 57:212–215, 1963

13. Evans EB, Eggers GW, Butler JK, Blumel J: Experimental immobilization and remobilization of rat knee joints. J Bone Joint Surg 42A:737–758, 1960

14. Frankel VH: Biomechanics of the knee. In Ingwersen O (ed): The Knee Joint. New York, Elsevier-Dutton, 1973

15. Frankel VH, Burstein AH: Orthopaedic Biomechanics. Philadelphia, Lea & Febiger, 1970

16. Frankel VH, Burstein AH, Brooks DB: Biomechanics of internal derangement of the knee: Pathomechanics as determined by analysis of the instant centers of motion. J Bone Joint Surg 53A:945–962, 1971

17. Freeman MAR (ed): Adult Articular Cartilage. London, Pitman and Sons, 1973

18. Freeman MAR: The fatigue of cartilage in the pathogenesis of osteoarthrosis. Acta Orthop Scand 46:323, 1975

19. Freeman MAR: The pathogenesis of primary osteoarthrosis. Mod Trends Orthop 6:40–90, 1972

20. Freeman MAR: Treatment of ruptures of the lateral ligament of the ankle. J Bone Joint Surg 47:661–668, 1965

21. Frymann, VM: A study of the rhythmic motions of the living cranium. J Am Osteop Assoc 70:928–945, 1971

22. Goodfellow J, Hungerford DS, Woods C: Patellofemoral joint mechanics and pathology, I and II. J Bone Joint Surg 58B:287, 1976

23. Johnell O, Telhag, H: The effect of osteotomy and cartilage damage and mitotic activity: An experimental study in rabbits. Acta Orthop Scand 48:263–265, 1977

24. Kellgren JH: On the distribution of pain arising from deep somatic structures, with charts of segmental pain areas. Clin Sci 4:35, 1939

25. Klineberg IJ, Greenfield BE, Wyke B: Contribution to the reflex control of mastication from mechanoreceptors in the temperomandibular joint capsule. Dent Pract 21:73, 1970

26. Knott M, Voss D: Proprioceptive Neuromuscular Facilitation: Patterns and Techniques. New York, Harper & Row, 1968

27. MacConnaill MA: The function of intra-articular fibrocartilage with special references to the knee and inferior radioulnar joints. J Anat 66:210–227, 1932

28. MacConnaill MA, Basjaian JV: Muscles and Movements: A Basis for Human Kinesiology. Baltimore, Williams & Wilkins, 1969

29. Mankin HJ: Biochemical and metabolic aspects of osteoarthritis. Orthop Clin North Am 2(1):19–31, 1971

30. Mankin HJ, Dorfman H, Lipiello L et al: Biochemical and metabolic abnormalities in articular cartilage from osteoarthritic human hips. J Bone Joint Surg 53:523–537, 1971

31. Mankin HJ: The reaction of articular cartilage to injury and osteoarthrosis: Part I. N Engl J Med 291:1284, 1974

32. Mankin HJ: The reaction of articular cartilage to injury and osteoarthrosis: Part II. N Engl J Med 291:1335, 1974

33. Mankin HJ, Thrasher AZ, Hall D: Characteristics of articular cartilage from osteonecrotic femoral heads. J Bone Joint Surg 59A(6):724–728, 1977

34. McCutcheon CW: Lubrication of joints. Br Med J 1:384–385, 1964

35. Meachim G: Articular cartilage lesions in osteoarthritis of the femoral head. J Pathol 107:199–210, 1972

36. Meachim G, Emergy IA: Cartilage fibrillation in shoulder and hip joints in Liverpool necropsies. J Anat 116:161–197, 1973

37. Meachim G, Emergy IH: Quantitative aspects of patellofemoral fibrillation in Liverpool necropsies. Ann Rheum Dis 33:39–47, 1974

38. Mennell J: Joint Pain. Boston, Little, Brown & Co, 1964

39. Neviaser JS: Adhesive capsulitis of the

shoulder: A study of pathological findings in periarthritis of the shoulder. J Bone Joint Surg 27:211–222, 1945

40. Paris SV: Cranial manipulation. Fysioterapeuten 39:310, 1972

41. Peacock EE: Comparison of collaginous tissue surrounding normal and immobilized joints. Surg Forum 14:440, 1963

42. Radin EL, Paul IL: A consolidated concept of joint lubrication. J Bone Joint Surg 54A(3):607, 1972

43. Radin EL, Paul IL: Does cartilage compliance reduce skeletal impact loads? Arthritis Rheum 13(2):138, 1970

44. Roach JE, Tomblin W, Eyring EJ: Comparison of the effects of aspirin, steroids and sodium salicilate on articular cartilage. Clin Orthop 106:350–356, 1975

45. Sammarco GJ, Burstein AH, Frankel VH: Biomechanics of the ankle: A kinematic study. Orthop Clin North Am 4(1):75–95, 1973

46. Seileg AJ, Gerath M: An in vivo investigation of wear in animal joints. J Biomech 8:169–172, 1975

47. Sherrington C: The Integrative Action of the Nervous System. New Haven, Yale University Press, 1906

48. Skogland S: Anatomical and physiological studies of knee joint innervation in the cat. Acta Physiol Scand (Suppl)124:1–100, 1956

49. Swanson SA: Lubrication of synovial joints. J Physiol 223:22, 1972

50. Warwick R, Williams P (eds): Gray's Anatomy, 35th ed. Philadelphia, W B Saunders, 1973

51. Weightman BO, Freeman MAR, Swanson SAV: Fatigue of articular cartilage. Nature 244:303–304, 1973

52. Woo SL, Mathews JV, Akeson WH et al: Connective tissue response to immobility. Arthritis Rheum 18(3):257–264, 1975

53. Wright V (ed): Lubrication and Wear in Joints. Philadelphia, J B Lippincott, 1969

54. Wyke B: The Neurology of joints. Ann R Coll Surg Engl 41:25, 1967

3 Pain

Maureen K. Lynch and
Randolph M. Kessler

It is not a fixed response to a noxious stimulus, its perception is modified by past experiences, expectations and even by culture. It has a protective function, warning us that something biologically harmful is happening, but anyone who has suffered prolonged severe pain would regard it as an evil, a punishing affliction that is harmful in its own right.

—Ronald Melzack

There are many reasons why the clinician should understand mechanisms of pain perception. We frequently see patients whose primary complaint is pain, which often leads to a loss of function. Usually, a careful assessment of pain behavior is invaluable in determining the nature and extent of the underlying pathology. Development of an appropriate treatment program and evaluation of progress may depend largely upon pain assessment. Therefore, it is important for those who see patients with pain complaints to have a basic understanding of the neurophysiology of pain, including mechanisms of pain perception and the phenomena of referred and projected pain. The clinician should understand how specific treatment modalities influence the nature of pain and how knowledge of pain mechanisms can be applied to its management.

PAIN OF DEEP SOMATIC ORIGIN

When examining a patient with pain of musculoskeletal origin, the clinician often finds that the site that the patient indicates as the most painful does not correspond well with the site of the lesion. The patient often gives a history of proximal or distal radiation of pain and may describe it as moving from one place to another. In addition, we often find cutaneous hyperalgesia or hypalgesia and tenderness to palpation at sites distant from—or at least not directly over—the site of pathology. For example, patients with shoulder problems often describe pain over the lateral brachial region, radiating to the elbow or hand. This type of radiation eliminates muscle spasm as a possible cause of pain since no muscle traverses the extent of this distribution. Similarly, the patient with a low-back problem often describes more pain in the buttock than in the lumbar region. In the past, a discrepancy between the site of the pathology and the site at which pain is perceived was often attributed to muscle spasm or sciatic nerve inflammation. These possibilities are unlikely, however, since the pain is often described as traveling distally down the leg and spiraling around the thigh to the front of the lower leg, a distribution that does not correspond to any nerve or muscle. Pain patterns that are associated

51

with deep somatic lesions relate to the embryological development of the musculoskeletal system (see Chapter 1, Embryology of the Musculoskeletal System). Kellgren and other researchers have clarified and supported this association by mapping areas of pain reference from stimulation of deep somatic structures, by determining the relative sensitivities of the various structures, and by describing the general qualities of pain of somatic origin.

EXPERIMENTAL DATA

In their series of studies, Kellgren and co-workers injected saline into various joint tissues, including the fibrous capsule, ligaments, tendons, muscle, fascia, menisci, synovia, and articular cartilage.[30,31] They also stimulated the periosteum with a Kirschner wire. These studies revealed several significant findings on the nature of musculoskeletal pain that, unfortunately, are still widely ignored clinically.

> The structures most sensitive to noxious stimulation are the periosteum and joint capsule. Subchondral bone, tendons, and ligaments are moderately pain sensitive, while muscle and cortical bone are somewhat less sensitive. Synovium, articular cartilage, and fibrocartilage are essentially insensitive to nociceptive stimulation.

Thus, cartilaginous erosion accompanying degenerative joint disease, synovitis, meniscus tears, and disc protrusions are not painful. Secondary or concomitant involvement of other tissues must occur in order for the patient to be aware of the problem. These, then, are pathologies that can be "silent" for a period, leading to insidious, and often significant, progression before being seen by the clinician.

Tendon and ligament injuries are likely to be most painful when their junction with the periosteum is affected. Too often muscle is implicated as the source of pain in patients with somatic pain complaints.

> Pain of musculoskeletal origin is usually delocalized; the site at which pain is perceived rarely corresponds exactly with the site of stimulation. Generally, the closer the tissue is to the body surface, the better the site of pain corresponds to the site of stimulation.

This finding deviates markedly from the way we are accustomed to thinking of pain, or sensation in general. Most common sensations affect the skin and are well localized to the site of stimulation. This, however, is not true of subcutaneous sensations, whether somatic or visceral. Thus, for example, pain from lesions about the glenohumeral joint is felt in the lateral brachial region, pain from cervical joints is felt in the scapular area, and pain from the hip joint is felt anywhere from the groin to the knee. These are common cases of deeply situated pathologies that cause delocalized sensations. On the other hand, pain from ligament sprains at the knee, ankle, or wrist, all of which are relatively superficial lesions, is quite well localized to the site of involvement.

Although documented years ago, this characteristic of pain of deep-tissue origin, still goes widely unrecognized by clinicians. Patients continue to receive injections, ultrasound, or massage about the scapulae for disorders arising from the neck; the sacroiliac joint or sciatic nerve is often blamed for pain originating in the lumbar spine; and on occasion, an adolescent presenting with slipped capital femoral epiphysis may receive treatment for "knee pain."

With increased stimulation, pain of deep somatic origin may radiate into a characteristic distribution. The pattern of distribution is always the same for a particular site of stimulation, and tends to follow a segmental, or sclerotomic, pathway. The extent of radiation is dependent upon the intensity of stimulation, and pain tends to radiate distally rather than proximally.

Recall that a sclerotome is defined as those deep somatic tissues that are innervated by the same segmental spinal nerve. These have been mapped by Inman and Saunders and are depicted in Figure 3-1. Note that they do not correspond exactly to dermatomes (Fig. 3-2 and 3-3). When a tissue of a particular sclerotome is irritated, the patient may perceive the resulting pain as arising from any or all of the tissues innervated by the same segmental nerve. This is a result of the lack of precision in central neural connections and is not related to abnormal impulses "spreading down a nerve"; in other words, the "problem" is central, not peripheral, and there is nothing wrong with most of the area from which pain seems to arise. Furthermore, it is crucial to realize that *radiating pain does not necessarily imply nerve irritation.*

Thus, patients with supraspinatus tendinitis often have pain referred down the lateral aspect of the arm and forearm to the wrist; disc protrusions may cause pain

(*text continues on page 56*)

Fig. 3-1. Sclerotomes

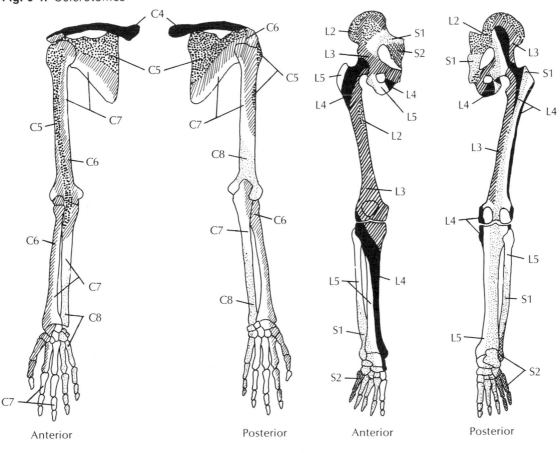

Anterior   Posterior   Anterior   Posterior

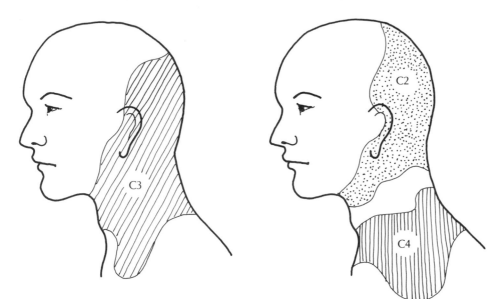

Fig. 3-2. Dermatomes of the head and neck

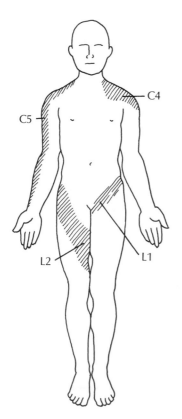

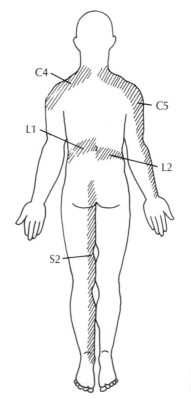

Fig. 3-3. Dermatomes of the body

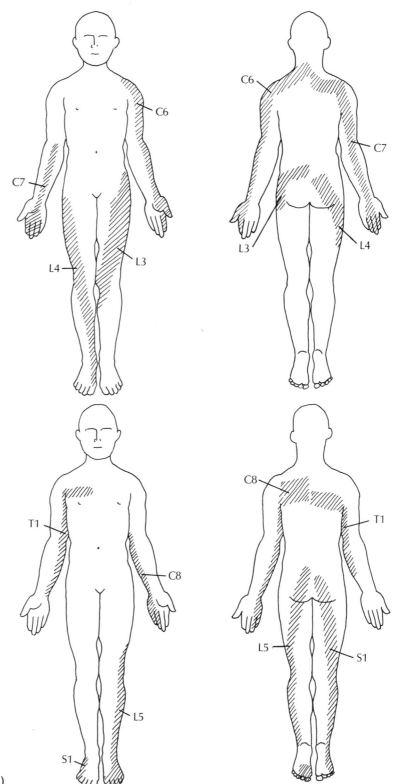

Fig. 3-3. (*Continued*)

to radiate into a limb without nerve-root pressure, and trochanteric bursitis is often mistaken for L5 nerve-root irritation or is diagnosed as fasciitis of the iliotibial band. Again, the clinical implications of referred pain cannot be overemphasized, and must be appreciated by the clinician seeing patients with musculoskeletal disorders.

> Pain of deep somatic origin is of a deep, aching, generalized quality as opposed to the sharp, well-localized pain that may arise from stimulation of the skin. In addition, deep somatic pain is often associated with autonomic phenomena such as increased sweating, pallor, and reduced blood pressure, and is commonly accompanied by a subjective feeling of nausea and faintness.

The terms *sclerotomic* and *dermatomic* are often used to distinguish between pain arising from deep somatic tissues and from the skin. Sclerotomic pain is typically deep, aching, and poorly localized whereas dermatomic pain is sharp, sometimes shooting, and well localized. In most clinical settings, pain arising from the surface of the skin is not commonly encountered, and therefore is insignificant. However, a very important source of both dermatomic and sclerotomic pain is direct irritation of nerve pathways projecting afferent input from a particular area. This is properly referred to as *projected* pain, rather than *referred* pain, and the most common site of irritation is the nerve root. Thus, an intervertebral disc protrusion or bony osteophyte may directly excite nerve fibers subserving sensory or motor functions, producing symptoms or signs confined to the relevant dermatome, myotome, or sclerotome. The symptoms or signs will vary, depending upon the fibers affected.

The largest myelinated nerve fibers are most sensitive to pressure, whereas small-diameter, unmyelinated fibers are least sensitive. It is generally agreed that eventual dissociation of the quality of sensation is, in part, related to fiber size, and that sensations may be arranged in order of decreasing fiber size, as follows:

Vibration sense, proprioception—Large, myelinated (A-alpha) fiber

"Fast" (dermatomic) pain, temperature—Small, myelinated (A-delta) fiber

"Slow" (sclerotomic) pain—Unmyelinated (C) fiber

Touch and pressure (not listed) travel over fibers spanning the entire range of diameters. Consistent with the above scheme is the clinical observation that patients presenting with nerve root irritation may complain of paresthesia (A-alpha stimulation); pain of a sharp, well-localized, dermatomic quality (A-delta irritation); or deep, aching, sclerotomic pain (C-fiber involvement). In any case, the sensation is perceived as arising from any or all of the tissues innervated by the involved nerve.

As an aside, it should be mentioned that projected pain rarely occurs clinically from nerve irritation at sites other than the nerve root. Pressure on nerves farther out in the periphery, as in the case of carpal tunnel syndrome, thoracic outlet syndrome, or ulnar nerve palsy, are subjectively manifested primarily by paresthesia—a "pins and needles" sensation.

Differences in central projections between large-fiber afferent input and small-fiber input are responsible for observed differences in associated motor and sensory phenomena. Small-fiber afferent nerves transmitting sclerotomic and visceral pain follow a multisynaptic pathway with diffuse projections to areas such as the hypothalamus, limbic system, and reticular formation. These projections may mediate autonomic changes, such as changes in vasomotor tone, blood pressure, and sweat gland activity, that may accompany the pain experience. They may also be responsible for associated affective phenomena, such as depression, anxiety, fear, and anger. Sensory modalities transmitted over large fibers, such as dermatomic pain and non-noxious sensations, project largely to the thalamus and cortex and skip areas of the brain involved with affective and autonomic mediation. They are thus less likely to be associated with emotional and behavioral changes.

HISTORY AND DEVELOPMENT OF PAIN THEORIES AND MECHANISMS

Inconsistencies in interpreting the experiential and behavioral aspects of pain complicate any discussion of the physiology of a nociceptive system. While some researchers attempt to discuss pain as a sensory experience, others define pain in terms of associated behavioral responses, both somatic and autonomic. One might argue that extreme pain may affect an individual as a sensory experience without being recognized by an observer. Another would counter that even were this possible, pain is insignificant unless it somehow alters the victim's bodily functions, behavior, or life-style.

Still another concern of those interested in the phenomenon of pain is the affective component, the suffering, hopelessness, despair, or depression that may accompany pain, especially long-standing pain. On the basis of experience, most would agree that a "painful event" might comprise any combination of sensory, behavioral, or affective components. We might prick our finger with a pin without significant despair or depression, and in the absence of subsequent shouting, sweating, or shaking of the part. However, smashing the thumb with a hammer is frequently followed by some verbal display of displeasure and significant motor activity, including flailing of the injured part as well as generalized increased sympathetic tone. But this event is not usually associated with depression or sorrow because we realize that the swelling will soon subside. On the other hand, loss of a loved one may lead to excruciating "pain" manifested as grieving and sorrow but without a painful sensation. It is often accompanied by diminished motor activity, loss of appetite, and weeping. Interestingly, the sufferer of chronic pain behaves similarly. While individuals in each of the above situations may well complain of pain, psychosocial rewards may condition an individual to complain of pain and manifest other pain-associated behaviors in the absence of prior nociceptive events. Suffice it to say that there seem to be areas in which the neural pathways involved with pain sensation, with certain affective phenomena, and with stereotyped skeletal and smooth muscle activation intersect. Activation of all or part of these pathways results in the experiential or behavioral events generally classified as pain. Which components of the system will be activated depends upon the nature of the stimulus as well as central modulation of information reaching the central nervous system (CNS). As we know, a given stimulus may or may not result in pain, and pain behavior may occur in the absence of nociception. We have all heard stories about those wounded in war who deny pain at the time of severe tissue damage. On the other hand, individuals with no demonstrable tissue damage may complain of pain and display disabling pain behaviors. In summary, nociception may occur without pain, and pain without nociception. Theories dealing with the neurophysiology of pain must explain these facts in terms of known mechanisms and their anatomical correlates.

Knowledge of the evolution of pain theory is interesting on a historical level and contributes to an appreciation of present pain research. Today's understanding of the nociceptive system is a composite of past and present research, hypotheses, and theories, each of which has emphasized different components of the nociceptive system. Therefore, one approach to understanding pain mechanisms would be to follow the evolution of pain theory and select and combine important contributions.

One of the first recorded pain theories was proposed by Aristotle. He postulated that pain occurs with every kind of stimulation whenever that stimulation became excessive. Therefore, anything too hot, too sharp, or abnormally loud causes pain. Excessive stimulation was carried from the periphery by blood vessels to the heart where it was perceived as a negative passion or absence of pleasure. Aristotle's proposal implied that the pain experience has emotional, psychological, and physiological dimensions. The proposed anatomical pathway for nociceptive input is of course, incorrect. Aristotle chose the heart—the center of emotion—as the organ receiving and interpreting painful stimulation, which suggests that he considered the affective or emotional component of pain to be of critical importance. It is interesting to note that the affective dimension of pain was not emphasized again until the development of modern theories.

SPECIFICITY THEORY

With the advent of the microscope, scientists became greatly preoccupied with morphological detail. Investigators in the early 1800s searched for precise anatomical evidence to support hypothesized pain mechanisms. Mueller and others found minute structures in the skin, viscera, and muscles that they believed were receptor end organs for various modalities of sensation.[41,51,52] The primary theory based on microscopic evidence was Von Frey's specificity theory proposed in 1895.[45,57] Von Frey proposed a specific relationship between the type of end organ stimulated and the nature of the resulting sensation. For example, pressure is perceived when the pacinian corpuscles are stimulated, whereas stimulation of free nerve endings causes pain.

It has since been found that such a precise one-to-one relationship between type of receptor and sensation does not exist. Weddell found, for example, that the cornea, which contains only free nerve endings, is sensitive to many types of sensory stimuli.[13,45] The specificity theory proponents demonstrated, however, that there are peripheral receptors that must be excited in order for pain sensation to be perceived. Unfortunately, the theory paid little attention to central pain modulation (the influence of spinal cord or brain on input) and considered only the sensory experience of pain. It ignored the associated emotional, psychological, or motor responses.

PATTERN THEORY

Several years later, investigators became interested in peripheral nerves. Head cut a peripheral nerve in his own arm, knowing that smaller nerve fibers regenerate before larger ones. With regeneration of the small nerve fibers, Head noted spontaneous tingling, dysesthesia, and other abnormal nociceptive sensations.[13,18,45] Not until the large nerve fibers regenerated, and light pressure, touch, and vibration sense returned, were the painful sensations abolished. From this information and from insight gained through their own research (including research on cornea sensation), Weddell and Sinclair proposed a pattern theory of pain.[13,18,45,51] The pattern theory emphasized that it is the anatomical variation in fiber size over which afferent impulses travel that leads to temporal and spatial summation of input in central receiving areas. The pattern theory suggested that variation in fiber size was related to both the site of central connections and the pattern of central excitation. For example, input traveling over small fibers ascends multisynaptically in the contralateral anterolateral tract with little cortical input, whereas large-fiber input ascends in the ipsilateral dorsal column to the thalamus, with subsequent projections to the cortex. Weddell also noted that signals traveling over larger fibers reach the spinal cord before small-fiber input. Weddell and Sinclair combined this information in a theory that stated that patterns of input over various fiber sizes are a major determinant of sensation and pain perception. Thus, large fiber stimulation may be felt as light touch or pressure, whereas small-fiber stimulation tends to cause noxious sensations. A mixture may result in a combination or cancellation of sensory input.

The pattern theory postulates that a specialized system exists that combines and modifies all peripheral sensory input before it ascends to higher brain centers, thereby modifying the nature of the resultant sensation. The theory also proposes that all stimulus information from the periphery must summate in the central nervous system (CNS) to allow determination and execution of a proper response. Weddell and Sinclair stated that major determinants of intensity and quality of experienced sensations are the discharge characteristics of afferent fibers and the sites of central connections. The weaknesses in the pattern theory are (1) that pain is again considered to be largely a sensory phenomenon, and little reference is made to associated affective phenomena; (2) that knowledge of the role of receptors was ignored or denied, and (3) that the influence of central modulation of input was not considered.

NEUROANATOMY

Before discussing the gate theory of pain, it is important to compare the pathways taken by large as opposed to small, or nociceptive, afferent nerve fibers. Upon entering the dorsal horn of the spinal cord, nociceptive afferents from both somatic and visceral tissues travel in the dorsolateral fasciculus (Lissauer's tract) a few segments rostrally and caudally before entering the gray matter of the dorsal horn.[13,35,57] They then relay with cells in the substantia gelatinosa (SG) (lamina II and III) and proceed to synapse ipsilaterally in the dorsal funicular gray (lamina V), a nuclear mass that lies at the base of the dorsal horn (Fig. 3-4). The second or third order fiber crosses by way of the anterior white commissure to ascend contralaterally in the anterolateral tract. This fiber tract continues rostrally to synapse in the ventroposterolateral and ventroposteromedial nuclei of the thalamus; collaterals also project to the medullary reticular formation, limbic system, and hypothalamus. The nociceptive afferents are small myelinated and unmyelinated, slowly transmitting nerve fibers, and the receptors for this system adapt slowly to the application or removal of the irritating stimulus. The final synapses are in regions where past experience, motivation, and emotion may influence the ultimate response to noxious stimulation.[13,35,57]

Large fiber afferents from proprioceptors and mechanoreceptors transmitting information concerning light touch, vibration, and joint and muscle position enter the dorsolateral fasciculus and send collaterals to segments several spinal levels above and below the level of entry. The collateral branches enter the dorsal horn and synapse on interneurons in the SG (see Fig. 3-4). The large myelinated fibers then enter the dorsal columns ipsilaterally and ascend to the medulla where they synapse, decussate, and ascend as the medial lemniscus to the VPL of the thalamus. The third order neuron leaves the thalamus and projects to the postcentral gyrus, the sensory cortex.[13,35,57]

Both large and small fiber systems send collaterals to the anterior horn of the spi-

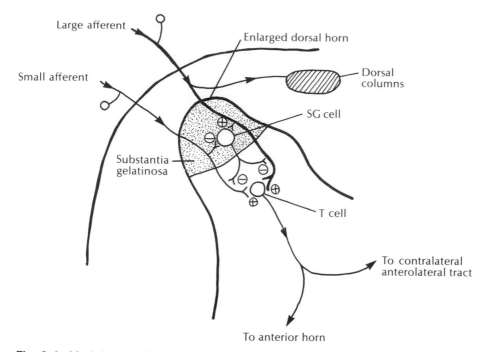

Fig. 3-4. Modulation of afferent input as proposed by the gate theory. Activation of the T cell results in ascending nociceptive input and reflex motor changes. The T cell is inhibited by SG cell input which is, in turn, inhibited by small-fiber input and facilitated by large-fiber input.

nal cord before entering ascending tracts. These projections mediate reflex motor activity associated with noxious and nonnoxious stimulation.

GATE THEORY

In 1965 Melzack and Wall proposed the gate theory of pain.[41,42,45,57] Several investigators studying the SG measured electrical potentials in some of the interneuron synapses. They found that with small-fiber input (C fibers mediating pain and temperature), hyperpolarization was recorded, and when large fibers were stimulated, depolarization was recorded. Melzack and Wall postulated that interneurons in the SG act as a "gate" to modulate sensory input (Fig. 3-5). They proposed that the SG interneuron projected to the second order neuron of the pain/temperature pathway located in the dorsal funicular gray (lamina V) which they

called the *transmission cell* or *T cell*.[41,42] If the SG interneuron were depolarized it would inhibit T-cell firing and thus decrease further transmission of input ascending in the spinothalamic tract. For example, nociceptive fibers enter the dorsal horn and send a collateral fiber into the SG, which hyperpolarizes the interneuron. The nociceptive afferent continues to lamina V where it synapses with the T cell. Upon reaching threshold levels of excitation, the T cell sends nociceptive input rostrally in the anterolateral spinal tract. Large-fiber input (joint movement, pressure, vibration) enters the dorsal horn sending a collateral into the SG, which depolarizes the SG interneuron. This interneuron projects to lamina V and presynaptically inhibits the T cell, preventing or decreasing ascending nociceptive input.[41,42,45,57] Melzack and Wall thus used concepts presented in the pattern theory and described a specific anatomic path-

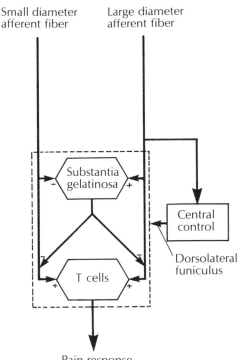

Small diameter
afferent fiber

Large diameter
afferent fiber

Substantia
gelatinosa

Central
control

T cells

Dorsolateral
funiculus

Pain response

Fig. 3-5. Scheme of dorsal horn pain-modulating system

way by which modulation of peripheral stimuli could occur. Essentially, the theory proposed an analogy to a gate, that allows ongoing transmission of painful input when opened. The position of the gate is determined by the balance between large-fiber and small-fiber input to the system and is regulated by interneurons in the SG of the dorsal horn.

The gate theory was, and is, supported by both practical and experimental evidence. When you hit your skin on the coffee-table corner, your immediate response is to rub the injured area; thus you increase large-fiber input that decreases the pain. Physical therapists use a large number of modalities to decrease pain by increasing large-fiber input. Hot packs, whirlpools, massage, vibrators, and joint mobilization all act to increase large-fiber input and, therefore, to decrease nociceptive transmission. There are also certain clinical pain states, such as alcoholic

neuropathy, in which preferential destruction of large fibers leads to chronic, relatively spontaneous pain.

Melzack and Wall also suggested that the gate could be modified by a descending inhibitory pathway from the brain or brain stem.[41,42,45,57] This was originally proposed largely on the basis of everyday experience. For example, it has been noted that people injured during stressful, life-threatening, or athletic events often do not realize the seriousness of the injury. Following frontal lobotomy or while on morphine, a patient knows when noxious stimulation is occurring, but it is no longer painful or worrisome. Melzack and Wall postulated that these observations could be explained by central inhibitory input descending to the spinal cord to decrease T-cell firing. Sometimes patients experience more pain than expected following a certain amount of noxious input. In this case it was speculated that learned or affective behavior prevented or decreased inhibition of T-cell activity.

Since the proposal of the gate theory, researchers have identified many clinical pain states that cannot be fully explained by the gate mechanism.[45,57] However, the theory has made several significant contributions to current pain research. First, it directed the attention of researchers to the importance of pain modulation by higher CNS centers. Secondly, it accomodated most past research findings dealing with receptors, peripheral nerves, the dorsal horn, and ascending sensory pathways. Thirdly, clinical applications of this theory are still useful, and many effective clinical procedures are based on the model provided by the gate theory. Transcutaneous nerve stimulation increases large-fiber input and abolishes or decreases pain to acceptable levels for many patients living with chronic pain. Clinics specializing in treatment for patients with chronic pain use behavior modification techniques to increase a patient's activity level. These techniques may act to increase large-fiber input and decrease pain or they may activate a central descending pathway which inhibits nociceptive input at the spinal cord level.[12,13,17]

CENTRAL MODULATION OF NOCICEPTIVE INPUT

Having started with Von Frey's research on peripheral skin receptors in 1850 we have now progressed to present day investigations delineating the nature of the nociceptive system in the brain. During the last decade there has been a wealth of research and discovery related to central pain modulation. Current research continues to explore the relationship between the anatomical and physiological components of central pain pathways. The spark for this research was provided by technical advancements that provide a better understanding of biochemical and neurohistological features of the nociceptive system. After years of studying morphine and other opiate derivatives, researchers discovered "endogenous opiates," peptides native to the CNS that are now thought to be involved in nociceptive modulation. More recently the role of other neurotransmitters in the nociceptive system has begun to be elucidated. Additionally, there is much more interest in the affective and behavioral components of the nociceptive system—a return to Aristotle's emphasis. It is becoming generally agreed that any comprehensive pain theory must explain pain as a sensory experience as well as its associated affective and motor (autonomic and somatic) phenomena.

OPIATES AND ENKEPHALINS

Research leading to the discovery of endogenous opiates, the enkephalins, began with studies of morphine and its mechanism of action. For years researchers and the medical community have searched for a nonaddictive opiate agonist. Because morphine exerts analgesic effects with very small doses, it was generally agreed that morphine might act as a neurotransmitter in the CNS. The subsequent prediction was that receptors for morphine must exist in the CNS.[52,53] Pert and Snyder, using advanced neurohistological and neurochemical techniques, were able to trace morphine receptor sites in the CNS. Kumar, Pert, and Snyder demonstrated the distribution of opiate receptors in many brain regions using direct receptor-binding techniques and autoradiography of brain sections containing radioactive morphine.[26,52] The receptor distribution pathway strikingly parallels the paleospinothalamic pathway (Fig. 3-6), which ascends along the midline of the brain, synapsing in the central gray matter of the brain stem, the reticular formation, and the central thalamus. This pathway mediates duller, more chronic, and less localized pain; it is the phylogenically older pain pathway, and contains many synapses and small-diameter, unmyelinated nerves.[13,32,52] Consistent with this is the observation that morphine exerts its analgesic effects on dull pain, whereas sharp, well-localized pain is poorly relieved by opiates.

Other brain areas with opiate receptors are the amygdala, the corpus striatum, and the hypothalamus, all of which are parts of the limbic system—a group of brain regions that largely mediate emotional phenomena.[52,58] These brain regions seem to be concerned with the affective components of pain, such as rage, anger, and depression, and perhaps the euphoric effects of morphine. Hypothalamic connections may mediate associated autonomic activity, such as sweating, palor, or blood pressure changes. Opiate receptors are also localized in lamina II in the SG of the dorsal horn of the spinal cord—an important synapse area for the upward conduction of nociceptive information—as

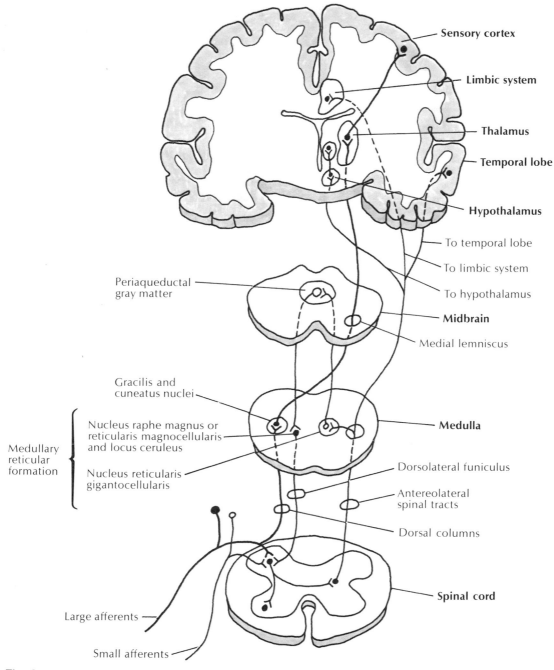

Fig. 3-6. Scheme of large- and small-fiber afferent systems and the ascending-descending inhibitory loop. The small-fiber system is often referred to as the paleospinothalamic tract and the large-fiber system as the neospinothalamic tract.

well as in lamina II of the caudal trigeminal nucleus, which receives nociceptive input from the face.[52,58]

With the discovery of morphine receptors, the search began for an endogenous substance with opiate activity. Several researchers simultaneously identified a morphinelike brain factor consisting of two closely related pentapeptides, which were named *enkephalins*.[26,52,57] It was found that naloxone, a morphine antagonist, also inhibited the analgesic effects of enkephalins.[5,15,16,38,57] Research in morphine addiction revealed that an increase in the presence of morphine is accompanied by a decrease in enkephalin production and release. It was speculated that opiate withdrawal symptoms occur from enkephalin depletion and subside as soon as enkephalin concentrations return to normal.[37,52] Several studies have also described decreased enkephalin levels associated with chronic pain.[7,33,34]

The mechanism of enkephalin action as a neurotransmitter is both interesting and speculative. Enkephalin is an excitatory transmitter thought to presynaptically inhibit the dorsal horn T cell of lamina V, and thus modulate input to ascending pain pathways in the spinal cord and the brain.[38,52,57] This has special significance for the gate theory, which 15 years ago suggested that descending inhibition occurred at the level of the dorsal horn in the spinal cord, and that perhaps the mechanism was presynaptic inhibition of the T cell in lamina V.[53]

STIMULUS-PRODUCED ANALGESIA

Following the discovery of enkephalins, researchers began to investigate possible mechanisms by which enkephalin-mediated circuits might be activated. Therefore, they have attempted to define the role of enkephalins in the nociceptive system. Opiate receptor sites (and synaptic vescicles of enkephalin) are located in the periventricular, periaqueductal, and mesencephalic central gray matter, dorsal horn, and in some limbic regions (*e.g.*, amygdala, corpus striatum) of the CNS.[38,52,57] It was found that electrical stimulation of the periaqueductal gray matter (PAG) in rats, cats, monkeys, and man produced profound analgesia.[8,13,19,32,36–39,47,49,52,57] Subsequently, researchers noted that this stimulus-produced analgesia (SPA) was partially reversed by administering naloxone.[1,4,37,38] Because SPA is only partially reversed by naloxone, it was concluded that SPA was the result of the release of both enkephalin and another unknown neurotransmitter. Investigators have measured in the cerebrospinal fluid a significant increase in enkephalin content following stimulation of the PAG in rats, and have found that injections of enkephalin into the central gray matter increase the animal's pain tolerance and produce a long-lasting analgesia to electrically evoked pain.[5,38,49,52,57] It was subsequently postulated that enkephalins were released in the PAG following noxious input. Researchers then administered radioactively labeled amino acids to experimental animals, in order to label enkephalins, which incorporate the amino acids. Following stimulation of A-delta nerve fibers (which mediate thermal and nociceptive input), the animals' brains were sectioned and analyzed for labeling. It was found that the areas where enkephalins were released overlapped the anatomical substrate for SPA.[52] This area appears to be concentrated in medial brain stem structures extending from the diencephalon (periventricular gray matter and PAG) caudally to the medullary raphe nuclei, which is part of the midbrain reticular formation.[7,8,19,21,36,38,39,48,58] It was subsequently noted that stimulation of A-delta nerve fibers also caused increased firing of nerve cells located in the medullary raphe nuclei.[7,38]

In man, stimulation of periventricular structures was effective in relieving diverse pain syndromes.[36,38] Electrical stimulation of the PAG was also shown to increase experimental pain tolerance to both painful heat and electrical shock.[38,57,58] Morphine injections into and electrical stimulation of the periventricular gray matter and PAG in cats clearly depress the discharge of neurons in lamina V of the dorsal horn (site of the first synapse in the afferent pain pathway) evoked by strong cutaneous and thermal stimulation.[19] Non-noxious stimulation was not affected by PAG stimulation or morphine injection. Finally, recent experiments have revealed that morphine injected into the amygdala produces analgesia as well as the characteristic euphoric behavior.[38,52]

The implications are fascinating. There are specific brain sites that when stimulated block pain; these areas mediate the response to morphine; a natural morphinelike substance exists exerting its influence in the same brain site as morphine; and finally, stimulation of these brain areas can prevent transmission of nociception at the level of the spinal cord.

CENTRAL DESCENDING INHIBITORY PATHWAY

The above findings strongly suggest that endogenous opiates are neurotransmitters in a nociceptive modulating system.[38,50,53] The physiological mechanism proposed is an "endogenous pain inhibitory system" or negative feedback loop[21,38] (Fig. 3-6). Specifically, peripheral nociception leads to activation of the PAG, and nuclei of the midbrain and medullary reticular formation. These nuclei then send descending inhibitory signals to the dorsal horn to reduce ongoing transmission of nociceptive input. The descending inhibitory system includes the rostral and caudal PAG, the medullary nuclei of the reticular formation, and connections in the dorsal horn. The descending limb of this feedback loop begins with neurons in the rostral PAG, an important area for SPA that is known to be rich in enkephalins.[8,38,58] The PAG neuron makes an excitatory synapse with the nucleus raphe magnus (NRM) of the medulla, near the caudal PAG, and with the adjacent nucleus reticularis magnocellularis (Rmc), perhaps using dopamine or enkephalin as a neurotransmittor. These two nuclei send fibers to the spinal cord by way of the dorsolateral funiculus that terminate among pain-transmission cells concentrated in lamina II and V of the dorsal horn.[11,12,38] Both the NRM and the nucleus Rmc exert an inhibitory effect specifically on pain-transmission neurons. The NRM uses serotonin as a transmittor; the Rmc transmittor is speculated to be enkephalin. The pain-transmission neurons (activated by substance P) following peripheral nociceptive stimulation) cross and project cranially in the anterolateral spinal tract.[14,25,39] As the anterolateral tract continues cranially, it contacts the cells of the descending analgesia system in the PAG through the nucleus reticularis gigantocellularis (RgC) of the medulla, thus establishing a negative feedback loop.[21,36,38,49] Norepinephrine-containing neurons of the locus ceruleus (LC) may also contribute to pain-modulating systems through the dorsolateral funiculus (DLF).

There is ample evidence supporting the existence of such a negative feedback loop. It has been shown that SPA readily suppresses spinal cord nociceptive reflexes.[38] Morphine injected into PAG can clearly depress the discharge of pain-transmission neurons in lamina V.[57] Stimulation of caudal PAG in the cat markedly inhibits the responses of most dorsal horn lamina V cells to noxious skin stimuli.[19] Furthermore, the analgesia due to PAG stimulation or systemic opiate administration is markedly reduced caudal to transection of the spinal DLF.[11,12] Central gray matter stimulation while inhibiting nociceptive input does not affect responses to gentle tactile stimulation.

The NRM's critical link in the descending nociceptive inhibitory system is also well supported experimentally. Stimulation of the NRM in cats results in analgesia.[47] Several investigators found that after PAG stimulation or morphine administration, they noted a significant increase in neuronal activity in NRM neurons.[46] Lesions of the NRM block opiate analgesia, while electrical stimulation of the NRM produces a potent analgesia reversed by the opiate antagonist naloxone.[7,48] Recent studies have demonstrated a population of neurons in NRM projecting to the spinal cord.[38] It was further found that this population of NRM neurons was excited by electrical stimulation of the PAG as well as by opiates administered systemically or by local injection into midbrain PAG. The PAG and NRM receive a large amount of input from the nucleus RgC, which in turn receives input from spinal cord pain-transmission neurons.[21,38] PAG stimulation in the rat has been shown to suppress the nociceptive responses of neurons in the nucleus RgC.[49] This could have been the result of supraspinal descending inhibition of the nucleus RgC or inhibition of incoming nociceptive input at the spinal cord level.

Bilateral lesions of the DLF in rats reverse the analgesic effects of systemically administered morphine.[11,12,38] Lesions of the DLF also abolish the analgesic effects of morphine injected into the PAG in rats.[11,12,36,38] Other researchers have documented that lesions of the DLF reverse both SPA and morphine-induced analgesia. This evidence implies that a descending pathway inhibits nociceptive input at the level of the spinal cord, and that this inhibition functions as part of a negative feedback loop.

MONOAMINERGIC NEUROTRANSMITTERS

It is interesting that naloxone administration only partially blocks SPA. From recent studies it now appears clear that monoaminergic neurotransmittors also play important roles in SPA and morphine analgesia.[2,20,29,42] These transmittors are serotonin, dopamine, and norepinephrine. Depletion of serotonin with p-chlorophenylalanine (p-CPA) has been shown to reduce SPA, but the analgesia can be restored by administration of the serotonin precursor, 5-hydroxytryptamine.[2,3] p-CPA is most effective in reducing SPA when the electrode stimulating sites are in the region of the NRM or dorsal raphe magnus (DRM). Both of these reticular nuclei contain serotoninergic neurons.[14,38] The NRM descends through the dorsal lateral funiculus to the dorsal horn. The DRM is part of the ascending nociceptive pathway that involves complex multisynaptic pathways first ascending to forebrain structures and then descending to the spinal cord in an as yet unknown circuit.[14] An inhibitor of serotoninergic neurons, LSD-25, has been shown to reduce the inhibitory effect that SPA has on dorsal horn lamina V neurons. Animals treated with p-CPA were found to be more reactive to electroshock presentations. Humans with migraine headaches who were treated with p-CPA experienced superficial and muscular algesias and pain with facial movement or with clothing friction—in short, fairly spontaneous pain.[38] In animals, injections of a serotonin uptake-blocking drug produces analgesia and will antagonize the hyperalgesia associated with injections of p-CPA.[29,43] Lesions of the NRM, DRM, medial forebrain bundle, or the septum produce large reductions in serotonin concentrations leading to increased pain sensitivity.[38,57] Destruction of the DRM or of the NRM and resultant loss of serotoninergic activity blocks the analgesic effect of systemically administered morphine, while increased serotonin levels potentiates morphine analgesia.[38,43] Another method of disrupting the pain inhibition pathway involves blocking the action of NRM fibers, as they synapse in the dorsal horn. Recent research documented that morphine-induced analgesia could be antagonized by administration of antiserotonin drugs to the dorsal horn. Other studies have shown that serotonin has an inhibitory effect on neurons located in the superficial laminae of the dorsal horn which respond to noxious stimuli.[28,29,43] These are also the laminae where NRM fibers terminate. In summary, it has been found that with increased serotonin levels, morphine and stimulus-produced analgesia are potentiated, while depletion of serotonin causes hyperalgesia and spontaneous pain, and blocks morphine analgesia and SPA.

Catecholaminergic neurotransmitters (*e.g.*, norepinephrine, dopamine) also appear to be involved in both SPA and morphine analgesia.[2,38,57] Compounds that deplete all monoamines almost completely abolish SPA. When compounds that deplete only catecholamines are used, a smaller reduction in SPA is found.[20] Increasing catecholamine levels with L-dopa, which leads to increased dopamine levels, potentiates SPA.[38] Recent research has found that blocking dopamine receptors inhibits SPA and morphine analgesia, whereas stimulation of dopamine receptors potentiates both. The reverse is true for norepinephrine.[20,38] Depletion of norepinephrine increases the effect of morphine and stimulus-produced analgesia; injections of excess norepinephrine block morphine and SPA.

The evidence for dopaminergic involvement in the nociceptive inhibitory pathway is less extensive than that for serotonin involvement. The only known dopamine systems ascend from the brain stem to forebrain structures, so that dopamine involvement necessitates complex ascending and descending pathways.[20,38,43] Even though the location of the dopamine pathway operating in the descending nociceptive inhibitory pathway is not known, it has been shown that dopamine plays some role. Norepi-

nephrine-containing neurons of the LC in rats and of the subceruleus parabrachialis in cats may contribute to pain modulating systems by sending fibers in the dorsolateral funiculus to lamina V of the dorsal horn.[38]

CENTRAL STRUCTURES MODULATING DESCENDING INHIBITION

Other CNS structures may play a role in nociceptive modulation. The PAG region of the midbrain receives diverse inputs from numerous brain areas and is involved in various emotional, motivational, and sensory systems.[38,49] The rostral PAG neurons integrate input from many brain areas, and the resulting output determines the level of nociceptive modulation at the midbrain and spinal cord. The PAG receives nociceptive input from the spinal cord by way of the RgC while simultaneously receiving thalamic, limbic, and cortical input. In this way, memory, learned responses, and affective components may all contribute to modulation and perception of ascending nociceptive input.

The reticular formation contains the NRM and DRM and a number of other ascending and descending pathways.[14,38] The major descending pathway concerned with nociception is that of the NRM and nucleus Rmc, which both send fibers to the dorsal horn. The ascending pathways include reticular formation (1) to the cortex—a direct pathway; (2) to several thalamic nuclei (posterior, ventral, and intralaminar); and (3) to the hypothalamus, limbic forebrain, and frontal cortex.[14] The pathway also includes a catecholamine system that arises in parts of the brain-stem reticular formation and passes through the medial forebrain bundle and septum to reach the neocortex.[14,38] This last pathway may be part of an ascending serotoninergic fiber tract.

These ascending pathways, activated by nociceptive input, excite regions of the brain involved in behavioral, affective, and motor responses to nociception. Output from these higher centers (frontal cortex, limbic regions, and thalamus) may in turn descend to the PAG to modulate ongoing nociception through the previously mentioned descending loop.[9,14,23,38] The higher cortical centers and PAG integration of input appear to determine each person's response to nociceptive input. This explains why some people perceive intense pain, others a mild discomfort, and some no noxious sensation at all in response to the same nociceptive stimulus.

There are several other brain areas that produce analgesia when electrically stimulated. One well-studied region is the medial forebrain bundle – lateral hypothalamic region.[38] Stimulation of this region in the rat has produced analgesia to pin prick, hot plate, and electric shock. For several reasons it appears that the medial forebrain bundle must produce analgesia by a pathway other than PAG → NRM → dorsal horn. Some evidence indicates that stimulation of the medial forebrain bundle can reduce clinical pain in humans.

Stimulation of the septal region also produces analgesia, again seemingly by a different pathway than the medial brain stem system. Septal region stimulation has been reported to be effective in relieving clinical pain syndromes in man.[38]

ENDORPHINS

Another class of polypeptides with endogenous opiate activity are the endorphins.[24,49] Beta-endorphin, with a chain of 30 amino acids, is among the most potent endogenous analgesics known. It has been found that a sequence of five amino acids on the amino terminal of the beta-endorphin molecule corresponds to the sequence of enkephalin. This may account for their similar analgesic properties. In fact, beta-endorphins have been shown to bind to some of the same sites in the brain,

such as the PAG, as the enkephalins. Endorphins do not appear to bind in the spinal cord, however. There is no evidence that enkephalins are products of endorphins; it is probable that enkephalins are primarily produced within neurons, to be used as neurotransmitters.

Immunochemical studies have demonstrated endorphins in the pituitary, brain, and intestinal tract. They seem to be released from the pituitary as part of a much larger polypeptide molecule, beta-lipotropin (Fig. 3-7), which may in turn be a product of a still larger "prohormone." Beta-lipotropin is also a precursor of adrenocerticotropic hormone (ACTH), and there is evidence that endorphins are released in response to the same stimuli that trigger ACTH release, for example, stress.[44]

The role of endorphins in pain modulation has not yet been elucidated. Intracerebral injections of endorphins produce profound and prolonged analgesia, but large doses administered into the peripheral blood stream have no analgesic effects. There is a tendency to want to attribute apparent cases of relative analgesia under stress, such as in the case of the war-injured or shark-bite victim, to massive endorphin release. However, there is no experimental evidence to demonstrate analgesia from endorphins released from the pituitary, and it is unlikely that they cross the blood-brain barrier. While speculation on the role of endorphins in mediating such phenomena as the "runner's high" are interesting, corroboration awaits further study. It is likely, however, that the endorphins do influence the maintenance of behavioral homeostasis, perhaps affecting the central nociceptive modulating system.[24]

SUMMARY OF SENSORY PATHWAYS

Nociceptive stimulation of free nerve endings is usually associated with concomitant stimulation of non-nociceptive recep-

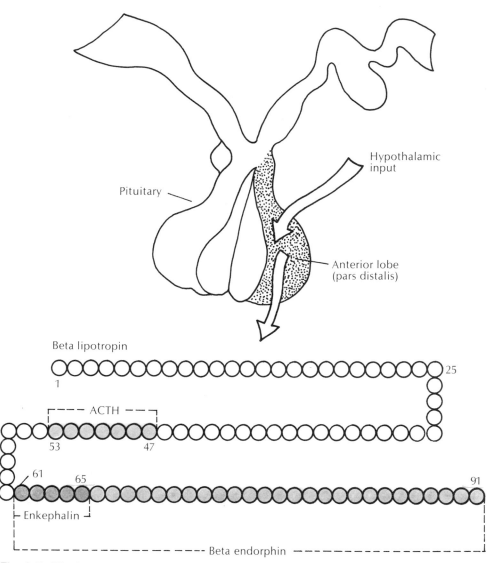

Pituitary

Hypothalamic input

Anterior lobe
(pars distalis)

Beta lipotropin

1

25

ACTH

53 47

61 65 91

Enkephalin

Beta endorphin

Fig. 3-7. The beta lipotropin hormone complex released from the anterior pituitary contains amino acid sequences corresponding to ACTH and beta endorphin. Beta endorphin, in turn, contains the sequence for enkephalin.

tors, such as mechanoreceptors. Touch and pressure input travels to the cord over large myelinated fibers and to the cortex by a dorsal column–medial lemniscus–thalamus–cortex pathway (see Fig. 3-6). It serves to localize the stimulus, including associated nociceptive input. Nociceptive signals travel by A-delta and unmyelinated C fibers to Lissauer's tract in the apex of the dorsal horn. There they bifur-

cate into short neurons and ascend or descend one to two segments before synapsing in the SG (lamina II). Cells of laminae I, IV, V and perhaps VI respond to nociceptive stimulation. Neurons in laminae V and VI project axons to the contralateral cord which ascend as the anterolateral tract. Some lamina V cells send axons to the ipsilateral anterolateral tract.

Recent evidence suggests that the

spinothalamic system is composed of two divisions, the neospinothalamic tract and the paleospinothalamic tract. The neospinothalamic tract is located laterally and is a more recent evolutionary development. It is composed of myelinated fibers that project directly to the ventrolateral and posterior thalamus, where they synapse. The third-order neuron then projects to the somatosensory cortex. Nociceptive input traveling over this pathway is perceived as sharp, well-localized pain with little or no accompanying affective component and a short latency between stimulus and perception. It travels over larger pain fibers (*e.g.*, A-delta fibers). The paleospinothalamic tract, on the other hand, is located medially and is an evolutionarily older pathway. It is composed of more unmyelinated fibers that make many synapses, so that input travels more slowly than in the neospinothalamic tract. The paleospinothalamic tract projects to the reticular formation (especially the nucleus RgC), to the lateral pons, to the limbic midbrain area, and then to the intralaminar thalamic nuclei. Fibers then continue rostrally and synapse ultimately with neurons in the hypothalamus, in the limbic forebrain structures, and with diffuse projections to many other parts of the brain. Nociceptive input traveling over this pathway is perceived as diffuse, poorly localized pain, with a strong affective component and a long latency between stimulus and perception. The paleospinothalamic tract mediates suprasegmental reflex responses, such as autonomic responses, as well as affective phenomena associated with pain. It is the more important system with respect to clinical pain states.

Nociceptive input to the medullary reticular formation, thalamus, cortex, and limbic regions activates neurons that feed back to the PAG integration center. The PAG in turn provides input to the NRM and the adjacent nucleus Rmc (Fig. 3-6). Each sends nerve fibers to the dorsal horn through the dorsal lateral funiculus fiber tract. These fibers presynaptically inhibit the nociceptive T cells in lamina I and V of the dorsal horn. As the paleospinothalamic tract ascends rostrally, it synapses and activates the nucleus Rgc in the medulla. The Rgc sends projections to the PAG and to the NRM. In some manner it also activates the DRM. The DRM (another reticular formation nucleus) forms a portion of the ascending serotoninergic pathway that eventually excites neurons in the hypothalamus, limbic forebrain areas, frontal cortex, and septum. Presumably, the DRM contributes to affective, memory, sensory, autonomic, and somatic motor responses to pain. Descending output from these areas impinges on the PAG, thereby modulating nociceptive input originating at spinal cord levels. The nature of modulation depends on the integration of ongoing activity in these areas.

CLINICAL APPLICATIONS

Knowledge of the gate theory and central modulation of pain enables us to make clinical applications with variable success. It has been known for centuries that counterirritants such as heat and massage reduce pain. More modern counterirritant techniques, such as transcutaneous nerve stimulation and dorsal column stimulation, may also relieve pain in patients with certain pain problems. All of these techniques stimulate pressure and touch receptors that send information to the dorsal horn through large, myelinated fibers. This large fiber input leads to partial or complete inhibition of nociceptive T-cell firing, and therefore to less transmission of nociceptive input to higher brain centers by way of segmental modulation.[40]

Some reports suggest that acupuncture-induced analgesia may be reversed by naloxone.[39] Generally, it is speculated that the opiate-system activation is involved in acupuncture analgesia, although some studies cast doubt on this.[38,39] It should be noted that acupuncture points, "trigger points," and motor points coincide closely; perhaps they are simply convenient sites for eventual activation of PAG and descending inhibition of nociceptive input by peripheral stimulation.

Behavior modification approaches to management of chronic pain patients often result in decreased pain behavior (fewer complaints, reduced drug dependency), increased activity level, and often a return to a more acceptable life-style.[22,50] Increasing activity, ignoring pain complaints, and replacing old behaviors with new ones may all lead to stimulation of the PAG and, therefore, activate the central descending pathway that inhibits nociceptive input at the spinal cord level. Increasing activity also increases large-fiber input. This may balance small fiber nociceptive input and lead to inhibition of the nociceptive T cell in lamina V of the dorsal horn. However, many chronic-pain patients have symptoms with apparently minimal somatic contribution but excessive affective components. After behavior modification, many patients claim that their pain is the same even though they are now able to engage in more activities and lead a more normal life. It is likely that more complex pathways are involved than have yet been described.

As more research is done, the evidence becomes highly suggestive that little difference exists between the biologic substrate and clinical manifestations of chronic pain and depression. Researchers have measured serotonin levels in severely depressed and suicidal patients and have found them to be markedly reduced. As you may recall, serotonin inhibitors administered to human subjects lead to hyperalgesia and spontaneous pain syndromes.[3,38] Decreased serotonin levels block morphine effects and SPA in labora-

tory animals.[20] Patients with chronic pain and depression often behave similarly. Both are generally less active, have altered appetite and sleep patterns, lose motivational and sexual drives, and may become self-abusive.[22] Perhaps the same component of the nociceptive system is involved in both kinds of patients. This may explain why chronic pain patients exhibit "depressive behaviors," and why depressed patients frequently complain of pain. Interestingly, tricyclic drugs, which inhibit serotonin depletion, have been found to be useful in treating depression as well as chronic pain. This suggests that serotoninergic pathways may be important in both disorders.

Of primary importance clinically is the understanding that pain involves much more than a simple relay of sensory input. Culture, past experience, emotional state, personality, motivation, role expectations, and learned behavior can all contribute to modulation of nociceptive stimuli and can influence the final pain experience. People with a strong will to complete a task (*e.g.*, athlete, soldier) undoubtedly receive a barrage of nociceptive input, but pain, suffering, or pain behavior may not accompany nociceptive input, presumably because segmental or central modulation creates a relatively analgesic state. On the other hand, pain can occur without nociceptive input, just as suffering, depression, grief, or other affective phenomena associated with pain can occur without pain or nociception. Many patients exhibit pain behaviors when nociception is no longer present. For clinicians treating patients with pain problems, it is essential to understand the nociceptive process and to consider possible contributing factors affecting nociceptive input. For this purpose, patient history and evaluation are invaluable. The patient with musculoskeletal pain may also be depressed, lonely, have a drug or alcohol problem, or be going through a difficult adjustment period. The clinician must consider these possibilities when the treatment program is established, as well as provide the appropriate treatment and all other necessary resources to enable the patient to deal with the pain problem most effectively.

REFERENCES

1. Adams JE: Naloxone reversal of analgesia produced by brain stimulation in the human. Pain 2:161– 166, 1976

2. Akil H, Liebeskind JC: Monoaminergic mechanisms of stimulation-produced analgesia. Brain Res 94:279– 296, 1975

3. Akil H, Mayer DJ: Antagonisms of stimulation-produced analgesia by p-CPA, a serotonin synthesis inhibitor. Brain Res 44:692– 697, 1972

4. Akil H, Mayer DJ, Liebeskind JC: Antagonism of stimulation-produced analgesia by naloxone, a narcotic antagonist. Science 191:961– 962, 1976

5. Akil H, Richardson DE, Hughes J, Barchas JD: Enkephalin-like material elevated in ventricular cerebrospinal fluid of pain patients after analgetic focal stimulation. Science 201:463– 465, 1978

6. Almay BG, Johansson F, Von Knorring L, Terenius L, Wahlstrom A: Endorphins in chronic pain: Differences in CSF endorphin levels between organic and psychogenic pain syndromes. Pain 5:153– 162, 1978

7. Anderson SD, Bausbaum AI, Fields HL: Responses of medullary raphe neurons to peripheral stimulation and to systemic opiates. Brain Res 123:363– 368, 1977

8. Balagura, S, Ralph T: The analgesic effect of electrical stimulation of the diencephalon and mesencephalon. Brain Res 60:369– 381, 1973

9. Barnes DC, Fung SJ, Adams WL: Inhibitory effects of substantia nigra on impulse transmission from nociceptors. Pain 6:207– 215, 1979

10. Basbaum AI, Marley N, O'Keefe J: Effects of spinal cord lesions on the analgesic properties of electrical brain stimulation. Presented at a symposium held at the First World Congress on Pain. Advances in Pain Research p 268, 1975

11. Basbaum AI, Marley N, O'Keefe J, Clanton C: Reversal of morphine and stimulus-produced analgesia by subtotal spinal cord lesions. Pain 3:43– 56, 1977

12. Black RG: The chronic pain syndrome. Surg Clin North Am 55:999– 1011, 1975

13. Bonica JJ: Neurophysiologic and pathologic aspects of acute and chronic pain. Arch Surg 112:750– 761, 1977

14. Bowsher D: Role of the reticular formation in responses to noxious stimulation. Pain 2:361– 378, 1976

15. Buchsbaum MS, Davis GC, Bunney WE: Naloxone alters pain perception and somatosensory evoked potentials in normal subjects. Nature 270:620– 622, 1977

16. Buscher HH, Hill RC, Romer D, Cardinaux F, Closse A, Hauser D, Pless J: Evidence for analgesic activity of enkephalin in the mouse. Nature 261:423– 425, 1976

17. Callaghan M, Sternbach RA, Nyquist JK, Timmermans G: Changes in somatic sensitivity during transcutaneous electrical analgesia. Pain 5:115– 127, 1978

18. Clark WC, Hunt HF: Pain. In Downey J, Darling R (eds): Physiological Basis of Rehabilitation Medicine, pp 373– 401. Philadelphia, W B Saunders, 1971

19. Duggan AW, Griersmith BT: Inhibition of spinal transmission of nociceptive information by supraspinal stimulation in the cat. Pain 6:149– 161, 1979

20. Fennessy MR, Lee JR: Modification of morphine analgesia by drugs affecting adrenergic and tryptaminergic mechanisms. J Pharm Pharmacol 22:930– 935, 1978

21. Fields HL, Anderson SD: Evidence that raphe-spinal neurons mediate opiate and midbrain stimulation-produced analgesias. Pain 5:333– 349, 1978

22. Fordyce WE: Behavioral Methods for Chronic Pain and Illness. St Louis, C V Mosby, 1976

23. Guilbaud G, Peschanski M, Gautron M, Binder D: Neurons responding to noxious stimulation in VB complex and caudal adjacent regions in the thalamus of the rat. Pain 8:303– 318, 1980

24. Guillemin R: Beta-lipotropin and endorphins: Implications of current knowledge. Hosp Pract 13(11):53– 60, 1978

25. Henry JL, Sessle BJ, Lucier GE, Hu JW: Effects of substance P on nociceptive and

non-nociceptive trigeminal brain stem neurons. Pain 8:33–45, 1980

26. Hughes J, Smith TW, Kosterlitz HW, Fothergill LA, Morgan BA, Morris HR: Identification of two related pentapeptides from the brain with potent opiate agonist activity. Nature 258:577–579, 1975

27. Inman VT, Saunders JB: Referred pain from skeletal structures. J Nerv Ment Dis 99:660–667, 1944

28. Johansson F, Von Knorring L: A double-blind controlled study of a serotonin up-take inhibitor (Zimelidine) versus placebo in chronic pain patients. Pain 7:69–78, 1979

29. Jordan LM, Kenshalo DR, Martin RF, Haber LH, Willis WD: Depression of primate spinothalamic tract neurons by iontophoretic application of 5-hydroxy-tryptamine. Pain 5:135–142, 1978

30. Kellgren JH: On the distribution of pain arising from deep somatic structures with charts of segmental pain areas. Clin Sci 4:35–46, 1939

31. Kellgren JH, Samuel EP: The sensitivity and innervation of the articular capsule. J Bone Joint Surg 32(B):84–92, 1950

32. Kerr FW, Wilson PR: Pain. Annu Rev Neurosci 1:83–102, 1978

33. Leavitt F, Garron DC: Psychological disturbance and pain report differences in both organic and non-organic low back pain patients. Pain 7:187–195, 1979

34. Lindblom U, Tegner R: Are the endorphins active in clinical pain states? Narcotic antagonism in chronic pain patients. Pain 7:65–68, 1979

35. Loeser JD, Black RG: A taxonomy of pain. Pain 1:81–84, 1975

36. Mayer DJ, Liebeskind JC: Pain reduction by focal electrical stimulation of the brain: An anatomical and behavioral analysis. Brain Res 68:73–93, 1974

37. Mayer DJ, Murphin R: Stimulation-produced analgesia (SPA) and morphine analgesia: Cross tolerance from application at the same brain site. Fed Proc 35:385, 1976

38. Mayer DJ, Price DD: Central nervous system mechanisms of analgesia. Pain 2:379–404, 1976

39. Mayer DJ, Price DD, Rafii A, Barber J: Acupuncture hypalgesia: Evidence for activation of a central control system as a mechanism of action. In Proceedings of the First World Congress on Pain. New York, Raven Press, 1976

40. Mayer DJ, Wolfle TL, Akil H, Carder B, Liebeskind JC: Analgesia from electrical stimulation in the brainstem of the rat. Science 174:1351–1354, 1971

41. Melzack R: The gate theory revisited. In LeRoy PL (ed): Current Concepts in the Management of Chronic Pain. Miami, Symposia Specialists, 1977

42. Melzack R, Wall PD: On the nature of cutaneous sensory mechanisms. Brain 85:331–356, 1962

43. Messing RB, Lytle LD: Serotonin-containing neurons: Their possible role in pain and analgesia. Pain 4:1–21, 1977

44. Millan MJ, Przewlocki R, Herz A: A non-B-endorphin adenohypophyseal is essential for an analgetic response to stress. Pain 8:343–353, 1980

45. Nathan PW: The gate-control theory of pain—A critical review. Brain 99:123–158, 1976

46. Oleson TD, Twombly DA, Liebeskind JC: Effects of pain-attenuating brain stimulation and morphine on electrical activity in the raphe nuclei of the awake rat. Pain 4:211–230, 1978

47. Oliveras JL, Woda A, Guilbaud G, Besson JM: Analgesia induced by electrical stimulation of the inferior centralis of the raphe in the cat. Pain 1:139–145, 1975

48. Proudfit HK, Anderson ED: Morphine analgesia: Blockade by raphe magnus lesions. Brain Res 98:612–618, 1975

49. Rhodes DL: Periventricular system lesions and stimulation-produced analgesia. Pain 7:51–63, 1979

50. Roberts AH, Reinhardt L: The behavioral management of chronic pain: Long-term follow-up with comparison groups. Pain 8:151–162, 1980

51. Sinclair DC, Weddell G, Feindel WH: Referred pain and associated phenomena. Brain 7:184–211, 1948

52. Snyder SH: Opiate receptors and internal opiates. Sci Am 240 (3):44–56, 1977

53. Stacher G, Bauer P, Steinringer A, Schreiber E, Schmierer G: Effects of the synthetic enkephalin analogue FK 33-824

on pain threshold and pain tolerance in man. Pain 7:159–172, 1979

54. Wall PD: The gate control theory of pain mechanisms—A re-examination and re-statement. Brain 101:1–18, 1978

55. Weddell G, Palmer E, Pallie W: Nerve endings in mammalian skin. Biol Rev 30:159–193, 1954

56. Wyke B: Neurological mechanisms in the experience of pain. Acupuncture and Electro-Therapeutical Research International Journal 4:27–35, 1979

57. Yaksh TL, Rudy TA: Narcotic analgetics: CNS sites and mechanisms of action as revealed by intracerebral injection techniques. Pain 4:299–359, 1978

58. Yeung JC, Yaksh TL, Rudy TA: Concurrent mapping of brain sites for sensitivity to the direct application of morphine and focal electrical stimulation in the production of antinociception in the rat. Pain 4:23–40, 1977

RECOMMENDED READINGS

Biedenbach MA, Van Hassel HJ, Brown AC: Tooth pulp-driven neurons in somatosensory cortex of primates: Role in pain mechanisms including a review of the literature. Pain 7:31–50, 1979

Browne RG, Segal DS: Alterations in B-endorphin-induced locomotor activity in morphine-tolerant rats. Neuropharmacology 19:619–621, 1980

Feinstein B, Langton JN, Jameson RM, Schiller F: Experiments on pain referred from deep somatic tissues. J Bone Joint Surg 36(A): 981–997, 1954

Fordyce WE: Evaluating and managing chronic pain. Geriatrics 33:59–62, 1978

Lewis T: Suggestions relating to the study of somatic pain. Br Med J, 1:321–327, 1938

Lewis T, Kellgran JH: Observations relating to referred pain, visceromotor reflexes and other associated phenomena. Clin Sci 49:470–471, 1939

Melzack R, Loeser JD: Phantom body pain in paraplegics: Evidence for a central "pattern generating mechanism" for pain. Pain 4:195–210, 1978

Melzack R, Wall PD: Pain mechanisms: A new theory. Science 150:971–979, 1965

Oleson TD, Liebeskind JC: Relationship of neural activity in the raphe nuclei of the rat to brain stimulation-produced analgesia. Physiologist 18:338, 1975

Procacci P, Maresca M, Zoppi M: Visceral and deep somatic pain. Acupuncture and Electro-Therapeutic Research International Journal 3:135–160, 1978

Vogt M: The effect of lowering the 5-hydroxytryptamine content of the rat spinal cord on analgesia produced by morphine. J Physiol (London) 236:483–498, 1974

Wall PD: On the relation of injury to pain. Pain 6:253–264, 1979

Weddell G, Sinclair DC: "Pins and needles": Observations on some of the sensations aroused in a limb by the application of pressure. J Neurol Neurosurg Psychiatry 10: 26–46, 1947

4 Assessment of Musculoskeletal Disorders

Randolph M. Kessler

RATIONALE

A comprehensive examination is, without question, the most important step in the physical therapist's management of patients with common musculoskeletal disorders. The physical therapist's role is to clarify the nature and extent of the lesion, to assess the extent of the resulting disability, and to accurately record significant data in order to establish a basis against which to judge progress. These activities must not be confused with or mistaken for the physician's diagnosis. A diagnosis, in addition to clinical evaluation, often requires the use and interpretation of laboratory tests, radiographs, and other data employing skills and knowledge not included in the physical therapist's training. A diagnosis must *differentiate* a particular disease state from other possible causes of the symptoms and signs. The therapist, in performing a *clarifying* examination, is not concerned with such differentiation, but with collecting qualitative and quantitative data on the existing lesion, so as to judge how best to apply certain treatment procedures and to assess their effectiveness.

Consider the case of a patient referred to the therapist with the diagnosis of "shoulder tendinitis." This is a condition easily managed by physical therapy over a rela-

tively short period of time. However, in order for an effective program to be instituted, several features of the problem must be clarified. The therapist must determine which tendon is at fault in order to know where to direct treatment. Similarly, he must know at what site on the tendon the lesion exists. Assessment of the lesion's chronicity will influence the choice of treatment procedures and their application. It is important to know whether secondary problems such as stiffness or weakness exist; if so, they must be dealt with as well. The therapist must obtain information concerning the possible behavioral effects of the lesion. Are the conditions accompanying the problem reinforcing in any way to the patient's disease behaviors or is the patient "highly motivated"? Daily activities must be assessed, not only to determine the existence of any functional deficit, but also to judge whether any present activity will aggravate or prolong the condition. Generally, such information does not accompany the referral, but it is precisely this information that is required in order to institute an effective treatment program. The physical therapist must perform a thorough initial examination on every patient to be treated.

As mentioned, information collected as part of the initial examination is used to set a baseline against which to judge progress and to assess the effectiveness of treatment. Therefore, not only must the therapist perform a complete initial examination, but he must assess certain key

75

signs before, during, and after each treatment session. In this way the clinician can determine whether, in fact, a particular procedure is effective and can quantitatively document the patient's progress. Progress must be judged on objective evidence. The patient's subjective report of the degree of pain must be considered, but not dwelt upon; in itself, it is not a valid measurement of progress. Instead, the therapist should be able to inform the patient as to whether or not he is better. Treatment sessions should begin less often with, "Hello, Mrs. Jones. How is your back today?" but rather with, "Hello, Mrs. Jones. Let's take a look at your back to see how it's doing." This approach is possible only after complete initial examination and continued assessment of objective signs.

There are, of course, several approaches to patient examination. However, it is most important that the examination of musculoskeletal disorders be systematized. This avoids the possibility of omitting a crucial test or step, which may prevent accurate interpretation. Perhaps no one has contributed more to systematization of soft tissue examination than James Cyriax. (His approach is well described in his book, *Textbook of Orthopaedic Medicine* and should be reviewed by anyone dealing with patients with common musculoskeletal disorders.)[1] The format set out here is fashioned after Cyriax's approach. It consists of the History, Physical Examination, and Correlation/Interpretation.

HISTORY

To help determine the nature and extent of the lesion and the resultant degree of disability, we must gather data from the patient that cannot be determined by physical examination. This subjective data is correlated with the findings of the physical exam.

In the case of common musculoskeletal disorders the lesion is usually manifested primarily by pain. Some of the routine questions suggested here as part of every history are directed at obtaining a complete account of the history of the pain and the present status of the pain as perceived by the patient. However, we must also inquire about other symptoms, such as paresthesias, feelings of weakness, feelings of instability, and autonomic disturbances. It is important to keep in mind that the patient's perception of pain and other symptoms offers valuable clues to the nature and extent of the lesion but does not alone serve as an indicator of progress. We must rely instead upon assessment of objective signs and examination of the patient's functional status.

Determination of the degree of disability does offer some data by which to legitimately judge progress. It also yields information concerning the nature and extent of the lesion. Needless to say, this is an important part of the history and is too often omitted. To determine the degree of disability we assess the patient's "health-state" behaviors and activity level (occupation, recreation, and other activities of daily life), by history, as well as the patient's "disease-state" behaviors and activity level. Documentation of the disease-state behaviors will set a baseline against which to judge progress; comparison with the patient's health-state behaviors may provide clues to the nature and extent of the problem. For example the patient with a shoulder problem who has been able to comb her hair all her life, but who is now unable to do this since the onset of the problem lacks full, pain-free active elevation and external rotation. This is very suggestive of a capsular restriction. In this example we have some data to compare with the physical findings that may help determine the nature and extent of the lesion. One treatment goal will naturally be restoring the patient's ability to comb her hair. We also have established a criterion by which to judge progress. Consequently, when judging progress we must be less concerned with whether Mrs. Jones had shoulder pain this morning and its extent or duration, and we must be more concerned with whether Mrs. Jones was able to comb her hair or fasten her bra.

Disability assessment and disease-state behavior assessment become especially important in evaluating patients with a chronic-pain state but no physical findings or pain that is out of proportion to physical findings, and in evaluating patients with a permanent functional deficit from some serious pathology. In the first two situations, it is often necessary to change from a "medical model," in which treatment is aimed at the lesion in order to change behavior, to an "operant model," in which treatment is aimed at altering the consequences to the disease state behaviors.[2-4] In the last situation, treatment is no longer directed at the primary lesion, such as a spinal cord lesion, but rather at improving residual function. There are some relatively common disorders in which pain complaints and functional disability are out of proportion to the extent of the pathology. Some of these abnormal pain states, such as reflex sympathetic dystrophy (see Chapter 14, The Wrist), have a physiological basis. Other cases, such as those involving pending

litigation, substantial monetary compensation, or welcomed time away from activities the patient finds undesirable, may have a psychosocial basis. The patient's pain or disability may promise rewards, which may in turn reinforce disease-state behaviors. It is essential that the presence of such abnormal behavior states be determined upon examination. In these cases, treatment aimed primarily at some physical pathology may only serve to maintain the patient's disability. Primary emphasis must be placed upon improved function by altering the consequences of the disabled state (Fig. 4-1).

Although this text emphasizes the assessment and treatment of the lesion itself, we must not lose sight of the fact that we are treating patients, and that our ultimate goal in any treatment program is rehabilitation of the patient. We do not rehabilitate a lesion. Even when treatment is aimed largely at the lesion, we must be careful not to reinforce the disease-state, especially pain behavior. Similarly, we must also be concerned with functional deficits associated with the disease state and see that they are resolved, when possible, along with the primary pathologic process. Thus, whether we approach patient management through a "medical model" or through an "operant model,"

Fig. 4-1. Disability scheme

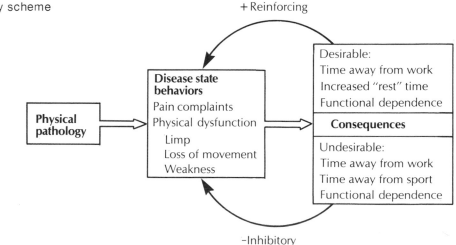

the primary goal is to restore health-state behaviors. When a well-defined pathology exists, and the consequences of the resulting disability appear to have a negative effect on the patient's attitude toward his disability, we can reasonably expect that resolving the pathologic process will restore health-state behavior. However, when the consequences of disability are rewarding to the patient, treatment of the physical pathology may have little or no effect.

The specific inquiries during the initial history are naturally going to vary according to the site of the lesion, nature of the lesion, and other factors. Questions that are particularly important for specific anatomical regions will be discussed in the respective chapters dealing with those regions. There are, however, certain routine inquiries that should be included in virtually every case.

The most efficient method of obtaining subjective information is to direct a list of specific, predetermined questions to the patient. However, this is not always the *best* method for eliciting certain important pieces of information, and it is certainly not the best method for developing the most effective patient–professional relationship. The direct-question approach is close-ended; it assumes that the relevant information will fall into predetermined categories, and it does not encourage consideration of factors outside these categories. It leads or directs the line of inquiry to specific categories. The patient often attempts to please the examiner by providing information related to these categories but not necessarily pertinent to the problem at hand. Alternatively, a more open-ended approach guides the discussion but does not restrict information to certain categories. Furthermore, it allows the patient the freedom to relate what he feels is important, in addition to what the examiner may feel is important. The open-ended patient interview is structured to be a discussion session rather than a question-and-answer period. The examiner structures the discussion carefully, however, to elicit the necessary information.

A close-ended, direct-question method of interviewing creates a patient–therapist relationship in which the therapist assumes the authoritarian role of "healer," while the patient assumes a passive role. Within this relationship the patient need only provide the requested information, after which the examiner will perform the appropriate tests, decide what the problem is, and correct it. Such an approach favors the assumption that there is a specific physical pathology that the therapist will treat while the patient assumes a relatively passive role in the treatment program. This is consistent with a medical model of patient management and excludes from the outset the possibility of an operant disease-state or an operant approach to management. In an open-ended interview, the therapist and patient discuss the patient's problem on a one-to-one basis. The therapist maintains his position as an expert in the field by virtue of the professional atmosphere in which the interview takes place. The patient is the expert with respect to the particular problem, since he is more familiar with it than anyone else. The interview serves as a forum in which the patient is encouraged to offer information and insight concerning his problem in return for advice and help in overcoming it. Both patient and therapist maintain distinct roles but remain equals. They establish an understanding that mutual co-operation and effort are required to execute an effective treatment program.

Practically speaking, there are appropriate uses for both the open-ended and closed-ended approaches to history taking. In all situations, it is important to begin the interview open-endedly to establish an effective professional relationship and to get a feeling for the patient's problem. But as the nature of the problem becomes more obvious, it is necessary to seek more detailed information by directing specific questions to the patient. However, even during a close line of questioning, we must avoid asking leading questions that may elicit irrelevant or inaccurate information. For example, instead of asking, "Does the pain travel down the arm?" we should ask, "Is the pain felt in any other parts?" Instead of, "Do you have a lot of pain in the morning?" we might ask, "When do you typically feel the pain?" The same is true when inquiring about disability. Rather than asking if a particular activity is painful or difficult, one should ask, "Which activities are particularly painful or difficult to perform?" In this way the patient is responsible for judging what information in a particular category is important, and he is less likely to provide information primarily for the purpose of satisfying the examiner.

The following list of questions is presented to indicate the type of information one should attempt to elicit. As much of the information as possible should be obtained through an open-ended discussion in an environment in which the patient feels free to discuss his problem and provide related information. The setting should be quiet, private, and free from disturbances. The examiner should be seated, and the patient should still be in his street clothes. Following a well-structured discussion, any information that has not come out should be sought through specific questions. The discussion should end with a fairly open-ended question, as indicated below, to re-establish an appropriate working relationship.

1. ***Tell me about your problem.***
   Do not assume anything. The patient sent down with a referral for a back problem may be more concerned with his prostatic neoplasm; some valuable information may be elicited by letting the patient discuss freely whatever he feels is most important.

On the other hand, the patient is likely to go on for as long as you allow, informing you about a third cousin twice removed who had a similar problem, and so on. Be prepared to politely interrupt by saying, for example, "I'm beginning to get an idea of the nature of your problem. Now I would like to obtain some specific information pertaining to it." The patient, having been allowed the opportunity to talk freely, is assured that you are interested in him as a person, and that you have begun to involve him in the therapeutic process by listening to his opinion.

2. ***Where, exactly, is your pain?***
   We are assuming that the problem is a common musculoskeletal disorder, for which the patient presents to the physician because of pain. Ask the patient to indicate with one hand or one finger the primary area of pain and then any areas to which it might spread. Be sure to determine whether in fact it does or does not spread.
   —If the patient points to one, small, localized area and claims that the pain does not spread from it, the lesion is probably not severe, or it is relatively superficial, or both.
   —If a diffuse area is indicated as the primary site, it suggests that the lesion is more severe or more deeply situated, or both.
   —If the pain spreads, determine if it is confined to a segment. If so, determine if it follows a well-delineated pathway, as in dermatomic radiation, or if it is more diffuse, as in scleratomic reference of pain. Well-delineated, radiating pain suggests pressure on a nerve root in which the A-delta fibers are irritated, but still transmitting. Diffuse, segmental referred pain may have its origin in the viscera, a deep somatic structure, or a nerve

root in which the large myelinated fibers are no longer conducting, but the small C fibers are. Cyriax proposes that some structures such as the dura mater and viscera will refer pain extrasegmentally.[1]

—Generally speaking, reference of pain is favored by a strong stimulus (a severe lesion), a lesion of deep somatic structures or nerve tissues, and a lesion lying fairly proximally (since pain is more often referred distally than proximally).

3. **When did the present pain arise? Was the onset gradual or sudden? Was an injury or unusual activity involved?**
   —An insidious onset unrelated to injury or unusual activity should always be viewed with suspicion since this history is typical of a neoplasm. However, degenerative lesions or lesions due to tissue fatigue are common and may also arise in this manner. If the patient blames some injury or activity, keep in mind that he may or may not be correct. Determine the exact nature of the event or mechanism of injury so that correlation can be made to symptoms and signs for interpretation. Determining the direction and nature of forces producing the injury may give some clues as to which tissues may have been stressed.

4. **What is the quality of the pain (sharp, dull, burning, tingling, aching, constant, boring, excruciating, etc.)? Has it changed at all in quality or intensity since its onset?**
   —Sharp, well localized pain suggests a superficial lesion.
   —Sharp, lancinating, shooting pain suggests a nerve lesion, usually at a nerve root, presumably affecting the A-delta fibers.

—Tingling suggests stimulation of nerve tissue affecting A-alpha fibers. A segmental distribution suggests a nerve root; a peripheral nerve distribution implicates that nerve. Tingling into both hands, both feet, or all four extremities suggests spinal-cord involvement or some other more serious pathology.

—Dull, aching pain is typical of pain of deep somatic origin.

—Excruciating pain, unrelenting pain, intolerable pain, and deep, boring pain all suggest some serious pathology.

—Change in intensity of the pain may offer some clue as to the progression of the problem. This must be considered when treatment begins. If the patient was getting worse prior to treatment and continues to worsen, once treatment has begun, then the treatment has probably not been effective. However it is probably not the cause of the worsening following initiation of treatment. On the other hand, if the patient had been improving but stops getting better or gets worse once treatment has begun, the treatment is probably at fault.

—Change in quality of the pain may offer many clues as to the nature and extent of the lesion. Progression of nerve-root pressure, such as from a disc protrusion, typically leads to rather marked changes in symptoms (see Chapter 3, Pain).

5. **What aggravates the pain? What relieves it? Is it any better or worse in the morning or evening? When do you typically feel pain?**
   —Pain *not* aggravated by activity or relieved by rest should be suspected as arising from some pathology other than a common musculoskeletal disorder. The ex-

ception is a disc problem that may be aggravated by sitting and relieved by getting up and walking.

—Morning *pain* is suggestive of arthritis, especially the inflammatory varieties. Morning *stiffness* is suggestive of degenerative joint disease or chronic arthritis.

—Pain awakening the patient at night is typical of shoulder or hip problems that may be aggravated by lying on the affected side. Otherwise, a more serious problem should be suspected, particularly if the patient is kept awake, and especially if he must get up and walk about.

—Arthritis in weight-bearing joints leads to pain on fatigue (long walks, etc.) in its early stages. In later stages, the pain is felt when beginning a walk, somewhat relieved once going, and returning after walking too far.

6. *Have you had this problem in the past? If so, how was it resolved? Did you seek help? Was there any treatment? Is the pain the same this time?*

Should you elicit a history of recurrence, you might inquire in depth about the first episode and the most recent episode, with an estimate of the number of intervening episodes. Recurrences are typical of spinal lesions, but many common extremity lesions such as ankle sprains, minor meniscus lesions or other internal derangements, minor degenerative joint problems, tendinitis, and frozen shoulder also may tend to recur.

By inquiring about previous management, some helpful information may also be obtained for treatment planning. However, the patient's judgment of the effectiveness or value of previous treatment must not be weighed too heavily. If an injection

helped before, for example in the case of supraspinatus tendinitis, it does not necessarily follow that another injection is necessary or indicated. If physical therapy—perhaps inadequately instituted—was unsuccessful in the past, do not assume that it will not be helpful on this occasion.

7. *Are there any other symptoms that you have or have had that you associate with the problem, such as grinding, popping, giving way, numbness, tingling, weakness, dizziness, or nausea?*

By concentrating on the patient's account of pain, you may well overlook some other important symptoms. A wide variety of responses may be elicited with this question, each of which must be carefully weighed and considered. A patient's description of "numbness" is very often not true hypesthesia but is actually referred pain. In most cases, considerable weakness must be present before the patient can accurately perceive it as such, and very often what the patient describes as "weakness" is actually instability or giving way. Symptoms inconsistent with musculoskeletal dysfunction must be viewed with some suspicion and medical consultation sought for interpretation.

8. *How has this problem affected your dressing, grooming, or other daily activities? Has it affected your ability to work at your job or around the house? Has it affected or altered your recreational activities? Is there anything that is difficult or impossible for you to do since the onset of this problem?*

Determine the patient's normal occupation and daily activity level. The existence of a functional deficit often contributes to interpretation of the problem by considering the demands placed on various musculoskeletal structures in performing the task. Later quantification of the deficit or residual function during physical examination will set a baseline against which to assess progress.

Any functional deficit must be correlated later with the apparent nature of the lesion, and any inconsistencies considered. In cases involving compensation or litigation, the disease-state may be reinforced in such a way that a functional deficit is no longer the result of the problem but rather its cause.

9. *What treatment are you having or have you had for the present problem? Are you taking any medications for this problem or for any other reason?*
   —Here again, it may or may not be helpful to determine whether certain attempts at treatment have had any good or bad effects, especially treatments involving physical agents.
   —You must determine whether pain medications, anti-inflammatories, or muscle relaxants are being taken. Symptoms or signs may be masked accordingly. Certain medications may produce rather marked musculoskeletal changes (in addition to effects on other tissues and functions). Most important, perhaps, is the long-term use of steroids, which produces osteoporosis; proximal muscle weakness; generalized tissue edema; thin, fragile skin; collagen tissue weakening; and increased pain threshold. These of course will affect findings on examination. More importantly, however, they must be considered when planning treatment.

10. *How is your general health?*
   —It is necessary to determine whether the patient has or has had any disease process or health problem that may have contributed to the present problem, or that may influence the choice of treatment procedures.

11. *Do you have any opinions of your own as to what the problem is?*
   You may elicit some useful information concerning what he has learned from others, what his insight is into the problem, and so on. If nothing else, you will reassure the patient that you are interested in him and his opinions, and that he is to be involved in the therapeutic program.

PHYSICAL EXAMINATION

A complete history performed by the experienced clinician will often be sufficient to determine the extent and nature of the lesion. Even so, the physical examination must not be excluded or cut short. Objective data is needed to facilitate or confirm the interpretation of subjective findings. It is equally important that every effort be made to precisely quantify objective data to allow documentation of a baseline and, therefore, accurate assessment of progress.

Specific tests and measurements will vary, of course, depending upon the area to be examined and to a certain extent upon the information obtained on the history. This chapter presents a systematic approach that can be applied to any region to be evaluated; tests specific to particular regions will be discussed in the respective regional chapters. This discussion will include general guidelines and statements meant to assist in interpretation of findings. It should be noted that the order of testing procedures presented here is for the sake of conceptual organization. Clinically, tests must be organized according to patient positioning. This point will be elaborated in the regional chapters.

Having discussed the phenomenon of referred pain, it should be apparent that at times we may be at a loss as to which region should be singled out as the primary area to be examined. For example, elbow pain may have its origin locally or at the neck or shoulder, but surely it is not necessary that we examine each of these areas in depth. Fortunately, the physician's referral, the history, or both, will often implicate the involved area. However, this is not always the case. When such a difficulty arises, it is often helpful to perform a brief *scan exam*. This is done by asking the patient to actively move each joint within the suspected areas and by applying some passive overpressure to the extremes of each motion. If pain or dysfunction is noted at a particular area, it may be examined in depth. Generally speaking, we must consider every structure derived embryologically from the same segment as the segment or portion of a segment in which the patient indicates the pain exists.

The physical examination will be organized as follows:

Observation
Inspection
Selective tissue tension
  Active movements
  Passive movements
    Range of movement
    Joint play
  Resisted movements
  Neuromuscular tests
  Palpation

OBSERVATION

Observe the patient's general appearance and functional status when he walks in, during dressing activities, during the examination and treatment session, and as he leaves. If specific functional disabilities are related during the history, the examiner may ask the patient to attempt to perform the involved activity in order to assess the exact degree and nature of the disability.

Note and record the patient's general appearance and body build—slim, obese, muscular, emaciated, short, tall, and so on. Note obvious postural deviations as well as abnormalities in positionings of body parts.

Record and describe as precisely as possible all functional abnormalities or deficits noted during the patient's visit. These might typically include observations relating to gait, guarding of particular movements, use of compensatory or substitution movements, or the use of certain aids or assistive devices.

INSPECTION

This part of the examination entails a closer assessment of the patient's physical status. It is usually performed in conjunction with palpation, which is discussed later in this section. To avoid excluding crucial assessments, it is convenient and helpful to organize inspection of body parts according to the following three layers: bony structure and alignment, subcutaneous soft tissue; and skin.

Bony Structure and Alignment

This is a critical component of the biomechanical examination, especially when correlated with specific functional abnormalities such as gait deviancies and altered range of motion. For example, a person with increased femoral anteversion is likely to present with a loss of external rotation at the hip, but with respect to his structure, a decrease in average external rotation is normal. If a careful assessment of static alignment were not made, one might make the mistake of attempting to restore external rotation in this case. Similarly, a common gait abnormality seen clinically is increased pronation of the hindfoot during stance phase. This often occurs secondary to structural malalignments elsewhere in the extremity, such as increased internal tibial torsion, increased femoral anteversion, or adduction of the first metatarsal. The ultimate cause of the pronation can only be determined through a careful structural examination. Assessment of structural alignment is likewise of utmost importance following the healing of fractures. A person who has sustained a Colles' fracture invariably ends up with some residual angulation dorsally and radially; restoration of full wrist flexion and ulnar deviation should never be expected. Thus, structural assessment becomes important in planning treatment as well as when setting treatment goals.

Assessment of a particular part in which some pathology may exist should often include structural assessment of biomechanically related parts. In the case of low-back disorders, you should examine the alignment of the lower extremities, and *vice versa*. The same is true for the cervical spine and upper extremities. Each part should be assessed with respect to frontal, sagittal, and transverse planes. Identify key bony landmarks and determine their relationships to fixed points of reference (*e.g.*, ground, wall, plumb-bob) as well as their relationships to each other. In judging whether malalignments exist, you must often rely upon your experience of what is normal, as well as upon comparison to a normal side in cases of unilateral problems. Malalignments should be documented through careful measurements when possible.

Specific assessments related to particular regions of the body will be discussed in the regional chapters. The following list includes some key bony landmarks that you must often identify when testing structural alignment, and with which the clinician must become familiar:

Navicular tubercles
Talar heads
Malleoli
Fibular heads
Tibular heads
Patellar borders
Adductor tubercles
Greater trochanters
Ischial tuberosities
Posterior and anterior iliac spines
Iliac crests
Spinous processes
Scapular borders
Mastoid processes
Clavicles
Acromial processes
Greater tubercles
Olecranons
Humeral epicondyles
Radial and ulnar styloid processes
Lister's tubercles
Carpal bones

Subcutaneous Soft Tissues

Inspect and palpate for abnormalities involving the soft-tissue regions of a part. Look for swelling or increase in the size of an area, wasting or atrophy of the part, and alterations in the general contours of the region. When an increase in size is noted, one should attempt to distinguish the cause, whether generalized edema, articular effusion, muscle hypertrophy, or hypertrophic changes in other tissues. Examine for localized cysts, nodules, or ganglia. In the presence of wasting, you should determine whether localized or generalized muscle atrophy exists, or whether there is perhaps some loss of continuity of soft tissues.

Measurements should be taken to carefully document soft tissue changes and to use as baseline measurements. Volumetric measurements of small parts, such as fingers, hands, and feet, can be made by measuring the displacement of water in a tub. Swelling or wasting elsewhere in an extremity can often be documented with circumferential measurements using a tape measure.

Skin and Nails

Note and document local or generalized changes in the status of the skin. These might include

- Changes in color either from vascular changes accompanying inflammation (erythema) or vascular deficiency (pallor or cyanosis)
- Changes in texture and moisture. These commonly accompany reflex sympathetic dystrophies, in which the sympathetic activity of the part becomes altered. Increased activity results in hyperhidrosis; smooth, glossy skin; cyanosis; atrophy of skin; and splitting of the nails. Decreased sympathetic activity may result in pink, dry, scaly skin.
- Local scars, distinct blemishes, abnormal hair patterns, calluses, blisters, open wounds, and other localized skin abnormalities. When a scar exists, whether surgical or traumatic, the type of surgery or injury should be determined because it may have some bearing on the present problem. Blemishes such as large, brownish, pigmented areas (*cafe au lait* spots) and localized hairy regions often accompany underlying bony defects, such as spina bifida. Calluses develop with increased shear or compressive stresses; blisters occur with increased shear between the skin and subcutaneous tissue. When an open wound is observed, determine whether it is of traumatic origin or of insidious origin, as often accompanies diabetes.

Describe local skin changes according to size and location. Size can be most precisely documented by outlining the borders of the defect on a piece of acetate, such as old x-ray film.

SELECTIVE TISSUE TENSION TESTS

This portion of the exam consists of specific active-, passive- and resisted-movement tests designed to assess the status of each of the component tissues of the physiological joint. When properly interpreted, findings from these tests can yield very specific information relating to both the nature and extent of the pathology. The organization and interpretation of these tests is largely the work of Cyriax, and is certainly a significant contribution to the field.[1]

I. **Active movements.** These yield very general information, relating primarily to the patient's functional status. They provide information concerning the patient's general willingness and ability to use the part. They offer no true indication of the range of motion or strength of a part. If a patient is asked to lift an arm overhead, and only lifts it to horizontal, it cannot be determined at that point whether the loss of function is due to pain, weakness, or stiffness.

Therefore, active movement tests are used primarily to assess the patient's ability to perform common functional activities related to the part being evaluated. For lower extremity and spinal regions, then, active movements should be performed while bearing weight. Upper extremity parts should be moved in functional directions. At the shoulder, for example, internal and external rotation are performed by asking the patient to reach behind him and to touch the back of his neck, rather than rotating the humerus with the arm to the side.

Note and document the following for the active movements tested:

A. The patient's account of the onset of, or increase in, pain associated with the movement, and at what point or points in the range of movement the pain occurs. The existence of a painful arc of movement is best detected on active, weight-bearing or antigravity movements. A painful arc of movement, in which pain is felt throughout a small arc of movement in the midrange of motion suggests an irritable structure being (1) pulled across a protuberance or (2) pinched between two structures. An example of the former is a nerve root pulled across a disc protrusion during straight leg raises. An example of the latter is an inflamed supraspinatus tendon squeezed between the greater tubercle and the acromial arch during abduction of the arm.

B. The range of motion through which the patient is able to move the part. This should be measured by some easily reproducible method.

C. The presence of crepitus. You can usually best detect this on active movements, with the forces of weight-bearing or muscle contraction maintaining compression of joint surfaces. Crepitus usually indicates roughening of joint surfaces or increased friction between a tendon and its sheath due to swelling or roughening of either the tendon or the sheath. Fine crepitus at a joint suggests early wearing of articular cartilage or tendinous problems, whereas more course crepitus implies considerable cartilaginous degeneration. A creaking sound, not unlike that which a large tree makes when swaying in the wind, often occurs when bones articulate in the late stages of joint-surface degeneration.

II. Passive movements.

A. Passive range of motion testing. The part is passively put through the major motions in the frontal, sagittal, and transverse planes that normally occur at the joint being moved. Very specific information concerning both the nature and extent of a disorder may be obtained by making the following assessments:

1. Range of movement. Determine whether movement is normal, restricted, or hypermobile. Carefully measure the degree of any abnormal movements. If there is restriction of movement at a joint, the first and foremost determination that should be made is whether the restriction is in a capsular or noncapsular pattern. (See the Appendix for a description of the capsular pattern of restriction at each joint.)

a. Capsular patterns of restriction indicate loss of mobility of the entire joint capsule from fibrosis, effusion, or inflammation. Differentiation can be made by assessing the "end-feel" at the extremes of movement (see below). Capsular restrictions typically accompany arthritis or degenerative joint disease (fibrosis, inflammation, or effusion), prolonged immobilization of a joint (fibrosis), or acute trauma to a joint (effusion).

b. Noncapsular patterns of joint restrictions typically occur with intra-articular mechanical blockage or extra-articular lesions. Common causes include

   i. Isolated ligamentous or capsular adhesion. A common example of isolated ligamentous adhesion is that of adherence of the medial collateral ligament at the knee to the medial femoral condyle during healing of a sprain. This results in restriction of knee flexion to about 90°, with extension being of full range. Isolated anterior capsular tightness at the shoulder often occurs following an anterior dislocation, resulting in a disproportionate loss of external rotation.

ii. Internal derangements, such as displacement of pieces of torn menisci and cartilaginous loose bodies. These typically produce a mechanical block to movement in a noncapsular pattern. The most common example is a "bucket handle" medial meniscus tear, resulting in blockage of knee extension, with flexion remaining relatively free in the absence of significant effusion.

iii. Extra-articular tissue tightness such as reduced lengthening of muscles from contracture (fibrosis) or myositis ossificans.

iv. Extra-articular inflammation or swellings, such as those accompanying acute bursitis and neoplasms.

2. End-feel at extremes of painful or restricted movements. This is the quality of the resistance to movement that the examiner feels when coming to the end point of a particular movement. Some end-feels may be normal or pathologic, depending upon the movement they accompany at a particular joint, and the point in the range of movement at which they are felt. Other end-feels are strictly pathologic.

a. End-feels that may be normal or pathologic include

i. Capsular end-feel. This is a firm, "leathery" feeling, felt, for example, when forcing the normal shoulder into full external rotation. When felt in conjunction with a capsular pattern of restriction, and in the absence of significant inflammation or effusion, it indicates capsular fibrosis.

ii. Bony end-feel. This feels abrupt as when moving the normal elbow into full extension. When accompanying a restriction of movement, it may suggest hypertrophic bony changes, such as those that occur with degenerative joint disease, or possible malunion of bony segments following healing of a fracture.

iii. Soft-tissue-approximation endfeel. This is a soft end-feel, as when fully flexing the normal elbow or knee. It may accompany joint restriction in the presence of significant muscular hypertrophy.

iv. Muscular end-feel. This more rubbery feel resembles what is felt at the extremes of straight-leg raising from tension on the hamstrings. It is less abrupt than a capsular end-feel.

b. End-feels that are strictly pathologic include

i. Muscle-spasm end-feel. Movement is stopped fairly abruptly, perhaps with some "rebound," due to muscles contracting reflexively to prevent further movement. It usually accompanies pain felt at the point of restriction. When occurring with a capsular restriction, it indicates some degree of synovial inflammation of the portion of the joint capsule being stretched during the movement.

ii. Boggy end-feel. This is a very soft, mushy end-feel that typically accompanies joint effusion in the absence of significant synovial inflammation. It will usually occur together with a capsular pattern of restriction.

iii. Internal derangement end-feel. This is often a pronounced, springy rebound at the end point of movement. It typically accompanies a noncapsular restriction from a mechanical block produced by a loose body or displaced meniscus.

iv. Empty end-feel. The examiner feels no restriction to movement, but movement is stopped at the insistence of the patient because of severe pain. This end-feel is relatively rare except with acute bursitis at the shoulder or a few other painful extra-articular lesions such as neoplasms. The muscles do not contract to prevent movement since this would cause compression at the painful site and further pain.

3. Pain on movement and the point in the range in which it is felt
   a. Pain at the extremes of a movement indicates
      i. A painful structure is being stretched. In this case, you should consider first a lesion of the joint capsule or a ligament, and secondly a lesion of a muscle or tendon. For biarticular muscles, the constant-length phenomenon can be used to differentiate the location. Otherwise one must correlate this finding with findings of resisted movement tests (see below) in order to differentiate between capsuloligamentous and musculotendinous lesions. If the lesion lies in a muscle or tendon, resistance to the movement opposite the direction of the painful passive movement will be painful, whereas resisted movements are painless with capsuloligamentous lesions.
      ii. A painful structure is being squeezed. This usually occurs with extra-articular lesions such as tendinitis and bursitis. An inflamed subdeltoid bursa is sus-

ceptible to impingement beneath the acromial arch; the trochanteric bursa is squeezed on abduction of the hip; the semimembranosus bursa, when swollen, is squeezed upon full knee flexion. With supraspinatus tendinitis, pain will be felt on elevation of the arm from squeezing of the involved part of the tendon between the greater tuberosity and the posterior rim of the glenoid cavity.

b. A painful arc may occur with passive movement tests. (See section on active movements for a discussion of its significance.)

4. Crepitus on movement. This is best detected by active movement testing but may be noted on passive movements as well. (See section on active movements for discussion.)

B. Passive joint play movement tests (capsuloligamentous stress tests) are designed to stress various portions of the joint capsule and major ligaments in order to detect the presence of painful lesions affecting these structures or loss of continuity of these structures. The method of performing the movements and the various movements performed at each joint are the same as the movements included in the section on specific joint mobilization techniques. Instead of being performed therapeutically as rhythmic oscillations, the movements are performed as examination procedures. In doing so, you assess

1. The degree of mobility (amplitude). The possibilities include

a. Hypermobility, suggesting a loss of continuity (partial tear or complete rupture) of the structure being tested

b. Hypomobility, suggesting fibrosis, as from increased laying down of collagen in the presence of chronic stresses and low-grade inflammation, or suggesting adhesion to adjacent structures, as may occur during healing of a sprain. Hypomobility may be due to protective muscle spasm, in which case some degree of inflammation of the structure or synovial lining is implied.

c. Normal mobility, implying normal status of the structure being tested.

2. Presence of pain or muscle guarding (irritability) at extremes of movement. Pain on joint play movement testing suggests the presence of a sprain or actual tear of the structure being stressed.

3. One must consider, then, six possible findings on joint play movement testing, and their probable interpretations.

a. Normal mobility—painless. There is no lesion of the structure tested.

b. Normal mobility—painful. There is a minor sprain of the structure tested.

c. Hypomobility—painless. There is a contracture or adhesion involving the tested structure.

d. Hypomobility—painful guarding. This may accompany a more acute sprain of the structure. If the hypomobility is due to muscle guarding, you cannot at this point, know whether an actual tear or rupture exists.

e. Hypermobility—painless. This suggests a complete rupture of the structure; there are no longer intact fibers from which pain can be elicited.

f. Hypermobility—painful. This will be found in the presence of a partial tear, in which some fibers of the structure are still intact and being stressed.

III. **Resisted tests.** These are tests designed to assess the status of musculotendinous tissue. Traditional muscle testing procedures that are included under Neuromuscular tests are used primarily to evaluate neurologic function, while here the intention is to determine whether there is some lesion, or loss of continuity, of the musculotendinous tissue itself. In order to do so, ideally we need to stress the muscle and tendon that we wish to test, without stressing other joint tissues. These tests are performed, then, as maximal, isometric contractions, disallowing any movement of the joint. Realistically, in most cases other tissues are going to be squeezed or compressed by the contracting muscles, but this seldom poses a problem when the test is done well. A particular muscle and tendon are tested in the position that best isolates them, and in a position in which they are at an optimal length for maximal contraction (usually a midposition). Maximal stabilization is required to prevent substitution and to minimize joint movement.

When performing resisted tests, determine whether the contraction is strong or weak, and whether it is painful or painless. Weakness may be due to a neurologic deficit or actual loss of continuity of muscle or tendon tissue; appropriate neurologic testing may be performed to differentiate. Keep in mind that few neurologic disorders result in isolated weakness of a single muscle. A painful contraction signifies the presence of some painful pathology involving the muscle or tendon tissues being tested. In the majority of cases the problem will be in the tendon, since muscle strains are rare except in sport-related injuries. Very often the patient feels the most pain as the contraction is released rather than during maximal contraction. When this occurs, it should be considered a positive test; the lengthening that occurs as a muscle relaxes apparently stresses the involved fibers sufficiently to cause more pain than does the shortening that occurs during contraction. Practically speaking, these resisted tests are often performed in conjunction with standard neuromuscular strength tests, discussed below.

There are four possible findings on resisted tests

A. Strong and painless. There is no lesion or neurologic deficit involving the muscle or tendon tested.

B. Strong and painful. A minor lesion of the tested tendon or muscle exists; usually the tendon is at fault. Occasionally auxiliary resisted tests must be performed to differentiate the involved structure from synergists.

C. Weak and painless.
   1. There may be some interruption of the nerve supply to the muscle tested. Correlate your findings with other muscle tests and neurologic tests.
   2. There may be a complete rupture of tendon or muscle; there are no

longer fibers intact from which pain can be elicited.

D. Weak and painful.

1. There may be a partial rupture of muscle or tendon in which there are still some intact fibers that are being stressed.
2. This may be the result of painful inhibition in association with some serious pathology, such as a fracture or neoplasm, or an acute inflammatory process.

NEUROMUSCULAR TESTS

If, at this point in the examination, you suspect that there may be a lesion interfering with neural conduction, the appropriate clinical tests should be performed in an attempt to detect loss of neurologic function. The common nerve lesions are extrinsic in nature. Loss of conduction usually resulting from pressure on a nerve from some adjacent structure or structures. In the common nerve disorders, the pressure is usually minor, intermittent, or both, and usually involves a single nerve or segment. For this reason, the manifestations of the disorder are often quite subtle; findings on evaluation are often largely subjective, and some objective signs may only be detected with more sophisticated electrotesting procedures.

When assessing neurologic function clinically, if you detect a deficit, you can estimate the approximate site of the lesion by correlating the extent of the deficit with peripheral nerve and segmental distributions. More central or serious lesions must be suspected when the extent of the deficit exceeds the distribution of a single segment or a single peripheral nerve. Peripheral nerve and segmental innervations are indicated in Table 4-1 and Figure 4-2. Key segmental distributions, both myotomal and dermatomal are listed in Table 4-2. These are the muscles and skin areas that are most likely to be affected by involvement of a particular segment. These are important to know, since segmental deficits, such as those that occur with disc protrusions, are very common neural disorders seen clinically. Because of the overlapping of dermatomes and myotomes in the extremities, lesions involving a single segment, even when conduction is completely interrupted, result in only subtle deficits.

The tests described below may be used when performing clinical neurologic assessment.

Strength Tests

Employ traditional muscle testing procedures. It is often necessary to repeat a test, comparing the strength carefully to a normal side if possible, since weaknesses resulting from common nerve lesions are usually subtle. Note weaknesses and asymmetries in strength.

Sensory Tests

A pin, wisp of cotton, and tuning fork may be used to assess conduction along sensory pathways. Pressure on a nerve will usually result in loss of conduction along the large myelinated fibers first, and the small unmyelinated fibers last. Therefore, minor deficits will often be manifested first by loss of vibration sense, with sensation to touch and noxious stimulation being reduced with more severe or long-lasting pressure.

When performing sensory tests, test a particular area on the normal side and ask the patient if he perceives the sensation. Then test the involved side and ask the patient again if it is felt. If sensation is intact on both sides, ask the patient if it felt the same on both sides. This procedure is followed when testing each key segmental sensory area and each peripheral nerve distribution. Note sensory deficits and asymmetries in perception.

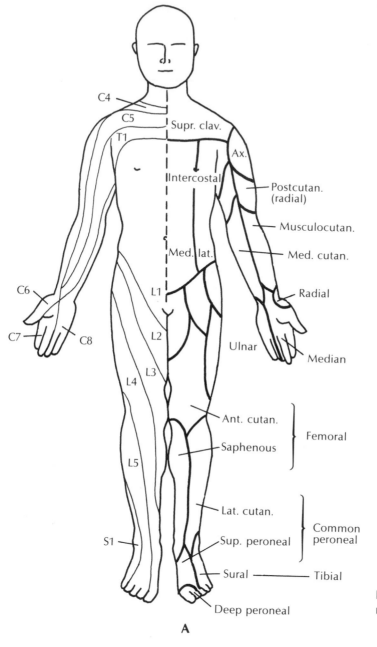

C4
C5
T1
Supr. clav.
Ax.
Intercostal
Postcutan. (radial)
Musculocutan.
Med. lat.
Med. cutan.
C6
L1
Radial
C7
C8
L2
Ulnar
Median
L3
L4
Ant. cutan.
Saphenous
Femoral
L5
Lat. cutan.
Common peroneal
S1
Sup. peroneal
Sural ——— Tibial
Deep peroneal
A

Fig. 4-2. Segmental and peripheral nerve distributions

Deep Tendon Reflexes

Lower motor-neuron lesions, such as segmental or peripheral nerve disorders, may result in diminution of certain deep-tendon reflexes, while more central, upper motor-neuron lesions may cause hyperreflexia. The important assessments to make when testing deep tendon reflexes are whether the responses at homologous

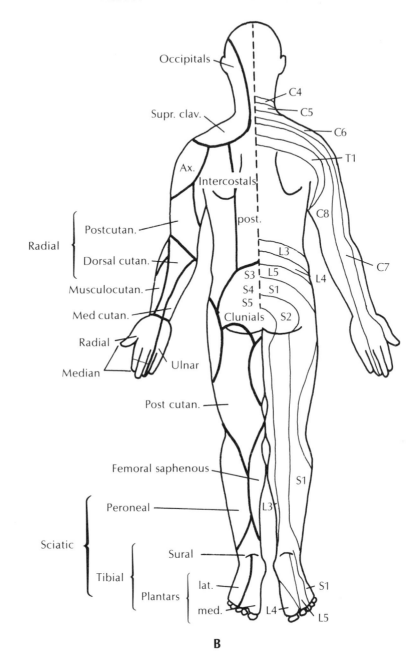

Fig. 4-2. (*Continued*)

B

tendons are symmetrical, and whether any responses are clonic. The presence of hyporeflexia is difficult to judge since some individuals normally have reflexes that are difficult to elicit. Generally speaking, if it is equally difficult to elicit responses at corresponding tendons, no significance can be attributed. However, if upper-extremity responses are difficult to elicit, but lower-extremity responses are

(*text continues on page 96*)

Table 4-1. Peripheral Nerves and Segmental Innervation

ACTION TO BE TESTED	MUSCLES	CORD SEGMENT	NERVES	PLEXUS
Shoulder Girdle and Upper Extremity				
Flexion of neck Extension of neck Rotation of neck Lateral bending of neck	Deep neck muscles (sternomastoid and trapezius also participate)	C1–C4	Cervical	Cervical
Elevation of upper thorax	Scaleni	C3–C5	Phrenic	
Inspiration	Diaphragm	C3–C5		
Adduction of arm from behind to front	Pectoralis major and minor	C5–C8 T1	Medial and lateral pectoral (from medial and lateral cords of plexus)	Brachial
Forward thrust of shoulder	Serratus anterior	C5–C7	Long thoracic	
Elevation of scapula	Levator scapulae	C5 (C3–C4)	Dorsal scapular	
Medial adduction and elevation of scapula	Rhomboids	C4–C5		
Abduction of arm	Supraspinatus	C4–C6	Suprascapular	
Lateral rotation of arm	Infraspinatus	C4–C6		
Medial rotation of arm Adduction of arm from front to back	Latissimus dorsi, teres major, and subscapularis	C5–C8	Subscapular (from posterior cord of plexus)	
Abduction of arm	Deltoid	C5–C6	Axillary (from posterior cord of plexus)	Brachial
Lateral rotation of arm	Teres minor	C4–C5		
Flexion of forearm Supination of forearm	Biceps brachii	C5–C6	Musculocutaneous (from lateral cord of plexus)	
Adduction of arm Flexion of forearm	Coracobrachialis	C5–C7		
Flexion of forearm	Brachialis	C5–C6		Brachial
Ulnar flexion of hand	Flexor carpi ulnaris	C7–T1	Ulnar (from medial cord of plexus)	
Flexion of terminal phalanx of ring finger and little finger Flexion of hand	Flexor digitorum profundus (ulnar portion)	C7–T1		
Adduction of metacarpal of thumb	Adductor pollicis	C8–T1	Ulnar	Brachial
Abduction of little finger	Abductor digiti quinti	C8–T1		
Opposition of little finger	Opponens digiti quinti	C7–T1		
Flexion of little finger	Flexor digiti quinti brevis	C7–T1		
Flexion of proximal phalanx; extension of two distal phalanges; adduction and abduction of fingers	Interossei	C8–T1		
Pronation of forearm	Pronator teres	C6–C7	Median (C6,C7 from lateral cord of plexus; C8,T1 from medial cord of plexus)	Brachial
Radial flexion of hand	Flexor carpi radialis	C6–C7		
Flexion of hand	Palmaris longus	C7–T1		
Flexion of middle phalanx of index finger, middle finger, ring finger, little finger Flexion of hand	Flexor digitorum sublimis	C7–T1		
Flexion of terminal phalanx of thumb	Flexor pollicis longus	C7–T1	Median	Brachial

Table 4-1. (*Continued*)

ACTION TO BE TESTED	MUSCLES	CORD SEGMENT	NERVES	PLEXUS
Shoulder Girdle and Upper Extremity				
Flexion of terminal phalanx of index finger, and middle finger Flexion of hand	Flexor digitorum profundus (radial portion)	C7–T1		
Abduction of metacarpal of thumb	Abductor pollicis brevis	C7–T1	Median	Brachial
Flexion of proximal phalanx of thumb	Flexor pollicis brevis	C7–T1		
Opposition of metacarpal of thumb	Opponens pollicis	C8–T1		
Flexion of proximal phalanx and extension of 2 distal phalanges of index finger, middle finger, ring finger, little finger	Lumbricals (the two lateral) Lumbricals (the two medial)	C8–T1	Median Ulnar	Brachial
Extension of forearm	Triceps brachii and anconeus	C6–C8	Radial (from posterior cord of plexus)	Brachial
Flexion of forearm	Brachioradialis	C5–C6		
Radial extension of hand	Extensor carpi radialis	C6–C8		
Extension of phalanges of fingers Extension of hand	Extensor digitorum communis	C6–C8		
Extension of phalanges of little finger Extension of hand	Extensor digiti quinti proprius	C6–C8		
Ulnar extension of hand	Extensor carpi ulnaris	C6–C8	Radial	Brachial
Supination of forearm	Supinator	C5–C7		
Abduction of metacarpal of thumb Radial extension of hand	Abductor pollicis longus	C7–C8		
Extension of thumb Radial extension of hand	Extensor pollicis brevis and longus	C6–C8		
Extension of index finger Extension of hand	Extensor indicis proprius	C6–C8		
Trunk and Thorax				
Elevation of ribs Depression of ribs Contraction of abdomen Anteroflexion of trunk Lateral flexion of trunk	Thoracic, abdominal, and back		Thoracic and posterior lumbrosacral branches	
Hip Girdle and Lower Extremity				
Flexion of hip	Iliopsoas	L1–L3	Femoral	Lumbar
Flexion of hip and eversion of thigh	Sartorius	L2–L3		
Extension of leg	Quadriceps femoris	L2–L4		
Adduction of thigh	Pectineus Adductor longus Adductor brevis Adductor magnus Gracilis	L2–L3 L2–L3 L2–L4 L3–L4 L2–L4	Obturator	Lumbar
Adduction of thigh Lateral rotation of thigh	Obturator externus	L3–L4		

Table 4-1. *(Continued)*

ACTION TO BE TESTED	MUSCLES	CORD SEGMENT	NERVES	PLEXUS
Hip Girdle and Lower Extremity				
Abduction of thigh Medial rotation of thigh	Gluteus medius and minimus	L4–S1	Superior gluteal	Sacral
Flexion of thigh	Tensor fasciae latae	L4–L5		
Lateral rotation of thigh	Piriformis	L5–S1		
Abduction of thigh	Gluteus maximus	L4–S2	Inferior gluteal	
Lateral rotation of thigh	Obturator internus	L5–S1	Muscular branches from sacral plexus	
	Gemelli	L4–S1		
	Quadratus femoris	L4–S1		
Flexion of leg (assist in extension of thigh)	Biceps femoris	L4–S2	Sciatic (trunk)	Sacral
	Semitendinosus	L4–S1		
	Semimembranosus	L4–S1		
Dorsal flexion of foot Supination of foot	Tibialis anterior	L4–L5	Deep peroneal	Sacral
Extension of toes II–V Dorsal flexion of foot	Extensor digitorum longus	L4–S1		
Extension of great toe Dorsal flexion of foot	Extensor hallucis longus	L4–S1		
Extension of great toe and the 3 medial toes	Extensor digitorum brevis	L4–S1		
Plantar flexion of foot in pronation	Peronei	L5–S1	Superficial peroneal	Sacral
Plantar flexion of foot in supination	Tibialis posterior and triceps surae	L5–S2	Tibial	Sacral
Plantar flexion of foot in supination Flexion of terminal phalanx of toes II–V	Flexor digitorum longus	L5–S2		
Plantar flexion of foot in supination Flexion of terminal phalanx of great toe	Flexor hallucis longus	L5–S2		
Flexion of middle phalanx of toes II–V	Flexor digitorum brevis	L5–S1		
Flexion of proximal phalanx of great toe	Flexor hallucis brevis	L5–S2		
Spreading and closing of toes	Small muscles of foot	S1–S2		
Flexion of proximal phalanx of toes				
Voluntary control of pelvic floor	Perineal and sphincters	S2–S4	Pudendal	Sacral

(Chusid JG: Correlative Neuroanatomy and Functional Neurology. Los Altos, CA, Lange Medical Publications, 1970)

strong, you should consider the presence of a myelopathy or some other more serious pathology.

Coordination, Tone, and Pathologic Reflexes

These should be assessed if myelopathy or other upper motor-neuron disturbances are suspected. For example, myelopathy resulting from cervical spondylosis may result in a mildly spastic gait, increased lower-extremity tone, lower extremity hyperreflexia, and perhaps a positive Babinski response (dorsiflexion of big toe in response to noxious stimulation along the sole of the foot).

Table 4-2. Key Segmental Distributions (Myotomal and Dermotomic)

SEGMENTS	KEY MOVEMENTS TO TEST
C4	Shoulder shrug, diaphragmatic function
C5	Shoulder abduction, external rotation
C6	Elbow flexion, wrist extension
C7	Elbow extension, wrist flexion
C8	Ulnar deviation, thumb abduction, small finger abduction
T1	Approximation of fingers
L2	Hip flexion
L3	Knee extension, hip flexion
L4	Knee extension, ankle dorsiflexion
L5	Ankle/large toe dorsiflexion, eversion of ankle
S1	Plantar flexion, eversion, knee flexion
S2	Knee flexion, ankle plantarflexion
	REFLEXES TO TEST
C5,C6	Biceps, brachioradialis
(C7),C8	Triceps
(L3–L4)	Patellar tendon (quadriceps)
S1–S2	Achilles tendon
	KEY SEGMENTAL SENSORY AREAS TO TEST **(distal part of segment)**
C6	Thumb and index finger, radial border of hand
C7	Middle three fingers
C8	Ring and small finger, ulnar border of hand
L2	Medial thigh
L3	Anteromedial, distal thigh
L4	Medial aspect of large toe
L5	Web space between large and second toes
S1	Below lateral malleolus
S2	Back of heel
S3–S4	Saddle, anal region

N.B. Others, *e.g.*, upper cervical, thoracic, and lumbar, are less definite due to overlapping

(Chusid JG: Correlative Neuroanatomy and functional Neurology. Los Altos, CA, Lange Medical Publications, 1970)

PALPATION

These tests are usually conveniently performed at the same time as the inspection tests discussed previously. As with inspection, palpation tests should be organized according to layers, assessing the status of the skin, subcutaneous soft tissues, and bony structures (including tendon and ligament attachments). Document significant findings.

Skin

Move the back of the hand lightly across the area of skin to be examined. The following should be noted:

Tenderness. Minor pressure on a nerve supplying a particular area of skin may result in dysesthesia that may be perceived as a painful burning sensation to normally non-noxious stimulation, such as light touch. A similar phenomenon may also occur in the presence of lesions involving other tissues innervated by the same segment. This is thought to be the result of summation of otherwise subthreshold afferent input to a segment of the spinal cord.

Moisture and Texture. These may be altered with changes in vascularity or changes in sympathetic activity to the part. In the presence of increased sympathetic activity, such as that which commonly occurs in the chronic stages of reflex sympathetic dystrophy, the skin will be abnormally moist and very smooth. With reduced sympathetic activity, sometimes preceding a reflex sympathetic dystrophy, the skin may be dry and scaly.

Temperature. Skin temperature will be elevated in the presence of an underlying inflammatory process or with reduced sympathetic activity. A reduction in skin temperature may accompany vascular deficiency or increased sympathetic activity.

Mobility. The skin should be moved relative to the underlying tissues to examine for the presence of skin adhesions. This is especially important following healing of surgical and other traumatic wounds.

Subcutaneous Soft Tissues

Palpate the soft tissues deep to the skin—fat, fascia, muscles, tendons, joint capsules and ligaments, nerves, and blood vessels. Use no more pressure than what is necessary. A common mistake is to press harder and harder in an attempt to distinguish deep structures. This only serves to desensitize the palpating fingertips and does not assist in determining the nature of the tissues being palpated. Soft tissue palpation may offer information concerning the following:

Tenderness. Tenderness to deep palpation is a very unreliable finding. In itself it is never indicative of the site of a pathology because of the prevalence of referred tenderness associated with lesions of deep somatic tissues. The phenomenon is similar in all respects to that of referred pain. In many common lesions, the area of primary tenderness does not correspond well to the site of the lesion. Thus, patients with low-back disorders are often most tender in the buttock, those with supraspinatus tendinitis are most tender over the lateral brachial region, and persons with trochanteric bursitis are most tender over the lateral aspect of the thigh. These "trigger points," or referred areas of tenderness, are found in some area of the segment corresponding to the segment in which the lesion exists. Generally, tenderness associated with more superficial lesions, such as medial ligament sprains at the knee, corresponds more closely with the site of the lesion than does tenderness occurring with more deeply situated pathologies.

Edema and Swelling. Note the size and location of localized soft tissue swellings.

Abnormal fluid accumulations should be differentiated as intra- or extra-articular. Articular effusion will be restricted to the confines of the joint capsule; pressure applied over one side of the joint may, therefore, cause increased distension observed over the opposite side. This type of "ballottement" test can be used with more superficial joints. Often articular effusion is distinguished by its characteristic distribution at a particular joint; these distributions are discussed in the regional chapters. Extra-articular swelling may accompany acute inflammatory processes, such as abscesses and those following acute trauma, because of protein and plasma leaking from capillary walls. Generalized tissue edema may accompany vascular disorders, lymphatic obstructions, and electrolyte imbalances.

Consistency, Continuity, and Mobility. Normal soft tissue is supple and easily moved against underlying tissue. Palpate for abnormalities such as indurated areas, loss of mobility, stringiness, doughiness, nodules, and gaps, and note them.

Pulse. Palpating for the pulse of various major arteries can assist in assessing the status of blood supply to the part. Heart rate may also be determined.

Bony Structures

Bony structures also include ligaments and tendon attachments. When palpating bony structures, note the following:

Tenderness.   As with deep, soft-tissue tenderness, tenderness at various bony sites may be referred, and is therefore often misleading. Lesions involving both ligaments and tendons commonly occur at the site where these structures join the periosteum. Typically, these are highly innervated regions and may be tender to palpation in the presence of tenoperiosteal or periosteoligamentous strains and sprains. Periosteal tenderness will also accompany specific bony lesions, such as stress fractures or other fractures.

Enlargements. Bony hypertrophy often accompanies healing of a fracture and degenerative joint disease. In the latter, the bony changes will be noted at the joint margins in more superficial joints.

Bony Relationships.   Structural malalignments, as discussed in the section on inspection, may be detected clinically by assessing the relationships, in the various planes of reference, of one bony structure to another. This is especially important following healing of fractures, and in cases of vague, subtle insidious disorders that may have a pathomechanical basis.

GUIDES TO CORRELATION AND INTERPRETATION

Judgments relating to the nature and extent of the disorder and the resultant degree of disability can be made by correlating the information obtained during a comprehensive initial patient examination. With respect to the nature of the problem, it is important to judge whether the disease state is a "medical" disorder,

or if perhaps operant behavior patterns have developed that may account for a significant part of the disability. We should consider if the degree of disability is consistent with the apparent nature and extent of the physical pathology, or is the patient exhibiting disability behaviors that are out of proportion to clinical findings. In the latter case we should consider the possibility that the disease state is being maintained by external consequences that have a reinforcing effect. It is essential that such determinations be made, since treatment directed at some physical pathology in the presence of an operant disease state will be futile and can further reinforce "learned" disability behaviors.

THE NATURE OF THE LESION

If it appears that some physical pathology is primarily responsible for the patient's disorder, the nature of the pathology should be estimated as precisely as possible. To do so, we must correlate the information obtained on examination with knowledge of anatomy, physiology, kinesiology, and pathology in order to identify the involved tissue or tissues. Some estimate should also be made concerning the extent to which these tissues are involved. A few common pathologies make up the majority of disorders affecting each musculoskeletal tissue. For each of these pathologies, there are also consistent key clinical findings. In developing judgements concerning the nature of common clinical disorders, it is helpful to be aware of the lesions common to each tissue, and how they are manifested clinically. The following descriptions are meant to guide the clinician in this respect but are not meant to be all-inclusive.

Bone

Fractures are best identified in the physician's examination through the use of radiographs. When examining a patient following healing of a fracture, it is important to determine the presence of bony malunion on inspection of bony structure and alignment. This may affect eventual functioning of the part. Dislocations are also best detected through the physician's interpretation of radiographs, although dislocations are often obvious on inspection.

Articular Cartilage

Degeneration from fatigue wearing is the most common lesion affecting this tissue. It causes roughening of the normally smooth surface layers of cartilage. Clinically this is manifested as crepitus on movements when opposition of joint surfaces is maintained by weight-bearing or other compressive forces. However, considerable degeneration must usually take place before crepitus is detected clinically.

A loose body is a fragment of articular cartilage that has broken away and lies free in the joint. This may occur in the late stages of cartilage degeneration or as a result of avascular necrosis of an area of subchondral bone (osteochondrosis). A loose body becomes symptomatic when it alters the mechanical functioning of the joint, usually causing a restriction of movement in a noncapsular pattern (joint block).

Intra-articular Fibrocartilage

The common disorder affecting intra-articular fibrocartilaginous discs and menisci is tearing, usually from traumatic injury. Forces sufficient to tear a meniscus or disc in the extremities will usually also cause some strain to the joint capsule to which these structures attach. This causes synovial inflammation in the acute stage. Thus, movement is likely to be restricted in a capsular pattern.

Minor displacement of a torn fragment of fibrocartilage may simply result in "clicking" of the joint on specific movements. Lower-extremity joints, namely the knee, may give way when a tag of a torn meniscus is caught between the articular surfaces, suddenly interfering with normal mechanics of the joint.

A major displacement of a torn fragment may grossly interfere with normal mechanics and block joint movement in a noncapsular pattern. The classic example is a "bucket-handle" tear of a medial meniscus.

When the annular ring of a vertebral disc is torn, secondary neurologic symptoms or signs may result from bulging of the nucleus against adjacent nerve tissue.

Joint Capsule

Fibrosis (see section on capsular tightness) typically occurs with prolonged immobilization of a joint, in association with a chronic, low-grade inflammatory process such as occurs with degenerative joint disease, and with resolution of acute inflammation of the synovium. Joint motion is limited in a capsular pattern, and there is a capsular end-feel at the extremes of movement.

Synovial inflammation is commonly caused by rheumatoid arthritis, acute trauma to the joint, joint infection, and arthrotomy. Joint motion is limited in a capsular pattern. There is a painful, muscle spasm end-feel at the points of restriction of movements.

Inflammation of the synovium results in an increased production of synovial fluid, causing capsular distension and loss of the capsular laxity necessary for full movement. In the more superficial joints, the articular swelling can be observed and palpated. If the effusion persists following resolution of the synovial inflammation, motion will continue to be limited in a capsular pattern, with a boggy end-feel to movement.

It is worthwhile to note that patients with capsular pathology typically have some combination of fibrosis, synovial inflamation, and effusion. Therefore, end-feels are not always distinct.

Forces sufficient to sprain a ligament usually cause some capsular disruption as well. Occasionally in traumatic injuries, a particular portion of a joint capsule is ruptured, such as the anterior capsule of the shoulder when the humerus dislocates anteriorly. Synovial inflammation and joint effusion usually follow capsular sprains.

In the case of a sprain, the joint play movement that stresses the involved portion of the capsule will be of normal amplitude. In more severe sprains, the joint may be slightly hypermobile, with a painful muscle-guarding end-feel.

Ligaments

The history of a sprain invariably gives a traumatic onset. In the case of a mild sprain, the joint-play movement that stresses the ligament is of normal amplitude and is painful. More severe sprains (partial ruptures) will present as somewhat hypermobile and painful on the associated joint-play test. The synovial lining of the adjacent aspect of the joint capsule will often become inflamed, resulting in capsular effusion in the acute stage. There is usually tenderness over the site of the lesion.

The onset of a rupture is also usually traumatic in origin. The associated joint-play movement test will be *hypermobile and painless* in the chronic stages. Even in the acute stage it is usually painless, since there are no fibers intact from which to elicit pain. If adjacent capsular tissue is also sprained, there may be some pain on stress testing in the acute stage. Capsular effusion often does not occur because fluid leaks through the defect. In the chronic stages the patient may give a history of instability. The joint gives way during activities that stress it in the direction that the ruptured ligament is supposed to check.

Bursae

The common disorder is inflammation, secondary to chronic irritation, infection, gout, or, rarely, acute trauma. Movement of the nearby joint will cause pain, restriction of motion, or both in a noncapsular pattern. There may be a painful arc of movement as well.

In acute bursitis, such as at the shoulder, the end-feel to movement is often empty and painful; protective muscle spasm would only serve to squeeze the inflammed structure, increasing the pain. There is usually tenderness over the site of the lesion.

Tendons

Tendinitis is a minor lesion of tendon tissue involving microscopic tearing and a chronic, low-grade inflammatory process. In most cases it is degenerative in nature; the pathology results from tissue fatigue rather than from acute injury. Since progression of the pathologic process will result in a partial tear (macroscopic) or rupture of the tendon, tendinitis should be considered on a continuum with more serious lesions.

The key clinical sign associated with tendinitis is a strong but painful resisted test of the involved musculotendinous structure. There may be pain at the extremes of the passive movement or movements that stretch the tendon. Seldom is there limitation of movement. There may be palpable tenderness at the site of the lesion, referred tenderness into the related segment, or both.

When the involved part of a tendon is that which passes through a sheath, two other terms are often used: *tenosynovitis* and *tenovaginitis*. Tenosynovitis is an inflammation of the synovial lining of a sheath resulting from friction of a roughened tendon gliding within the sheath. This will present similarly to tendinitis, but there is often pain on active movements that produce movement of the tendon within the sheath. Thus, active movement in the direction or opposite the direction of pull of the tendon may be painful. In tenovaginitis, a tendon gliding within a swollen, thickened sheath causes pain. The classic example occurs with rheumatoid arthritis. The clinical signs are essentially the same as those for tenosynovitis. There may be palpable and visible swelling of the tendon sheath.

In the case of a partial tendon tear, actual loss of continuity of tendon tissue will cause the resisted test for the musculotendinous complex to be weak and painful. The passive movement that stretches the tendon may be painful.

When the tendon has torn completely, the related resisted test will be weak and painless. In some cases, for example, rupture of the achilles tendon, there may be a palpable gap at the site of the rupture.

Muscles

Muscle strains and ruptures are relatively rare. When they do occur they are invariably the result of acute trauma, and are therefore most prevalent in sports-medicine settings. Muscle, being well vascularized and resilient, does not commonly undergo fatigue degeneration as do tendons.

In the case of a strain, a minor tear of muscle fibers will result in a strong and painful finding on the resisted test that stresses the involved muscle. There may be pain on full passive stretch of the muscle, as well as palpable tenderness. In the case of a rupture, the associated resisted test will be weak and painless. A gap may be palpable, or occasionally visible, at the site of the defect.

Nerves

The common conditions affecting nerves are those in which some extrinsic source of pressure results in altered conduction along some or all of the nerve fibers—the so-called *entrapment syndromes*. The most common sites of pressure are the points of exit of the lower cervical and lower lumbar spinal nerves from the intervertebral foramina. Here pressure is usually from a protruding disc or projecting osteophyte. There are other common sites of pressure further out in the periphery that affect the nerves to the extremities. As indicated in Chapter 3, Pain, pressure tends to alter conduction first along the largest fibers, and last along the smallest. Altered nerve conduction is usually manifested subjectively before any objective clinical evidence of neurologic dysfunction can be detected. In fact, in the case of the common entrapment syndromes, objective clinical findings are rare, and when present they are usually quite subtle. Often more sophisticated electrodiagnostic tests are required to objectively detect changes in nerve conduction.

The subjective complaints associated with common entrapment disorders can generally be classified as paresthesia (pins-and-needles), dysesthesia (altered sensation in response to some external stimulus), and pain. Although some patients may describe paresthesia and dysesthesia as painful, pain is usually not a primary complaint when there is pressure on a nerve farther out in the periphery rather than at the nerve-root level. Thus, patients with thoracic outlet syndrome, ulnar nerve palsy, and carpal tunnel syndrome, as well as those who have sat too long with the legs crossed, do not complain of pain but of a pins-and-needles sensation. Pain is a common complaint, however, in cases in which there is pressure on a nerve at nerve-root level. With initial pressure, when the larger, myelinated, "fast pain" fibers are stimulated, patients describe a sharp, shooting dermatomic quality of pain. With prolonged or increased pressure, when the larger fibers cease to conduct and the small, unmyelinated, C fibers are stimulated, a dull, aching scleratomic type of pain will be perceived.

Paresthesia, the primary subjective complaint with pressure farther out in the periphery, may occur either with the onset of pressure, or when the pressure is released, or both. For example, a person usually feels little or nothing when sitting with legs crossed, applying pressure to the tibial or peroneal nerve. It is not until the person uncrosses the legs, releasing the pressure, that he feels the pins-and-needles sensation of the foot being "asleep." A similar situation holds true for pressure on the lower cord of the brachial plexus from depression of the shoulder girdle; the patient invariably describes the onset of pins-and-needles in the early morning hours (1:00 or 2:00 A.M.) some time after the pressure is released. It seems that the interval between the release of pressure and the onset of paresthesia is in some way proportional to the length of time during which the pressure was applied. In other common nerve problems, the onset of symptoms occurs when the pressure is applied. For example, many patients with carpal tunnel syndrome describe paresthesia felt primarily during fine finger-movements; the tension on the finger flexor tendons produces pressure on the median nerve sufficient to cause symptoms. Similarly, when an individual sits or lies with pressure over the ulnar groove, pins-and-needles are usually felt in the ulnar side of the hand while the pressure is applied, and relieved after the pressure is released.

As mentioned, more objective findings associated with common nerve-pressure disorders are usually very subtle when present. They are more common with nerve-root pressure from a disc protrusion than with more peripheral entrapment syndromes. The earliest evidence of decreased conduction will be related to those functions mediated by the largest myelinated fibers, since these fibers are most sensitive to pressure. Therefore, reduced vibration sense is often the earliest deficit detected by clinical testing. With increased or prolonged pressure, diminished deep-tendon reflexes may be noted, followed by reduced muscle strength. Finally, there is reduced sensation, first to light touch, then to noxious stimulation. Because of overlapping dermatomes and myotomes, and because each muscle and skin area typically receives innervation from more than one segment, even completely severing a nerve root will usually cause only a minor deficit.

THE EXTENT OF THE LESION

When clinicians speak of "acute" and "chronic" lesions, it is often unclear whether they are referring to the length of time that the pathology has existed, the severity of the disorder, or the nature of the inflammatory process. There are relatively few consistent clinical findings related to either the duration or severity of common musculoskeletal problems. However, there are certain symptoms and signs that are consistently present with acute inflammatory processes, and others that are pathognomonic of lesions in which a more chronic inflammatory state exists. *Acute inflammation* is that stage or type of inflammatory process in which hyperemia, increased capillary permeability with protein and plasma leakage, and an influx of granulocytes and other defense cells take place. *Chronic inflammation* is characterized by an attempt at repair, with increased numbers of fibrocytes and other "tissue building" cells, and the presence of granulation tissue. An acute lesion is characterized by the following clinical findings:

Pain is relatively constant.

On passive range of motion of the related joint, there is a muscle spasm end-feel or an empty end-feel to movement.

Pain is likely to be referred over a relatively diffuse area of the related segment.

There may be a measurable skin-temperature increase over the site of the lesion.

There is often difficulty in falling asleep, difficulty in sleeping, or both.

In the presence of chronic lesions, the patient is likely to present with the following symptoms or signs:

Pain is increased by specific activities and relieved by rest.

On passive movement of the related joint, there is no muscle spasm or empty end-feel.

Pain is likely to be felt over a relatively localized area, close to the site of the lesion, though often not directly over the site of the lesion.

There is little or no temperature elevation over the involved part.

Unless the lesion involves the shoulder or hip, there is little or no difficulty in sleeping.

REFERENCES

1. Cyriax J: Textbook of Orthopedic Medicine, Vol I, The Diagnosis of Soft Tissue Lesions. Baltimore, Williams & Wilkins, 1969
2. Fordyce W, Fowler RS, Lehmann JF, DeLateur BJ, Sands PL, Trieschmann RB: Operant conditioning in the treatment of chronic clinical pain. Arch Phys Med Rehabil 54:399–408, 1973
3. Fordyce WE: Behavioral Methods for Chronic Pain and Illness. St Louis, CV Mosby, 1976
4. Fordyce WE: Evaluating and managing chronic pain. Geriatrics 33:59–62, 1978

RECOMMENDED READINGS

Cyriax J: Textbook of Orthopedic Medicine, Vol I, The Diagnosis of Soft Tissue Lesions. Baltimore, Williams & Wilkins, 1969

Endow AJ, Swisher SN: Interviewing and patient care. New York, Oxford University Press, 1972.

Hoppenfeld S: Physical Examination of the Spine and Extremities. New York, Appleton-Century-Crofts, 1976

Stolov WC: Evaluation of the Patient. In Krusen FH, Kottke FJ, Ellwood PM (eds): Handbook of Physical Medicine and Rehabilitation. Philadelphia, W B Saunders, 1971

Part Two
SELECTED TECHNIQUES

5 *Concepts of Management*

Randolph M. Kessler

This section on selected techniques will discuss only those procedures that may not be well understood or are new to most professional training programs. It is assumed that the reader is familiar with many basic therapeutic procedures and modalities, such as therapeutic exercise, use of assistive devices, massage, and electrotherapy. The application of these forms of treatment, in conjunction with traditional therapies, to specific pathologies affecting the various extremity regions will be discussed in Part Three.

REHABILITATION

The correlation and interpretation of findings from a comprehensive initial patient examination is the basis for developing a treatment plan. As mentioned in Chapter 4, Assessment of Common Musculoskeletal Disorders, during the initial examination we seek to elicit information that relates to the nature and extent of the physical pathology as well as to the degree of disability. The choice of therapeutic procedures depends upon this information.

When we speak of the nature of the physical pathology, the primary considerations are the site of the lesion and the type of tissue involved. Once the nature of the pathology has been determined, there is often a tendency to direct treatment primarily at the site of the lesion with the expectation that resolving the physical pathology will alleviate any resultant physical dysfunction, and will in turn restore the patient to his normal "health state." There are many potential fallacies to this approach that make it unsuitable as a reliable treatment model.

First, such an approach ignores the secondary effects that a lesion involving a particular structure may have upon the normal functioning of other related structures. It calls for treatment of "anatomical structures" rather than "physiological units." By considering the synovial joints as the basic physiological—rather than anatomical—unit of the musculoskeletal system, we are better prepared to respect the interactions of the various components of this system under normal and abnormal conditions. This is essential, since an alteration in one component of a functional unit often leads to dysfunction of other components of the same or neighboring units; this may act to maintain the primary pathology, predispose to recurrence, or result in secondary pathologies. Thus, even in the case of relatively localized lesions, we must respect such interactions and be prepared to deal with them therapeutically.

For example, a painful lesion of the supraspinatus tendon tends to result in reflex inhibition of the supraspinatus and other rotator-cuff muscles. This will predispose to subacromial impingement from abnormal movement of the head of the humerus during elevation activities, which may further traumatize the supraspinatus tendon as well as the subdeltoid bursa. Also, muscles such as the deltoid and the trapezius may reflexively contract

107

abnormally during movement of the arm, secondary to abnormal afferent input from the site of pathology to the lower cervical segments. This may further interfere with normal joint mechanics at the shoulder, as well as at the neck, to which the trapezius attaches. It should be clear that effective treatment of this problem involves more than resolution of the pathologic process affecting the tendon. The rotator-cuff muscles must, at some time, be strengthened; excessive elevation of the arm must be temporarily avoided; and relaxation of abnormally contracting muscles should be promoted. If we were to treat only the lesion of the tendon, it is likely that treatment would be ineffective or take much longer than necessary to be effective. Continued subacromial impingement would enhance the chance of recurrence. The patient would also be predisposed to developing a coexistent cervical pathology from increased stresses to the neck due to abnormal muscle activity.

Secondly, an approach in which treatment is aimed exclusively at some discrete pathology tends to ignore etiologic considerations. Temporary amelioration may ensue without true resolution of the problem. Unless underlying etiologies, such as biomechanical abnormalities, are recognized and dealt with, chronic recurrent problems can be expected. Thus, a patient with chondromalacia patellae resulting from abnormal foot pronation may temporarily do very well on a program of reduced activity and strengthening of the vastus medialis. However, he is likely to experience similar problems with the resumption of normal activity levels unless the alignment of his foot and leg is corrected. Similarly, the patient with trochanteric bursitis caused by a tight iliotibial band usually responds well to ultrasound over the site of the lesion, but if extensibility of the iliotibial band is not increased, relief will be short-lived. The clinician should implement the concept that prevention is the ultimate cure by attempting to identify etiologic factors and by employing appropriate measures to deal with them. This should be a major consideration in chronic, fatigue disorders, which will tend to be self-resolving once the cause of the abnormal stresses is corrected. (See the discussion of treatment of chronic disorders in this chapter.)

Thirdly, and most importantly, when treatment is directed only at a physical pathology, the psychosocial implications of the problem are not given due respect. Comprehensive rehabilitation requires restoration of an optimal level of function. Although a physical pathology may have been the original cause of physical dysfunction or other "disease behaviors," such as complaints of pain, there are often other factors that may serve to maintain or inhibit the disability behaviors. Such "motivational factors" may eventually assume a greater influence upon the disability state than the original pathology (see Fig. 4-1). These factors must be recognized since they often determine whether or not treatment is successful, whether an optimal level of function is restored, and whether disability behaviors (pain complaints, physical dysfunction, and functional dependence) are resolved. If being disabled carries excessively negative consequences for the patient, such as often occurs in sports-medicine settings, these consequences will strongly inhibit the disability state. As a result, the patient often attempts to do more than is appropriate and imposes deleterious effects on the physical pathology. This may counteract any beneficial effects of other treatment procedures. On the other hand, if the patient stands to gain in some way from being disabled, such as time away from work, financial compensation, or welcomed dependence, the potential for gain may have a significant reinforcing effect upon the disability state. The patient is not likely to improve in spite of otherwise effective treatment of the physical pathology. In both of the above situations, the psychosocial, motivational influences are likely to have a greater effect upon the disease state than the physical pathology itself. Unless they are dealt with, the patient cannot be truly rehabilitated. To estimate the relative influence of such factors, we must determine whether the degree of disability is consistent with the symptoms and signs manifested by the pathology. If there are inconsistencies, we should suspect that significant psychosocial influences are affecting the nature of the disability state.

TREATMENT OF
PHYSICAL PATHOLOGIES

Although the principle of "treating the patient, not the disease" has become somewhat of a cliché, its application to patients with common musculoskeletal disorders is too often overlooked. The first and foremost consideration when devising a therapeutic program should always be how the patient's ability to function normally has been compromised. We must ask, what conditions are responsible for the dysfunction and are these conditions reversible? If reversible, what would be the most appropriate means of intervening therapeutically so as to affect these conditions? If the conditions at fault appear irreversible, what can be done to optimize residual function? And finally, what can be done to prevent recurrences, secondary problems, and progression of the existing disorder? With such an approach, therapy is disability-oriented rather than pathology-oriented. The primary goal of management becomes restoration of an optimal level of functioning rather than simply resolution of some pathologic process. Resolution of a physical pathology does not necessarily lead to restoration of function, reduction in pain behavior, or other necessary signs of improvement.

In the case of many common musculoskeletal disorders, in which the degree of disability appears to be consistent with the nature and extent of the lesion, physical treatment will constitute a major component of the therapeutic program. When this is the case, the clinician must choose, among the various forms of intervention at his disposal, the procedures and modalities most appropriate for the specific disorder. Treatment must be individualized for each patient and according to the nature and extent of the pathologic process. The tendency to incorporate "standardized" programs of exercises and other treatments, usually for the sake of efficiency, should be avoided. The controversies over and misconceptions about so many forms of treatment (*e.g.*, massage, manipulation, traction, and certain exercises) stem largely from their having been advocated or misconstrued as panaceae for disorders affecting certain regions.

CLASSIFYING PATHOLOGIES:
ACUTE VS. CHRONIC

As a preface to discussing specific types of treatments and their respective applications, we should consider some general concepts that are related to the overall approach to physical treatment. As mentioned above, approaches to treating physical pathologies should depend on the nature and extent of the disorder. The two common terms used clinically to classify pathologies according to their nature and extent are *acute* and *chronic*. As suggested in Chapter 4 on assessment these terms should not be used to refer to the severity or duration of a disorder, since when used in these contexts they have little relationship to symptoms and signs. A patient with a relatively severe lesion such as a ligamentous rupture, for example, may present with much less pain and dysfunction than one who has sustained a minor sprain. It is well known, even to those outside the health professions, that a sprained ankle may be more painful and disabling shortly after injury than a fractured ankle. With respect to duration, disorders of fairly recent onset often present with subtle symptoms and signs when compared to certain long-standing problems. If we are presented with two patients, one with recent onset of aching in his shoulder but no gross loss of function, and the other with long-standing severe pain and dysfunction, which condition do we call *acute* and which *chronic*?

The terms *acute* and *chronic* do have some significance when used to refer to the nature of the symptoms and signs with which a patient presents, as differentiated in Chapter 4. This is because symptoms and signs reflect the nature of various pathologies, and more specifically, they tend to reflect the nature of the inflammation or repair process that accompanies any physical pathology. Because these symptom—sign complexes do relate to the nature of pathologic processes, we will use them as a basis for a discussion of general approaches to management. The following scheme is based upon the definitions of *acute* and *chronic*.

TREATMENT OF ACUTE AND CHRONIC DISORDERS

I. **General concepts**
   A. Consider the nature and extent of the disorder, whether *acute* or *chronic*.
      1. The terms are sometimes used to refer to duration of the problem and not to symptoms and signs.
      2. They should be used to refer to the nature of the inflammatory process
         a. Acute hyperemic phase
            i. Pain is felt at rest and aggravated by activity;
            ii. pain is felt over a relatively diffuse area, and may be referred into any or all of the related segment (scleratome);
            iii. passive movement of related joints when, limited, is restricted by pain or muscle guarding, or both;
            iv. the skin temperature over the site of the lesion is often elevated.
         b. Chronic/reparative phase
            i. There is no pain at rest and pain is felt only with specific activities;
            ii. pain is felt over a fairly localized area, close to the site of the lesion (often not directly over the site of the lesion, however);
            iii. movement of related joints, when limited, is restricted by soft tissue tightness—pain is felt only at the extremes of movement or through a small arc of movement.
      3. The terms are not useful in describing the severity of the lesion. For example, a patient with a complete rupture of a ligament may present with less pain and disability and with fewer cardinal inflammatory signs than an individual with only a partial tear of a ligament.
   B. Assess, control, and monitor the patient's functional status.
      1. Assessment of disability. Determine by history and physical examination the degree of disability. Compare disease (injury) status to health (normal) status, and compare to other symptoms and signs.
         a. Is the degree of disability consistent with the appar-

ent nature and extent of the disorder? This yields important information relating to the patients "motivational" status, and is a major consideration in treatment planning.

   i. The "well-motivated" patient is one for whom the consequences of injury (disability) are punishing. For example, they imply time away from desirable situations or possibility of financial loss. It can be presumed that resolution of the pathology will lead to resolution of the disability state. A medical approach to treatment is appropriate.

   ii. The "poorly motivated" patient is one for whom the consequences of disability are *reinforcing.* For example, they offer time away from undesirable situations or the possibility of financial gain. It cannot be presumed that treatment of the pathology will result in resolution of the disability state. Rehabilitation must include attempts to alter the consequences to disability. An operant approach must be incorporated into the treatment program.

   b. Record and use information as a baseline by which to judge progress.

2. Control functional status (see below under techniques of management).

a. Inappropriate activities must be restricted to prevent prolongation or recurrence of the disorder.

b. Appropriate activities must be resumed as the physical pathology resolves. *This is the ultimate goal of management.*

3. Monitor functional status to accurately judge improvement. The patient is not rehabilitated until an optimal level of function is restored, regardless of the state of the physical pathology.

II. Treatment of acute inflammatory disorders (traumatic). The primary goal is to promote progression to a chronic state while minimizing dysfunction.

A. Physiological intervention to control the acute inflammatory response

   1. Ice—to reduce blood flow

   2. Compression—to prevent and reduce swelling

   3. Elevation—to prevent and reduce swelling and hyperemia

   4. Relaxation—to reduce pain and muscle spasm

B. Avoidance and prevention of continued trauma and irritation by reducing loading of the part

   1. Braces, slings, splints, assistive devices, strapping

   a. Lower extremity—Crutches or canes to reduce forces of weight bearing; splints, braces, or strapping to reduce forces of movement

   b. Upper extremity—Slings to reduce forces of gravity and therefore, postural muscle tone; splints, braces, or strapping to reduce the forces imposed by movement

2. Control of activities causing undesirable loading of the part. This requires careful, well-understood instructions to the patient.

C. Maintaining optimal levels of function and preventing unnecessary dysfunction.
   1. Isometric resistive exercises to maintain muscle function, but avoid undesirable movement of the part
   2. Gentle active or passive movement (when appropriate according to the nature of the disorder) to avoid pain and muscle guarding

III. **Chronic disorders**

A. Causative factors. These constitute the majority of disorders seen in most clinical settings. The two primary causes are
   1. Abnormal modeling of tissue during resolution of an acute disorder. The following are examples:
      a. Malunion of fractures resulting in a change in the direction or magnitude of forces acting on the part during use (increased stress)
      b. Abnormalities in collagen maturation or production (scarring, fibrosis, adhesions). An excess amount of collagen may be produced, and that which is produced may not be oriented along the normal lines of stress. Abnormal collagen cross-links are formed, and the tissue may adhere to adjacent structures. The net result is reduced extensibility, and therefore reduced capacity to attenuate energy by deforming when stressed.

2. Fatigue response of tissues. Following are the two types of response:
   a. Tissue breakdown—the rate of attrition exceeds the rate of repair (*e.g.*, stress fractures, cartilage degeneration). The tissue becomes "weaker" and begins to yield under loading conditions. It occurs with mild to moderately increased stress levels in tissues with low regenerative capacity (*e.g.*, articular cartilage); with higher stress levels in other tissues (*e.g.*, tendon, bone); under conditions of altered tissue metabolism (*e.g.*, hypovascularity).
   b. Tissue hypertrophy (*e.g.*, fibrosis and sclerosis) occurs with mild to moderately increased stress levels in tissues with good regenerative/repair capacity, acting over a prolonged period of time. Tissue becomes stiffer, with reduced energy attenuation capacity. Individual fibers or trabeculae begin to yield under loading conditions, resulting in low-grade inflammation, pain, increased tissue production, and so on.

B. Treatment planning
   1. Reduce stresses to involved tissue over time
      a. Reduce magnitude of loading (control of activities)
      b. Reduce magnitude of stresses by altering direction or magnitude of forces acting on the part through control of activities; use of protective/assistive devices;

and use of orthotic devices to control position or the part.

c. Increase surface area of loading (*e.g.*, foot orthosis).

d. Provide for external energy attenuation (*e.g.*, pads, helmets, cushioned heels).

2. Increase energy-attenuating capacity of the part

a. Increase compensatory muscle strength/activity with strengthening exercises; increase neuromuscular facilitative (afferent) input (*e.g.*, taping, coordination training)

b. Increase tissue extensibility (ability to deform without loss of structural integrity) by

  i. Active stretching;

  ii. Passive stretching, using passive range of motion stretching for musculotendinous tightness, and specific joint mobilization for capsuloligamentous tightness;

  iii. Use of ultrasound in conjunction with stretch;

  iv. Use of transverse friction massage to increase interfiber mobility and to prevent or reduce fibrous adhesion without longitudinally stressing the tissue.

c. Promote increase in structural integrity of the part (increased "strength"). This requires tissue hypertrophy, without loss of extensibility from overproduction of immature collagenous tissue, and so on; and maturation of collagen—orientation of fibers along normal lines of stress and development of appropriate cross-links.

The necessary stimulus is stress to the part. This means gradual, controlled participation in high-stress-level activities (training).

3. Resumption of optimal activity levels and prevention of recurrence. Judgments are based on

a. Clinical evidence of having accomplished above objectives

b. Awareness of the nature of stresses imposed by various activities, and an estimate of the capacity of the part to withstand those stresses. This requires biomechanical assessment and analysis, and familiarity with research related to biomechanical properties of musculoskeletal tissues under various conditions of loading and healing.

c. Extrinsic "motivational" factors—the consequences of disability for the patient.

RECOMMENDED READINGS

Abraham WM: Heat vs cold therapy for the treatment of muscle injuries. Athletic Training 9:4, 1974

Adams A: Effects of exercise upon ligament strength. Res Q 37 (2):163– 167, 1965

Akeson WH, Amiel D, LaViolette D, Secrist D: The connective tissue response to immobility: An accelerated aging response? Exp Gerontol 3:289– 300, 1968

Clayton ML, James SM, Abdulla M: Experimental investigations of ligamentous healing. Clin Orthop 61:146, 1968

Darling RC: Exercise. In Dawney JA, Darling RC (eds): Physiological Basic of Rehabilitation Medicine. Philadelphia, W B Saunders, 1971

DeLateur BJ, Lehmann JF, Fordyce WE: A test of the DeLorne Axiom. Arch Phys Med Rehabil 49:245– 248, 1968

DeLateur BJ, Lehmann JF, Giaconi R: Mechanical work and fatigue: Their roles in the development of muscle work capacity. Arch Phys Med Rehabil 57:321– 324, 1976

DeLateur BJ, Lehmann J, Stonebridge J, Warren CG: Isotonic vs isometric exercise: A double-shift transfer-of-training study. Arch Phys Med Rehabil 53:212– 217, 1972

Fordyce WE, Fowler RS, Lehmann JF, DeLateur BJ, Sands PL, Trieschmann RB: Operant conditioning in the treatment of chronic clinical pain. Arch Phys Med Rehabil 54:399– 408, 1973

Fordyce WE: Behavioral Methods for Chronic Pain and Illness. St Louis, C V Mosby, 1976

Frankel VH, Hang Y: Recent advances in the biomechanics of sport injuries. Acta Orthop Scand 46:484– 497, 1975

Kennedy JD, Hawkins RJ, Willis RB, Danylchuk KD: Tension studies in human knee ligaments. J Bone Joint Surg 58 A(3):350– 355, 1976

Knight K: The effects of hypothermia on inflammation and swelling. Athletic Training 11:1, 1976

Lehmann JF, DeLateur BJ, Stonebridge JB, Warren CB: Therapeutic temperature distribution produced by ultrasound as modified by dosage and volume of tissue exposed. Arch Phys Med and Rehabil 48:12:662– 666, 1967

Lehmann JF, Warren CG: Therapeutic heat and cold. Clin Orthop 99:207– 245, 1974

Noyes FR, Edward SG: The strength of the anterior cruciate ligament in humans and rhesus monkeys. J Bone Joint Surg 58 A(8):1074– 1082, 1976

Noyes FR, Grood ES, Nussbaum NS, Cooper SM: Effects of intro-articular corticosteroids on ligament properties. Clin Orthop 123:197– 209, 1977

Noyes FR, Torvik DJ, Hyde WB, Delucas JL: Biomechanics of ligament failure: An analysis of immobilization, exercise and reconditioning effects in primates. J Bone Joint Surg 56 A(7):1406– 1418, 1974

Olson MA, Stravino VD: A review of cryotherapy. Phys Ther 52:8, 1972

Radin EL, Paul IL: A comparison of the dynamic force transmitting properties of subchondral bone and articular cartilage. J Bone Joint Surg 52 A(3):444– 456, 1970

Stolov WC: Evaluation of the patient. In Krusen FH, Kottke FJ, Ellwood PM (eds): Handbook of Physical Medicine and Rehabilitation. Philadelphia, W B Saunders, 1971

Warren CG, Lehmann JF, Koflanski JN: Heat and stretch procedures: An evaluation using rat tail tendons. Arch Phys Med Rehabil 57:122– 126, 1976

6 The Use of Heat and Cold in the Treatment of Common Musculoskeletal Disorders

C. Gerald Warren

Heat and cold can be valuable adjuncts to the treatment of musculoskeletal disorders when applied with a defined rationale, with proper technique, and with an understanding of the expected outcome. This chapter discusses

Physiological principles for using heat to treat musculoskeletal disorders
Heat and stretch techniques
Application of heating modalities
Ultrasound as a modality of choice for treating musculoskeletal disorders
Physiological principles and techniques for using cold in the treatment of musculoskeletal disorders

Heat is used primarily to promote healing, to change the physical properties of tissue, and in some cases to reduce pain. Cold is most commonly used to reduce swelling, spasm, and spasticity, as well as pain. These modalities can be used effectively in combination with other techniques to produce various desired effects in the treatment of musculoskeletal disorders. [23]

PHYSIOLOGICAL PRINCIPLES IN THE USE OF HEAT

The response of the body to applications of heat is governed primarily by the temperature achieved in the tissues and the duration of temperature elevation. Mild heating that does not exceed 40°C usually produces only mild responses. These responses are usually considered therapeutic, since they produce relaxing or soothing effects and initiate moderate increases in blood flow. These observed responses to superficial application of mild heat fall into the counterirritant classification of treatment. In this treatment reflex activity can result in overall relaxation and quieting of the muscle tone.

Localized vigorous heating has a major effect on blood flow, producing substantial increases in vasodilation. A localized increase in temperature increases metabolic rate, capillary pressure and flow, clearance of metabolites, and oxygenation of tissue. These are the basic physiological responses that can occur as a result of local inflammation caused by the body's efforts to initiate healing. Because the body responds naturally to acute inflammation and to trauma, vigorous local heating is only appropriate when such natural responses have subsided. When augmentation of these responses is desired to promote healing in a subacute or chronic state, heat is indicated.

Since collagenous tissue is a major factor in joint contracture, a method for elongating or stretching this tissue is an important part of a program to increase range of motion. Elevating the temperature of collagenous tissue has been shown to increase its extensibility; when com-

115

bined with stretching procedures, it can produce a permanent elongation. Experiments to determine the response of collagenous tissue to various heat and stretch regimens were conducted using rat tail tendon as a model. [19,41,42] Figure 6-1 shows the effect of heating a sample of rat tail tendon being held under tension. [19] The tension in the heated tendon decreased substantially during the treatment. The effect of combining heat and stretch to produce a length increase is shown in Figure 6-2.[19] The combined application was found to be more effective in producing a permanent increase in the length of the tissue than either heat or stretch alone.

Further research defined some considerations for the optimal method for combining heat and stretch. Because it is viscoelastic, collagenous tissue can be permanently elongated by several methods of force application. If a constant load is applied to the tissue, using a force great enough to overcome tissue elasticity, the tissue will slowly increase in length. This is refered to as "creep." The rate of increase in length is controlled by the magnitude of the force applied. In a second method, the tissue can be stretched rapidly to a given length and held at that length. The tension or stress in the tissue will tend to decay as viscous flow in the

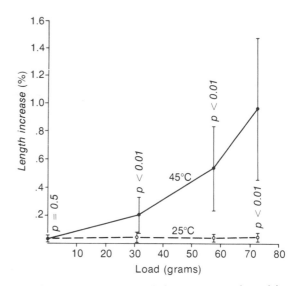

Fig. 6-2. Residual length increase produced in collagenous tissue after loading at indicated levels at 25°C and 45°C

tissue releases tension. A third method is to produce a constant rate of elongation by using a slow, steady force.

The effectiveness of treatment methods combining heat and load was evaluated by measuring the permanent length increase produced in the rat tail tendons as well as the damage caused to the treated tissue. Length change was determined by measuring the length of the tendon under a given load before and after the treatment procedure. Damage to the tissue produced by the treatment was evaluated by comparing the maximum load and elongation the tendon could sustain when stretched to rupture after treatment with the maximum load and elongation of untreated tissue.

The data in Figure 6-3 [41] illustrate a comparison of tendon samples that were elongated to the same length at two load levels and at four temperatures. The group categorized as "full load" had force applied at a relatively high level exceeding the working range of the tendon, defined as one quarter of its maximum load of rupture. [39] The other group, categorized

Fig. 6-1. Effect of temperature elevation on extensibility of collagenous tissue, using rat tail tendon as the tissue model

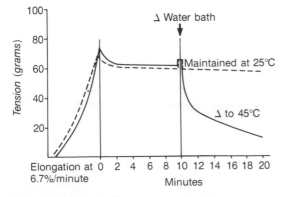
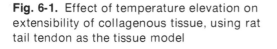

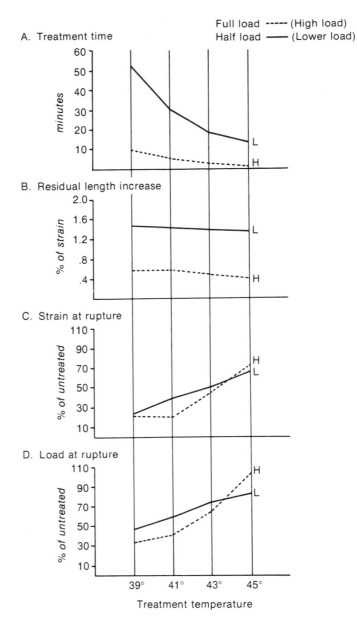

Fig. 6-3. Effect of load level and temperature on elongation of collagenous tissue: (A) represents time to achieve an elongation of 2.64%; (B) represents length increase produced by treatment procedures; (C) strain at rupture and (D) load at rupture are expressed as percent of untreated tissue length and load.

as "half load," had force applied that was in the middle of the working-range of the tendon. At this load level, the longer duration of treatment took greater advantage of the viscous properties of the heated tendon. Half load produced the greatest residual elongation as well as the least damage to the tissue. The effect of temperature is demonstrated by the increase in

the rate of elongation at higher temperatures and a reduction in the damage sustained by the tissue.

The sequence of applying heat and load was evaluated by comparing the results of loading before the temperature was elevated with the results of loading after the temperature was elevated. Both treatments produced similar elongations of the

Table 6-1. Comparison of Heating Before and After Loading at 45°C and 39°C with 10 Samples in Each Treatment Group

	RESIDUAL LENGTH INCREASE % GAUGE LENGTH		LOAD AT RUPTURE (% OF UNTREATED)		ELONGATION AT RUPTURE (% OF UNTREATED)	
Temperature During Treatment	45°C $\bar{x}$ S.D.	39°C $\bar{x}$ S.D.	45°C $\bar{x}$ S.D.	39°C $\bar{x}$ S.D.	45°C $\bar{x}$ S.D.	39°C $\bar{x}$ S.D.
Loaded Before Heating	0.43 ± 0.13	0.54 ± 0.21	74 ± 18	31 ± 11	59 ± 18	22 ± 5
Loaded After Heating	0.56 ± 0.11	0.61 ± 0.28	113 ± 31	67 ± 23	97 ± 20	50 ± 29
p-Value (Vertical Comparison)	$p = 0.113$	$p = 0.282$	$p = 0.001$	$p = 0.001$	$p = 0.001$	$p = 0.010$

tissue, but there was significantly less damage to the tissue when the temperature was elevated before stretch was applied. The data in Table 6-1 show the results of this comparison at 45°C and at 39°C.

Another factor considered was whether stretch should be maintained after treatment while the tissue cooled. Table 6-2 shows that a greater residual elongation was produced when stretch was maintained during the cooling process, as compared with tissue in which the load was removed prior to cooling.

When all these factors are taken into account (*i.e.,* using the highest therapeutic temperature, applying low loads, heating the tissue prior to applying the load, and cooling the tissue in the extended state), it was possible to produce changes in tissue length of up to 2% of the original length. Since in Figure 6-4 the curve for the treated tissue parallels that for untreated tissue and shows a similar failure strength within the working load range of the tissue, the elongation apparently is achieved without any significant tissue damage.

Further study was performed to establish whether these changes could be considered permanent. Figure 6-5 shows how the residual increase in length achieved in two samples changed after treatment. The tissue treated at 45°C had a greater increase in residual length; however, in both cases, with no load on the tissue over a 3-hour period, each lost little of the elongation produced by the treatment. Extrapolating to 24 hours would indicate

Table 6-2. Percent Length Increase Comparing Cooling of Tendons Under Loaded and Unloaded Conditions

PERCENT LENGTH INCREASE		
Load Maintained	No Load	
Mean & Standard Deviation 0.71% ± 0.20	Mean & Standard Deviation 0.48% ± 0.26	p-Value 0.0104

(Warren CG, Lehmann JF, Koblanski JN: Heat and stretch procedures: An evaluation using rat tail tendon. Arch Phys Med Rehabil 57:122–126, 1976)

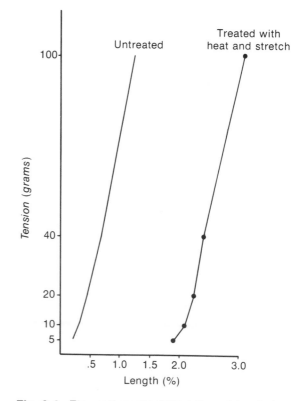

Fig. 6-4. Elongation characteristics of treated and untreated collagenous tissue

Fig. 6-5. Residual length increase achieved in collagenous tissue after low load stretch at 45°C and at 39°C

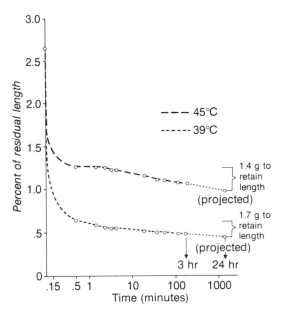

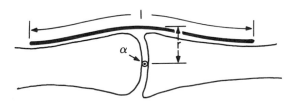

If: l = 10 cm

r = 2 cm

$\Delta l_1 = 0.1$ cm (1%)

$\Delta l_2 = 0.2$ cm (2%)

$\Delta \text{R.O.M.} = \alpha = \text{Arc Tan } \dfrac{\Delta l}{r}$

$\alpha_1 = \text{Arc Tan } \dfrac{.1}{2} = 2.9°$

$\alpha_2 = \text{Arc Tan } \dfrac{.2}{2} = 5.7°$

Fig. 6-6. Schematic representation of a joint, in which range of motion is limited by contracted tendon of length *l*. Calculations show angular increase in range of motion produced by 1% and 2% increases in tendon length.

that multiple treatment might be cumulative.

The clinical significance of the 1% to 2% increases is schematically represented in Figure 6-6. If the soft tissue crossing the joint has a length of 10 cm, and the joint has a radius of 2 cm, an increase in length of 1% or 1 mm will produce an increase of motion of 2.9° If the tissue length increase is 2%, the increase in range of motion is 5.7°.

THE APPLICATION OF THERAPEUTIC HEAT

The studies performed show that it is possible to produce a permanent length increase in collagenous tissue by combining heat and stretch. In clinical applications it is important first to determine the cause of the limitation in joint range of motion. When motion is limited by collagenous tissue crossing the joint, the combined application of heat and stretch may be a very useful modality if the following considerations are observed:

Stretch should be combined with the highest tolerable therapeutic temperature that can be achieved in the area to be treated.

The application of stretch should be of long duration.

Moderate forces should be used to take advantage of the viscous nature of the tissue.

The tissue temperature should be elevated prior to applying stretch to reduce the amount of tissue damage.

The tissue elongation achieved during the treatment should be maintained while the tissue is allowed to cool. This takes approximately 8 to 10 min.

The application of superficial heating modalities is governed primarily by the temperature tolerance of the tissues. The purpose for using various forms of energy to produce localized vigorous heating is to raise the tissue temperature to therapeutic levels and maintain those levels for significant periods of time. It is important when applying energy to the human body to consider that this energy is dissipated in the body in many ways, including convection by blood, conduction to adjacent tissues, and radiation from the body surface. If treatment is to be vigorous, it is important to maintain therapeutic temperatures in the tissue. This will force the body to maintain an increased blood flow to the treated area and will allow maximum tissue extensibility.

The technique of application must take into account the rate at which energy is to be applied to the tissue. The rate of application can be controlled either by varying the rate of energy input or by varying the volume of tissue to which energy is being applied. Figure 6-7 shows schematically the results of applying energy to tissue at various rates. If the rate of energy input to a fixed volume is too high, the temperature in the tissue will rise very rapidly, soon exceeding pain tolerance. This usually causes treatment to be discontinued before significant therapeutic effects are produced. If the energy input rate is too low, however, energy is dissipated more quickly than it is absorbed, and therapeutic temperatures are never achieved. Optimally, the rate should be such that the tissue reaches a maximum temperature just at or below pain tolerance and remains within the therapeutic range for the desired duration.

Infrared, electromagnetic radiation, and ultrasound are three sources of energy used for therapeutic heating. The choice of energy source depends on the treatment objective, since each of the three sources produces a different heating pattern in tissue. For example, in areas where there is very little soft-tissue cover, such as in the small joints of the hand or foot, infrared sources such as lamps, hot packs, paraffin, and immersion baths may adequately elevate tissue temperatures. When the treatment objective is to heat muscle tissue, the most effective modality currently avail-

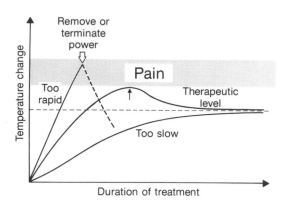

Fig. 6-7. Effect of rate of energy application on the production of therapeutic temperature levels in tissue

able is shortwave diathermy using induction applicators operating at 27 MHz. This modality provides vigorous heating of the superficial musculature, elevating temperatures 2 to 3 cm deep into the therapeutic range. [16] When applying diathermy with induction coils, adequate cooling from the surface of the tissue must be provided to avoid excessive heating of the skin surface. The combination of heating superficial tissues and heating of the applicator head itself tends to cause the peak temperature to occur near or at the surface, rather than deep in the muscle. Radiation from the surface and convection between the tissue and the applicator surface will reduce this problem if there is adequate air space between the applicator and the tissue. If the surface temperature is kept relatively cool, the traditional practice of using terry-cloth toweling is not needed, since the patient will not perspire. The air-spacing method has been shown experimentally to produce the highest temperatures deep in the tissue.

Microwave applicators operating at 2450 MHz have been shown to heat superficially and are not currently considered to be the modality of choice for deep heating. [10] Experimental applicators operating at 915 MHz that use built-in cooling of contact surfaces produce the most uniform muscle-heating.[6] Further development of these new microwave diathermy applicators will not proceed until federal standards and regulations on safety and effectiveness of microwave modalities are finalized.[21]

ULTRASOUND

Ultrasound is selectively absorbed by bone. Therefore, if the treatment objective is to perform vigorous heating, bone should be a focal point in the treatment field.[18,22] Because this technique produces the peak temperature in the bone, sensation of temperature can be used as a dosimetry for vigorous heating.

Ultrasound is somewhat attenuated in the soft tissue; therefore, the thickness of soft-tissue covering must be compensated for, usually by varying the intensity of the energy input.[17] The technique of application most commonly used at present relies on the threshold of pain or sensation in the periosteum as a guideline to maximizing the temperatures at the interface of soft tissue and bone. Either by adjusting the size of the field or by adjusting the intensity, the rate of energy input to a volume of tissue can be controlled to establish the pain or sensation thresholds. If the field size is to be held constant, the intensity can be increased until the patient senses pressure or mild pain in the periosteum, indicating maximum temperature. At that point, the intensity can be reduced to 15% to 20% in order to maintain the tissue temperature within the therapeutic range. Another way to achieve the same effect is to hold the intensity constant and increase the field size to decrease the volume of tissue being exposed. This serves to concentrate the energy in a smaller volume of tissue and elevates local temperatures.

Early experiments in evaluating ultrasound as a heating modality used various baths, if the ultrasound treatment was given in a mineral-oil bath at 24°C, the highest temperature in the distribution was produced on the surface of the tissue.[15] This finding suggested that perhaps ultrasound should be applied prior to superficial heating to prevent the highest temperature from occuring in superficial tissues. Further studying of this question evaluated the effect of applying hot packs prior to ultrasound.[20] Hot packs were applied for 8 min until the temperature had stabilized on the surface. They were then removed and ultrasound was applied, during which time the temperature distribution in the deep tissue was measured. It was found that superficial temperatures dropped rapidly. The decrease may have been enhanced by the surface application of the room-temperature ultrasound head. The study concluded that applying hot packs before ultrasound had no effect on temperature distribution in deep tissues as long as the source of heat was removed, and the surface tissue was allowed to cool prior to or during the ultrasound application. Therefore, the traditional regime of hot packs followed by ultrasound was shown to be acceptable.

Coupling Media

Those who use ultrasound often ask about the relative effectiveness of various coupling media. The purposes of coupling media are to eliminate air between the transducer and the tissue, to effectively transmit ultrasound into the tissues, and to serve as a lubricant in contact applications. Warren and co-workers conducted a study to determine the effectiveness of various coupling media in a situation that closely simulated their use in contact applications in which very thin layers of coupling media are used.[40] To prevent near-field effects from biasing the results, they measured the power transmitted through the medium in the far field of a tank of distilled degassed water. Common coupling media of mineral oils, gels, and creams were measured and were compared to distilled degassed water. Some variation in the transmissivity of the various media was recorded. However, variations of approximately three tenths of a pound in transducer force on the simulated tissue were found to cause a variance in transmissivity that far exceeded the differences between the various coupling media.

Various ointments and creams used in phonophoresis were evaluated. Pharmaceutically prepared hydrocortisone ointment and two of the commercially prepared ointments commonly used were compared. Their percentage of transmissivity ranged between 25% and 60%, which was attributed to their method of manufacture. Because hydrocortisone is soluble only in alcohol, it must be prepared as an emulsion; this requires that the solution of hydrocortisone be blended or beaten into the ointment or cream. This process may incorporate microscopic amounts of air into the medium. Measuring the transmissivity of the base of the ointment, and then beating it in a blender for several minutes confirmed this theory. Measurement of the blended base showed a similar reduction in transmissivity.

When using water-soluble coupling media, the skin must be cleansed of oil to assure that the medium can adequately wet the skin surface and not allow air to be entrapped in follicles or between the water-based media and skin oils. Cleansing the skin prior to treatment is less important when oil-based media are used. A similar situation exists when using a water-immersion technique. As when using water-based gels, the skin should be cleansed of oils, and air bubbles must be brushed from the surface of the skin and the transducer surface to assure maximum transmission of energy.

In summary, when coupling media are used in thin films, the energy absorption in the media is insignificant. However, air trapped microscopically in a medium reduces its capability to transmit ultrasound. Small pressure variations on the transducer cause variations in transmissivity. The variations are greater than the differences measured between any of the common coupling media. This variation in pressure is extremely difficult for the therapist to prevent during clinical application. Therefore, the therapist should choose a coupling medium for its economy and convenience, rather than according to claims of ultrasound transmissivity.

Contraindications

Contraindications to the use of ultrasound are those common to all vigorous heating. It especially should not be used over an acute inflammatory site or in areas where sensation of temperature and pain are limited. Recently, developments in prosthetic joint implants have introduced to the body several compounds, namely polymethyl methacrylate and high-density polyethylene, that selectively absorb ultrasonic energy. A recent study of the properties of these materials indicates that selective absorption of ultrasound in polymethyl methacrylate is equivalent to that of bone, and therefore peak temperatures could occur in the polymethyl methacrylate. This could potentially cause destruction of adjacent tissue, since the material lacks the safeguard of temperature or pain sensation.[24]

THE USE OF COLD IN MUSCULOSKELETAL DISORDERS

Cold applications are very important in treating musculoskeletal disorders. They are usually applied to minimize the swelling or edema in the acute phase of injury; to reduce the pain associated with injury or with neuromuscular involvement; and to increase neuromuscular function, to reduce spasms and spasticity, and to enhance muscle contraction.

The ability to achieve these clinical objectives depends on several interactive physiological responses to cold application. Where localized cooling is used, the anticipated physiological responses are initial vasoconstriction, reduction of tissue metabolism, decrease in nerve conduction velocity, reduced response of muscle afferents, secondary vasodilation, and an increase in muscle strength after treatment. Cold applications that do not depress localized tissue temperatures can produce remote effects such as a generalized vasodilation and a reduction in the overall sensation of pain. Recent reviews on the use of cryotherapy point out the need for understanding clearly the rationale prior to the use of cold therapy. [28,34]

ACUTE TRAUMA

The use of cold therapy in acute trauma is probably one of the most common and effective uses of this modality. In treating trauma, the mnemonic ICE (Ice, Compression, Elevation) is an excellent guide to acute injury management.[4] The same reasons for using cold therapy in acute trauma may be applied in treating the acute phases of inflammatory conditions. The primary mechanism of vasoconstriction decreases blood flow, decreases the inflammatory response, and blocks the release of histamine responsible for vasodilation and exudate formation, thereby reducing localized edema and further hemorrhage.[5,12] Cold-treatment regimes for ankle sprains have been shown to produce accelerated recovery when used over prolonged periods. Cooling has also been shown useful in treating ankle sprains of recent origin, especially when the ligaments are only stretched or are partially torn.[2,37]

When cold applications are used, they should be integrated into a complete treatment program that combines acute care with posttreatment care. It is also important that the level of temperature depression in the tissues be controlled. In cases of complete rupture or fracture when there may be extensive and severe trauma, the use of cold may have only limited effects, and it should be used prudently with appropriate posttreatment care. This may include compression, elevation, or both to avoid secondary, cold-induced swelling.[30] Vasodilation and increased profusion as a result of cooling should be avoided, because when tissue temperatures approach 15°C, vasodilation can occur as a survival response; the tissue attempts to increase in temperature to avoid necrosis.[25] Therefore, in the use of cold in acute or inflammatory conditions, care must be taken to avoid excessive cooling, which will induce vasodilation and swelling, thus counteracting the desired effects. Posttreatment management of the injury site by compression and elevation is necessary to maintain the desired effects of the cold application.

PHYSIOLOGICAL EFFECTS OF COLD TREATMENT

The effects of cold in the treatment of pain can be divided into the effects produced by localized cooling and those produced by remote cooling. Specific localized effects include reduced nerve conduction velocities in both motor and sensory nerves produced by a depression in the temperature of the nerve.[14] This effect can be considered to influence the transmission of pain sensation; however, it has not been clearly documented that reduced nerve conduction velocities directly affect the perception of pain. Conduction in the tissue can be eliminated by depressing tissue temperatures to 10°C or 15°C.[8]

The use of cold in treating muscle spasms is probably one of the most effective yet least understood applications of cold. The classic model for muscle spasms is so closely related to pain and the splinting phenomenon that the two cannot be easily separated when discussing the effects of cold application.

Vigorous localized cooling, as previously discussed, depresses nerve conduction velocity, possibly producing an analgesic effect by reducing the excitability of muscle afferents.[7,26] The classic model of spasm is that of localized pain, caused by pathology or trauma, inducing muscle spasms that are intended to immobilize and thus protect the injured area. Muscle spasm is usually an involuntary sustained contraction that utilizes a large amount of nutrient substances and simultaneously creates ischemic areas because of compression of intramuscular blood vessels. The muscle ischemia produces further tissue damage, which in turn causes additional pain that produces more muscle spasms. Eliminating either the pain or the spasm usually improves the physical condition of the patient. It has been theorized that simultaneous application of both deep and superficial cooling bombards the central pain receptor areas with such a barrage of cold impulses that the pain impulses and the pain are obliterated.[23,33,38]

This type of application falls into the category of noxious stimulus. Cold has also been shown to be specifically effective in reducing spasticity through a reduction in the excitability of muscle afferents. This, however, has not been shown to have long-term effects on spastic conditions. Wolf and co-workers have shown that the motor outflow can be altered in muscle tissue underlying the specific thermal stimulus.[45] They showed that during the application of cold, single motor unit activity tended to decrease during the first minute of cold application, and its activity was significantly reduced during continued application. It has also been demonstrated that the level of excitation of the central nervous system plays a significant role in determining how the cutaneous cooling information is processed to affect motor changes.[32,44,45] The effect of cold on spasticity has also been attributed to a reflex sympathetic influence on the muscle spindle, which decreases spasticity. The analgesic effects have been attributed to the ability of cold to depress the excitability of free nerve endings and peripheral nerve fibers, thereby increasing the pain threshold.[11]

Cold has also been used as a stimulus to increase muscle function. Several studies have documented the influence of cold on increased activity after application.[13,35] The application of superficial cooling substantially modifies activities within muscles. The mechanisms are not fully understood; however, cold is recognized as a valuable adjunct in interfering with pathophysiological functions such as swelling, spasm, and spasticity.

THE APPLICATION OF COLD THERAPY

In order to apply cold effectively, the thermodynamics of the procedure must be considered. A heat absorber must be placed in physical contact with the tissue to conduct heat from the body. This conduction of heat from body tissues over a period of time causes the local cooling effect. It is therefore important to understand the relationship of the heat capacity of the body to that of the cooling medium. Because the body is as a large heat source with the capacity to compensate for heat loss by modifying patterns of blood circulation, the cooling medium must have a substantial heat capacity if vigorous cooling is desired. Otherwise, the cooling effect of the medium will soon be overwhelmed or compensated for by the heat generated by the body. When a cooling medium of sufficient heat capacity is used, time must be allowed for heat to be conducted from the body, especially if vigorous cooling of deep tissues is desired.

Temperature depression is highly dependent on the thickness of overlying soft-tissue layers, especially fat layers. The insulating property of fat significantly modifies the ability to depress muscle temperatures. Both Lowden and Wolf showed the effectiveness of this fat layer, indicating an order of magnitude of difference in the rate of cooling where excessive fat layers were present.[27,43]

Bierman measured deep temperature in the human calf muscle with a continuous application of ice bags.[3] He showed that a reduction in deep-tissue temperatures occurred only after prolonged periods, on the order of 60 min of continuous application. McMaster evaluated the following cooling sources: an ice pack consisting of ice chips in a plastic bag; a "snap-pack" endothermic chemical reaction cooling pack; an inflatable plastic envelope through which the gaseous refrigerant Freon was pumped; and a frozen, flexible gel pack.[29] The ice pack produced the greatest change in temperature, achieving as much as an 11°C depression in temperature in the tissue within 60 min. The next most efficient was the gel pack, which produced an 8°C depression in tissue temperatures within 60 min. The chemical snap pack produced only a 3°C reduction in tissue temperature, followed by the refrigerant pack, which produced a 1.7°C reduction. These temperatures were measured in adult mongrel dogs and in human quadriceps, adjacent to the femur; however, no specific depth in the tissue was reported.

Ice massage has been considered, in most literature, to be a superficial cooling technique. However, Lowdon measured temperature depressions of up to 17°C in short applications of ice massage across the biceps.[27] These findings are not consistent with other reported studies and do not quite fit the thermodynamic model. The use of ice massage provides a considerable temperature decrease on the surface and is effective in producing local analgesia. It is also useful as a stimulus in the treatment of pain, similar to the use of ethyl chloride sprays in treating acute pain. Menell and Travell have developed techniques for establishing the location of "trigger points" in patterns of pain. They have attempted to eliminate pain and in-crease range of motion through the application of intermittent sprays of ethyl chloride just below the level of "frosting" the skin, combined with gentle stretch.[31,38]

Contraindications

Specific caution should be used when cold therapy is applied to ischemic and anesthetic tissues. Its use is specifically contraindicated in several collagenous diseases where rheumatoid conditions may increase the symptoms of pain and joint stiffness.[1] In Raynaud's phenomenon, the application of cold can result in excessive digital arterial spasms, and ischemic necrosis has been reported, resulting in subsequent amputation and extensive loss of tissue.[9] Cold allergies, which manifest themselves in giant hives and joint pain, have also been described.[36] In the case of athletic injuries, cold is often applied in situations where athletes may want to re-enter the playing scene. Caution should be exercised, since the anesthetic effect of cold may mask pain that provides the athlete with a protective mechanism.

REFERENCES

1. Backlund L, Tiselius P: Objective measurement of joint stiffness in rheumatoid arthritis. Scand J Rheumatol 13:275, 1967
2. Basur RL, Shephard E, Mouzas GL: A cooling method in the treatment of ankle sprains. Practitioner 215:708–711, 1976
3. Bierman W, Friedlander M: The penetrative effect of cold. Arch Phys Med Rehabil 21:585–592, 1940
4. Brown A: Physical medicine in rehabilitation. Md State Med J 19:61, 1970
5. Clark R, Hellon R, Lind A: Vascular reactions of the human forearm to cold. Clin Sci 17:165, 1958
6. DeLateur BJ, Lehmann JG, Stonebridge JB, Warren CG, Guy AW: Muscle heating in human subjects with 915 MHz microwave contact applicator. Arch Phys Med Rehabil 51:147–151, 1970

7. Eldred E, Lindsley DF, Buchwald JS: The effect of cooling on mammalian muscle spindle. Exp Neurol 2:144– 157, 1960

8. Fox RH: Local cooling in man. Br Med Bull 17:14– 18, 1961

9. Goldberg EA, Pittman DR: Cold sensitivity syndrome. Ann Intern Med 50:505, 1959

10. Guy AW, Lehmann JF, Stonebridge JB: Therapeutic applications of electromagnetic power. Proc IEEE 62:55–75, 1974

11. Haines J: A survey of recent developments in cold therapy. Physiotherapy 53:222– 229, 1967

12. Janssen CW Jr, Waaler E: Body temperature, antibody formation and inflammatory response. Acta Pathol Microbiol Scand 69:555– 566, 1967

13. Johnson DJ, Leider FE: Influence of cold bath on maximum handgrip strength. Percept Mot Skills 44:323– 326, 1977

14. Lee JM, Warren MP, Mason SM: Effects of ice on nerve conduction velocity. Physiotherapy 64:2– 6, 1978

15. Lehmann JF, DeLateur BJ, Silverman DR: Selective heating effects of ultrasound in humans. Arch Phys Med Rehabil 47:331– 339, 1966

16. Lehmann JF, DeLateur BJ, Stonebridge JB: Selective muscle heating by shortwave diathermy with a helical coil. Arch Phys Med Rehabil 50:117, 1969

17. Lehmann JF, DeLateur BJ, Stonebridge JB, Warren CG: Therapeutic temperature distribution produced by ultrasound as modified by dosage and volume of tissues exposed. Arch Phys Med Rehabil 48:662– 666, 1967

18. Lehmann JF, DeLateur BJ, Warren CG, Stonebridge JB: Heating produced by ultrasound in bone and soft tissue. Arch Phys Med Rehabil 48:397– 401, 1967

19. Lehmann JF, Masock AJ, Warren CG, Koblanski JN: Effect of therapeutic temperatures on tendon extensibility. Arch Phys Med Rehabil 51:481– 487, 1970

20. Lehmann JF, Stonebridge JB, DeLateur BJ, Warren CG, Halar E: Temperatures in human thighs after hot pack treatment followed by ultrasound. Arch Phys Med Rehabil 59:472– 475, 1978

21. Lehmann JF, Stonebridge JB, Wallace JE, Warren CG, Guy AW: Microwave therapy: Stray radiation, safety and effectiveness. Arch Phys Med Rehabil 60:578– 584, 1979

22. Lehmann JF, Warren CG, Guy AW: Therapy with continuous wave ultrasound. In Fry (ed): Ultrasound: Its Applications in Medicine and Biology, Part II, Vol 3, Methods and Phenomena: Their Applications in Science and Technology, pp 561– 587. Amsterdam, Elsevier Scientific Publishing Co, 1978

23. Lehmann JF, Warren CG, Scham SM: Therapeutic heat and cold. Clin Orthop 99:207– 245, 1974

24. Lehmann JF, Warren CG, Wallace JE, Chan A: Considerations for the use of ultrasound in the presence of prosthetic joints (Abstr). Arch Phys Med Rehabil 60:531, 1979

25. Lewis T: Observations on some normal and injurious effects of cold on the skin and underlying tissues. Br Med J 2:795– 797, 1941

26. Lightfoot E, Verrier M, Ashby P: Neurophysiological effects of prolonged cooling of the calf in patients with complete spinal transections. Phys Ther 55:251– 258, 1975

27. Lowdon BJ, Moore RJ: Determinants and nature of intramuscular temperature changes during cold therapy. Am J Phys Med 54:223– 233, 1975

28. McMaster WC: Literary review on ice therapy in injury. Am J Sports Med 5:124– 126, 1977

29. McMaster WC, Liddle S, Waugh TR: Laboratory evaluation of various cold therapy modalities. Am J Sports Med 6:291– 294, 1978

30. Matsen FA, Questad K, Matsen AL: The effect of local cooling on post-fracture swelling. Clin Orthop 109:201– 206, 1975

31. Mennell JM: The therapeutic use of cold. J Am Osteopath Assoc 74:1146– 1158, 1975

32. Miglietta O: Action of cold on spasticity. Am J Phys Med 52:198– 205, 1973

33. Nielsen AJ: Spray and stretch for myofascial pain. Phys Ther 58:567– 569, 1978

34. Olson JE, Stravino VD: A review of cryotherapy. Phys Ther 52:840– 853, 1972

35. Ricker K, Hertel G, Stodieck S: The influence of local cooling on neuromuscular transmission in the myasthenic syndrome of Eaton and Lambert. J Neurol 217:95– 102, 1977

36. Shelley WB, Caro WA: Cold erythema, a new hypersensitivity syndrome. JAMA, 180:639–642, 1962

37. Starkey JA: Treatment of ankle sprains by simultaneous use of intermittent compression and ice packs. Am J Sports Med 4:142–144, 1976

38. Travell J: Ethyl chloride spray for painful muscle spasm. Arch Phys Med Rehabil 33:291–298, 1952

39. Walker LB Jr, Harris EH, Benedict JV: Stress-strain relationship in human cadaveric plantaris tendon: Preliminary study. Medical Electronics and Biological Engineering 2:31–38, 1964

40. Warren CG, Koblanski JN, Sigelmann RH: Ultrasound coupling media: Their relative transmissivity. Arch Phys Med Rehabil 57:218–222, 1976

41. Warren CG, Lehmann JF, Koblanski JN: Elongation of rat tail tendon: Effect of load and temperature. Arch Phys Med Rehabil 52:465–474, 484, 1971

42. Warren CG, Lehmann JF, Koblanski JN: Heat and stretch procedures: An evaluation using rat tail tendon. Arch Phys Med Rehabil 57:122–126, 1976

43. Wolf SL, Basmajian JV: Intramuscular temperature changes deep to localized cutaneous cold stimulation. Phys Ther 53:1284–1288, 1973

44. Wolf SL, Letbetter WD: Effect of skin cooling on spontaneous EMG activity in triceps surae of the decerebrate cat. Brain Res 91:151–155, 1975

45. Wolf SL, Letbetter WD, Basmajian JV: Effects of specific cutaneous cold stimulus on single motor unit activity of medial gastrocnemius muscle in man. Am J Phys Med 55:177–183, 1976

The author wishes to thank John Imre for his assistance in preparing this chapter.

7 Joint Mobilization Techniques

Randolph M. Kessler and Darlene Hertling

HISTORY

Although specific mobilization techniques are just being introduced in physical therapy curricula in this country, their use in the management of patients with musculoskeletal disorders is certainly not new. It seems somewhat odd that physical therapists have been so slow in adopting joint mobilization techniques. After all, therapists have been delegated the duty of passive movement for years, and joint mobilization simply a form of passive movement. Some time in the past this important method of treatment was lost from medical practice and is just beginning to emerge again. The explanation for its disappearance probably lies in the fact that early users of mobilization techniques based their value on purely empirical evidence of their effectiveness; there was no scientific basis for their use. Later, specific joint mobilization was practiced only by more esoteric "professions" that claimed beneficial effects on all disease processes, usually from manipulations of the spine. This tended to further alienate orthodox medical practitioners, with the result that the use of any and all forms of joint mobilization, other than movement in the cardinal planes, became somewhat taboo. Our approach to the management of many joint conditions is still largely influenced by the teachings of the early orthopaedic surgeons, who advocated strict rest in the management of all joint conditions. While scientific proof of the effectiveness of specific joint mobilization is still largely lacking, our expanded knowledge of joint kinematics at least provides a scientific *basis* for its use. It is becoming evident that in order to deal with mechanical joint dysfunctions effectively and safely, a knowledge of joint kinematics as well as skill in the use of joint examination and mobilization techniques is required.

EARLY PRACTITIONERS

The use of specific mobilization techniques did not arise with the emergence of osteopathy and chiropractic. Some of the earliest recorded accounts of the use of joint manipulation and spinal traction are from Hippocrates, a physician in the fourth century B.C. In fact, Hippocrates proposed refinements in some of the techniques used in his time. For example, one traction technique required that the patient be tied to a ladder and dropped 30 feet, upside down, to the ground. Hippocrates suggested that ropes be tied to the ladder so that two people could shake it up and down, thus affecting an "intermittent" traction. Hippocrates also developed many of the methods of reducing dislocations that are still in use today. Accounts of the use of manipulation by Cato, Galen, and other physicians during the time of the Roman Empire also exist.[1]

Little is known of the practice of joint manipulation during the disintegration of the Roman Empire and the beginning of the Middle Ages. During this time most hospitals were attached to monasteries, and treatment was carried out by members of the religious orders. Friar Moulton, of the order of St. Augustine, wrote *The Complete Bonesetter*. The text, which was revised by John Turner in 1656, suggests that manipulation was practiced in medical settings throughout the Middle Ages and early Renaissance. With the reign of Henry VIII in England and the subsequent dissolution of the monasteries, medicine lost its previous "mystic" influences and became the practice of "art and science." The English orthopaedic surgeons of the late 1700s and early 1800s, such as John Hunter and John Hilton, advocated strict rest in the early management of joint trauma.[5] This view was emphasized by Hugh Owen Thomas in the late 1800s. For two centuries this influence prevailed, and joint manipulation remained in the hands of "bonesetters." Bonesetting was practiced by lay people, and the art was passed down over the centuries within bonesetting families. The bonesetters had no basis for the use of their manipulations other than past experience. The successful bonesetters were those who remembered details of cases in which ill-effects had resulted and avoided making the same mistakes over again. Bonesetters tended to guard their techniques, keeping them secret among family members. A few bonesetters, because of their success, became quite famous. One such bonesetter, a Mrs. Mapp, was called upon to treat nobility and royalty.

Bonesetters vs. Physicians

During this particular period there was extreme rivalry and animosity between physicians and bonesetters. Physicians were well aware of disastrous effects that bonesetting had at times on tuberculous joints or other serious pathologies. It is interesting that Thomas, who was particularly outspoken against bonesetters, was the son and grandson of bonesetters. Thomas, who gave his name to the *Thomas splint*, was the originator of many of the orthopaedic principles concerning immobilization of fractures and joint injuries still adhered to today. It goes without saying that medical opinion of joint manipulation has changed very little since his time.

Despite medical opinion, Sir James Paget, a famous surgeon and contemporary of Thomas in England, recognized the value of judiciously applied bonesetting techniques. His lecture entitled "Cases that Bonesetters Cure," which appeared in the *British Medical Journal* in 1867, spoke of the rivalry between bonesetters and physicians. He described types of lesions for which manipulation may be of value and advised that physicians "imitate what is good and avoid what is bad in the practice of bone-setters." Unfortunately, the medical profession at the time, and for years to come, ignored this advice.

The first medical book on manipulation since Friar Moulton's work was published in the 1870s. It was written by Dr. Wharton Hood whose father, Dr. Peter Hood, treated a bonesetter, a Mr. Hutton, for a serious illness. Dr. Hood did not charge Hutton since he was aware of Hutton's free services to many poor people. In repayment, however, Hutton offered to teach Hood all he knew of bonesetting. The elder Hood was too busy to accept the offer, but his son, Wharton did. In his paper on the subject, published in *Lancet* in 1871, Hood describes Hutton's techniques of spinal and peripheral manipulation.[6] He lists the conditions that Hutton was willing to treat as primarily postimmobilization stiffness, displaced cartilages and tendons, carpal and tarsal subluxations, and ganglionic swellings; he also states that Hutton avoided working on acutely inflamed joints. Hutton usually applied heat before manipulating, especially to the larger joints. Hood describes Hutton's manipulations as being very precise as to the direction and amplitude of motion. They were always of a high-velocity thrust. The illustrated descriptions of some of the common manipulations used by Hutton show them to be essentially identical to the manipulations used by manual therapists and even some orthopaedists and physiatrists today. Hutton admitted to knowing nothing of anatomy and felt that in all of his cases a bone was "out." Of his techniques he says that forced pushing and pulling are useless; "the twist is the thing."

OSTEOPATHY AND CHIROPRACTIC

Meanwhile in the United States, Dr. Andrew Taylor Still was practicing medicine in Kansas.[19] It happened that Still's children contracted meningitis and all three died. Still, being frustrated and angered by the failure of current medical practices to save his children, set out to find a solution. For a time he spent his days studying the anatomy of exhumed Indian remains, paying special attention to the relationships of bones, nerves, and arteries. In 1874, through a "divine relation," Still claimed he had discovered the cause of all bodily disease. His "law of the artery" claimed that all disease processes were a direct result of interference with blood flow through arteries that carried vital nutrients to a part. If normal blood flow to the part could be restored, then the body's natural substances would resolve the disease process. In 1892, Still founded the first school of osteopathy in Kirksville, Missouri, offering a 20-month course. By 1916 the osteopathic course was extended to 3 years, and by 1920 the United States Congress granted equal rights to osteopaths and M.D.s.[15] In the early 1900s, the osteopathic profession gradually became aware that some of Still's original proposals were incorrect. Over the years they incorporated traditional medical thought with the practice of joint manipulation. Especially during the last decade, osteopathic schools have de-emphasized the practice of manipulation, and have attained essentially the same standards as medical schools. Osteopaths now qualify for residency programs in all medical and surgical fields.

In 1895 a grocer named D. D. Palmer, who had been a patient of Still, founded the Palmer College of Chiropractics in Davenport, Iowa. No prior education was required, and one of the first graduates was Palmer's 12-year-old son, B.J. Chiropractic theory evolved around the "law of the nerve" which stated that "vital life forces" could be cut off from any body part by small vertebral subluxations placing pressure on nerves. Since this could cause disease in the part to which the nerve ran, most, if not all, disease could be prevented or cured by maintaining proper spinal alignment through manipulation. Chiropractic was a "drugless" remedy that often supplemented manipulative treatment with various herbs, vitamins, and so forth. The chiropractic profession was fraught with internal turmoil from the outset.[16] (B.J. apparently grew up hating his father, and later bought him out. When the father died, he stipulated that B.J. was not to attend his funeral.) Unlike osteopathy, most chiropractors adhered to their original concept, the law of the nerve, although the profession has always been divided into two or more schools of thought. They have received bitter opposition from the medical profession, which views them as charlatans and quacks. Today there remains some division in chiropractic philosophy. The "straights" continue to follow the "law of the nerve," claiming to treat most disease by manipulating the spine or other body parts. The "mixers" tend to accept the limitations of this practice and use local application of ultrasound, massage, exercises, and so on, to supplement their manipulative treatment. It is significant that due to a strong lobbying force and the realization by chiropractors that, in order to survive, professional standards and education must be upgraded, chiropractors are rapidly gaining acceptance by governing bodies, the public, and even some medical physicians. It will be interesting to see if the profession of physical therapy keeps abreast of this trend.

CURRENT SCHOOLS OF THOUGHT

In spite of efforts by Paget and Hood to emphasize the value of bonesetting techniques, manipulation was not readopted as a method of treatment by medical doctors until this century. The earliest physicians to practice manipulation were Englishmen. Books on the subject were published by A. G. Timbrell Fisher, an orthopaedic surgeon, in 1925, and by James Mennell in 1939. [5,11] Mennell was a doctor of physical medicine at St. Thomas' Hospital. Both he and Fisher often performed their manipulations with the patient anesthetized. In 1934 Mixter and Barr published an article in the *New England Journal of Medicine*, and T. Marlin published *Manipulative Treatment for Medical Practitioners*. [10,13,14] These works have had a powerful effect on medical thought, stimulating much interest and leading to a series of excellent publications since then. Later in the century books advocating manipulative treatment were published by Alan Stoddard and James Cyriax. [3,17] Cyriax was to succeed Mennell at St. Thomas'. Cyriax advocates manipulations performed without anesthesia. Most of allopathic medicine's knowledge of manipulations can be traced to Mennell and Cyriax; the former made contributions in the field of synovial joints, the latter in the area of the intervertebral disc. Cyriax's examination approach is considered superb and contains a wealth of medical logic.

Presently, a school of thought that has attracted some attention (especially in Europe) is being led by Robert Maigne, who has postulated the "concept of painless and opposite motion." [8] This concept states that a manipulative maneuver should be administered in the direction opposite to the movement that is restricted and causing pain. Maigne, like Cyriax, has worked hard to focus medical attention on manipulative therapy as an effective modality in the relief of pain.

The driving force behind a school of thought that has flourished in Scandinavia is F. M. Kaltenborn. [7] Under his leadership, a systematic postgraduate education program that requires passage of practical and written exams leads to certification in the specialty of manual therapy. The philosophy behind Kaltenborn's technique is a fusion of what he has considered the best in chiropractic, osteopathy, and physical medicine. He uses Cyriax's methods to evaluate the patient and employs mainly specific osteopathic techniques for treatment. Disc degeneration and facet joint pathologies are the two main spinal pathologies that the Scandinavians theorize are amenable to physical therapy.

Maitland, an Australian physical therapist whose approach is currently being taught in Australia, has a non-pathologic orientation to the treatment of all joints. [2,9] His techniques are fairly similar to the "articulatory" techniques used by osteopaths, involving oscillatory movements performed on a chosen joint. To increase movement of a restricted joint, movement is induced within the patient's available range of movement tolerance. He distinguishes between mobilizations and manipulations, but puts heavy emphasis on mobilization. A meticulous examination is essential to this method because examination provides the guideline to treatment.

A prominent figure in the United States has been Dr. John Mennell, the son of the late James Mennell, who came to practice in this country. His work on the spine and extremities has been described in several publications and is particularly well known in this country. He has made a significant contribution to a better understanding of joint pain and its treatment by placing stress on the function of small involuntary movements within a joint. He refers to these small movements as *joint play*; a disturbance of these movements is termed *joint dysfunction*. He states that full, painless, voluntary range of motion is not possible without restoration of all joint-play motions. [12]

In spite of their efforts, Mennell, Cyriax, Stoddard, and Maigne remain among the very few medical physicians to practice joint manipulation. As a result, manipulative treatment was not—and still is not—available to most patients seeking help from the medical profession. The original reasons for avoiding the practice of manipulation stemmed from the teachings of Hilton, Thomas, and Hunter, and the occasional disasters that occurred at the hands of bonesetters and other manipulators. Today many more medical physicians accept the value of judiciously applied manipulative treatment. However, the majority are kept more than busy with handling more serious pathologies, due to a shortage of physicians and the sophistication of medical practice. Since effective manipulative treatment requires considerable time for evaluative and therapeutic management, most physicians simply do not have the time to learn or practice manipulative technique.

THE ROLE OF THE PHYSICAL THERAPIST

Physical therapists are the logical practitioners to assume the responsibility for manipulative treatment. They work closely with physicians, who are capable of ruling out serious pathology. They tend to develop close and ongoing rapport with patients because the nature of their work requires close patient contact. They are taught to evaluate and treat by use of the hands. The advantages of the physician/physical therapists team in orthopaedic manual therapy are perhaps best described by Cyriax: "Between them they have every facility: informed selection of cases, a wide range of different types of treatment, alternative approaches when it is clear that manual methods cannot avail." [4]

The United States, which has lagged far behind other countries in the development of orthopaedic manual therapy, is gradually catching up. Thanks to the efforts of Mennell and Stanley Paris, a therapist originally from New Zealand, American therapists have at least had the opportunity to take postgraduate courses and to gain some competency in manual therapy and the management of orthopaedic patients. The formation of the Orthopaedic Section of the American Physical Therapy Association in 1974 and education will hopefully improve this situation. Undergraduate courses in the physical therapy schools, clinically oriented long-term courses, postgraduate apprenticeships, and orthopaedic specialization in master's degree programs are still needed.

INTRODUCTION TO JOINT MOBILIZATION TECHNIQUES

GENERAL RULES

The following rules and considerations should guide the therapist when performing joint mobilization techniques:

1. **The patient must be relaxed.**
   This requires that he be properly draped, and that the room be of comfortable temperature without distracting noises, and so on. Joints, other than the joint to be mobilized, must be at rest and well supported.
   The operator's handholds must be firm but comfortable. He must remove

watches, jewelry, and so forth, and be sure buttons and belt buckles are not in contact with the patient.

2. ***The operator must be relaxed.***
This requires good body mechanics — especially in regards to the spine. The operator should attempt to create a situation in which his body and the part to be treated "act as one." This requires close body contact between the operator and patient for optimal control and mobilization.

3. ***Do not move into or through the point of pain.***
One must be able to determine the difference between the discomfort of soft-tissue stretch, which is at times desirable, and the pain and muscle guarding that are a signal to ease up lest damage be done.
The advanced manual therapist at times will move into or through the point of pain, but only in highly selective circumstances. These techniques are not to be taught, nor are they expected to be learned in a basic-level course.

4. ***When performing any of the joint mobilization techniques, one hand will usually stabilize while the other hand performs the movement.***
At times the plinth, the patient's body weight, and so on, are used for external stabilization. This allows both hands to assist in the movement. The therapist uses his hand or a belt to fix or stabilize one joint partner against a firm support. The fixation is maintained close to the joint space without causing pain. The mobilizing hand grips the joint structure to be moved as close to the joint space as possible.

5. ***The operator must consider***
 —Direction of movement — almost always parallel to or perpendicular to a tangent across adjoining joint surfaces

 —Velocity of movements — slow stretching for large capsular restrictions; faster oscillations for minor restrictions
 —Amplitude of movement — graded according to pain, guarding and degree of restriction.

6. ***Compare accessory joint movement to opposite side (extremity), if necessary, to determine presence or degree of restriction.***

7. ***One movement is performed at a time, at one joint at a time.***

8. ***Each technique can be used as***
 —An examination procedure by taking up the slack, only, to determine the existing range of accessory movement and the presence or absence of pain.
 —A therapeutic technique in which a high-velocity, small-amplitude thrust or graded oscillations are applied to regain accessory joint movement and relieve pain.

9. ***Reassessment***
This should be done at the beginning of each treatment session, as well as during the treatment session. A selection of a few important "markers" for assessment enables a quick estimate of progress to be made without repeatedly going through the whole examination procedure.

INDICATIONS

That is, joint mobilization techniques are indicated in cases of joint dysfunction; restriction of accessory joint motion causing pain or restriction of motion during normal physiological movement. However, as discussed in Chapter 2, Arthrology, there may be numerous causes of loss of accesory joint movement. The most common of these include capsuloligamentous tightening or adherence; internal derangement, as from a cartilaginous loose body or meniscus displacement; reflex muscle guarding; and bony blockage, as from hypertrophic degenerative changes. From this it should be clear that the proper indication for using specific mobilization techniques is loss of accessory joint motion (joint-play movement) due to capsular or ligamentous tightness or adherence. Other causes of joint dysfunction are relative contraindications. Refer to the section on capsular tightness in Chapter 3, Pain.

CONTRAINDICATIONS

1. Absolute
—Bacterial infection, neoplasm, recent fracture

2. Relative
—Joint effusion or inflammation
—Arthrosis (*e.g.*, degenerative joint disease) if acute, or if causing a bony block to movement to be restored
—Rheumatoid arthritis
—Osteoporosis
—Internal derangement
—General debilitation (*e.g.*, influenza, pregnancy, chronic disease)

GRADING OF MOVEMENT

Gaining a feel for the appropriate rate, rhythm, and intensity of movement is perhaps the most difficult aspect of learning to administer specific joint mobilization. Generally, rate, rhythm, and intensity must be adjusted according to how the patient presents—whether acute or chronic—and according to the response of the patient to the technique. When significant pain or muscle spasm are elicited, the rate of movement must be adjusted, or the intensity reduced, or both.

The type of movement performed ultimately depends upon the immediate effect desired. These techniques, in the majority of cases, are used to provide relief of pain and muscle guarding, to stretch a tight joint capsule or ligament, and, rarely, to

reduce an intra-articular derangement that may be blocking movement.

1. Relief of pain and muscle guarding
This is desirable in relatively acute conditions, as a treatment in and of itself, and in chronic conditions to prepare for more vigorous stretching. The techniques in this case are performed to increase proprioceptive input to the spinal cord so as to inhibit ongoing nociceptive input to anterior horn cells and central receiving areas (see Chapter 3, Pain). They are what Maitland refers to as Grade I and II techniques.[9] Movement is performed at the beginning or midpoint of the available joint play amplitude, avoiding tension to joint capsules and ligaments. A rhythmic oscillation of the joint is produced at a rate of perhaps 2 to 3 cycles per second.

In the case of acute joint conditions, these may constitute the only passive mobilization techniques used until the acute manifestations subside. In more chronic cases, these techniques should be used at the initiation of a treatment session, between stretching techniques, and at the end of a session in order to promote relaxation of muscles controlling the joint. Here they are used on a continuum with stretching techniques, gradually increasing in intensity as the patient relaxes.

2. Stretching techniques
Since we use these techniques primarily in cases of capsular tightness or adherence, our goal is ultimately to apply an intermittent stretch to the particular aspect of the capsule that we wish to mobilize. In doing so, we must move the joint up to the limit of the pathologic amplitude of a particular joint play movement and attempt to increase the amplitude of movement. These techniques must be applied rhythmically—no abrupt changes in speed or direction—to pre-

vent reflex contractions of muscles about the joint that might occur from overfiring of joint receptors. They must also be applied slowly in order to allow for the viscous nature—resistance to quick change in length—of connective tissue. The slack that is taken up in the joint play movement is not released as the movement is performed. In effect, one is applying a prolonged stretch with superimposed rhythmic oscillations of small amplitude. The rationale is two-fold. A prolonged stretch is the safest, most effective means of increasing the extensibility of collagenous tissue. Rhythmic oscillations reduce the amount of discomfort and facilitate maximal relaxation during the procedure presumably by increasing large-fiber input to the "gate."

STOPS

When stretching at the limits of a particular osteokinematic movement in the presence of a tight capsule, it is usually helpful to provide a rigid "stop" against which the oscillation is made. It is best for the practitioner to arrange one of his body parts, such as the thigh, forearm, or trunk as a stop. In this way the stop is easily moved to allow progressively increased range of movement. Such a stop also gives the patient an indication of exactly how far the therapist is going to move the part during a particular series of oscillations. This will reduce anticipatory muscle guarding to a minimum. If a greater range of movement is desired, the patient is informed where the stop will be made. The therapist rearranges the stop so as to allow a small increase in motion, and the oscillations are resumed. Such a technique seems to be most effective if the patient's part is brought up rather firmly against the stop with each oscillation. See Figure 7-3,*B* for the shoulder, in which the therapist's thigh is brought up onto the plinth to act as a stop for external rota-

tion, while the therapist simultaneously applies a posterior glide at the glenohumeral joint.

Note: For the sake of simplicity, the operator will be referred to as the male, and the patient as the female. All of the techniques described apply to the patient's left extremities, except where indicated. (P—patient; O—operator; M—movement)

TECHNIQUES FOR THE UPPER EXTREMITY

THE SHOULDER

Techniques performed with the arm at the side of the body are primarily used to promote relaxation of the muscles controlling the joint, to relieve pain, and to prepare for more vigorous stretching techniques. In relatively acute cases of adhesive capsulitis, they may constitute the primary techniques used until resolution of the acute state allows more aggressive mobilization. In more chronic cases, they are typically used at the initiation of the mobilization session, between techniques, and at the end of the session to prevent and reduce reflex muscle-cramping. As these techniques are performed, the arm may be gradually moved from the side of the body toward positions in which more vigorous techniques may be applied. For chronic conditions, these techniques should be used on a continuing basis in conjunction with the stretching techniques described.

1. *The Shoulder Joint*—Techniques for elevation and relaxation
   a. *Inferior Glide*—with the arm at the side of the body (Fig. 7-1,*A*)
      P—Supine, with arm resting at side of body
      O—Stabilizes the scapula with the left hand at the patient's axilla. The web of the hand contacts the inferior aspect of the neck of the glenoid. The right hand grasps the patient's forearm as proximally as possible. **Note:** The patient's arm and the oper-

ator's forearm are essentially parallel. The patient's wrist rests across the antecubital fossa of the operator's stabilizing hand.

M—The scapula is held fixed while the humerus is moved caudally. The movement is performed initially with the patient's arm to the side and resting on the plinth. As the patient relaxes, the arm may gradually be moved toward abduction or flexion. **Note:** This is an important technique for relaxation of spasm and relieving pain, to be used before and after a treatment session and between other techniques. For greater ranges of elevation, see Techniques 1,*b*–*e*.

b. *Progressive Long Axis "Distraction"*—moving toward abduction (Fig. 7-1,*B*)

P—Supine, with the arm resting at the side

O—Stabilizes the inferior neck of the glenoid with the web space of his left hand. The forearm is pronated and the elbow is straight. The other hand grasps the humerus just above the elbow, gaining a purchase on the humeral epicondyles. **Note:** The operator stands with his body facing away from the patient. The patient's forearm is tucked between the therapist's arm and trunk, and the therapist fixes the patient's arm against his trunk.

M—With the scapula held stable and the patient's arm fixed against the operator's trunk, the humerus is moved distally along its long axis. To perform the movement, the therapist shifts his trunk into outward rotation. As the patient relaxes, the arm may be gradually

moved toward abduction. When about 60° abduction is obtained, the therapist must shift his stabilizing hand to contact the lateral border of the scapula with the heel of the supinated hand.

This may be performed up to about 80° abduction. For greater ranges of abduction see Techniques 1,*d* and *e*.

c. *Inferior Glide*—moving toward flexion (Fig. 7-1,*C*)

P—Supine, with the humerus flexed to 60°–100° and the elbow bent, with the wrist resting across the clavicular region

O—Grasps the proximal humerus with both hands, the fingers interlaced. The patient's elbow region is contacted with the clavicular region of the operator's shoulder closest to the patient.

M—The operator pulls caudally with his trunk to produce a movement of combined flexion of the humerus and inferior glide at the glenohumeral joint.

The arm is gradually moved toward greater ranges of flexion up to about 110°. For greater degrees of flexion see Technique 1,*e*.

d. *Inferior Glide*—in abduction (Fig. 7-1,*D*)

P—Supine, elbow bent. The arm is close to the limits of abduction and external rotation, but comfortable.

O—Approaches the arm superiorly. He supports the elbow with the left hand at the distal humerus. The patient's forearm is tucked and supported between the operator's arm and trunk. The right hand contacts the superior aspect of the proximal humerus with the heel of the hand, with the forearm supinated and elbow bent.

M—Inferior glide of the humeral

head is produced by the right hand. As the patient relaxes, the arm can be guided into gradually increasing degrees of abduction with the stabilizing hand.

This may be performed up to about 90°. The choice of position is guided by the ease with which a relaxed movement can be produced. This technique is used to increase abduction allowing stretching into abduction while avoiding impingement of the greater tuberosity on the acromial arch.

e. *Inferior Glide*—in more than 90° of elevation (Fig. 7,1*E*)

P—Supine, with arm elevated comfortably, but close to the limits of full elevation in a somewhat horizontally abducted position, between flexion and abduction. The elbow is bent. **Note:** When moving into ranges past 90°, the patient's forearm may be supported on her forehead or on a pillow above her head, or the operator may support it (as shown).

O—Approaches the arm superiorly. He supports the elbow with the left hand, supporting the patient's arm on his right arm. The operator contacts the superior aspect of the proximal humerus with the right hand, with the thumb positioned ventrally just distal to the acromion.

M—Inferior glide of the humeral head is produced with the right hand. The arm can be guided into gradually increasing degrees of elevation. **Note:** The direction of movement is performed caudally and in a somewhat lateral direction in keeping with the relationship of the joint surfaces in this position.

Movements in elevation beyond 90° are particularly useful as stretching techniques and may be used even when only a few degrees of elevation are restricted. They have no place in the treatment of a very painful shoulder.

2. *The Shoulder Joint*—Techniques for internal rotation

a. *Posterior Glide*—with the arm in various degrees of abduction (10° to 55°), (Fig. 7-2,*A*)

P—Supine, with the arm slightly abducted

O—Stands between the patient's arm and body, and supports the patient's elbow with the right hand. The hand, wrist, and forearm are supported by tucking them between his elbow and side. The left hand contacts the anterior aspect of the upper humerus with the heel of the left hand, with the forearm pronated and elbow straight.

M—A posterior glide is produced by leaning forward slightly and flexing the knees, transmitting the force through the straight arm.

This technique is used to increase joint play necessary for internal rotation and flexion.

b. *Anterior Glide*—arm close to the limits of internal rotation (Fig. 7-2,*B*)

P—Lies on uninvolved side with the arm behind the back so it rests comfortably, but close to the limits of internal rotation.

O—Stands behind patient with both thumb pads over the posterior humeral head. The finger of the right hand grasps around anteriorly to stabilize at the anterior aspect of the acromion and clavicle. Elbows remain almost fully extended. The left knee may be brought up onto the plinth to support the patient's arm.

M—An anterior glide is produced by leaning forward with the upper trunk, transmitting the force through the thumbs. Internal rotation is gradually increased by progressively moving the patient's hand up the back.

This technique results in a posterior capsular stretch, stretching into internal rotation while avoiding posterior impingement of the humeral head on the glenoid labrum. A similar technique may be performed in prone (Technique 2,*c*).

c. *Anterior Glide*—alternate technique in prone (not shown)

P—Prone, with the arm abducted to approximately 45° to 60°. The flexed forearm extends over the edge of the plinth. The upper arm is supported on the plinth. A towel roll or pad is

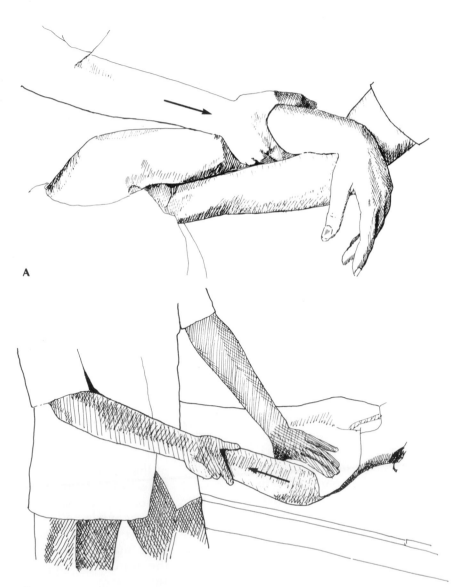

A

B

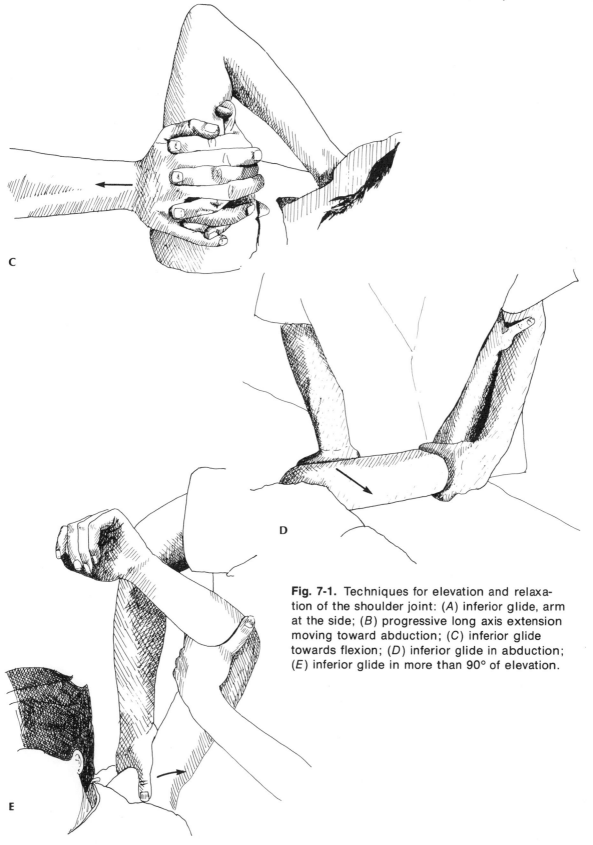

Fig. 7-1. Techniques for elevation and relaxation of the shoulder joint: (*A*) inferior glide, arm at the side; (*B*) progressive long axis extension moving toward abduction; (*C*) inferior glide towards flexion; (*D*) inferior glide in abduction; (*E*) inferior glide in more than 90° of elevation.

placed under the anterior aspect of the shoulder girdle.

O—Stands between the patient's arm and trunk. He supports the patient's elbow against his body with one hand, maintaining the arm in abduction and neutral rotation. The posterior aspect of the upper humerus is contacted with the opposite hand, using the heel of the hand. The forearm is pronated, and the elbow is straight.

M—An anterior glide is produced by leaning forward with the trunk, transmitting the force through the straight arm and flexion of the knees. **Note:** By shifting the supporting hand to the patient's wrist, internal rotation may be gradually increased by simultaneously rotating the arm internally. The operator's body provides a stop to internal rotation. This is an oscillatory technique.

d. *Internal Rotation Technique*—arm close to 90° of abduction (Fig. 7-2,*C*)

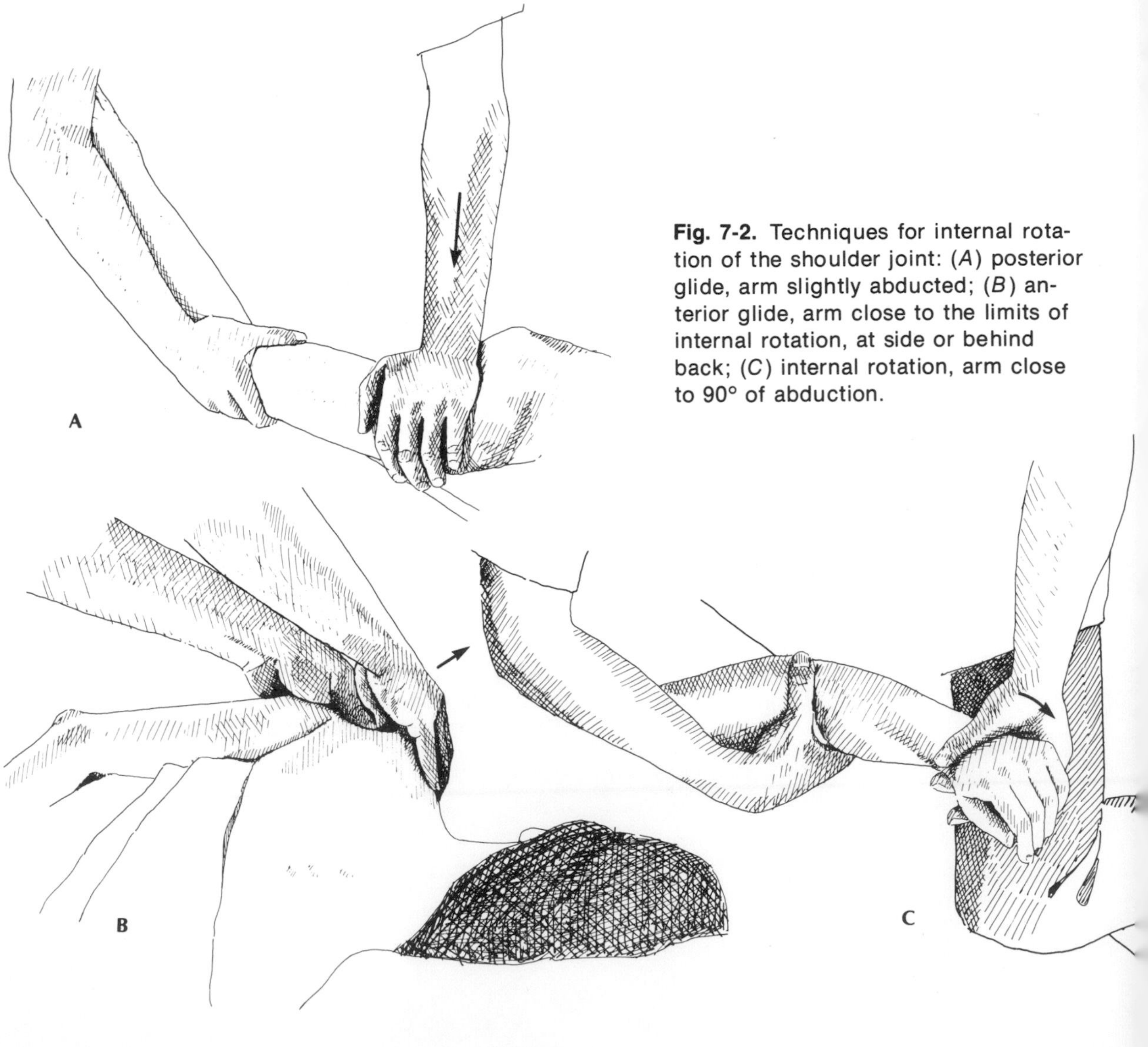

Fig. 7-2. Techniques for internal rotation of the shoulder joint: (*A*) posterior glide, arm slightly abducted; (*B*) anterior glide, arm close to the limits of internal rotation, at side or behind back; (*C*) internal rotation, arm close to 90° of abduction.

P—Supine, with the arm resting comfortably, but as close to 90° of abduction as possible, the elbow bent to 90°, and forearm pronated.

O—Supports the wrist with the left hand; supports under the elbow with the fingers of the right hand from the medial side. He positions the right upper arm in front of and just medial to the shoulder. The left knee is brought up onto the plinth to act as a stop.

M—The right upper arm provides only enough counterpressure to the shoulder to prevent lifting of the shoulder girdle; the hand maintains the arm in abduction. The left hand simultaneously rotates the arm internally. The left thigh provides a stop to internal rotation. The stop is close to the limit of movement so as to minimize anticipatory guarding by the patient. The stop is progressively moved as motion increases. This is an oscillatory movement.

Methods for internal rotation are useful for restoring necessary joint play movements with the arm near the side, or in various degrees of abduction (see 2,*a*), or as stretching techniques in functional positions (see 2,*b–d*).

3. *The Shoulder Joint*—Techniques for external rotation
   a. *Anterior Glide*—arm at the side (Fig. 7-3,*A*)
      P—Supine, arm at the side, elbow bent, forearm supported by operator's arm
      O—Stabilizes with the right hand, grasping the distal humerus just proximal to the elbow. He grasps around medially to the posterior aspect of the humerus with the left hand, as far proximally as possible.
      M—An anterior glide is affected with the left hand, after the "slack" in the shoulder girdle has been take up. This is an oscillatory mobilization.

   This technique is used to increase the joint play movement necessary for external rotation.

   b. *Posterior Glide*—arm close to 90° of abduction (Fig. 7-3,*B*)
      P—Supine, with the arm resting comfortably, but as close to 90° of abduction as possible; elbow bent to 90°
      O—Supports the wrist with his right hand. He contacts the anterior aspect of the proximal humerus with the heel of the left hand. The right knee is brought up onto the plinth to act as a stop.
      M—Posterior glide is produced with the left hand, while the right hand simultaneously rotates the arm externally. The right thigh provides a stop to external rotation close to the limit of movement. This minimizes anticipatory guarding by the patient. The stop is progressively moved as motion increases. This is an oscillatory movement, produced synchronously with posterior glide.

   This method results in an anterior capsular stretch, stretching into external rotation while avoiding anterior impingement of the humerus on the glenoid labrum.

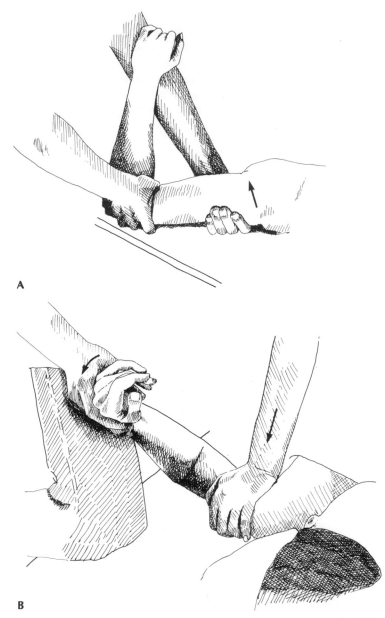

A

B

Fig. 7-3. Techniques for external rotation of the shoulder joint: (*A*) anterior glide, arm at the side; (*B*) posterior glide, arm close to 90° of abduction.

4. *The Shoulder Joint*—Techniques for horizontal adduction and general capsular stretch

  a. *Lateral Glide*—arm at side (glenohumeral distraction), (Fig. 7-4,*A*)

    P—Supine, arm at the side with the elbow bent and the hand resting on her stomach or on the forearm of the operator.

    O—Stabilizes with the right hand at the lateral aspect of the patient's elbow. The left hand grasps the humerus medially, as far proximally as possible. The forearm is brought around over the patient's thorax, in line with the direction of movement.

    M—A lateral glide is affected by moving the upper humerus laterally with the left hand. The elbow should be allowed to move laterally through the same excursion as the humeral head, avoiding a tilting maneuver, unless it is specifically intended to stretch the superior joint capsule.

  This technique (performed at the side of the body) is used to promote relaxation, to relieve pain, to prepare for more vigorous stretching techniques, and as a general capsular stretch. As the last, it may be useful in increasing movement toward the close-packed position by helping to prevent premature compression of the joint.

  b. *Lateral Glide*—in flexion (Fig. 7-4,*B*)

    P—Supine, with the arm flexed comfortably to 90° and elbow bent so that the hand rests on the upper chest

    O—Stabilizes distal humerus with his right hand at the elbow. The left hand is placed against the medial surface of the upper end of the humerus. By bending

forward the arm is placed in a horizontal position in line with the movement.

    M—The proximal humerus is moved laterally.

  This technique is used to restore joint play necessary for horizontal adduction. It results in separation of the joint surfaces (lateral distraction).

  c. *Lateral and Backward Glide*—in flexion (Fig. 7-4,*C*)

    P—Supine, with the arm flexed comfortably to 90° and elbow bent so that the hand rests on the upper chest

    O—Stabilizes distal humerus and elbow by resting them against his trapezial ridge. He grasps the medial aspect of the proximal humerus with both hands, interlacing the fingers.

    M—The proximal humerus is moved backward, toward the plinth, and outward simultaneously in a rocking forward and downward movement of the operator's trunk.

  The arm may be progressively moved toward increased horizontal adduction, as the patient relaxes. This technique is used to increase joint play necessary for horizontal adduction by employing lateral glide with a backward glide simultaneously.

Scapulothoracic, acromioclavicular, and sternoclavicular mobilizations may also be performed in certain circumstances. However, these are rarely necessary in cases of glenohumeral capsular tightness, because these joints tend to become hypermobile by compensating for the restriction at the glenohumeral joint. They may be useful following immobilization of the entire shoulder complex or in other disorders.[7,8,9,18]

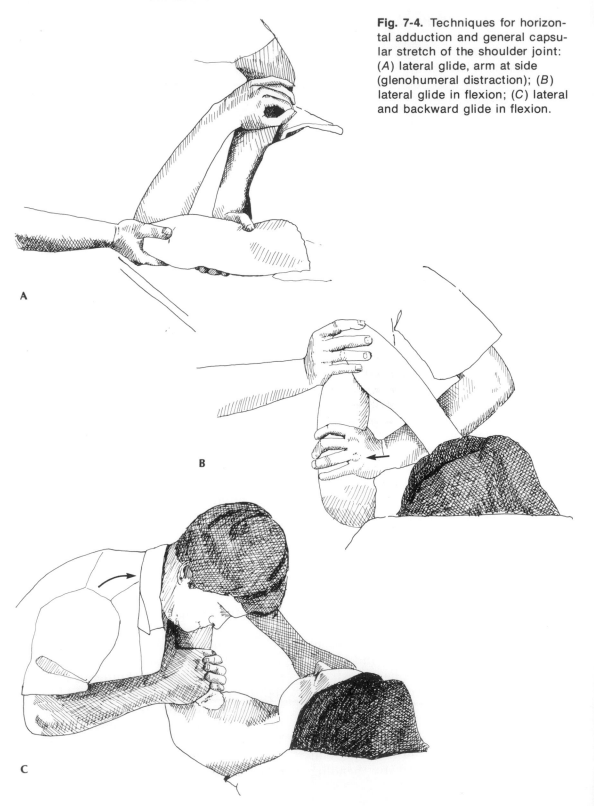

Fig. 7-4. Techniques for horizontal adduction and general capsular stretch of the shoulder joint: (A) lateral glide, arm at side (glenohumeral distraction); (B) lateral glide in flexion; (C) lateral and backward glide in flexion.

THE ELBOW AND FOREARM

1. *The Humeroulnar Joint*—Techniques for distraction
   a. *Joint Distraction*—in flexion (Fig. 7-5,A)
      P—Supine with the arm at the side, elbow bent, and forearm supinated
      O—Stabilizes the wrist with the left hand. He grasps the proximal forearm high up in the antecubital space with the right hand in a pronated position, using the web of the hand for contact.
      M—The proximal ulna is moved inferiorly, affecting a joint distraction, with perhaps some inferior glide. As movement increases, the elbow can be progressively flexed.
      This technique is used as a general capsular stretch primarily to increase elbow flexion (see Alternate Technique 5,*b*).
   b. *Joint Distraction*—in flexion; alternate technique (Fig. 7-5,B)
      P—Supine, with the arm at the side, forearm supinated, and the elbow flexed
      O—Stabilizes the upper arm by holding the distal humerus at the elbow down against the plinth with the right hand. With the left hand, he grasps the back of the supinated wrist.
      M—The proximal ulna is moved superiorly, affecting joint distraction. **Note:** By holding the forearm against his body, the operator can combine distraction with increasing flexion (oscillatory movement) by a rocking motion of his body while maintaining constant stabilization of the humerus.
   c. *Joint Distraction*—moving toward extension (Fig. 7-5,C)
      P—Supine, with the arm at the side, elbow bent, and forearm in neutral position

O—Stabilizes the distal humerus against the plinth with the left hand, forearm pronated. He grasps the distal ulna with his right hand, using primarily the thumb and index finger.
M—Ulnar distraction is affected as a distal pull and by a little outward rotation of the operator's entire body. The elbow may be gradually extended as movement increases.
This technique may be considered an inferior glide of the coronoid on the trochlea or, in a sense, a joint distraction. When used at the limit of extension it becomes an anterior capsular stretch.

2. *The Humeroulnar Joint*—Medial-lateral tilt (Fig. 7-6)
   P—Supine, with arm at the side, forearm supinated; the elbow is close to the limit of extension.
   O—Supports the wrist with his left hand; grasps the humeral epicondyles, supporting the olecranon in the palm of his hand.
   M—Keeping the patient's wrist stationary, the right hand moves medially or laterally, affecting a medial or lateral (valgus or varus) tilt of the patient's humeroulnar joint. The elbow is gradually extended as movement increases.
   This technique is used only when the elbow lacks a few degrees of extension. It is intended to increase a joint play movement necessary for full elbow extension.

3. *The Proximal Radioulnar Joint*—Distal glide of radius on ulna (Fig. 7-7)
   P—Supine, with arm resting at the side, elbow bent, and forearm in neutral position.
   O—Stabilizes the distal humerus against the plinth with his left hand, forearm pronated. He grasps the distal radius with his right hand, using primarily the thumb, index, and long fingers.
   M—The radius is pulled distally with

(*text continues on page 148*)

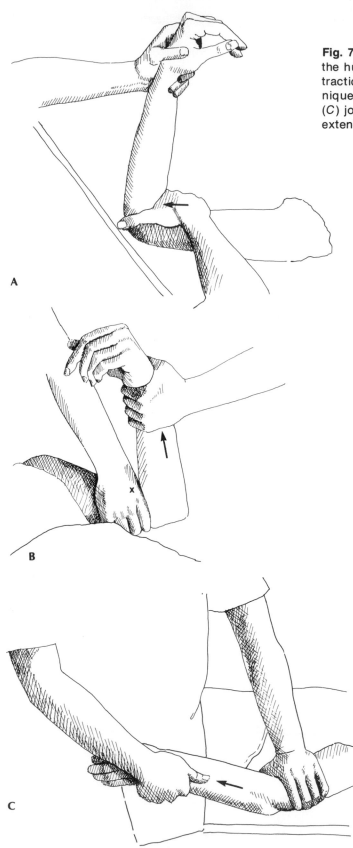

Fig. 7-5. Techniques for distraction of the humeroulnar joint: (*A*) joint distraction in flexion; (*B*) alternate technique for joint distraction in flexion; (*C*) joint distraction, moving toward extension

Fig. 7-6. Medial-lateral tilt of humer-oulnar joint

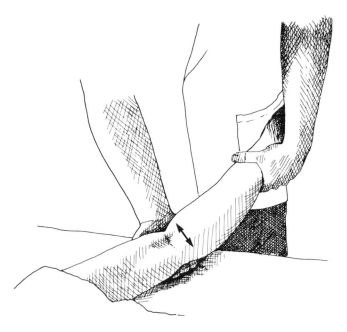

Fig. 7-7. Distal glide of radius on ulna for proximal radioulnar joint

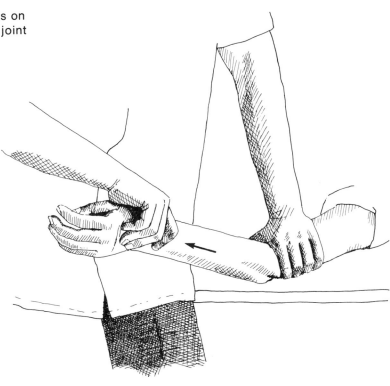

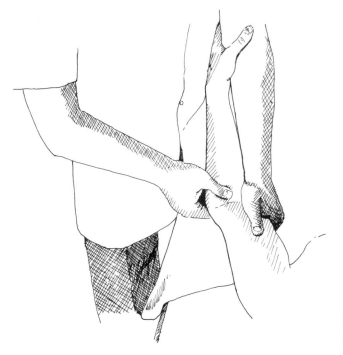

Fig. 7-8. Dorsal-ventral glide of proximal radioulnar joint

the right hand and by a little outward rotation of the operator's entire body. The elbow may be gradually extended as movement increases.

This technique may also be considered distraction at the radiohumeral joint and is intended to increase joint play movement necessary for full elbow extension.

4. *The Proximal Radioulnar Joint*—Dorsal-ventral glide (Fig. 7-8)

  P—Supine, with the arm at the side, elbow slightly flexed, and forearm in slight supination. The patient's forearm is supported by placing her hand lightly on the operator's left forearm.

  O—Supports the medial aspect of the distal humerus and proximal surface of the upper forearm with his left hand. The right hand holds the ventral surface of the proximal radius with the thumb and the dorsal surface with the crook of the flexed proximal interphalangeal (PIP) joint of the index finger.

M—The radial head may be moved dorsally or ventrally as separate motions. These movements can be performed in varying degrees of elbow flexion, extension, supination, or pronation.

This technique may also be considered a movement at the radiohumeral joint. It is used to increase joint movement necessary for pronation and supination.

5. *The Proximal Radioulnar Joint*—Technique to regain pronation (after Mennell[12]) (Fig. 7-9)

  P—Supine, with the arm in full supination and slightly abducted

  O—With his left hand, he supports the wrist with his fingers over the ventral aspect and his thumb on the dorsal aspect. He places the thenar eminence of his right hand over the anterior aspect of the head of the radius and maintains the patient's upper arm on the plinth. The position of the head of the patient's radius is maintained with his thenar eminence.

  M—The carrying angle of the patient's

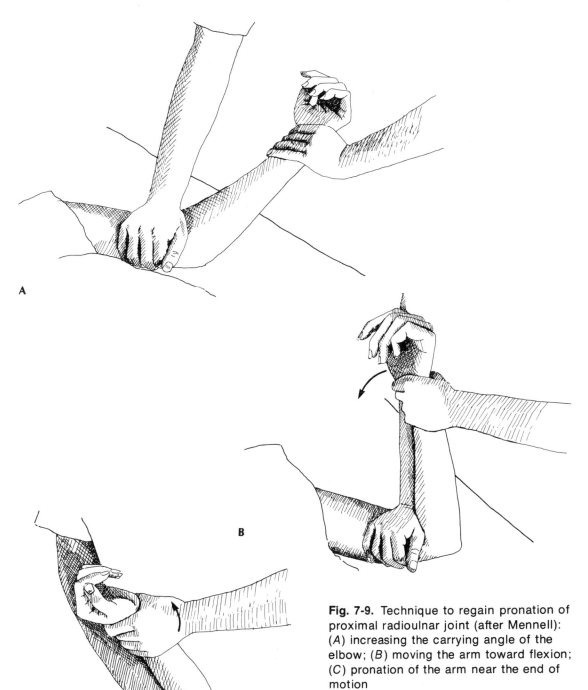

Fig. 7-9. Technique to regain pronation of proximal radioulnar joint (after Mennell): (*A*) increasing the carrying angle of the elbow; (*B*) moving the arm toward flexion; (*C*) pronation of the arm near the end of motion

elbow is increased by the operator's hand at the wrist while maintaining full supination (Fig. 7-9,*A*). While maintaining both supination and the carrying angle of the forearm, the operator flexes the patient's elbow until the head of the radius is felt to press firmly against his right thenar eminence (Fig. 7-9,*B*). While maintaining the forearm in this position with firm pressure against the radial head, the forearm is moved into pronation (Fig. 7-9,*C*). **Note:** This technique requires considerable practice to be effective. If early supination, flexion, and pressure of the thenar eminence throughout the technique are not maintained, the proper movement will not be achieved. The angle of flexion should not be altered while the forearm is moved from supination to pronation.

This is a most valuable technique in regaining joint play movements necessary for pronation and supination.

6. *The Distal Radioulnar Joint*—Dorsal-ventral glide (Fig. 7-10)

P—Supine, with arm somewhat abducted and elbow bent, so that the forearm may rest on the plinth in a neutral position with respect to pronation and supination.

O—Stabilizes the distal radius against the plinth, grasping it between the heel of his hand and the pads of the second through fifth fingers. He grasps the distal ulna dorsally with the thumb pad and ventrally with the pads of the index and long fingers.

M—The distal ulna may be moved dorsally or ventrally relative to the distal radius. These motions should be performed separately. **Note:** Alternatively, the distal ulna may be stabilized and the distal radius moved, by reversing the handholds. The movement may also be performed with the forearm vertical. These techniques are used to increase joint play motions necessary for pronation and supination.

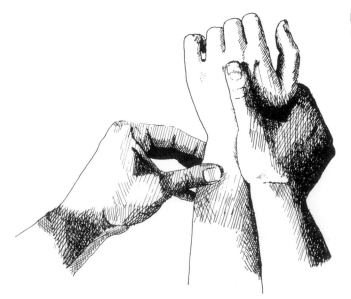

Fig. 7-10. Dorsal-ventral glide of distal radioulnar joint

THE WRIST AND HAND

1. *The Ulnomeniscotriquetral Joint*—Dorsal glide (Fig. 7-11)

   P—Supine or sitting, with the elbow resting on the plinth or table, and the forearm vertical

   O—Stabilizes the radial side of the wrist and hand with his left hand. The right hand contacts the dorsal aspect of the head of the ulna with the thumb, and the palmer aspect of the triquetrum and the pisiform with the radial aspect of the crook of his flexed PIP joint of his index finger.

   M—A dorsal glide of the pisiform and triquetrum on the ulna is produced by a squeezing action between the thumb and the crook of the index finger.

   This technique is used to increase a joint play movement necessary for pronation and supination.

2. *The Radiocarpal Joint* (*and ulnomeniscotriquetral joint*)—Joint distraction (Fig. 7-12)

   P—Sitting or supine, with the elbow bent and resting on the plinth, and the forearm in neutral pronation and supination

   O—Stabilizes the distal humerus and elbow against the plinth with his right hand at the antecubital space. The left hand grasps around the proximal row of carpals, just distal to the styloid processes.

   M—A distraction is produced with the left hand, paying particular attention to the radiocarpal joint.

   This technique is used as a general mobilization procedure to increase joint play at the radiocarpal joint. Distraction tends to occur with palmar flexion of the wrist. By increasing the amount of joint distraction, movement toward the closed-packed position dorsiflexion) may be increased. This prevents premature compression of joint surfaces.

3. *The Radiocarpal Joint*—Dorsal-palmar glide (Fig. 7-13)

   P—Sitting with the arm somewhat abducted, the elbow bent, and the forearm resting on the plinth in pronation. The hand extends over the edge of the table or plinth.

   O—Stabilizes the distal end of the forearm with his right hand, just proximal to the styloid processes. He grasps the proximal row of carpals with his left hand using the styloid processes and pisiform for landmarks.

   M—The proximal row of carpals may be moved dorsally or palmarly, paying particular attention to the radiocarpal joint. Dorsal glide and palmar glide should be performed as separate techniques. **Note:** Dorsal glide may be performed more effectively with the arm in full supination, the hand extended over the edge of the plinth or table.

   Palmar glide is used to increase joint play movements necessary for dorsal flexion. Dorsal glide is used to increase joint play movements necessary for palmar flexion.

4. *The Radiocarpal Joint* (*and ulnomeniscotriquetral joint*)—Radioulnar glide (or tilt) (Fig. 7-14)

   P—Sitting, with the arm near the side, the elbow bent, and the forearm resting on the plinth in neutral pronation and supination. The radial aspect of the forearm faces superiorly.

   O—Stabilizes the distal end of the forearm with the left hand, just proximal to the styloid processes. He grasps the proximal row of carpals with the right hand.

   M—The proximal row of carpals may be glided radially or ulnarly on the distal ends of the radius and ulna (articular disc). Alternatively, a radial tilt or ulnar tilt may be produced.

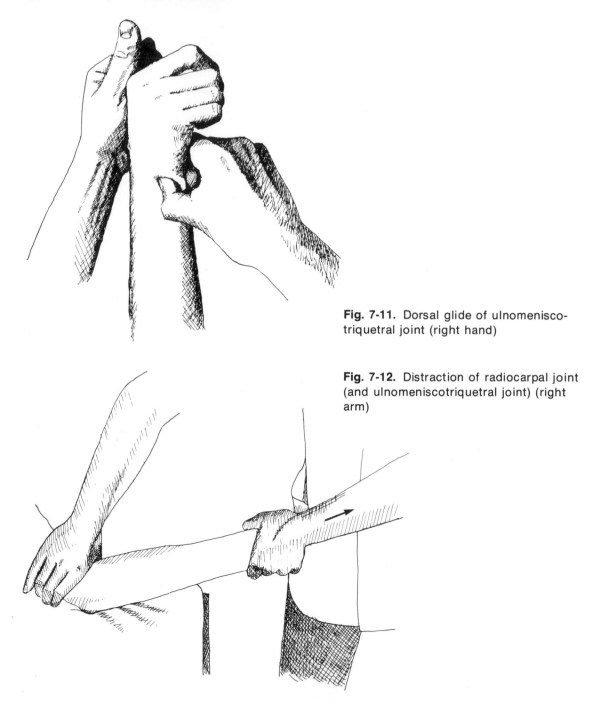

Fig. 7-11. Dorsal glide of ulnomenisco-triquetral joint (right hand)

Fig. 7-12. Distraction of radiocarpal joint (and ulnomeniscotriquetral joint) (right arm)

Radial glide and ulnar tilt are joint play movements necessary for ulnar deviation. Ulnar glide and radial tilt are joint play movements necessary for radial deviation.

5. *Midcarpal Joint*—Joint distraction (not illustrated)

This technique is produced in exactly the same way as that for the radiocarpal joint except the left handhold moves distally to grasp the distal row of carpals. (See Technique 2 for distraction of the radiocarpal joint and Fig. 7-12.)

This technique is used as a general mobilization to increase joint play at the midcarpal joint.

6. *Midcarpal Joint*—Dorsal-palmar glide (not illustrated)

This technique is produced in exactly the same way as that for the radiocarpal joint except the left handhold moves distally to grasp the distal row of carpals (See Technique 3 for dorsal-palmar glide of the radiocarpal joint and Fig. 7-13.)

Palmar glide is used to increase joint play movements necessary for dorsal flexion. Dorsal glide is used to increase joint play movements necessary for palmar flexion.

7. *The Midcarpal Joint*—Palmar glide of the distal row of carpals on the proximal row of carpals (Fig. 7-15).

 P—Sitting or supine, with the elbow resting on the plinth and the forearm vertical

 O—Approaches from the ulnar aspect. The thenar eminence of his left hand contacts the distal row of carpals dorsally. The thenar eminence of his right hand contacts the proximal row of carpals palmarly. The fingers are interlaced over the radial aspect of the wrist. The forearms are directed outward, perpendicular to the plane of the palm.

 M—A palmar glide of the distal row of carpals on the proximal row is produced by a squeezing motion between the thenar eminences. **Note:** This is a more effective method of palmar glide than that described in Technique 6 for dorsal-palmar glide. The performance of this movement depends upon the accurate placement of the operator's thenar eminences over

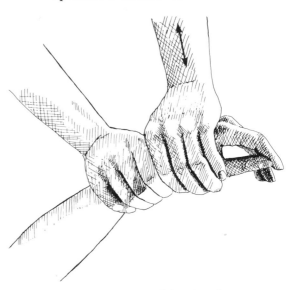

Fig. 7-13. Dorsal-palmar glide of radiocarpal joint

Fig. 7-14. Radioulnar glide (or tilt) of radiocarpal joint (and ulnomeniscotriquetral joint)

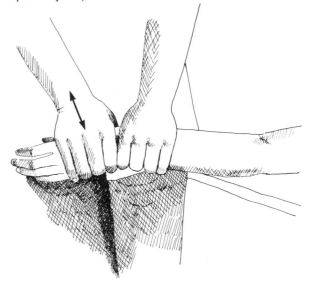

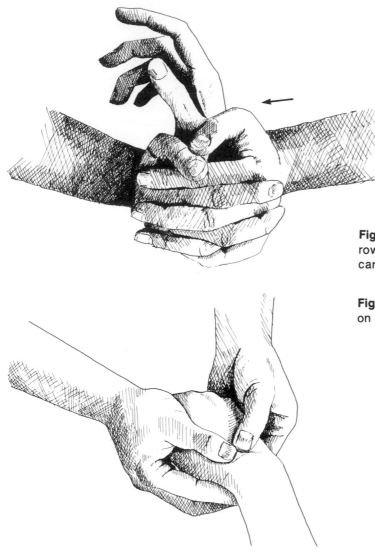

Fig. 7-15. Palmar glide of the distal row on the proximal row for midcarpal joint (right hand)

Fig. 7-16. Palmar glide of scaphoid on radius for intercarpal joints

the correct bones. Extension and spreading of the patient's finger should take place when this movement is elicited correctly.[12]

This technique is used to increase joint play motion necessary for dorsal flexion of the wrist.

Specific movements between adjacent bones of the wrist and carpal joints may be indicated. Mobility between triquetrum and lunate, lunate and radius, or capitate and lunate, for example, can be tested and mobilized. In general, one joint partner is always fixated while the other is moved. The individual carpal bones can be mobilized by placing the thumb and index finger on the volar and dorsal sides respectively. The thumbs may mobilize while the index fingers stabilize, or *vice versa*. The reader is referred to detailed descriptions of these advanced techniques by Kaltenborn and others.[7,12,18] Only one example will be described.

8. *The Intercarpal Joints*—Palmar glide of the scaphoid and radius (Fig. 7-16)

P—Sitting or supine, with the forearm resting on the table, or with the arm held forward by the operator.

O—Stands or sits facing the hand. Both hands hold the patient's thenar and hypothenar eminence. The index fingers are placed on the proximal palmar surface of radius, stabilizing in this position. The thumbs contact the scaphoid dorsally.

M—The scaphoid is moved palmarly relative to the distal end of the radius.

This technique is used to increase joint play motion necessary for dorsal glide of scaphoid on radius.

9. *The Intermetacarpal Joints*—Dorsal-palmar glide (Fig. 7-17) (These joints between the metacarpal heads are not true synovial joints, but movement must occur here during grasp and release as described in the Appendix.)

 P—Sitting or supine, with the elbow resting on the plinth, the forearm pronated.

 O—Approaches from the dorsal aspect. The left hand stabilizes the head and neck of the third metacarpal. The thumb pad contacts dorsally, and the pads of the index and long

fingers palmarly. The left hand grasps the head and neck of the fourth metacarpal in a similar fashion.

M—The head of the fourth metacarpal can be moved palmarly or dorsally with respect to the third metacarpal. Similarly, the right hand can stabilize the third metacarpal, while the left hand moves the second metacarpal. Note that the third metacarpal is the "center of movement" as the hand flattens and arches during release and grasp. It is always stabilized, while the other metacarpals are moved relative to it.

These techniques are used to increase joint play movements necessary for the arching and flattening of the hand that occur with grasp and release.

THE FINGERS

1. *The Metacarpophalangeal (MP) or Interphalangeal (IP) Joints*—Distraction (Fig. 7-18)

 P—Sitting or supine

Fig. 7-17. Dorsal-palmar glide of inter-metacarpal joints

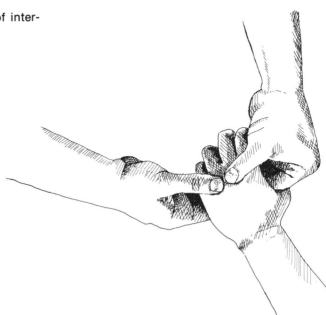

O—Supports the forearm and elbow by tucking them between his forearm and side. To treat the more radial joints, the operator approaches from the ulnar side for the thumb, index, and long fingers, and from the radial side for the ring and small fingers. He grasps the head of the proximal bone dorsally with the thumb pad and palmarly with the crook of the index finger. He grasps the base of the distal bone in a similar manner.

M—Keeping the joint in slight flexion (avoiding close-packed position), a long axis distraction is produced with the operator's more distal hand.

These techniques are used for general joint mobilization to increase joint play. Distraction is necessary especially during extension at the MPs and flexion at the IPs, since these are movements toward the close-packed position. Pre-mature compression of joint surfaces will result if sufficient joint play into distraction cannot occur.

2. *The Metacarpophalangeal or Interphalangeal Joints*—Dorsal-palmar glide (Fig. 7-19)

P—Supine or sitting

O—The handholds are essentially the same as those for distraction, except during dorsal glide the palmar contact of the more distal hand is with the pad of the index finger.

M—The base of the distal bone may be moved palmarly or dorsally.

Palmar glide is necessary for flexion. Dorsal glide is a joint play movement necessary for extension.

3. *The Metacarpophalangeal or Interphalangeal Joints*—Radioulnar glide (or tilt) (Fig. 7-20)

P—Supine or sitting

O—The handholds are similar to those used for distraction except that the

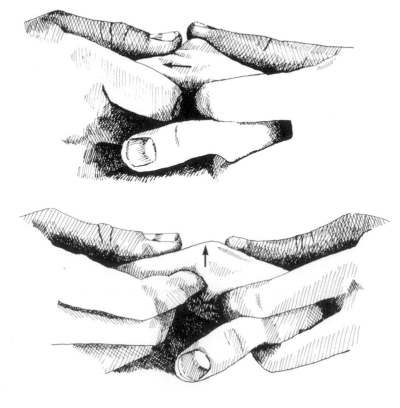

Fig. 7-18. Distraction of metacarpophalangeal or interphalangeal joints (right hand)

Fig. 7-19. Dorsal-palmar glide of metacarpophalangeal or interphalangeal joints (right hand)

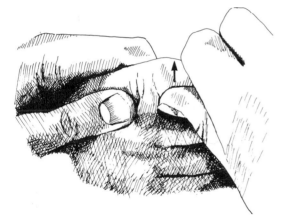

Fig. 7-20. Radio-ulnar glide of metacarpophalangeal or interphalangeal joints (right hand)

thumbs are brought around to the aspect of the bones closest to the operator, and the crooks or pads of the index fingers are brought around to the aspect of the bone farthest from the operator. The contacts are then made on the radial and ulnar sides of the joint.

M—Radial or ulnar glide or tilt may be produced by the thumb pad, in one direction, and by the index pad in the other. While one pad is producing the movement, the other moves to the more distal part of the bone. Ulnar glide (or ulnar tilt) is necessary for extension at the IP joints. Radial glide, or radial tilt, is necessary for flexion at the IP joints. The same is true, but to a lesser extent, at the MP joints.

4. *The Metacarpophalangeal or Interphalangeal Joints*—Rotation (pronation and supination) (Fig. 7-21)

   P—Supine or sitting

   O—The proximal handhold is the same as that for distraction. The distal handholds are also similar to those used for long axis distraction, except the operator may gain some leverage by holding the more distal segment of the digit, semi-flexed, in his remaining fingers. This must be performed with caution.

M—A pronation or supination of the distal end of the bone is produced by the operator's more distal hand. Supination is a joint play movement (conjunct rotation) necessary for flexion, especially at the IPs. Pronation occurs during extention. **Note:** The same techniques may be used at the carpometacarpal joint of the thumb. As for their specific uses in this case, consider the convex-concave rule and how it applies to this sellar joint.

TECHNIQUES FOR THE LOWER EXTREMITY

Note: All of the techniques described in this section apply to the patient's *right* extremities, except where indicated.

THE HIP

Like the shoulder joint, techniques performed with the hip in a neutral position are primarily used to promote relaxation of the muscles controlling the joint, to relieve pain, and to prepare for more vigorous stretching techniques. The hip joint is, however, much more stable than the shoulder joint.

Fig. 7-21. Rotation (pronation and supination) of metacarpophalangeal or interphalangeal joints (right hand)

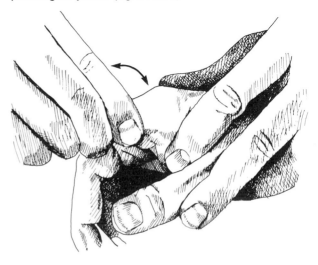

1. *The Hip Joint*—Techniques for elevation and relaxation

    a. *Inferior Glide*—in neutral (Fig. 7-22, *A*)

      P—Supine. A belt may be used to keep the upper body from sliding inferiorly on the plinth. The leg is in slight abduction, external rotation, and flexion.

      O—Grasps the patient's ankle just proximal to the malleoli with his left hand, behind his back. He grasps the femur distally, just proximal to the condyles and from the medial aspect, with the right hand. **Note:** If the patient has a knee disorder, both handholds may be shifted proximal to the knee or use Technique 1,*b* with the hip in about 30° of flexion.

      M—The operator's arms remain fixed. An inferior glide is imparted by leaning backward with the trunk. This may be done through various degrees of abduction.

This technique is used as a general mobilization to increase joint play. Inferior glide is a joint play movement necessary for hip flexion and abduction. It is also used for relaxation of spasm and pain relief and may be used before and after a treatment session and between other techniques. This procedure should be used on a continuing basis

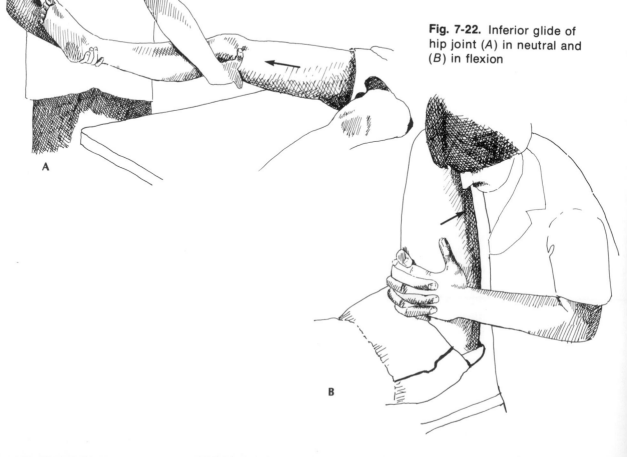

Fig. 7-22. Inferior glide of hip joint (*A*) in neutral and (*B*) in flexion

A

B

and in conjunction with the stretching techniques described below (Techniques 1,*b* and *c*).

b. *Inferior Glide*—in flexion (Fig. 7-22,*B*)

P—Supine, with hip and knee each flexed to 90°. A strap may be used to stabilize the upper body.

O—Supports the lower leg by letting it rest on his shoulder. He grasps the anterior aspect of the proximal femur as far proximally as possible, using both hands with the fingers interlaced.

M—An inferior glide is imparted with the hands. This may be performed while simultaneously rocking the thigh into flexion.

This technique is used to increase joint play movement necessary for hip flexion.

c. *Inferior Glide*—in extension (not illustrated)

P—Supine. A belt may be used to keep the upper body from sliding inferiorly on the plinth. The leg is extended over the side of the plinth and positioned in various degrees of abduction and internal rotation.

O—Same as that for Technique 1,*a*.

M—The operator's arms remain fixed. An inferior glide is imparted by leaning backward with the trunk. The leg may be progressively moved into various degrees of abduction and internal rotation combined with extension, working towards the close-packed position of the hip joint.

This technique is of particular use as a stretching technique.

2. *The Hip Joint*—Anterior glide techniques

a. *Anterior Glide*—in supine (Fig. 7-23,*A*)

P—Supine. A strap may be used to stabilize the pelvis.

O—Grasps around posteriorly with both hands to the posterior aspect of the proximal femur, level with the greater trochanter. The fingers are interlaced or overlapping. The operator stabilizes the distal thigh and knee against the plinth with his trunk.

M—The slack is taken up, and an anterior glide of the proximal femur is imparted with the hands.

This technique is used to increase the joint play movement necessary for external rotation.

b. *Anterior Glide*—in prone (Fig. 7-23,*B*)

P—Prone, with the knee bent to 90°. An inch thickness of towelling may be placed under the anterior aspect of the pelvis, just proximal to the acetabulum, for extra stabilization.

O—Supports the knee with the right hand by grasping around medially to the anterior aspect of the distal femur. He supports the lower leg by tucking it between his elbow and side. The left hand contacts the posterior aspect of the proximal femur with the heel of the hand. It is level with, and medial to, the greater trochanter.

M—The left hand imparts an anterior glide to the proximal femur. The right hand may simultaneously guide the leg into internal rotation or abduction.

This technique is considered more progressive than Technique 2,*a*. It is used to increase joint play necessary for external rotation. It also serves

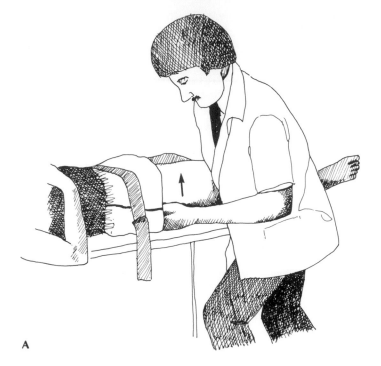

A

Fig. 7-23. Anterior glide of hip joint (*A*, right hip) in supine and (*B*, left hip) in prone positions

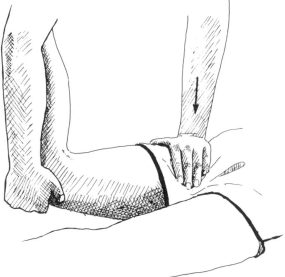

B

as a specific capsuloligamentous stretch by internally rotating the femoral head while simultaneously preventing its impingement on the acetabulum.

3. *The Hip Joint*—Posterior glide (Fig. 7-24)

P—Supine. An inch of padding is placed beneath the pelvis just proximal and medial to the acetabulum.

O—Supports the knee and distal thigh with the right hand by grasping around medially to the posterior aspect. He contacts the anterior aspect of the proximal femur with the heel of his left hand, with the forearm supinated.

M—A posterior glide is imparted with the operator's left hand by leaning forward with the trunk.

This technique is used to increase a joint play movement necessary for internal rotation.

4. *The Hip Joint*—Backward glide (Fig. 7-25)

P—Supine, with the hip flexed to 90° and the lower leg supported comfortably on the crook of the operator's elbow

O—Both hands contact the distal end of the femur. He places one hand over the other to provide reinforcement.

M—A backward (dorsal) glide is imparted by leaning forward with the trunk, and is assisted by the operator's body weight.

This technique is used to increase joint play movement necessary for horizontal adduction of the thigh.

THE KNEE AND LEG

1. *The Femorotibial Joint*—Distraction (Fig. 7-26)

P—Sitting on the edge of the plinth, with several layers of towelling supporting the underside of the distal thigh

O—Stands with his back to the patient so as to direct his forearms

Fig. 7-24. Posterior glide of hip joint

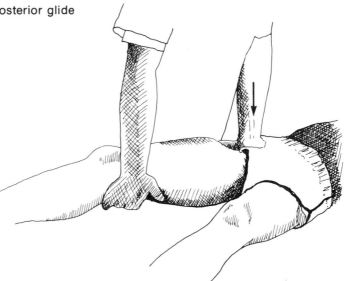

in the line of force. Both hands grasp the tibia proximal to the malleoli to gain a purchase on them.

M—A long axis distraction is imparted by leaning forward with the trunk. This may be performed through varying degrees of flexion and extension.

This technique is used as a general mobilization to increase femorotibial joint play. Distraction at this joint tends to occur when moving into flexion (out of close-packed position). As with any joint, if normal distraction does not occur, premature compression of joint surfaces will result when moving toward the close-packed position.

2. *The Femorotibial Joint*—Posterior glide techniques

    a. *Posterior Glide*—of tibia on femur with the knee flexed (Fig. 7-27,*A*)

        P—Supine, with the knee flexed to about 90°, the foot flat on the plinth.

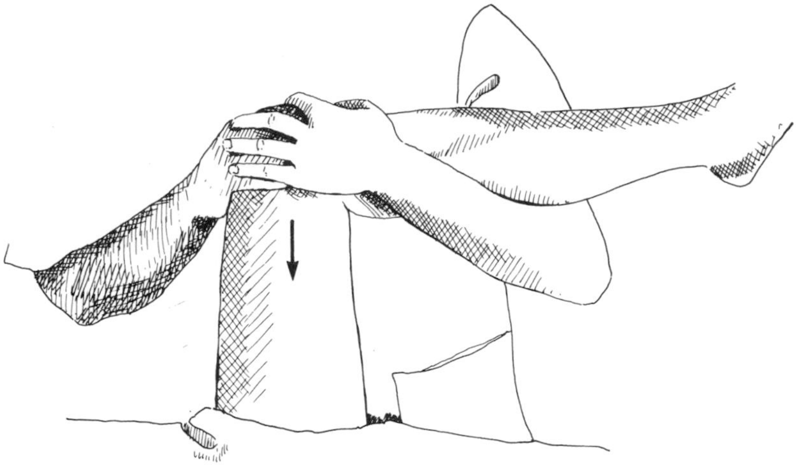

Fig. 7-25. Backward glide of hip joint (left hip)

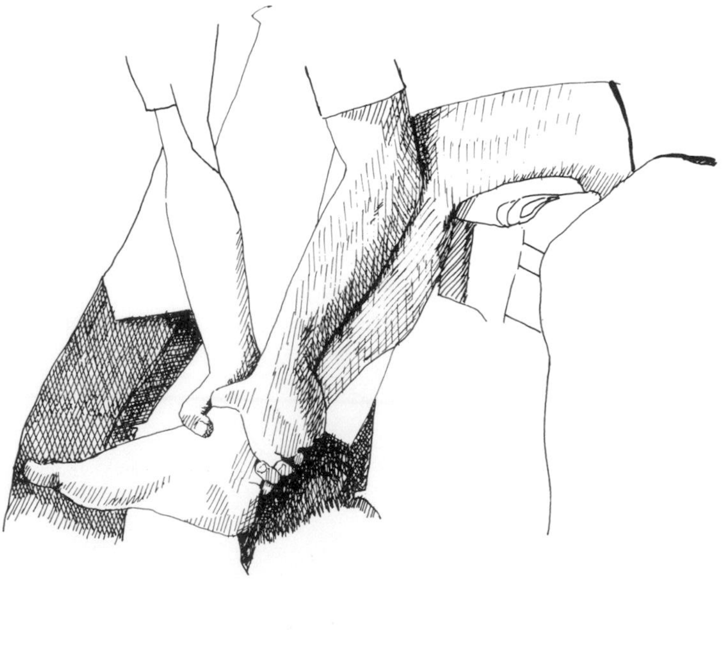

Fig. 7-26. Distraction of femorotibial joint

O—Stabilizes the anterior aspect of the distal femur by contacting it with his entire left hand. The forearm is directed horizontally. The operator contacts the tibial tuberosity with his right hand so that the tuberosity lies in the groove between the thenar and hypothenar eminences. The forearm is directed horizontally.

M—The right hand imparts a posterior glide of the tibia, while the left hand stabilizes the femur.

This technique is used to increase a joint play movement necessary for knee flexion.

b. *Posterior Glide*—of tibia on femur with the knee approaching full extension (Fig. 7-27,*B*)

P—Supine, with the knee slightly flexed from the limit of extension. An inch thickness of towelling may be placed under the posterior aspect of the distal femur.

O—Supports the knee with the right hand placed under the distal femur. He uses the forearm of the right extremity to

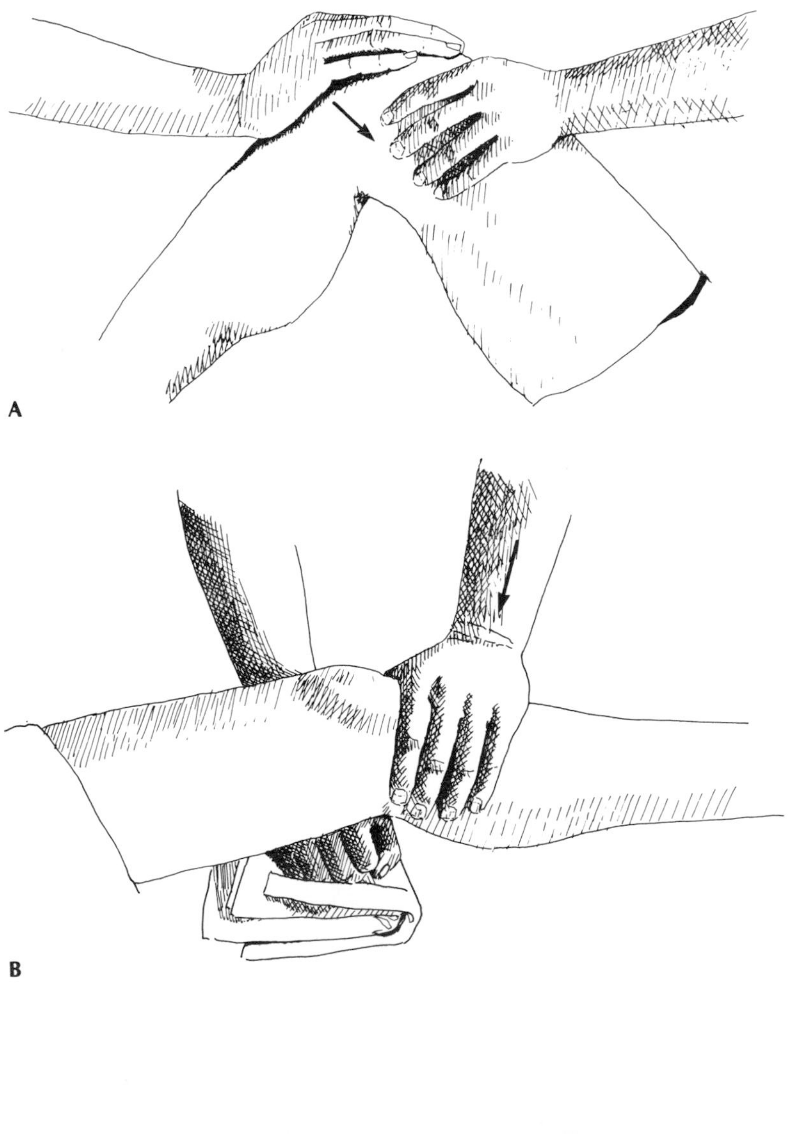

Fig. 7-27. Techniques for posterior glide of the femorotibial joint, tibia on femur: (*A*) with the right knee flexed to about 90°; (*B*) with the knee—here, the left knee—approaching full extension

A

B

support and control the femur. The left hand is placed on the proximal aspect of the tibia just distal to the joint space.

M—A posterior glide is produced with the left hand by moving the lower leg dorsally.

This technique is used to increase joint play movement necessary for knee flexion. Since the knee is approaching full extension (close-packed position), it is considered more vigorous than Technique 2,*a*.

3. *Femorotibial Joint*—Anterior glide techniques.

a. *Anterior Glide*—of the tibia on the femur with the knee flexed to about 90° (Fig. 7-28)

P—Supine, with the knee flexed to about 90° and the foot flat on the plinth.

O—Stabilizes the foot and lower leg by partway sitting on the plinth, placing the proximal thigh over the dorsum of the patient's foot. He grasps the proximal tibia by wrapping the fingers of both hands around posteriorly and contacting the tibial tuberosity with both thumbs anteriorly.

M—Anterior glide is produced by

keeping the arms fixed and leaning backward with the trunk.

This technique is used to increase a joint play movement necessary for knee extension.

b. *Anterior Glide*—of the tibia on femur (or femur on tibia) with the knee approaching full extension (not illustrated)

This is performed in the same manner as Technique 2,*b*. See Fig. 7-27,*B* for anterior glide of tibia on femur. However, the handholds are reversed. The right hand contacts the anterior surface of the distal femur, just proximal to the condyles. The operator reaches around medially with the left hand to grasp the posterior aspect of the proximal tibia. Both elbows are only slightly flexed. An anterior glide of the tibia on the femur is produced by leaning to the left. The right hand prevents movement of the femur. **Note:** Often the operator will find it better to stabilize the tibia with the left hand (hand underneath the tibia) and to use the right hand to mobilize the femur dorsally on the tibia. This takes advantage of gravity

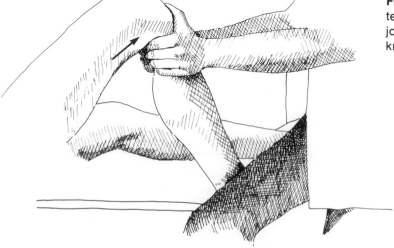

Fig. 7-28. Technique for anterior glide of the femorotibial joint, tibia on femur, with the knee flexed to about 90°

and the concave-convex rule. With this approach the femur is moved dorsally, resulting in an anterior glide of tibia on femur.

This technique is used to increase a joint play movement necessary for knee extension.

4. *The Femorotibial Joint*—Internal rotation techniques
   a. *Internal Rotation*—with the knee flexed to about 90° (Fig. 7-29,*A*)

   P—Supine, with the knee flexed to 90°, the foot flat on the plinth.

   O—Stabilizes the foot by sitting on the plinth, placing the proximal thigh over the dorsum of the patient's foot. The left hand grasps the proximal tibia laterally, with the fingers wrapped around posteriorly, the thumb contacting the lateral aspect of the tibial tuberosity so as to gain a purchase against it. The right hand grasps the tibia anteriorly and medially, just distal to the left hand, gaining a purchase on the tibial crest.

   M—Both hands rotate the proximal tibia medially (internal rotation), gaining purchase on the tibial tuberosity and lateral tibial condyle with the left hand, and the tibial crest and medial tibial condyle with the right hand.

   This technique is used to increase a joint play movement necessary for knee flexion.

   b. *Internal Rotation*—at varying degrees of flexion and extension (Fig. 7-29,*B*)

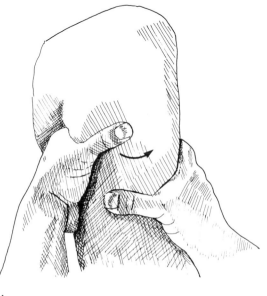

A

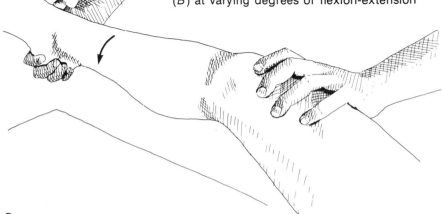

B

Fig. 7-29. Internal rotation of femorotibial joint: (*A*) with the knee flexed to about 90° and (*B*) at varying degrees of flexion-extension

P—Supine

O—Controls the distal thigh with the left hand grasping from the lateral aspect, the thumb wrapping around posteriorly and the fingers anteriorly. The right hand grasps the heel of the foot. He must place the ankle in close-packed position by fully dorsiflexing it so that the rotary force is transmitted to the tibia rather than to the ankle joint. The operator's forearm is kept in close alignment with the patient's tibia.

M—The right hand rotates the entire foot medially, transmitting the movement to the tibia through the close-packed ankle. Starting with the knee slightly flexed, the movement can be applied at various degrees of flexion and extension. Do not, however, rotate and simultaneously flex or extend. This technique is considered more vigorous than Technique 4,*a*. It increases joint play movement necessary for flexion.

5. *The Femorotibial Joint*—External rotation techniques

   a. *External Rotation*—with the knee flexed to about 90° (Fig. 7-30,*A*)

   This is performed in the same manner as Technique 4,*a*. The handholds are reversed, however, so that the right thumb contacts the tibial tuberosity medially, while the left hand grasps the tibial crest and lateral aspect of the proximal tibia.

   This technique is used to increase a joint play movement necessary for knee extension.

   b. *External Rotation*—applied in various positions approaching full extension (Fig. 7-30,*B*)

   P—Supine

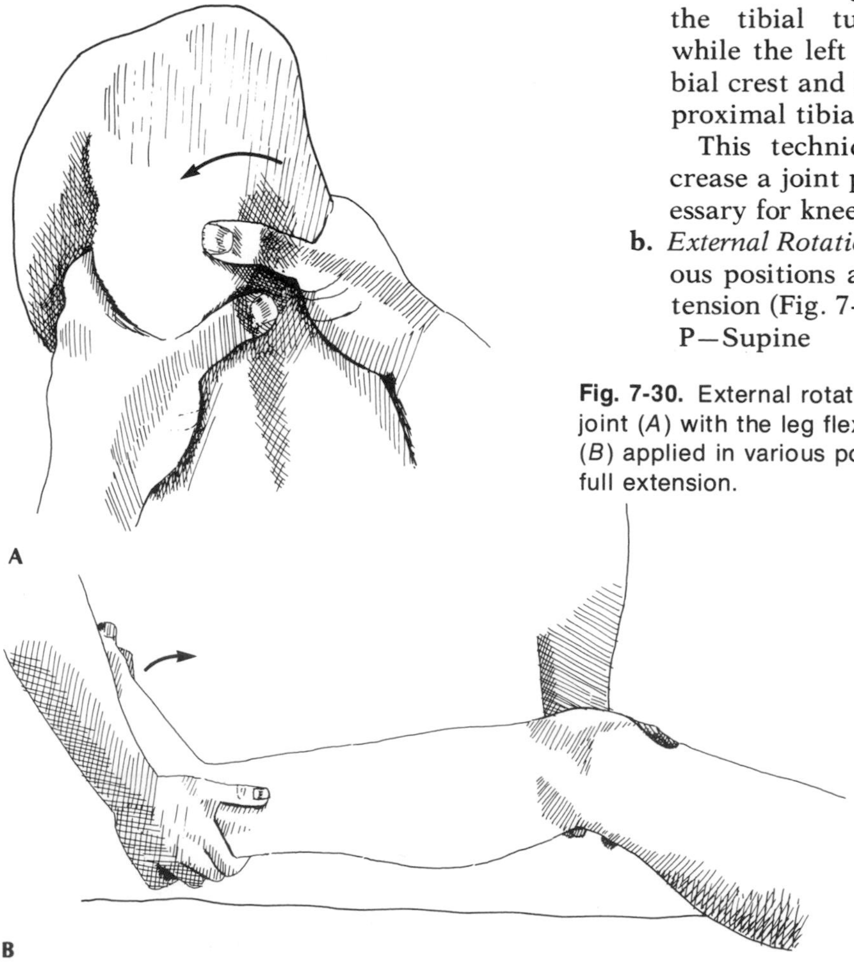

Fig. 7-30. External rotation of femorotibial joint (*A*) with the leg flexed to about 90° and (*B*) applied in various positions, approaching full extension.

A

B

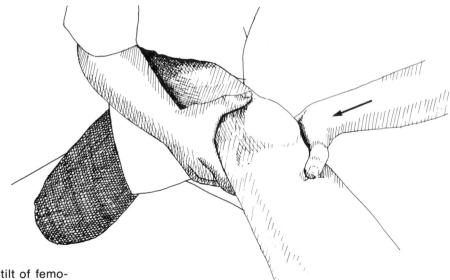

Fig. 7-31. Valgus tilt of femo-rotibial joint

O—Supports the knee and distal end of the thigh with his left hand from the lateral aspect, wrapping the fingers around posteriorly. The left hand primarily controls the position of the knee, keeping it from dropping into extension. He grasps the ankle and foot with the right hand, wrapping the fingers around the calcaneous and the achilles tendon posteriorly from the medial side. The forearm contacts the entire medial border of the foot. The ankle must be kept in close-packed position so as to transmit the rotatory force to the tibia rather than to the ankle joint.

M—The right hand and forearm rotate the foot and ankle externally (lateral rotation), keeping the ankle in close-packed position. The left hand controls the position of the knee. This may be performed at various positions approaching full extension. *Do not ro-*tate and simultaneously flex or extend the knee.

This technique is used to increase a joint play movement necessary for knee extension. It is considered more vigorous than Technique 5,*a*.

6. *The Femorotibial Joint*—Valgus tilt (Fig. 7-31)

P—Supine

O—Supports the foot and lower leg by resting the ankle on his proximal thigh. His knee is placed up onto the plinth. He tucks the leg between his elbow and side. The operator supports the proximal tibia and knee with his right hand from the medial side, wrapping the fingers around posteriorly and the thumb anteriorly. The left forearm is supinated and in line with the direction of force. The heel of the left hand contacts the lateral aspect of the femoral and tibial condyles. The fingers wrap around posteriorly for additional support. The patient's knee is kept slightly flexed.

M—The left hand gently moves the knee into valgus tilt, taking care

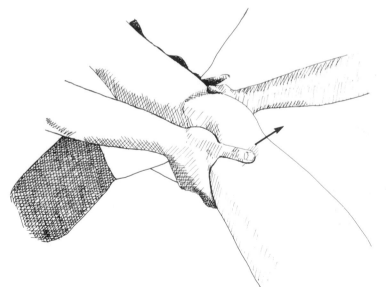

Fig. 7-32. Varus tilt of femoro-tibial joint

to avoid any flexion or extension of the knee. (The operator's right hand supports the knee, but yields with the valgus movement.)

This technique is used to increase joint play at the knee. As with any joint play movement, it must not be moved past normal anatomical limits.

7. *The Femorotibial Joint*—Varus tilt (Fig. 7-32)

This is performed in a similar manner as Technique 6. The handholds are reversed so that the left hand supports the proximal tibia and the knee. The right hand contacts the medial condyles. The right forearm comes around and is in line with the varus force to be produced.

8. *The Patellofemoral Joint*—Medial-lateral tilt (Fig. 7-33)
   P—Supine, with the knee slightly flexed over a firm support of towelling
   O—Contacts the lateral or medial patellar border with his thumb pads. The remaining fingers rest over the anterior aspect of the patient's leg to help support the

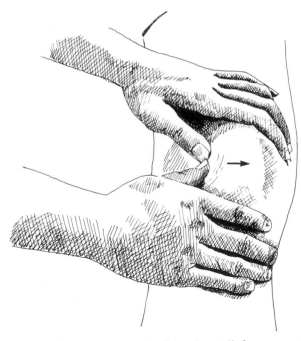

Fig. 7-33. Medial-lateral glide of patellofemoral joint

operator's hands. He keeps the elbows close to full extension.
   M—A medial glide of the patella can be imparted by leaning forward with the trunk. The movement should *not* be performed by pushing with the thumbs, radially de-

viating the wrists, or extending the elbows. A lateral glide can be imparted using the pads of the index fingers.

This technique is used for general patellar mobilization, in the presence of restricted patellar movement.

9. *The Patellofemoral Joint*—Superior-inferior glide (Fig. 7-34)

   This is performed in the same manner as Technique 8. The thumb pads contact the patella superiorly or inferiorly. The fingers rest over the medial and lateral aspect of the knee joint. The forearms are in line with the direction of force.

   The patella must glide superiorly during knee extension, and inferiorly on knee flexion.

10. *The Proximal Tibiofibular Joint*—Anterior-posterior glide (Fig. 7-35)

    P—Supine, with knee flexed to about 90°, the foot flat on the plinth

    O—Stabilizes the knee with the right hand contacting the medial aspect of the knee area. He grasps the head and neck of the proximal fibula with the left hand, the thumb contacting anteriorly, the index and long finger pads contacting posteriorly. The operator must take care to avoid direct pressure to the common peroneal nerve.

    M—The left hand may move the proximal fibula posteriorly or anteriorly. This should be performed through a movement of flexion and extension at the shoulder, rather than through finger or wrist movements.

    This technique is used to increase joint play at the tibiofemoral joint. The fibular head must move forward on knee flexion and backward on knee extension.

11. *The Distal Tibiofibular Joint*—Anterior-posterior glide (Fig. 7-36)

    P—Supine

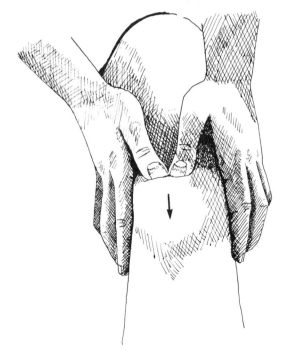

Fig. 7-34. Superior-inferior glide of patellofemoral joint (left knee)

O—Cradles the ankle in his right hand, fixing it to the plinth, so that the fingers wrap around the heel posteriorly. The medial malleolus rests over the palmar aspect of his dorsiflexed wrist. The left hand contacts the lateral malleolus anteriorly with the heel of the hand.

M—While the right hand prevents downward movement of the medial malleolus, the left hand glides the lateral malleolus posteriorly in relation to the medial malleolus. The handholds may be reversed to move the medial malleolus posteriorly on the lateral malleolus.

These techniques are used to increase joint play at the distal tibiofibular joint. This joint must spread slightly during ankle dorsiflexion, since the talus is wider anteriorly than posteriorly. Although spreading cannot be performed passively by the operator,

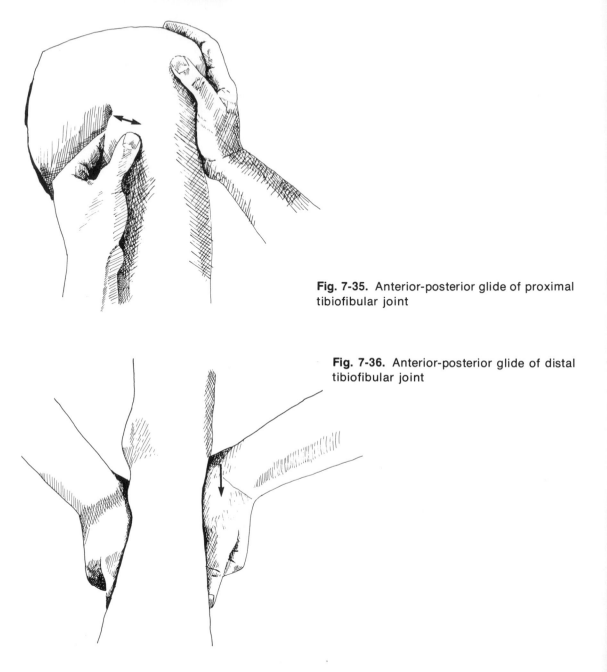

Fig. 7-35. Anterior-posterior glide of proximal tibiofibular joint

Fig. 7-36. Anterior-posterior glide of distal tibiofibular joint

increasing anterior-posterior movement is likely to increase other joint play movements such as spreading.

THE ANKLE

1. *The Ankle Mortice Joint*—Distraction (Fig. 7-37)

   P—Supine, with the knee flexed to about 90°, the hip flexed and somewhat abducted

   O—Half sits on the edge of the plinth, with his back to the patient. He wraps the patient's leg around his rightside to support the knee on his iliac crest, tucking the lower leg between his elbow and side (Fig. 7-37,A). The operator grasps the ankle with both hands so that the thumbs wrap around medially and the fingers laterally. The web of his right hand contacts the neck of the talus dorsally, the web of his left hand contacts the calcaneus pos-

Fig. 7-37. Distraction of ankle mortice joint: (A) position of the operator; (B) view of the operator's grip at the ankle.

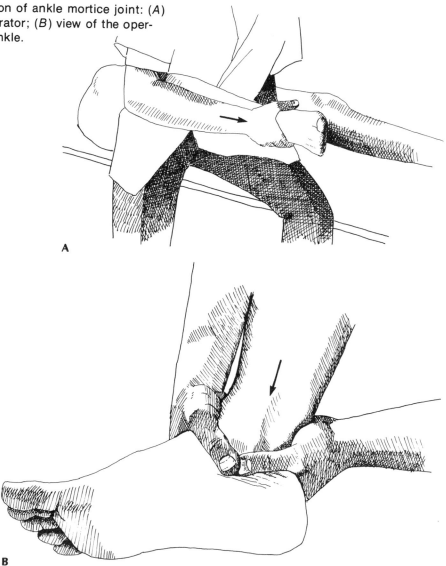

teriorly. The forearms are kept in line with the direction of force (Fig. 7-37,*B*).

M—A distraction is imparted with both hands. The ankle may be slightly everted to help lock the subtalar joint.

This technique is used to increase joint play at the ankle mortice joint. Distraction must occur here during plantar flexion, and is necessary for full movement toward the close-packed position, which is dorsiflexion.

2. *The Ankle Mortice Joint*—Posterior glide of the tibia on talus (or anterior glide of talus on tibia) (Fig. 7-38)

   P—Supine

   O—Stabilizes the talus and foot by grasping around medially to the posterior aspect of the calcaneus with the left hand. He contacts the distal tibia by placing his right hand over the anterior distal aspect of the tibia, just proximal to the malleoli.

   M—The tibia is glided posteriorly on the talus with the right hand. **Note:** An anterior glide of the talus on the tibia may be performed by stabilizing the tibia with the right hand and moving the talus anteriorly. When this technique is used, it is

important to keep the subtalar joint slightly everted to lock the calcaneus on the talus. The talus is glided anteriorly on the tibia via the calcaneus at the ankle mortice. This is a slightly more difficult technique since the operator must work against gravity.

Both of these techniques are used to increase joint play movements neces-

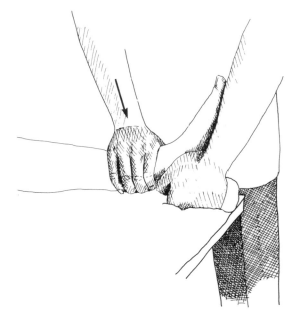

Fig. 7-38. Posterior glide of the tibia on talus of ankle mortice joint (left foot)

Fig. 7-39. Posterior glide of the talus on tibia of ankle mortice joint

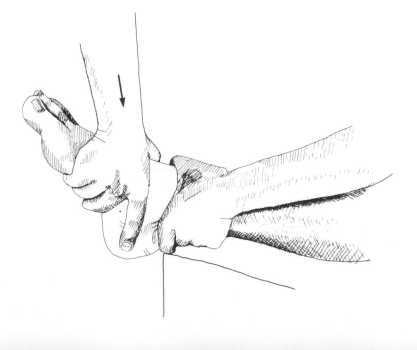

sary for plantar flexion at the ankle mortice joint.

3. *The Ankle Mortice Joint*—Posterior glide of the talus on the tibia (Fig. 7-39)

P—Supine, with the calcaneus hanging over the end of the plinth

O—Stabilizes the distal tibia against the plinth by grasping it with the left hand, wrapping the fingers around posteriorly. The left forearm rests over the dorsum of the patient's lower leg to prevent it from rising up from the plinth during the movement. He contacts the neck of the talus dorsally with the web of the right hand, bringing the thumb around laterally and the index finger medially. The remaining three fingers of the right hand wrap around the sole of the foot for support and control of the degree of plantar flexion.

M—The right hand moves the talus posteriorly on the tibia.

This technique is used to increase a joint play movement necessary for ankle dorsiflexion.

4. *The Subtalar Joint*—distraction (not illustrated)

This is performed in the same manner as distraction at the ankle mortice (see Technique 1), except the dorsal handhold moves distally to contact the navicular. In this way the calcaneus is distracted from the talus via the navicular and cuboid.

5. *The Subtalar Joint*—Valgus tilt (eversion) (Fig. 7-40)

P—Supine, with the knee flexed to about 90°, the hip flexed and somewhat abducted

O—Assumes the same position as for distraction (Fig. 37-A) and grasps the ankle so that the thumb pads contact the medial aspect of the calcaneus and the remaining finger pads contact laterally, just proximal to the calcaneus and level with the sinus tarsi.

M—A valgus tilt of the calcaneus is imparted by ulnar deviation of the wrists, transmitting the force through the thumb pads. The finger pads act as a fulcrum about which the movement occurs.

This technique is used to increase eversion at the subtalar joint.

6. *The Subtalar Joint*—Varus tilt (inversion) (Fig. 7-41)

This is carried out in the same manner as valgus tilt (see Technique 5). The operator's thumb pads move just prox-

Fig. 7-40. Valgus tilt (eversion)

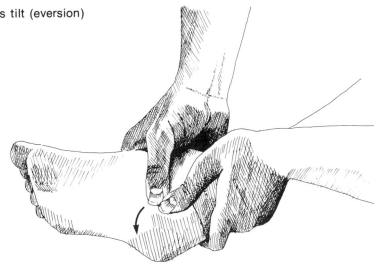

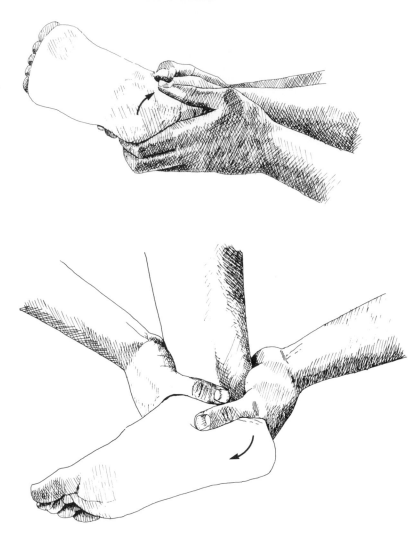

Fig. 7-41. Varus tilt (inversion) of subtalar joint

Fig. 7-42. Dorsal rock of the calcaneus on the talus of subtalar joint

imal to the calcaneus; the finger pads move distally to contact the calcaneus laterally. The finger pads move the calcaneus into inversion about a fulcrum created by the thumb pads.

This technique is used to increase inversion at the subtalar joint.

7. *The Subtalar Joint*—Dorsal rock of the calcaneus on the talus (Fig. 7-42)

   P—Supine, with the knee flexed to about 90°, the hip flexed and somewhat abducted

   O—Assumes the same position as for distraction (Fig. 37-A) and stabi-

lizes the talus dorsally with the web of the right hand, wrapping the thumb around medially and the fingers laterally. He contacts the upper border of the calcaneus posteriorly with the web of his left hand in a similar fashion.

M—While the right hand stabilizes the talus, the left hand rocks the calcaneus forward and dorsally. **Note:** According to Mennell, a small amount of movement must occur at the subtalar joint at the extremes of plantar flexion and dor-

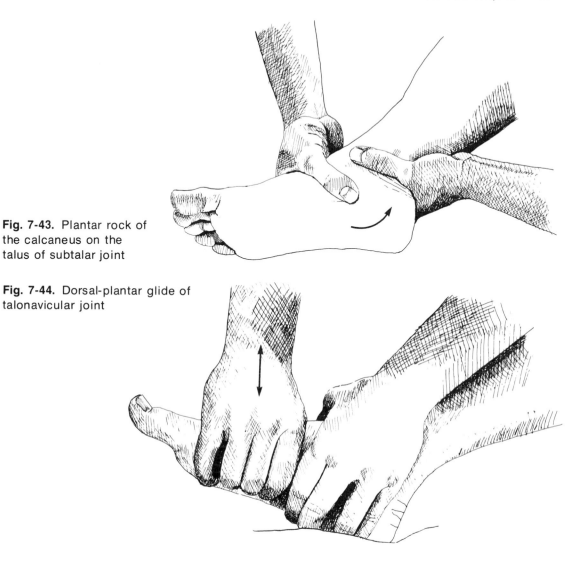

Fig. 7-43. Plantar rock of the calcaneus on the talus of subtalar joint

Fig. 7-44. Dorsal-plantar glide of talonavicular joint

siflexion. This, and the following technique, have been developed to restore that movement. [12]

8. *The Subtalar Joint*—Plantar rock of the calcaneus on the talus (Fig. 7-43)

This is carried out in the same manner as dorsal rock (see Technique 7), except the handholds are changed so that the right hand moves down to contact the navicular. The navicular tubercle is used as a landmark. The left hand moves just proximal to the posterior aspect of the calcaneus. The right hand rocks the calcaneus backward and plantarly via the navicular and cuboid. The web of the left hand acts as a fulcrum about which movement occurs.

THE FOOT

1. *The Talonavicular Joint*—Dorsal-plantar glide (Fig. 7-44)

P—Supine, with the knee bent to about 60°, the heel resting on the plinth

O—The left hand fixes the calcaneus and talus to the plinth by grasping dorsally at the level of the talar neck, the thumb wrapping around laterally, and the rest of the fingers medially. The right hand grasps the navicular, using the navicular tubercle as a landmark. The web and the thumb contact dorsally, and the hand and fingers wrap around the foot medially and plantarly.

M—As the left hand stabilizes and prevents movement at the ankle, the right hand may move the navicular dorsally or plantarly on the talus.

This technique is used to increase joint play at the forefoot.

2. *The Naviculocuneiform Joint*—Dorsal-plantar glide (Fig. 7-45)

This is performed in the same manner as dorsal-plantar glide at the talonavicular joint (see Technique 1) with the handholds moved distally. The left hand stabilizes the navicular while the right hand moves the cuneiforms.

This technique is used to increase joint play at the forefoot.

3. *The Cuneiform-Metatarsal Joints*—Dorsal-plantar glide (not illustrated)

This technique is also performed in the same manner as for the talonavicular joint with the handholds shifted

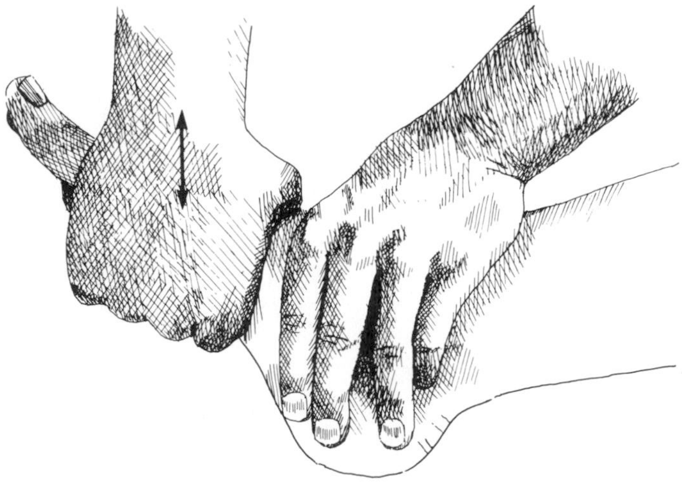

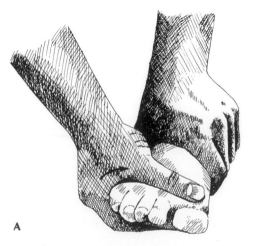

Fig. 7-45. Dorsal-plantar glide of naviculocuneiform joint

Fig. 7-46. (Below) Rotation of cuneiform-metatarsal and cuboid-metatarsal joints: (*A*) pronation and (*B*) supination

A

B

distally. The right hand grasps the cuneiforms and provides stabilization while the left hand moves the metatarsal joints.

This technique, like the Techniques 1 and 2 for the talonavicular and naviculocuneiform joints, is used to increase joint play of the forefoot.

4. *The Cuneiform-Metatarsal and Cuboid-Metatarsal Joints*—Rotation (pronation and supination) (Fig. 7-46)

P—Supine, with the knee bent to about 70°, the heel resting on the plinth

O—Stabilizes the cuneiforms and cuboids with the left hand, the thumb wrapping around the foot dorsally, the fingers plantarly.

a) For pronation, the operator's right hand grasps the proximal metatarsal shafts from the lateral aspect, with the thumb contacting dorsally and the fingers plantarly. His forearm is supinated. (See Fig. 7-46,*A*)

b) For supination, the operator's right hand grasps the proximal metatarsal shafts from the medial aspect, with the thumb contacting dorsally and the fingers plantarly. His forearm is pronated. (See Fig. 7-46,*B*)

M—The right hand rotates the metatarsals, as a unit, into pronation or supination.

These techniques are used to restore pronation and supination to the forefoot.

The remaining joints of the foot—the intermetatarsals, the metatarsal-phalangeals, and the interphalangeals may be mobilized in the same manner as that described for the corresponding joints of the hands. Specific intertarsal movements, *e.g.*, between cuboid and calcaneus, cuboid and navicular, etc., may be produced in a similar manner as specific intercarpal movements used for the hand.[7,18]

REFERENCES

1. Burke GL: Backache from Occiput to Coccyx. Vancouver, MacDonald, 1964
2. Cookson JC, Kent BE: Orthopedic manual therapy—An overview. Phys Ther 59:136–146, 1979
3. Cyriax J: Textbook of Orthopedic Medicine, Vol 1, Diagnosis of Soft Tissue Lesions, 5th ed. Baltimore, Williams & Wilkins, 1969
4. Cyriax J: Textbook of Orthopedic Medicine, Vol 2, Treatment by Manipulation, Massage and Injection, 8th ed., Baltimore, Williams & Wilkins, 1971
5. Fisher AGT: Treatment by Manipulation, 5th ed. New York, Paul B. Hoeber, 1948
6. Hood W: On so-called bone-setting: Its nature and results. Lancet 7:344–349, 1871
7. Kaltenborn FM: Manual Therapy for the Extremity Joints, 2nd ed. Oslo, Olaf Norlis Bokhandel, 1976
8. Maigne R: Orthopedic Medicine. Springfield, IL, Charles C Thomas, 1972
9. Maitland GD: Vertebral Manipulations. London, Butterworth & Co, 1964
10. Marlin T: Manipulative Treatment for the General Practitioner. London, Edward Arnold & Co, 1934
11. Mennell JB: The Science and Art of Joint Manipulation. London, J & A Churchill, 1949
12. Mennell JMcM: Joint Pain. Boston, Little, Brown & Co, 1964
13. Mixter WJ, Barr JS: Rupture of the intervertebral disc with involvement of the spinal canal. New Engl J Med 211:210–215, 1934
14. Nwuga VC: Manipulation of the Spine. Baltimore, Williams & Wilkins, 1976
15. Paris SV: The Spinal Lesion. Christ Church, New Zealand, Pegasus Press, 1965
16. Smith RL: At Your Own Risk: The Case Against Chiropractice. New York, Trident Press, 1969
17. Stoddard A: Manual of Osteopathic Technique. London, Hutchinson, 1978
18. Svendsen B: Joint Mobilization Laboratory Manual. Loma Linda, CA, Loma Linda University, 1979
19. Webster GV: Concerning Osteopathy. Norwood, MA, Plimpton Press, 1921

8 Automobilization Techniques of the Extremities

Darlene Hertling

Automobilization (self-mobilization) techniques are specific joint mobilization procedures that the patient himself performs. These passive exercises to maintain or increase joint mobility must be carefully taught to the patient.

Automobilization techniques of the spine were well known prior to 1975 through the work of Kaltenborn and his school. Then in 1975 the first of a series of articles by Rohde on automobilization techniques of the extremities appeared in East Germany. Automobilization techniques were first investigated and developed at the Fochkrankenhaus und Forschungsinstitut für Physiotherapie, Mahlow. [12-15] The extremity techniques described place emphasis on increasing capsular extensibility in order to restore painless range of motion to a joint. The primary indication for these techniques is painful limitation of joint movement due to loss of capsular extensibility.

Traditional home programs have, for the most part, stressed active or passive motions (performed at times with a wand or pulley) that are often poorly controlled by the patient, thus leading to further pain and stiffness. [3,11] According to Rohde, these techniques often compress the joint surfaces while having little or no effect on the joint capsule. [12,14] The logical and most effective approach in the management of capsular restriction is increasing capsular extensibility through techniques applied directly to the joint. Among the advantages cited by Rohde are the following:

—Major emphasis is placed on a pain-free position at the end of a range, in which mobilization can be most effective with regards to capsular stretch.
—Often the patient can control pain more easily than the therapist can.
—The patient can perform automobilizations several times a day independently. This reduces the time and expense of formal treatment sessions in a physical therapy department.
—Increased range of motion is possible without excessive force.
—No—or minimal—equipment is required, but if needed, is usually available in the home.
—The techniques are simple, easy to apply, and are not time consuming.

Furthermore, it is probable that the oscillatory nature of the techniques reduces pain by increasing proprioceptive input to "the gate." [1,9,10] (See Chapter 3, Pain.)

Some of the disadvantages of automobilization techniques would appear to include the following:

—Some of the positions that the patient must assume in order to employ automobilizations are awkward and often difficult if there is limitation or pain elsewhere (*e.g.*, spine or other joints).
—The variety of techniques is somewhat limited for some joints, such as the hip, because of poor accessibility. Some techniques may not be possible or are poorly managed at certain joints.
—Automobilization techniques of the finger joints require that the patient be able to stabilize one part and mobilize another with the same hand. This is somewhat difficult though not impossible.
—The movements cannot be observed once the patient is independent, and he may fail to carry out the techniques correctly.

ROHDE'S PRINCIPLES FOR AUTOMOBILIZATION OF THE EXTREMITIES

For most automobilization techniques, the patient either holds one part of the extremity from movement or provides a fulcrum over which movement can take place. Mobilization is carried out by the patient's hand, or in some cases, by use of his body weight. Rohde's approach is a form of oscillatory treatment, similar to Maitland's approach (9). It employs movements that are smooth and regular. These gentle rhythmic oscillations are performed at the end of motion 10 to 20 times (1 or 2 oscillations per second, or up to 3 to 4 per second in chronic conditions) without using excessive force. The basic rules for automobilizations are essentially the same as those for other mobilization tech-

niques. (See the descriptions in Chapter 7, Joint Mobilization Techniques.)

—The part must be completely relaxed if treatment is to be effective.
—The handgrip (or stabilizing belt) should be firm but should not produce pain.
—The patient's position must be comfortable, easy to maintain, and must allow complete control of the movements.

According to Rohde it is also important that

—The patient know the goals and principles of automobilization thoroughly.
—The patient be well motivated.
—The techniques be precise, easy to understand, and simple in nature.[12,14]
—The patient be seen periodically to determine if the techniques are being carried out correctly and are effective. They should be discontinued once normal range is achieved.

In general, automobilization is indicated in subacute or chronic painful conditions of the joints that have resulted in a capsular pattern of restriction, and for which restoration of range of motion appears possible. Rohde lists the following indications and contraindications:[12]

Indications
Arthrosis (*e.g.*, degenerative joint disease)
Chronic inflammatory diseases of the joints (*e.g.*, chronic polyarthritis or monarticular rheumatoid arthritis)
Sudeck-Leriche syndrome (reflex sympathetic dystrophy)
Postimmobilization stiffness (*e.g.*, following casting)
Capsular atrophy (*e.g.*, hemiplegia)

Contraindications
Hypermobility
Acute inflammatory conditions or very painful conditions in which the end point cannot be reached without pain. (Gentle tractions may be useful, however.)

Patients with limited intelligence or who are very awkward

Advanced cerebrosclerosis

PRACTICAL PROCEDURE

It is important that both the history and the physical examination be carried out (see Chapter 4, Assessment of Musculoskeletal Disorders). The examination might include the neighboring joints as well as relevant spinal levels. From this examination you should determine where to place emphasis in treatment and the general treatment approach (*e.g.*, mobilizations, manipulations, and/or soft-tissue techniques).

Automobilizations are usually started after the acute phase, but this will vary somewhat with the nature of the pathology. Usually a 2-week training period is required, after which the patient can become independent. Frequent re-evaluations are necessary. The frequency and intensity of automobilizations should correspond to the patient's condition and clinical picture. In chronic conditions, it is recommended that these techniques be carried out one to two times initially. They may be increased gradually to three or more times daily. In subacute conditions, three times weekly is suggested. [12]

Prior to automobilization, some form of heat or cold may be used, such as mild moist heat for subacute conditions, and more intense heat for chronic conditions (*e.g.*, hot packs if given at home). For certain joints, such as those of the hand and foot, the elbow or the knee, some of the techniques may be carried out in a warm bath. This is not practical for the shoulder or hip joint. Frequently, additional treatment of the soft tissue may be indicated. Rohde suggests the following: [12]

Self-massage (*e.g.*, the upper trapezius in shoulder joint problems)

PNF techniques (*e.g.*, hold-relax techniques to reduce muscle tightness and encourage relaxation) [7]

Isometric exercises (*e.g.*, for muscle weakness)

Pendulum or free swinging exercises with a weight, as advocated by Rössler and Kohlrausch, to increase range of motion and permit relaxation. [8,16] Although these exercises are somewhat similar to Codman's pendulum exercises for the shoulder, exercises for the trunk and lower extremity are also described. [2] In addition they incorporate relaxation techniques similar to those of Jacobson. [5]

In general, automobilization techniques should begin with distraction or inferior glide techniques. These are particularly useful in the early stages for managing pain (gentle traction may even be started in the acute phase) and prior to other automobilization techniques. A particularly effective variation is the use of hold-relax techniques applied directly before a specific automobilization. [7] These techniques, in which the patient performs an isometric contraction of the antagonists in order to reflexively inhibit a particular muscle group, are particularly useful just before shoulder automobilizations into internal and external rotation. Automobilization techniques are gradually added to the patient's program, based on the ongoing clinical evaluation. For example, following distraction or inferior glide techniques at the shoulder, the patient would incorporate flexion, extension, and internal rotation techniques. Finally abduction and external rotation techniques, which are more likely to produce pain and spasm, would be added.

Once the basic principles of mobilization and automobilization techniques are understood, the therapist can create any number of automobilization techniques and exercises. [4] Examples of shoulder joint techniques that you can design follow. In general, you should begin with inferior glide or distraction, emphasizing caudal shift of the humeral head in the glenoid cavity. Although automobilization techniques of the foot and hand have been described by Rohde, we will limit our discussion to those of the major large joints.[13] Only a few of the more important techniques of the elbow, knee, and hip will be described.

AUTOMOBILIZATION TECHNIQUES FOR THE SHOULDER

1. *Inferior Glide*—Long axis extension (Fig. 8-1)
    E—A high back chair that is well padded with a blanket or towel on the back of the chair
    P—Sitting, with the right arm over the back of the chair, the axilla firmly fixed over the back of chair
    MH—grasps the arm just proximal to the humeral epicondyles so as to gain a purchase on them. An alternate handhold would be to grasp the forearm just above the styloid processes.
    M—An inferior glide is produced by pulling directly downward toward the floor while employing rhythmic oscillations (Fig. 8-1A).
    Note: A variation of this technique, which Rohde tested, is to use a weight in the hand (*e.g.*, a bucket of sand) and to perform gentle pivotlike motions at the end (Fig. 8-1,*B*).
2. *Inferior Glide*—Shoulder adduction with distraction ventrally (Fig. 8-2)
    E—A firm pillow or towel roll placed in the axilla
    P—Standing, with the arm positioned across the chest
    MH—Grasps the forearm just above the styloid processes. MH pulls the arm rhythmically across the chest (into adduction) and downwards, resulting in a slight separation of the head of the humerus in the glenoid cavity (Fig. 8-2,*A*).
    Note: Distraction dorsally may be carried out in a similar fashion if the patient has sufficient internal rotation to place his forearm behind his back. In this case, the elbow is flexed and the MH employs rhythmic oscillations behind the patient's back in a downward direction dorsally (Fig. 8-2,*B*).
3. *Inferior Glide*—Shoulder abduction when the patient has less than 90° of abduction (Fig. 8-3)
    P—Sitting sideways to a table, the right arm is positioned comfortably at the end of painless abduction with the muscles relaxed.

Note: For the sake of simplicity, all of the techniques to be described in this chapter are applied to the patient's *right* extremity, except where indicated. In the automobilization techniques, the left hand usually will be performing the mobilizations. (E—equipment; P—patient; MH—mobilizing hand; M—movement)

Fig. 8-1. Inferior glide (long axis extension) of glenohumeral joint may be performed (*A*) manually or (*B*) by using a weight.

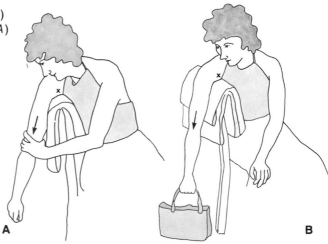

A   B

The elbow is extended with the hand, and the forearm is fixed on the table.

MH—Contacts the anterior, superior aspect of the proximal humerus below the acromion

M—An inferior glide is produced by pushing directly downward toward the floor, with rhythmic oscillations.

4. *Inferior Glide*—Shoulder abduction when the patient has more than 90° of abduction (Fig. 8-4)

P—Standing with the right side facing a wall. The arm is positioned, comfortably, in abduction so that the forearm rests on the wall, with the elbow in 90° of flexion.

MH—Contacts the anterior, superior aspect of the proximal end of the humerus below the acromion.

M—An inferior glide is produced by pushing directly downward toward the floor, with rhythmic oscillations. A stronger capsular stretch can be employed by bending the knees and using body weight to assist in the movement.

5. *Inferior Glide* (shoulder flexion)—When the patient has less than 90° of flexion (Fig. 8-5)

P—Sitting facing a table. The right

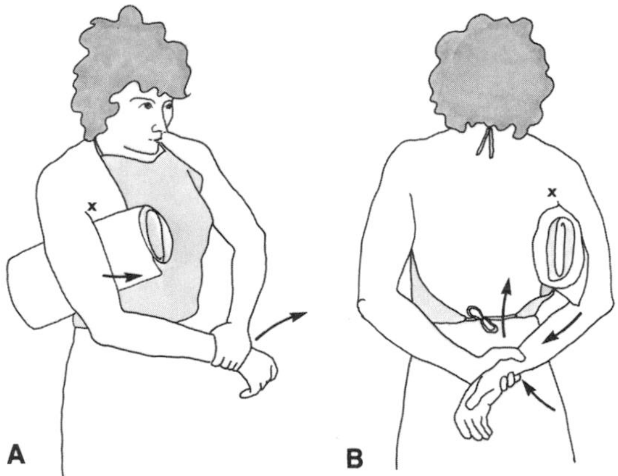

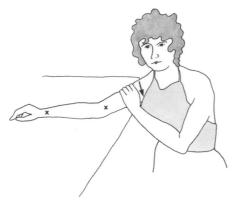

A **B**

Fig. 8-2. Inferior glide of glenohumeral joint: (*A*) shoulder adduction with distraction ventrally; (*B*) shoulder adduction with distraction dorsally

Fig. 8-3. Inferior glide (shoulder abduction for 90° or less abduction) of glenohumeral joint

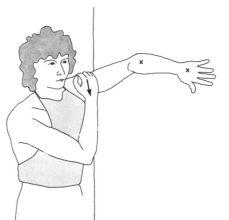

Fig. 8-4. Inferior glide (shoulder abduction for 90° or more abduction) of glenohumeral joint (left arm)

Fig. 8-5. Inferior glide (shoulder flexion for 90° or less flexion) of glenohumeral joint

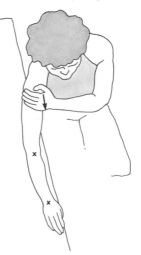

forearm is positioned comfortably at the end of painless flexion with the muscles relaxed. A pillow wedge is used under the forearm to provide fixation of the hand and forearm.

MH—Contacts the anterior, superior aspect of the proximal humerus below the acromion.

M—An inferior glide is produced by pushing directly downward toward the floor, with rhythmic oscillations.

6. *Inferior Glide* (shoulder flexion)—When the patient has more than 90° of flexion (Fig. 8-6)

P—Standing facing a wall. The right forearm, with the elbow bent to 90° of flexion, is positioned at the end of range on the wall for fixation.

MH—Contacts the anterior superior aspect of the proximal end of the humerus below the acromion.

M—An anterior glide is produced by pushing directly downward toward the floor, with rhythmic oscillations. A stronger capsular stretch may be employed by lowering the body weight.

7. *Anterior Glide*—Shoulder extension (Fig. 8-7)

P—Sitting, with the back to a table.

The right arm is positioned comfortably at the limits of painless extension with the muscles relaxed. The elbow is extended with the right hand fixed on the table. The trunk is in a flexed position.

MH—Contacts the posterior superior aspect of the proximal humerus just below the acromion.

M—An anterior glide is produced by moving the arm in a ventral caudal direction, with rhythmic oscillations.

8. *Shoulder Internal Rotation* (Fig. 8-8)

P—Sitting sideways to a table. The right upper arm is positioned so that its entire extent is braced against the table. To do this the patient bends his trunk to the side toward the upper arm. The elbow is bent to 90° of flexion.

MH—Grasps the dorsal aspect of the wrist with the thumb, and the fingers wrapped around the ventral aspect.

M—The arm is internally rotated as far as possible with rhythmic oscillations carried out at the end of range.

9. *Shoulder External Rotation* (Fig. 8-9)

P—Sitting sideways to a table. The right upper arm is positioned so

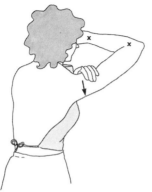

Fig. 8-6. Inferior glide (shoulder flexion for 90° or more flexion) of glenohumeral joint

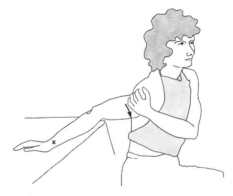

Fig. 8-7. Anterior glide (shoulder extension) of glenohumeral joint

that its entire extent is braced against the table. To do this the patient bends his trunk to the side toward the upper arm. The elbow is bent to 90° of flexion.

MH—Grasps the ventral aspect of the wrist.

M—The forearm is externally rotated, and rhythmic oscillations carried out at the end of range.

Note: Hold-relax techniques are particularly useful with rotation techniques of the shoulder.

AUTOMOBILIZATION TECHNIQUES FOR THE ELBOW

1. *Humeroulnar Joint* —Medial-lateral tilt (sidebending oscillations) (Fig. 8-10)

    P—Standing in a doorway with the right forearm and hand fixed against the wall. The elbow is in slight flexion or close to the limit of extension.

    MH—Grasps the upper arm near the humeral epicondyles.

    M—Keeping the forearm stationary, the MH moves the humerus medially or laterally, affecting a medial or lateral tilt of the humeroulnar joint.

2. *Humeroulnar Joint Distraction in Flexion* (Fig. 8-11)

    P—Sitting, with the shoulder abducted to 90°. The upper arm is supported on a table (kitchen counter is usually a good height). The elbow is flexed over a firm pillow or towel roll.

    MH—Is placed over the lower arm and dorsum of hand

    M—Slow, gentle, oscillating movements are performed downward in the direction of flexion.

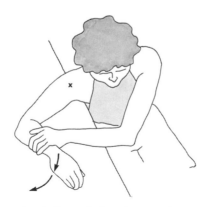

Fig. 8-8. Internal rotation of glenohumeral joint

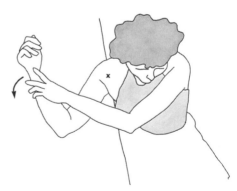

Fig. 8-9. External rotation of glenohumeral joint

Fig. 8-10. Medial-lateral tilt (sidebending oscillations) of humeroulnar joint

Fig. 8-11. Distraction in flexion of humeroulnar joint

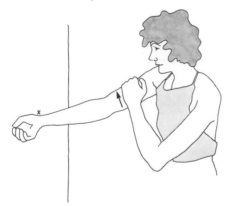

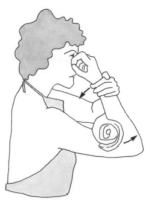

AUTOMOBILIZATION TECHNIQUES FOR THE KNEE

1. *Femorotibial Joint*—Valgus tilt (Fig. 8-12)

    E—A study couch or chair moved slightly away from a wall

    P—Stands on the right side of the chair with his back to the wall. The right foot is placed on the seat of the chair with support on the medial aspect of the foot to provide fixation. The posterior aspect of the thigh should be in contact with the back of chair, and the buttocks in contact with the wall for additional support. The hip should be in slight flexion so that it is not locked in extension.

    MH—The patient leans his trunk well forward so that his left forearm will be in line with the direction of movement. The forearm is supinated, with the heel of the left hand contacting the lateral aspect of the femoral and tibial condyles. The fingers wrap around the knee posteriorly for additional support.

    M—The left hand gently moves the knee into valgus tilt, taking care to avoid any flexion or extension of the knee.

Note: Varus tilt may be carried out in the reverse fashion.

2. *Femorotibial Joint*—Forced (gentle) flexion (Fig. 8-13)

    P—Supine, lying with the hip flexed slightly above 90°. The knee is flexed over a firm pillow or towel roll which acts as a fulcrum.

    MH—Both hands contact the lower leg over the anterior aspect with the fingers interlaced.

    M—Gentle flexion, with oscillations, is performed.

Note: Forced flexion may also be done in a sitting position. The right hip is completely flexed so that the thigh is supported on the chest. The knee is flexed over the right forearm, which now acts as a fulcrum and gives additional support. The left MH contacts the lower leg over the anterior aspect and carries out gentle flexion of the knee.

3. *The Patellofemoral Joint*—Medial-lateral glide (not illustrated)

    P—Long-sitting on a firm cot or the floor, with the knee slightly flexed over a firm pillow or towel roll. (A sitting position in a chair may be used, with the leg ex-

Fig. 8-12. Valgus tilt of femorotibial joint

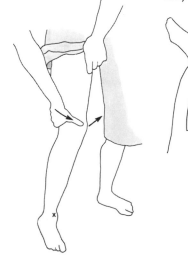

Fig. 8-13. Posterior glide (gentle forced flexion) of femorotibial joint (left leg)

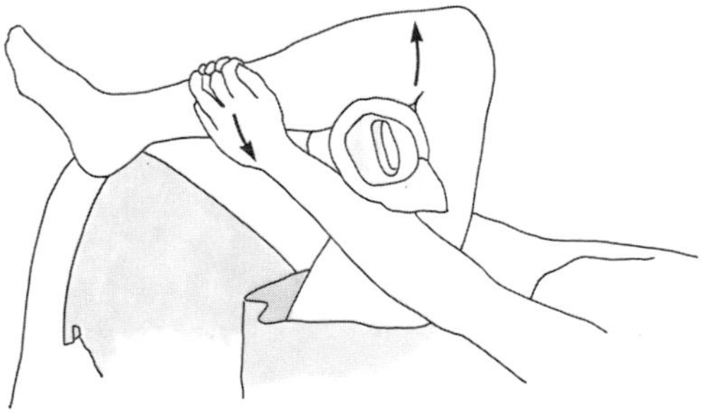

tended and the knee slightly flexed and the foot fixed to the floor.)

MH—Both thumb pads contact the lateral or medial patellar border. The remaining fingers rest over the anterior aspect of the patient's leg. The elbows are extended as much as possible.

M—A medial or lateral glide of the patella can be imparted by leaning the trunk forward and to one side. The movement is performed by movement of the trunk rather than any part of the hand. (See the description in Chapter 7, Joint Mobilization Techniques.)

Note: Superior-inferior glide may also be performed by contact of the thumb pads on the superior or inferior borders of the patella, with the rest of the hand resting over the medial and lateral aspects of the knee.

AUTOMOBILIZATION TECHNIQUES FOR THE HIP

1. *Inferior Glide or Long Axis Extension* (Fig. 8-14)

E—A comfortable, snug-fitting ankle strap and a stationary wall- or table-hook for attachment to the ankle strap.

P—Supine, the right leg extended, and the ankle strap attached to the end of table- or wall-hook. The left lower extremity is flexed, with the foot on the table or floor.

M—The left leg pushes downward and upward to push the body away from the fixed point, thus transmitting a traction force on the right lower extremity.

2. *Distraction in Sidelying* (Fig. 8-15)

This particular technique, described by Rohde, represents a combination of distraction and a muscle strengthening exercise.[12] In this case, the gluteus medius, which is commonly weak in most hip conditions, is exercised.

P—Lying on the right side, close to one side of a table. A firm pillow or blanket roll is placed between the legs in the groin area. The left hip is extended at the hip with the lower leg off the edge of the table. A sandbag or ankle cuff with a weight is applied to the left ankle.

M—The left leg is actively raised against the pull of the weight and held for a few seconds; the patient then relaxes, allowing the leg to fall into adduction, with the hip in slight extension, over the edge of the table. Slight oscillatory motion will occur naturally at the end of range.

Fig. 8-14. Inferior glide (long axis extension) of hip joint

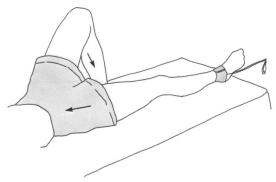

Fig. 8-15. Distraction (sidelying) of hip joint (left leg)

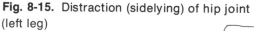
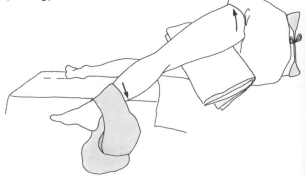

PASSIVE EXERCISE

Additional exercises that are particularly useful in a home program for painful extremity joints have been advocated by Dontigny and Grimsby. [3,4] They allow the patient to passively stretch his own joints by moving the body in relationship to the stabilized extremity. The principle of moving the body in relationship to the stabilized extremity affords an excellent stretch, minimizes incorrect movements by the patient, and allows for a greater degree of pain-free movement. Grimsby maintains that when used for the hip, shoulder, and ankle, the patient uses the concave surface of the joint to mobilize. By so doing, the patient avoids considerable pain and achieves a greater range of motion, since rolling and gliding occur in the same direction. [4] It would also appear—if we compare these exercises to the traditional approach of movement of the extremity in relationship to the body—that using a closed kinetic chain (through the stabilized extremity) provides greater stability of the joint as well as a more normal pattern of movement. Examples of these types of exercises are described for the shoulder.

PASSIVE SHOULDER EXERCISES

1. *Shoulder Flexion*
   a. *Sitting* (Fig. 8-16)
      P—Sits at side of table with the forearm resting on table
      M—Patient flexes trunk and head while sliding the arm forward along the edge of table so that the shoulder is moved passively into flexion.
   b. *Standing* (Fig. 8-17)
      P—Stands facing a high counter top (or high window ledge or bookshelf). He rests his hand,

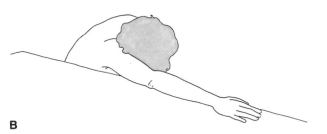

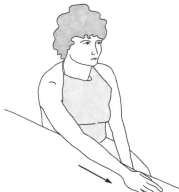

Fig. 8-16. Passive shoulder flexion (sitting): (*A*) starting position; (*B*) end position

Fig. 8-17. Passive shoulder flexion (standing): (*A*) starting position; (*B*) end position

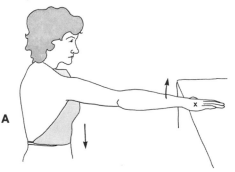

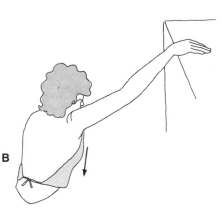

palm down, on the edge of the counter with the elbow extended.

M—The patient lowers his body weight to move the shoulder passively into flexion.

2. *Shoulder Extension* (Fig. 8-18)

P—Stands with his right side to the table and positions the right hand on the table, with the arm at the side and the elbow extended.

M—Maintaining the right hand in a fixed position on the table, he walks forward to impart shoulder extension through the painless range of motion available.

Alternate Technique (Fig. 8-19)

P—Stands with his back to table and grasps the edge of table with both hands.

M—The patient then lowers his body weight as he allows the elbows to flex and the shoulders to extend.

3. *Shoulder Abduction*

a. *Sitting* (Fig. 8-20)

P—Sits at side of a table and rests his forearm on the table, with the forearm supinated and the shoulder slightly abducted.

M—The patient sidebends the upper trunk to the left from the waist while sliding the arm across the

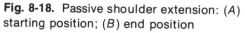

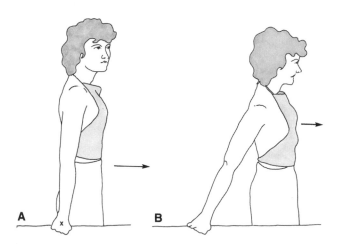

Fig. 8-18. Passive shoulder extension: (*A*) starting position; (*B*) end position

Fig. 8-19. Alternate technique for passive shoulder extension: (*A*) starting position; (*B*) end position

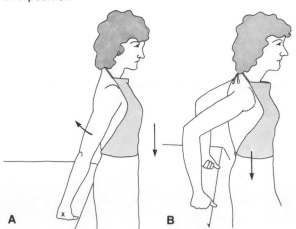

Fig. 8-20. Passive shoulder abduction (sitting): (*A*) starting position; (*B*) end position (left arm)

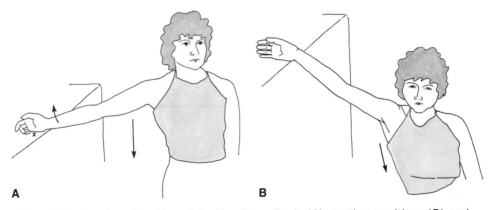

Fig. 8-21. Passive shoulder abduction (standing): (*A*) starting position; (*B*) end position

table so that the shoulder is moved into abduction as the lower trunk moves away from the table.

b. *Standing* (Fig. 8-21)

　P—Stands with his right side facing a high counter top (or high window ledge or bookshelf). He rests his hand on the surface with the forearm slightly supinated, elbow extended, and shoulder abducted through partial range.

　M—The patient lowers his body weight, allowing his shoulder to move passively into abduction and external rotation.

4. *Shoulder Internal Rotation* (Fig. 8-22)

　P—Stands with his left side toward a door frame. He places the back of his hand against the frame so that it will remain fixed with his elbow flexed to 90°. The upper arm remains at the side with the elbow held close to the trunk.

　M—The patient then walks forward as he rotates toward his left forearm to impart passive internal rotation to the shoulder.

Alternate Technique (Fig. 8-23)

　P—Stands with his back to the table and grasps the edge of the table with both hands

　M—The patient lowers his body weight

slowly, allowing the elbows to bend and the shoulders to abduct and internally rotate.

5. *Shoulder External Rotation*

　a. *Sitting* (Fig. 8-24)

　　P—Sits at the side of the table with the forearm resting on the table, the shoulder abducted, and the elbow flexed

　　M—The patient flexes his trunk and head forward toward the table allowing the shoulder to be moved passively into external rotation.

　b. *Standing* (Fig. 8-25)

　　P—Stands facing a door frame. He

Fig. 8-22. Passive internal rotation of shoulder: (*A*) starting position; (*B*) end position (left arm)

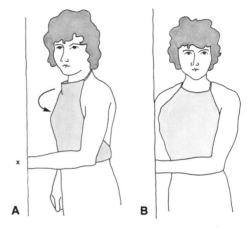

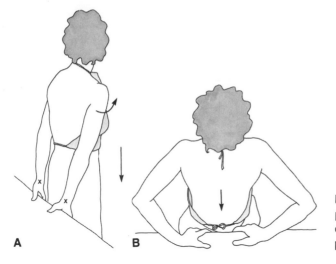

A   B

Fig. 8-23. Alternate technique for passive internal rotation of shoulder: (*A*) starting position; (*B*) end position

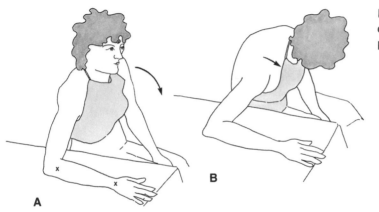

B

A

Fig. 8-24. Passive external rotation of shoulder (sitting): (*A*) starting position; (*B*) end position

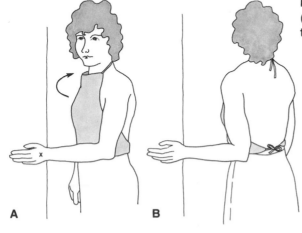

A   B

Fig. 8-25. Passive external rotation of shoulder (standing): (*A*) starting position; (*B*) end position (left arm)

places the palmar surface of his hand against the frame so that it will remain fixed. The elbow is flexed to 90°. The upper arm remains at the side with the elbow held close to the trunk.

M—The patient walks backwards, rotating his body away from his left arm to impart passive external rotation to the shoulder.

Similar exercises can be designed for the hip (such as in the "all fours" or crawling position) and for other extremity joints.

REFERENCES

1. Casey KL, Melzack R: Neural Mechanism of Pain: A Conceptual model. In Way EL (ed): New Concepts in Pain and Its Clinical Management. Philadelphia, F A Davis, 1967
2. Codman EA: The Shoulder. Boston, Thomas Todd Co, 1934
3. Dontigny RL: Passive Shoulder Exercises. Journal of the American Physical Therapy Association 50:1707, 1970
4. Grimsby O: Personal communication, 1977
5. Jacobson E: Progressive Relaxation. Chicago, University of Chicago Press, 1938
6. Knott M, Voss D: Proprioceptive Neuromuscular Facilitation. New York, Harper & Row, 1973
7. Kohlrausch W, Kohlrausch A: Bewegungstherapie and Rehabilitation bei Erkrankungen der Extremitätengelenke. In Grober J, Stieve FE (eds): Handbuch der Physiokalischen Therapie, BD II/1. Stuttgart, Gustav Fischer Verlag, 1971
8. Lewit K: Manuelle Therapie (im Rahmen der ärtlichen Rehabilitation). Leipzig, J A Barth, 1973
9. Maitland G: Peripheral Manipulation. Butterworth & Scarborough, Ont., 1976
10. Melzack R, Wall PD: Pain Mechanisms: A New Theory. Science 150:971, 1965
11. Robins V: Should patients with hemiplegia wear a sling. Journal of the American Physical Therapy Association 49:1029, 1970
12. Rohde J: Die Automobilisation der Extremitätengelenke (I). Zeitschrift für Physiotherapie 27:57, 1975
13. Rohde J: Die Automobilisation der Extremitätengelenke (II). Zeitschrift für Physiotherapie 28:51, 1976
14. Rohde J: Die Automobilisation der Extremitätengelenke (III). Zeitschrift für Physiotherapie 28:121, 1976
15. Rohde J: Die Automobilisation der Extremitätengelenke (IV). Zeitschrift für Physiotherapie 28:427, 1976
16. Rössler H: Die Physikalische Therapie. Stuttgart, Gustav Fischer Verlag, 1968

9 Friction Massage

Randolph M. Kessler

Massage, as is true of most forms of manual therapy, is a method of treatment that has been viewed with considerable controversy by the medical community. The "Laying on the hands" of any sort tends to be associated with charlatanism. Its value, if any, is frequently felt to be of a psychological nature or the result of the placebo phenomenon. This attitude is not necessarily unfounded, for several reasons. First, those who have advocated the use of massage have often done so on the basis of nonscientific or nonphysiological mechanisms that the medically oriented professional cannot always accept. Reflex zones, trigger points, fibrocystic nodules, and meridians have all been identified as areas to which massage may be directed, but have never been identified as true anatomical or physiological entities. Secondly, there is little empirical or direct scientific evidence for the efficacy of massage. It tends to be used on the basis that it "seems to work"; it makes the patient feel better. So, while there is little question among clinicians who employ massage as a therapeutic measure that it has some value, its value is not well documented. This is primarily because massage is often used for the relief of painful conditions in which there are few associated pathological signs. This makes reliable measurement of the possible effects of treatment a difficult problem in research design and technology. Finally, the use of massage by lay practitioners, especially in situations of questionable moral standards, has contributed to the adverse connotations often associated with its use.

The result of the prevailing attitudes toward massage is that it is often not used in the treatment of some conditions for which it might have a significant therapeutic effect. Furthermore, massage is time-consuming, occasionally strenuous, often boring, and relatively costly. Therefore, the clinician as well as the patient may at times avoid it. On the other hand, massage is often employed in circumstances in which it is unnecessary or its therapeutic effect is questionable.

In order to avoid the inappropriate use of any treatment, the clinician should consider not only the objectives but how these objectives fit into the overall plan of management. Although for many conditions seen clinically our primary goal is long-term relief of pain we cannot necessarily justify the use of massage solely on the basis that it helps relieve pain. While massage may certainly provide *temporary* pain relief in many conditions, it does not necessarily contribute to the *long-term* relief of pain, which requires resolution of the pathologic state. The use of massage may meet objectives (*i.e.*, relief of pain) on a short-term basis, but may not contribute to meeting overall objectives since the temporary relief of pain may have little relationship with resolution of the pathology. When this is true, massage should not be used. Not only will it not help the patient to feel better, but because of its often pleasurable effects it may help reinforce the disease state. We suggested here that massage should be used only when the clinician can rationalize that its use contributes to resolving the physical pathology. Such a rationale should have a well-accepted physiological basis. The therapist can better expect that treatment of the pathology will relieve pain, rather than that relief of pain will improve the patient's condition.

There are several types of conditions for which a particular form of massage, when appropriately administered, may have a direct or indirect effect upon the pathological state. Deep stroking in the presence of certain edematous conditions may assist in the resolution of fluid accumulations. A variety of massage techniques can be used as a means of reflexly promoting muscle relaxation to allow for more effective mobilization of a part. This may certainly be useful when abnormal muscle tension is an important factor in the perpetuation of the pathology (see Chapter 10, Relaxation). Deep frictions and kneading types of massage may assist in restoring mobility between tissue interfaces or may increase extensibility of individual structures. Deep massage also tends to increase circulation to the area treated, which may be desirable in certain cases. These effects are generally well described in traditional massage textbooks, along with descriptions of related massage techniques.[2-4]

DEEP TRANSVERSE FRICTION MASSAGE

A particularly important massage technique in the management of many common musculoskeletal disorders is deep transverse friction massage. Its importance and the rationale and technique of application have not been well described in the traditional literature.

RATIONALE

As discussed under pathological considerations in Chapter 2, Arthrology, many of the chronic musculoskeletal disorders seen clinically are manifestations of the body's response to fatigue stresses. Tissues tend to respond to fatigue stresses by increasing the rate of tissue production. Thus, prolonged abnormal stresses to a tissue will be met with tissue hypertrophy, provided that the nutritional status of the tissue is not compromised and provided that the stress rate (the rate of tissue breakdown) does not exceed the rate at which the tissue can repair the microdamage. Under continuing stress, if nutrition to the tissue is effected or if the rate of tissue breakdown is excessive, the tissue will gradually atrophy and weaken to the point of eventual failure. Tissues that normally have a low metabolic rate—usually those that are relatively poorly vascularized—are most susceptible to such degeneration. Such tissues include articular cartilage, intra-articular fibrocartilage, tendons, and some ligaments. On the other hand, those tissues with good vascularity and a normally high rate of turnover, such as cancellous bone, muscle, capsular tissue, and some ligaments, are more likely to respond by undergoing hypertrophy. This results in increased density of the structural elements. Of course, even these structures may not be able to keep up with the rate of tissue breakdown if the stress rate is too high or under conditions of reduced nutrition (*e.g.*, hypovascularity).

Under conditions of mildly increased stress rates, the body has the ability to adapt adequately, and no pathological state (pain, inflammation, or dysfunction) results. Such conditions might even include situations of high-magnitude stresses if the high stress levels are induced gradually and the stresses are intermittent enough to allow an interval for adequate repair to take place. A typical example is the individual engaging in vigorous athletic activities who goes through a period of gradual training. The training period allows for adequate maturation of new tissue so that structural elements become oriented in ways that best attenuate energy without yielding. Such energy attenuation requires that there be a sufficient mass of tissue to provide some resistance to deformation, but it also requires that the structure be adequately extensible to minimize the strain on individual structural elements. To increase the ability of a structure to attenuate the energy of work done on it (a force tending to deform the structure), new collagen is produced to increase the tissues' total ability to resist the force. However, this new collagen must be sufficiently mobile to permit some deformation. The less it deforms, the greater the resistance the tissue must offer. The greater the resistance it must offer, the greater will be the internal strain on individual collagen fibers or bony trabeculae. The greater the strain on individual structural elements, the greater the rate of microdamage. As the rate of microdamage increases, so does the likelihood of pain and inflammation. As you can see, a more massive tissue is not necessarily one that will permit normal functioning under increased stress. It must also be deformable, and deformability requires time for the new structural elements (collagen fibers and bony trabeculae) to assume the proper "weave."

The effect of the weave, or orientation, of structural elements in contributing to the extensibility of a structure as a whole can be appreciated by examining a Chinese "finger trap" (Fig. 9-1). You can lengthen and shorten the finger trap without changing the length of any of the individual fibers composing it. Its extensibility is due entirely to the weave of the fibers and interfiber mobility. Thus, you can apply an extending force to the structure without inducing internal strain on any of the individual fibers. If the fibers were not in the proper weave or if they were to stick to one another, the deforming force would be met with greater resistance by the structure and greater internal strain to individual fibers. The body adapts to mildly increased stress rates by laying down collagen precursors which, in response to imposed stresses, polymerize into collagen fibers. The fibers become oriented in the

Fig. 9-1. A Chinese finger trap before and after being extended illustrates the extensibility of structural elements.

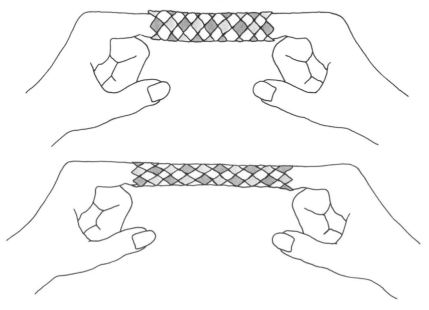

proper weave to allow deformability of the tissue.

Under abnormally high stress levels or under altered nutritional conditions, the body's attempt to adapt may be inadequate. The particular tissue may not be able to produce new tissue fast enough, or the new tissue that is produced does not have sufficient time, or is not properly induced, to mature. In the former situation, the tissue will degenerate, whereas in the latter, pain and inflammation are likely to result if stresses continue. Tissue degeneration must be treated by reducing stress levels, increasing nutrition to the tissue, or both, depending on the underlying cause. Typical examples of such tissue degeneration would include the degradation of articular cartilage in degenerative joint disease, and the lesions that commonly affect the soft tissues of the diabetic foot. Articular cartilage, being avascular and having a normally low metabolic turnover, does not adapt well to increased stress levels and is thus susceptible to fatigue degradation. The diabetic foot may have a nutritional deficit because of vascular changes, and possibly, increased stresses due to reduced sensory feedback, leaving it abnormally susceptible to tissue breakdown.

Situations in which the new tissue does not mature adequately are typically those in which the stress levels are not sufficient to cause degeneration but are too excessive to allow time for normal tissue modeling. In bone, the condition is referred to as *sclerosis*; in capsules, ligaments, and tendons, it may be referred to as *fibrosis*. In both situations there is often a normal or increased amount of tissue, but the tissue is not sufficiently deformable to attenuate the energy of loading from use of the part. This causes pain, inflammation, increased stresses to adjacent tissues, or some combination of these results. Correction of such conditions requires that stress levels be reduced while stresses sufficient to stimulate normal tissue modeling are maintained. In addition, normal extensi-

bility of the structure must be restored. This requires that interfiber mobility be increased. The nutritional status of the tissue must also be considered.

There are many common musculoskeletal disorders that might be considered pathologies related to abnormal or inadequate tissue modeling. Bony sclerosis typically occurs in degenerative joint disease when there are abnormal compressive stresses to a joint. Most tendinitis can be considered situations in which continued abnormal stresses to a tendon preclude adequate tissue modeling, creating a structure that is not sufficiently deformable. This is especially true of the condition often referred to as *tennis elbow*, in which the origin of the extensor carpi radialis brevis becomes fibrosed, and a chronic inflammatory process arises. Rotator cuff tendinitis, usually involving the supraspinatus or infraspinatus regions of the tendinous cuff, is a very common disorder in which normal modeling is compromised by hypovascularity to the area of involvement. Often these lesions at the shoulder progress to a stage at which gradual degeneration, and eventual failure ensue. It is likely that the capsular fibrosis associated with "frozen shoulder" is a similar disorder of tissue modeling; the joint capsule hypertrophies in response to increased stress levels, but in doing so loses its extensibility. Abnormal tissue modeling will also result when a tissue is immobilized during the repair phase of an inflammatory process. Thus, a fracture may "heal," but normal modeling of bony trabeculae requires resumption of normal stress levels. Similarly, a joint capsule will become fibrosed when the joint is immobilized following arthrotomy; collagen is layed down in response to the traumatic inflammatory process affecting the synovium, but the lack of movement permits an unorganized network of fibers that form abnormal interfiber bonds (adhesions) and that do not extend normally when the part is moved.

The approach to treatment of conditions in which continued stresses have not allowed the structure to mature adequately must include measures to reduce stresses to the part. We must consider means of reducing loading of the part as well as means of preventing excessive internal strain. Reduced loading might be accomplished through control of activities, the use of orthotic devices to control alignment or movement, or the use of assistive devices such as crutches. Also, to reduce loading of a particular tissue, the capacity of other tissues to attenuate more of the energy of loading might be increased. This is often done by increasing the strength and activities of related muscles. Thus, if we wish to reduce the likelihood of excessive loading of the anterior talofibular ligament, the peroneal muscles should be strengthened. However, we can also strap the ankle to provide additional afferent input to reflexly enhance the ability of the peroneals to contract.

Reduction of stress levels alone, however, will not assure that adequate maturation will take place. As mentioned earlier, stress to the part is a necessary stimulus for the restoration of normal alignment of structural elements. This apparent paradox is understood when we consider that reducing stress is necessary in order to allow new tissue to be layed down and reconstituted, while at the same time some stress is necessary to optimize the nutritional status of the part and to effect proper orientation and mobility of the new tissue. Consequently, in the case of most chronic musculoskeletal disorders, resolution is not likely to take place with complete rest of the part nor is it likely to take place with unrestricted use. A judgment must be made, then, as to what is the appropriate activity level for a particular disorder, and at what rate normal activities can be resumed. This judgment must be based upon data gained on examination that reflects the nature and extent of the pathology as well as etiologic con-

siderations. Knowledge of the healing responses of musculoskeletal tissues and of their responses to various stress conditions must also be applied.

In situations in which significant reduction of activities is necessary in order to allow for healing to occur, there are measures that the therapist can, and should, take. The therapist must help prevent undue dysfunction that may result from a mass of tissue being layed down as an unorganized, adherent cicatrix, and from the atrophy of related muscle groups that is likely to take place. There are few conditions, even of an acute inflammatory nature, in which some gentle range of motion exercises and isometric muscle exercises cannot be performed during the healing process without detrimental effects.

Some of the chronic disorders that tend to be the most persistent are minor lesions of tendons and ligaments. These are often refractory to such treatments as rest and anti-inflammatant therapy because they are not chronic inflammatory lesions *per se*, but pathologies resulting from abnormal modeling of tissue in response to fatigue stresses. Therefore, while rest allows new tissue to be produced, that which is produced is not of normal extensibility because of lack of a proper orientation of structural elements, abnormal adherence of structure elements to one another, and adherence to adjacent tissues. In some situations, most notably rotator cuff tendinitis at the shoulder, inadequate nutrition is also a factor. Because of the lack of extensibility that accompanies "healing" of these lesions, the structure becomes more susceptible to internal strain when stresses are resumed; it becomes less able to attenuate the energy of loads applied to it. The result is recurrence of a low-grade inflammatory process each time use of the part is resumed. The most common of these disorders are supraspinatus tendinitis at the shoulder, tendinitis of the origin of the extensor carpi radialis brevis (tennis elbow), tendinitis of the abductor pollicis longus or extensor pollicis brevis tendons at the wrist (de Quervain's disease), coronary ligament sprain at the knee, and anterior talofibular ligament sprain.

In such chronic, persistent lesions of tendons and ligaments—and occasionally muscle—procedures to promote normal mobility and extensibility of the involved structure are important, and often essential, components of the treatment program. Passive or active exercises that impose a longitudinal strain on the involved structure may be incorporated. However, in doing so we are faced with the danger of maintaining the weakened or unresolved state of healing by contributing to the rate of tissue microdamage. That is probably why these disorders tend not to resolve spontaneously with varying degrees of activity. Too little activity results in loss of extensibility; too much activity does not allow for adequate healing. The appropriate compromise is difficult to judge.

Another method of promoting increased extensibility and mobility of the structure, while stress levels are reduced and allowing healing to take place, is the use of deep transverse friction massage. This is a form of treatment advocated primarily by Cyriax, but unfortunately not widely adopted to date.[1] It involves applying a deep massage directly to the site of the lesion in a direction perpendicular to the normal orientation of fibrous elements. This maintains mobility of the structure with respect to adjacent tissues and probably helps to promote increased interfiber mobility of the structure itself without longitudinally stressing it. It may also help promote normal orientation of fibers as they are produced. This effect might be likened to the effect of rolling your hand over an unorganized pile of toothpicks; eventually the toothpicks will all become oriented perpendicular to the direction in which the hand moves. In some pathologies, such as rotator cuff ten-

dinitis, in which the etiology may be related to a nutritional deficit arising from hypovascularity, the hyperemia induced by the deep friction massage may also contribute to the healing response.

Although these effects of friction massage are highly conjectural, they are based upon sound physiological and pathologic concepts. Further support is provided by the often dramatically favorable results obtained clinically when friction massage is appropriately incorporated in a treatment program. Studies are needed, however, to substantiate the physiological effects and the clinical efficacy of friction massage in these chronic disorders. Designing a legitimate clinical study would be difficult because most of the disorders for which friction massage seems to be effective do not present with measurable objective signs, and documentation of subjective improvement is usually unreliable. Basic studies of the effects of friction massage, however, may be fashioned after previous investigations into the effects of exercise, immobility, and other variables on the healing and maturation of collagen tissue. Until we have more concrete evidence of the value of friction massage, its use must be justified on the above considerations combined with "educated empiricism."

CLINICAL APPLICATION

INDICATIONS FOR FRICTION MASSAGE

Friction massage is indicated for chronic conditions of soft tissues—usually tendons, ligaments, or muscles—arising from abnormal modeling of fibrous elements in response to fatigue stresses or accompanying resolution of an acute inflammatory disorder. The intent is to restore or maintain the mobility of the structure with respect to adjacent tissues and to increase the extensibility of the structure under normal loading conditions. The goal is to allow for increased energy-attenuating capacity of the part with reduced strain to individual structural elements. Typical conditions in which friction massage is often indicated include

Tendinitis
Supraspinatus or infraspinatus at the shoulder
Tennis elbow
de Quervain tendinitis at the wrist
Peroneal tendinitis at the ankle or foot

Subacute or chronic ligamentous sprains
Intercarpal ligament sprains at the wrist
Coronary ligament sprain at the knee
Minor medial collateral ligament sprains at the knee
Minor anterior talofibular or calcaneo-cuboid ligament sprains

Acute signs and symptoms should be resolved at the time at which friction massage is used (see criteria for acute versus chronic conditions in Chapter 4, Assessment of Musculoskeletal Disorders).

TECHNIQUE OF APPLICATION (REFER TO Figs. 9-2, 9-3)

The part should be well exposed and supported so as to reduce postural muscle tone. The structure to be treated is usually put in a position of neutral tension. It should be positioned so that the site of the lesion is easily accessible to the fingertips. If adherence between a tendon and its sheath is suspected, then the tendon should be kept taut to stabilize it while the sheath is mobilized during the massage.

The therapist should be seated, if possible. His elbow should be supported to reduce muscle tension of more proximal parts. The pad of the index finger, middle finger, or thumb is placed directly over the site of the pathology. Fingers that are not being used at the time should be used to provide further stabilization of the therapist's hand and arm. *No lubricant is used;* the patient's skin must move along with the therapist's fingers.

Beginning with light pressure, the therapist moves the skin over the site of the lesion back and forth, in a direction perpendicular to the normal orientation of the fibers of the involved part. The amplitude of movement is such that tension against the skin at the extremes of each stroke is minimal. This is necessary in order to avoid friction between the massaging fingers and the skin, which might well produce a blister. Friction may be further avoided by using the thumb and finger of the opposite hand to gather the skin in somewhat toward the area being massaged. The rate of movement should be about two or three cycles per second and rhythmical.

At the beginning of the massage, the patient may feel mild to moderate tenderness. This should not be a deterrent. However, after 1 or 2 minutes of treatment with light pressure, the tenderness should have subsided considerably. If it has not, or if tenderness has increased, treatment is stopped. At that point the therapist should consider whether pressure used at the initiation of the massage was excessive. Continuing or increasing tenderness is very rare, however; more often the massage has an anesthetic effect. As the tenderness subsides after 1 or 2 minutes, the pressure should be increased somewhat. The patient may feel some tenderness again. After about two more minutes, the therapist should again determine if the tenderness has subsided. If it has not, he should discontinue for that session; if it has subsided, he again increases the pressure and massages for about two more minutes. During the final 2 minutes of massage, the therapist should feel that the depth of massage is sufficient to affect the involved structure.

During the first treatment, the massage should be stopped after 5 or 6 minutes, and the key signs reassessed. If it is a muscular or tendinous lesion, the painful resisted movement is checked; if it is a ligamentous lesion, the painful joint play movement is retested. The patient should feel some immediate improvement. If he has not, the therapist should consider whether the technique of treatment was appropriate, assuming that the disorder is one for which friction massage is indicated.

With successive treatments, the depth massage is always gradually increased, as described above, and the length of treatment is gradually increased by about 3 minutes in each session, working up to 12 or 15 minutes each session. However, treatment should not be continued during a particular session nor should the depth of massage be increased if the tenderness to massage increases or does not subside during treatment. Responses will vary, of course, with the patient and with the nature of the disorder. In some cases the duration of treatment must be increased more slowly than in others. There are few conditions that do not resolve after 6 to 10 sessions over 2 or 3 weeks, provided that other components of the treatment program are appropriately carried out and provided that friction massage is indicated.

It is not unusual for a patient to feel some increased "soreness" following the first or second sessions, but it must be distinguished from exacerbation of symptoms. Some skin or soft-tissue tenderness and soreness are to be expected. This would occur whether the patient did or did not have an underlying pathology and should not be misconstrued by the therapist or patient as worsening of the condition, so long as key symptoms and signs related to the patient's pathology are no worse.

A common mistake during treatment by friction massage is the development of skin blisters or abrasions. These result either from fingernails that are too long or from poor technique that causes friction between the massaging finger and skin. Another common mistake is for the therapist to apply the massage to the area of pain rather than to the site of the lesion. The two areas do not necessarily coincide.

In addition, the therapist must avoid overstressing the more distal joints of his thumb and fingers when performing the massage. This is especially important if friction massage is being used frequently. Such stresses can be reduced by stabilizing the distal interphalangeal joint of the massaging finger with a free finger, as shown in Figure 9-3, and by alternating fingers during a particular treatment session.

Friction massage should be avoided when the nutritional status of the skin is compromised and in cases of impaired vacular response. These would typically include patients on long-term, high-dose, steroid drug therapy, and patients with known peripheral vascular disease.

EXAMPLES OF FRICTION MASSAGE TECHNIQUES

Supraspinatus Tendon (Fig. 9-2)

Light to deep transverse frictions are given over the tendon. The patient sits comfortably on a chair, and the arm is put in a neutral or somewhat extended position with the lower arm supported. The therapist sits at the patient's side. A position of neutral or slight humeral extension brings the tendon forward into a position in which the site of the lesion is easily accessible to the fingertip. The therapist identifies the site of the tendon lying between the greater tubercle of the humerus and the acromion process. It is essential that the tendon be accurately located by knowledge of anatomy; it cannot be distinguished by palpation. The pad of the therapist's middle finger, reinforced by the index finger (or *vice versa*), is placed

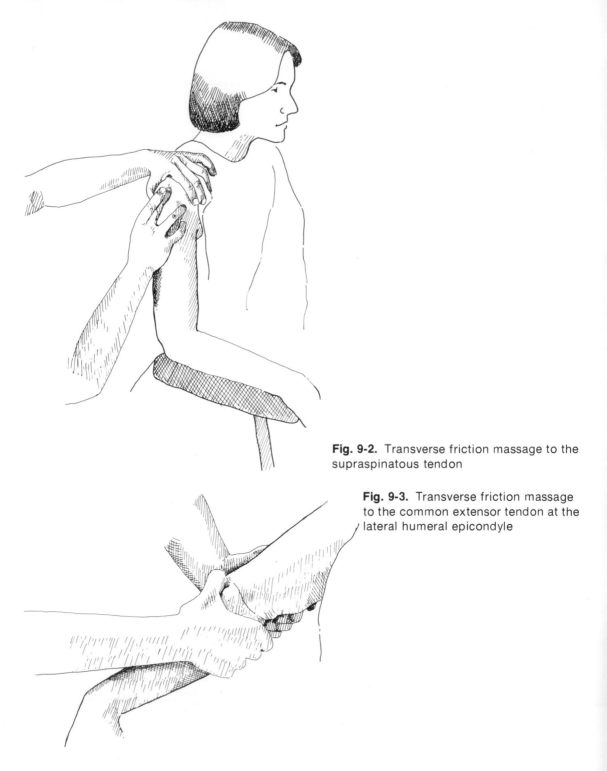

Fig. 9-2. Transverse friction massage to the supraspinatous tendon

Fig. 9-3. Transverse friction massage to the common extensor tendon at the lateral humeral epicondyle

directly over the site of the lesion, which is always just proximal to the tendon insertion on the greater tubercle. The thumb is used to stabilize the arm. The therapist applies frictions in a direction perpendicular to the normal orientation of the tendon, using the thumb both as fulcrum and to maintain pressure. The thumb and fingers of the opposite hand support and gather the skin over the shoulder in order to avoid friction between the massaging finger and skin.

This is the most valuable treatment in the management of supraspinatus tendinitis and is a key component of the treatment program (see Chapter 12, The Shoulder). A similar technique is used for the other tendons of the rotator cuff.

"Tennis Elbow" (Fig. 9-3)

Light to deep frictions are given to the affected fibers of the extensor carpi radialis brevis at the anterior aspect of the lateral humeral epicondyle. The patient sits with the lower arm supported; the elbow is flexed and the forearm is supinated to allow easy access of the massaging finger or thumb. The therapist sits at the side, facing the patient. One hand sup-

ports at the elbow. The massaging hand is placed so that the thumb is over the affected fibers. Counterpressure is applied by the fingers lying against the medial proximal aspect of the forearm. The thumb is drawn across the site of the lesion in a direction perpendicular to the fibers by alternate supination and pronation of the forearm, using the fingers as a fulcrum. The therapist may also use the index or long fingers for massage, as described for friction massage to the supraspinatus tendon.

REFERENCES

1. Cyriax J: Textbook of Orthopaedic Medicine, Vol II, Treatment by Massage, Manipulation and Injection, pp 8–32. Baltimore, Williams & Wilkins, 1971
2. Rogoff JB (ed): Manipulation, Traction and Massage, 2nd ed. Baltimore, Williams & Wilkins, 1980
3. Tappin FM: Healing Massage Techniques: A Study of Eastern and Western Methods. Reston, VA, Reston Publishing, 1978
4. Wood EC: Beard's Massage: Principles and Techniques. Philadelphia, W B Saunders, 1974

10 Relaxation

Darlene Hertling and Daniel Jones

THE REVIVAL OF RELAXATION TECHNIQUES AND THE DEVELOPMENT OF RELATED TECHNIQUES

Relaxation techniques are being used by physical therapists and other health professionals more than ever before. The concept of relaxation has had a long and varied history. In the early part of this century, Jacobson introduced a form of therapy based on muscular quiescence known as *progressive relaxation*. [21] American interest in the topic of relaxation waned during the 1940s and 1950s. It was not until the introduction of systematic desensitization by Wolpe in 1958, in which progressive relaxation played an important role, that American interest in this topic was once again renewed. [56]

Systematic desensitization is one of the most widely used behavioral therapy techniques to employ relaxation. It is a method used for breaking down neurotic anxiety-response habits in a step-by-step fashion. [55] Relaxation is used as a physiological anxiety-inhibiting state. The subject is first exposed to a weak anxiety-arousing stimulus, which is repeated until the stimulus progressively loses its ability to evoke anxiety. Successively stronger stimuli are applied and similarly treated until the habit is overcome, or the trainee gains some control over it. Relaxation training has since become an integral part of many behavioral procedures; the prin-

ciples of behavioristic psychology, behavior modification, stress management, and related techniques often employ relaxation training.

Relaxation techniques and related techniques have also found their way into the newly established pain clinics. The prototype, and now probably the largest and best-organized clinic, was begun in 1961 by Bonica and White, of the University of Washington Medical School. [38] Other pain clinics have been formed at other hospitals and clinics both here and abroad. There is evidence that many psychological approaches are able to produce some measure of pain relief. According to Sternbach, these include desensitization techniques (in which exposure to pain and the opportunity to gain some kind of control over it helps to relieve it or to make it bearable), hypnotic suggestion techniques, and progressive relaxation. [47]

Interest in relaxation and related techniques has been further augmented by increased self-awareness and by what has been called the "body boom" of the 1960s and 1970s. [30] It has led to increased concern with relaxation, posture, getting in touch with one's body, and thereby one's emotions. Ultimately, it has to do with healing the body and, hopefully, the mind as well. According to Kruger, "The body boom has begot a widely assorted, though in many ways a cohesive, family of both medical and nonmedical therapists who do body work—the father of the breed, Reich, the mother, Yoga, and the family estate Esalen, California, which is considered the mecca of the American Human Potential Movement." [30]

Recent research demonstrates that we

are more capable of controlling our bodily and psychological processes than was previously believed.[5,22,34,42-44,55] The defining mark of the "new body therapies" is their attention to exercise, relaxation, massage, and body and human potential.

Theoretical principles include an understanding of the relationship between the body and characture structure (first developed by psychoanalyst Wilhelm Reich), existentialist, physiological, behavioral, and sociological theories.

Therapeutic practices include a variety of psychophysiological methods for making use of bodily processes to reduce tension and anxiety. Among them are the following methods:

—The revival of ancient Asian disciplines such as yoga, T'ai Chi, and Zen awareness training, and their western modifications
—Principles of behavioristic psychology and behavior modification
—Sophisticated instrumentation of Western technology, such as biofeedback
—The neo-Reichian approach of bioenergetics, best known through the work of Lowen and of Kelemann.[32,33] Body movements and verbalization are used to release blocked or repressed energy and reintegrate body and mind.
—The Alexander Technique, which changes body alignment by increasing awareness of posture and by the use of suggestion and gentle repositioning of the limbs.[1,2]
—The rediscovery of dance therapy. An example is the Feher School of Dance and Relaxation, which works extensively with back problems. It is considered a form of dynamic or active distraction used for relaxation purposes.[30]
—A variety of massage techniques, including massages for different parts of the body to promote relaxation and well-being, and more recently,

acupressure massage and acupuncture.[4,14,15,49,54] Chapman of the University of Washington Pain Clinic has experimented with acupuncture. He believes that one of its effects is to bring about relaxation very quickly, and that it may tend to reduce physiological stress reactions.[38]
—The revival of the Jacobson Relaxation Technique, including newer techniques such as the Lamaze Technique (associated with natural childbirth), Autogenic Training (a medical therapy based on sensory awareness devised by J. H. Schultz, a German neurologist), and the Relaxation Response or Benson's Technique (meditation on a single word or color).[5,34,42,48]
—Differential relaxation techniques of body parts and systems through respiration exercises, such as Fuchs' Functional Relaxation and Jencks' Respiration Exercises for use in daily-life activities and coping with stress.[26,27]

COMPONENTS OF THE STRESS RESPONSE

Research during the past decade in the management of stress and the application of relaxation and related techniques has received an increasing amount of attention. The existing literature on relaxation and related states is extremely diverse. The foundations upon which this body of research rests range from age-old meditative disciplines of Asia to contemporary research on behavior modification, and the newest approach, biofeedback, which is often combined with relaxation techniques.

Components of the stress response identified by theorists include physiological, psychosomatic, psychological, and sociological aspects. Selye, has spent almost four decades of laboratory research on the physiological mechanism of adaptation to the stress of life. [43,44] From his studies on overstressed animals, he observed non-specific changes, which he called the *general adaptation syndrome*, and specific responses that depend on the kind of stressor and on the part of the organism involved. He established a stress index that comprises some major pathologic results of overstress, including enlargement of the adrenal cortex, atrophy of lymphatic tissues, and bleeding ulcers. He has further defined certain pathologic consequences of long-term stress as *diseases of adaptation*. Among these he classified stomach ulcers, cardiovascular disease, high blood pressure, connective tissue disease, and headaches.

Mason, one of the most distinguished investigators of the psychological and psychiatric aspects of biological stress, suggests that emotional stimuli are the most common stressors.[37] They are reflected in the endocrine, autonomic, and musculoskeletal system (Fig. 10-1). We know that every individual will not elicit the same syndrome even with the same degree of stress. Likewise, it is known that the same stressor can cause different lesions in different individuals, which can selectively enhance or inhibit one of the stress effects. Conditioning may be internal (*i.e.*, genetic predisposition, past experience, age, sex) or external (*i.e.*, treatment with certain hormones, drugs, dietary factors). Under the influence of such conditioning factors a normally well-tolerated degree of stress may be pathogenic and may cause disease of adaptation that selectively affects predisposed areas of the body. Any kind of activity sets our stress mechanism in motion. However, whether the heart, gastrointestinal tract, or musculoskeletal system will suffer most depends largely on accidental conditioning factors. Although all parts of the system are exposed equally to stress, it is the weakest link that breaks down first.

Sternbach has described a scheme for the onset of stress-related disorders and the resultant failure in the homeostatic mechanism to prevent the body from returning to a baseline level of function in many cases.[46] For example, frequent stressors cause an increase in blood pressure. Often, as the result of failure in the homeostatic mechanism, the system readjusts to a new level of increased blood pressure (Fig. 10-2). Similarly, Brown has pointed out that muscle behavior under stress is translated into muscle holding or tension.[6] If stressors are frequent, the following two muscle events occur: (1) muscle tension becomes sustained at higher levels, and (2) the tightness of the muscles causes them to be hyperactive. Under normal conditions, an appropriate adjustment is made by the central muscle control system. Special nerve cells in the muscle tissue sense when a fiber is contracting, how fast it is tensing, and other complex aspects of muscle contraction. The system seems to become inefficient, however, with continued stress or rumination about the stress, since the length of time muscle fibers have been tense does not seem to be relayed to the central muscle control system. As a result, the muscles

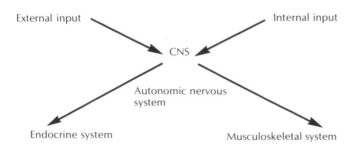

Fig. 10-1. Common stresses

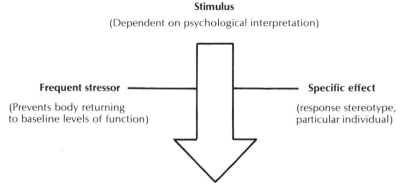

Stimulus
(Dependent on psychological interpretation)

Frequent stressor ———— **Specific effect**

(Prevents body returning
to baseline levels of function)

(response stereotype,
particular individual)

Fig. 10-2. Scheme illustrating onset of stress-related disorders

Failure in homeostatic mechanism

have little chance to recover from increased tension. Tension becomes sustained at higher levels and may continue to increase. If muscles are not given relief from tension by relaxation or a change of activity, the muscle fibers physiologically "adapt" to states of increased tension.

Hess produced the changes associated with the fight-or-flight response by stimulating a part of the cat's brain within the hypothalamus.[16,19] By stimulating another area within the hypothalamus, he demonstrated a response whose physiological changes were similar to those measured during the practice of relaxation, that is, a response opposite the fight-or-flight response (ergotropic response). He described it as a protective mechanism against overstress that belongs to the trophotropic system and promotes a restorative process (Fig. 10-3).

Benson believes the trophotropic response described by Hess in cats is the relaxation response in humans.[5] Both of these opposing responses are associated with physiological changes, and each appears to be controlled by the hypothalamus. Because the fight-or-flight response and the relaxation response are in opposition, one counteracts the effects of the other. This is why Benson and Wallace feel the relaxation response is so important; through its use the harmful effects of inappropriate elicitation of the fight-or-flight response are counteracted. They indicate that most of the relaxation therapies evoke the same physiological changes as the relaxation response.

Fig. 10-3. Effects of the ergotropic and trophotropic responses. BP—blood pressure; HR—heart rate; R—respiration; GI gastrointestinal

Ergotropic response	Trophotropic response
Primarily sympathetic	Primarily parasympathetic
Excitement, arousal	Relaxation
Mobilization of body	Energy conservation
↑ HR, BP, R	↓ HR, BP, R
↑ Blood sugar	↑ GI function
↑ Muscle tension	↓ Muscle tension
Pupil dilatation	Pupil constriction
↑ O_2 consumption	↓ O_2 consumption
↑ CO_2 elimination	↓ CO_2 elimination

ROLE OF PHYSICAL THERAPY

One of the common symptoms physical therapists see in many of their patients today is tension pain related to neuromuscular hypertension. Many feel that muscle tension or stress is actually a partial or complete cause of heart attack, cerebrovascular accident, peripheral and neurovascular syndromes, chronic musculoskeletal problems, and the common headache. Most physical therapists would agree that a chronic pain patient who is tense will invariably take much longer to treat and need more time to recover. Experience seems to indicate that many musculoskeletal disorders have more severe and/or more prolonged symptoms when muscular tension is a factor. Since this appears to be true, then certainly we should be aware of tension symptoms in the evaluation process and should develop skills to treat the tension factor in these patients.

Tension may not only prolong a condition but may be the primary factor in the causation of dysfunction. Tension tends not only to aggravate the condition, thus compounding the pathology, but it may actually bring to light what would otherwise have been a subclinical pathology. Holmes and Wolff believe that in many instances the primary local cause of backache is minimal, but the muscle tension produced by anxiety and emotional stress causes secondary pain in the back that may outlast and exceed the primary pain.[41] In any event, both the cause of the habitual holding—the tension itself—and the sublinical pathology will need treatment.

NEUROMUSCULAR HYPERTENSION

What is neuromuscular hypertension? Certainly we contract muscles isotonically or isometrically all day long, be it small muscle movement of the eyes, or the action of the quadricep, hamstring, and gastrocnemius muscles when running, or some normal activity that requires muscle contraction between the two extremes. This involves normal muscular effort, or normal energy expenditure. We also seem to have a remarkable ability to recruit muscular effort when faced with an emergency situation. Humans, however, are creatures of habit and can become accustomed to contracting these muscles subconsciously. This is when problems occur. One gets used to bracing or holding or continuous movement and then carries that muscular effort over into activities that should require a small amount of effort. This is learned behavior. Excess tension may even carry over into periods in which there should be minimal effort, such as lying down or sleeping.

Should some medical condition develop, this tension factor immediately prohibits the natural healing process. Jacobson says, "Acute conditions may occur after intense or prolonged pain or distress from whatever source, whether physical, as a trauma, angina or colic, or mental, as a fright, bereavement, quarrel or loss."[22] Our society probably perpetuates this holding or contracting habit. The pressures of occupation, family, church, and friends contribute to the overuse of muscle tissue, increased neuromuscular excitability. Whatmore and Kohli describe it as a pathophysiological state made up of errors in energy expenditure.[53]

The chronic musculoskeletal problems that therapists are confronted with are seldom found to be associated with only one factor but with a number of factors. Emotional tension, physical trauma, infection, immobilization, or various combinations may lead to joint dysfunction resulting in a sustaining cycle of pain, muscle guarding, retained metabolites, and restricted motion (Fig. 10-4).

Physical therapy plays an important role in the local relief of tension pain associated with neuromuscular hypertension. Often localized tension may be relieved by heat and massage. Joint mobilization of the involved part is often the most effec-

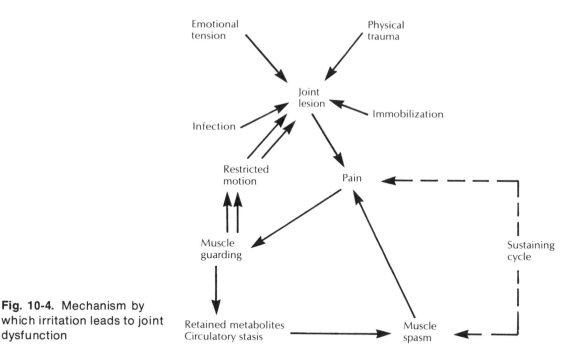

Fig. 10-4. Mechanism by which irritation leads to joint dysfunction

tive line of treatment for breaking up this sustaining cycle. But physical therapy can also act at a deeper level to relieve underlying muscle holding or tension by teaching the tense individual to relax his body and mind through conscious relaxation during normal daily activities.

A SURVEY OF RELAXATION AND RELATED TECHNIQUES

For habitual holding itself, Jacobson's approach has been used in physical therapy almost since its beginning. Jacobson's approach to instructing relaxation has been found to be very suitable in our work and certainly is the most well known in the United States. However, a large number and variety of techniques, and combinations of techniques, are now being used by physical therapists, as well as other medical practitioners. These include Benson's Relaxation Response, Transcendental Meditation, Schultz and Luthe's Autogenic Training, among others. It is generally felt that individual differences and the diversity of needs require a wide

choice of techniques. A review of clinical reports indicates a judicious mix of techniques may obtain the best results.[6] Of the many techniques now available to us, most carry similar requirements, most notably the need for practice, a quiet atmosphere, a comfortable position, and a passive and receptive attitude.

Indications are numerous. Jacobson cites some of the following:[22]

—Acute neuromuscular hypertension
—Chronic neuromuscular hypertension
—States of fatigue and exhaustion
—States of debility
—Various preoperative and postoperative conditions
—Sleep disturbances
—Alimentary spasms and peptic ulcers

Some of the most common conditions treated by physical therapists include

—Tension headaches
—Migraine headaches
—High blood pressure
—Pulmonary disease (asthma and emphysema)[45]
—Muscle guarding

—Spasticity
—Arthritis and related disorders
—Bell's palsy
—Cerebral palsy
—Burn patients (before debridement and range of motion)
—Various chronic pain conditions associated with muscle tension (*e.g.,* cervical strain, adhesive capsulitis, and others)

Types of relaxation and related techniques are difficult to pigeonhole but basically there are two types—the somatic or physical approach, and the cognitive or mental approach. Many techniques employ a combination of both of these approaches. Such a great variety of psychophysiological methods are available to us that only a general survey will be made here, with detail given to some of the more familiar ones. Physical approaches may primarily emphasize passive distraction (*e.g.,* Jacobson's Technique, Praskauer Massage, and respiratory techniques) or active or dynamic distraction (*e.g.,* Feldenkrais's Awareness Through Movement, T'ai Chi, or the Alexander Technique). Those that stress the mental or cognitive approach include meditation, sensory awareness techniques, autogenic training, and sentic cycles. The outline of Psychophysiological Methods of Relaxation and Related Techniques lists only a few of the more commonly used methods of relaxation and related techniques that are practiced in the United States and Europe today. Many excellent techniques have been omitted.

The two major techniques used by physical therapists in the United States are progressive relaxation and autogenic training. Various types of meditation, massage, breathing, and sensory awareness techniques are also employed and are often combined with other techniques. With the exception of self-hypnosis, hypnosis is used primarily by other health professionals in the management of pain-

ful conditions of the musculoskeletal system, as well as cancer, alcohol and drug abuse, natural child birth, and others.

RELAXATION AND MASSAGE

An invaluable tool in the management of common musculoskeletal disorders is massage. However, since World War II, there seems to have been a general decrease in the use of massage for these conditions, perhaps because massage is time consuming, sometimes strenuous, and demands skill on the part of the person giving the treatment. It is also possible that increased knowledge and sophistication of equipment has made basic massage too simple to use. Another reason is, unfortunately, that the basis for its use has been empirical rather than scientific. However, many therapists, including these authors, believe that experience has shown massage to be an extremely important and beneficial tool. Surely it is not the total answer, but as with heat or cold, exercise, relaxation, mobilization, and electrical stimulation, massage as part of our repertoire helps us treat our patients more effectively.

When discussing massage we could talk about stroking and effleurage, petrissage and kneading, friction, percussion, ice, mechanical virbration, or connective tissue massage. We could cover direction (centrifugal versus centripetal or proximal versus distal), pressure, rate and rhythm, media, positions of patient and person giving the massage, duration, and frequency. However, we have chosen to let you review this basic material and its history in the literature, what little there seems to be. One of the better sources is *Massage: Principles and Techniques*, by Beard and Wood.[3]

As mentioned earlier, much has been written about massage, although little scientific study has been done to tell us what physiological effects massage has on various body tissues. In one study of injured muscle, animal muscle tissue was subjected to a crushing injury and later examined microscopically. One group of the animals was left untreated, while another group received massage. The untreated group showed the following results:

1. Dissociation into fibrillae of muscular fibers as shown by well-marked longitudinal striation
2. Hyperplasia (sometimes simple thickening of the connective tissue)
3. Increase, in places, of the number of nuclei in the connective tissue
4. Interstitial hemorrhages
5. Enlargement of blood vessels, with hyperplasia of their adventitious coats
6. Sarcolemma was usually intact, but in one section, a multiplication of nuclei was seen, resembling somewhat an interstitial myositis.

The treated group, on the other hand, showed the following results:

1. Appearance of muscle was normal
2. No secondary fibrous bands separated the muscle fibers
3. No fibrous thickening around the vessels
4. General bulk of the muscle was greater
5. No signs of hemorrhages

It has been concluded, from this study and others that masssage may lessen the amount of fibrosis that inevitably develops in immobilized, injured, or denervated muscle. Even when there has not been injury, there are innumerable situations that will cause a metabolic imbalance within the soft tissue. Observation, and particularly palpation, will reveal abnormal muscle tissue that is often hard, well defined, stringy, and painful. Massage will benefit this uninjured but abnormal tissue, too.

Clinical Application

Massage should usually follow application of heat or cold, and should be done in a relaxing rhythm, with media of the therapist's choice. One should have good hand contact, but most importantly, the massage should be deep. That means we must feel for abnormal tissue (hard and tender) during the palpation portion of massage, and gradually restore that tissue to its normal soft, elongated, nontender state. This appears to increase circulation, decrease pain sensitivity, and promote relaxation; it certainly reduces tension or stress to the tissues with which the muscle comes in contact.

Since muscle is the only tissue in the body that contracts, it follows that excessive or continuous contraction, especially for prolonged periods of time, can only lead to abnormality. It is interesting to note that over the years many patients, after a few treatments of vigorous deep massage, experience considerable relief from arthritis, adhesive capsulitis, tension headaches, and so forth. Patients also tend to become unhappy if there is a change in personnel to someone who gives a gentler massage. From a practical standpoint, we must realize that acute conditions cannot tolerate deep massage immediately. Occasionally, there will be patients who never tolerate deep massage. Usually the extremely tense individual who is unwilling to change his daily habits is in this category. However, it is important to realize that some muscles become so tense that the patient has a very difficult time relaxing the tissue without some massage. If mobilization is used, it is common sense that the least amount of force used will add to the safety of patient treatment. Therefore, massage prior to mobilization can be extremely useful. On the other hand, a joint restriction can sometimes cause localized protective spasm, and by restoring the normal mobility to the joint by mobilization the muscle spasm will be relieved.

In 1963 Kopell and Thompson discussed various surgical procedures for the relief of certain peripheral entrapment

(*text continues on page 212*)

Psychophysiological Methods of Relaxation and Related Techniques

Active Tonus Regulation (Stokvis, Netherlands)

Ideomotor movements are used to prove the influence of mind over body. Suggestions for relaxation of muscles, respiration, and mind are used to induce an altered state of consciousness.[27]

Alexander Technique (Alexander, England)

Kinesthetics is the key word in the Alexander lexicon. The core of this technique is helping people to become aware of when and where their bodies are tense. Proper alignment of head on spine is used to correct physical misalignments, attitudes, and behavior.[1,2]

Autanalysis (Bezzola, Switzerland)

A simple technique in which the body serves as its own excellent biofeedback instrument through attention to and verbalization of successive internal sensations to induce deep mental and physical relaxation.[27]

Autogenic Training (Schultz, Germany)

One of the four major relaxation techniques now being used that developed directly from the therapeutic practice of hypnosis for relaxation. The complete program is divided into three categories of exercises: autosuggestion about relaxation; single-focus meditation (as in yoga); and, meditation on abstract qualities. The first series of exercises are primarily used by physical therapists, and occasionally the second.[34,42]

Awareness through Movement (Feldenkrais, Israel)

Sensory awareness involving movements of limbs, breathing, facial expressions, and self-massage for balance of tension and postural alignment. Feldenkrais, an expert body therapist from Israel, is now living in California and offers courses to health professionals.[14,15]

Functional Relaxation (Fuchs, Germany)

Slow, relaxed exhalations and breathing rhythms are used for differential relaxation of the body parts and systems. Gentle hand contact by the therapist and later by the patient is used to detect inhibiting tension. It is considered a medical therapy requiring a therapist's guidance.[27]

Hatha Yoga (India)

Hatha yoga exercises require both physical manipulation and concentration on awareness of body activities. Assumption of certain postures and controlled breathing are used to induce altered states of consciousness.[12,50]

Meditation Techniques

Whether of Hindu, Zen, Buddhist, or other origin, meditation behavior usually entails concentration of attention and awareness of a single idea, object, or point inside or outside the body. Many Western modifications have been developed for their usefulness as antidotes to the stress of ordinary living. Although meditative practices were not originally designed to be relaxation techniques, the experience of relaxation is a by-product of most such techniques.[11,52,54]

Muscular Therapy (Benjamin, U.S.)

An approach to tension relief that combines deep massage, tension-release exercises, body-care techniques, and postural re-education. The tension-release exercises make use of the neo-Reichian approach of Bioenergetics.[4]

Nyingma System (India)

A system of physical exercises, posture, breathing, and massage is used as a basis for sensory awareness and relief of emotional tension. The Nyingma Institute is located in Berkeley, California, and workshops are offered for psychotherapists. physical therapists, and other health professionals.[54]

Passive Movements (Michaux, France)

Passive movement of relaxed body parts, without the active participation of the subject, to induce both physical and mental relaxation.[27]

Progressive Relaxation (Jacobson, U.S.)

Most widely known of the four major relaxation techniques. Alternate tensing and relaxing of skeletal, respiratory, and facial muscles are used to induce physical and mental relaxation.[20-25]

Proskauer Massage (Proskauer, U.S.)

Also called *breath therapy.* Exhalation and inhalation are coupled with an extremely light and delicate massage to different muscle groups so that the massage is timed with the rhythm of the breathing exercise. Meditation and imagery are used to enhance physical and mental relaxation.[30,54]

Relaxation Response (Benson, U.S.)

From the collected writings of the East (meditation) and the West (autogenic training), Benson has devised a simplified method of eliciting the relaxation response. It consists of two basic categories of exercises: autosuggestion about relaxation, and single-focus meditation usually on the mantra "one."[5]

Respiration of Special Accomplishment (Jencks, U.S.)

Self-suggesting technique coupled with breathing rhythm to enhance relaxation or invigoration, warmth or coolness, for use in daily life activities and coping with stress. Jencks' exercises can easily be adapted for use in physical therapy as well as in psychotherapy.[26,27]

Self-Hypnotism (Pierce, U.S.)

Attention, with closed eyes, to tensing the skeletal muscles of the body part to a point of fatigue. Attention is then shifted to another body part to bring about automatic complete relaxation. This is followed by a series of eye exercises. Finally, imagery is used as a method of distracting attention to further enhance relaxation.[40,54]

Sensory Awareness Training (Grindler, Germany)

Sensory awareness training originated about 100 years ago in Europe as part of training methods for the performing arts. Several of the teachers later emigrated to the United States. The earliest and perhaps most significant work with sensory awareness training was done by Elsa Grindler (1885–1961).[27] A large number and variety of exercises have evolved, including autogenic training. Most of the therapeutic techniques are used for inducing physical relaxation through sensory awareness of muscle tension and inhibited breathing.

Sentic Cycles (Clynes, U.S.)

A behavioral therapy technique composed of eight sentic states or self-induced emotional states. Clynes, a psychophysiological researcher, has demonstrated the close relationship between emotional states and predictable physiological change.[9]

Systematic Desensitization (Wolpe, U.S.)

A behavioral therapy technique in which progressive relaxation is used (following Jacobson) in conjunction with behavioral management techniques. The client develops a series of "scenes" or "visualizations" which he calls forth in a hierarchial order based on their fear-evoking ability while he attempts to remain relaxed.[55,56]

Transcendental Meditation (T.M.) (Maharishi Mahesh Yogi, United States)

A form of meditation adapted to Western concepts and philosophic background most often used as an adjunct to therapeutic relaxation techniques, including EMG biofeedback.[35,51] Graduates are required to meditate for twenty minutes per day using a mantra that has been assigned to them. Credited courses in T.M. have been given in dozens of colleges and universities in the United States and abroad.

neuropathies.[28] It has been found that massage, stretching, mobilization, and exercise can provide relief from symptoms in these same conditions. This seems to indicate the tense, spasmodic, or contracted muscle is at least partly the cause of the symptoms in some of these entrapment conditions.

MUSCLE RE-EDUCATION

Although massage is a valuable tool in relieving tension in muscle, it is imperative that the patient be taught how to relax his muscles in order to achieve prolonged good results. This requires a learning process like that for any other skill we have learned—riding a bike, tying our shoes, reading, playing a sport, or driving a car. It is essentially muscle re-education, a skill physical therapists have used in their practice for years. To teach relaxation, we must develop a muscle awareness in the student. This means practice on the part of the patient.

One way for the patient to develop muscle awareness is to lie down in a comfortable position in a quiet place and practice, in an easy way, three things, the Basic Three. The first is belly or abdominal breathing. Explain to the patient that chest breathing requires contraction of various muscles from neck to chest. Since relaxation of muscle tissue is the desired result, and not contraction, abdominal breathing is the method of choice. As the lungs expand with inspiration, their normal space is taken up in the chest cavity. More space can be given to the expanding lungs by allowing the diaphragm, which separates the chest from the abdominal cavity, to be pushed down into the abdominal cavity. Consequently, the external appearance and feel is that the abdomen rises. With exhalation the pressure is reversed; the air is expelled easily, and the diaphragm returns to its normal position. The normal habit of tension is rapid, shallow, chest breathing or sighing types of patterns. Abdominal breathing with a slow, rhythmical, average amount of air is extremely important for relaxation.

Secondly, the patient should "let all the muscles go." Explain that this means no movement and no holding or bracing. Instruct the patient that it is best to have a couple of pillows under the knees to protect the low back. The legs must roll outward, that is, be externally rotated, in order to relax the various hip muscles. One or two pillows may be placed under the head to support the mid-cervical area. The arms may be flexed with the hands resting on the abdomen but not touching or interlocked, since the muscle will tend to contract. Or they may be extended and externally rotated if the bed or plinth allows complete support of the arms.

Several key areas should be pointed out for the patient to "let go." For example, the eyes should not be closed quickly, since this is a contraction, but be closed gradually after a few minutes have passed. Muscle relaxation can never be forced or done with determined effort because relaxation is a negative effort rather than a positive effort of contraction. Point out the various forms of muscle that contract or relax for facial expression and the contraction of the tongue with speech. The neck, upper back, arms, legs, and low back can all be pointed out again as areas where the patient "lets go" or "turns the power off."

The third aspect of the Basic Three is thinking about letting go without hard concentration. Learning, of course, requires some mental energy, and relaxation as a means of combating tension is definitely a learning process. So, by having the patient think—not concentrate hard—about letting go of that residual tension in the various areas of the body mentioned above, he can learn to relax. As Jacobson states, "The mind and body are one operating unit, not two, and this operating unit is based on muscle contractions."[23] Thus, letting the muscle go in itself will help to put the mind at ease.

PROGRESSIVE RELAXATION

One of the most widely accepted tools used in learning relaxation is the control-relax method commonly known as Jacobson's Progressive Relaxation. By teaching the patient to contract a muscle and develop recognition of the tension signals, or effort, he can begin to recognize tension as it occurs in daily life. This is followed by a period of "letting go," "turning the power off," "going negative," or whatever term one chooses, or more significantly, that is most meaningful to a particular patient. In other words, effort is discontinued, and the fibers of that muscle lengthen as relaxation takes place.

The patient is asked to practice 60 minutes each day in a quiet room free from intruders and phone calls. The following eight instructions for steps to be followed consecutively during the first period are adapted in part from Jacobson's *Self-Operations Control*.[23]

Arm Practice
1. Lying on your back with arms at sides, leave eyes open 3 to 4 minutes.
2. Gradually close eyes and keep them closed during the entire hour.
3. After 3 to 4 minutes with eyes closed, bend left hand back. Observe the control sensation 1 to 2 minutes, and how it differs from the strains in the wrist and in the lower portion of the forearm.
4. Go negative for 3 to 4 minutes.
5. Again bend left hand back and observe as described in **3**.
6. Go negative once more for 3 to 4 minutes.
7. Bend left hand back a third and last time, observing the control sensation 1 to 2 minutes.
8. Finally, go negative for the remainder of the hour.

Eight similar steps are taken in the second period, except that the left wrist is flexed instead of extended. The same eight instructions apply during every period of the entire course except that the motion performed will vary with the number of the period. The motion indicated for a period is usually performed three times at intervals of several minutes.

It should be noted that this does not apply to every third period of practice. During these sessions all motion is omitted, and the patient simply relaxes for the entire hour ("zero period"). In this way he avoids forming the bad habit of tensing a part before relaxing it.

The sequence of the movements performed each day and the periods for relaxation of the left arm are as follows:

Periods	Left Arm
1	Bend hand back (wrist extension
2	Bend hand forward (wrist flexion)
3	Relax only (no contraction at all)
4	Bend at elbow (elbow flexion)
5	Straighten arm (elbow extension)
6	Relax only
7	Progressive tension and relaxation of whole arm

Day seven, and each subsequent period of progressive tension and relaxation of the entire part, involves slowly tightening the entire part—a gradual and continuous increase in the amount of muscle contractions. When the part has become moderately tense, the patient gradually and slowly relaxes, contracting less and less for the remainder of the 60 minutes.

Periods eight through 14 follow exactly the same procedures as periods one through seven, except with the right arm. The periods then continue to other areas of the body as follows:

Periods	Left Leg
15	Bend foot up (dorsiflexion of foot)
16	Bend foot down (plantar flexion of foot)
17	Relax only
18	Raise foot (knee extension)

Periods   Left Leg
19   Bend at knee (knee flexion)
20   Relax only
21   Raise knee (hip flexion)
22   Press lower thigh down (hip extension)
23   Relax entire leg
24   Progressive tension and relaxation of entire leg

Following the pattern described above, Periods 15 through 24 are the left leg, and Periods 25 through 34 are the right leg.

Periods   Trunk
35   Pull in abdomen (contraction of abdominals)
36   Arch back slightly (spinal extension)
37   Relax abdomen, back, and legs
38   Observe a deeper breathing pattern
39   Bend shoulders back (contraction of interscapular muscles)
40   Relax only
41   Lift left arm forward and inward (pectorals)
42   Lift right arm forward and inward
43   Relax only
44   Elevate shoulders (upper trapezius and levator scapulae)

Periods 45 through 50 are neck practice.

Periods   Neck
45   Bend head back
46   Bend chin toward chest (neck flexion)
47   Relax only
48   Bend head left (left side flexion)
49   Bend head right
50   Relax only

Finally, Periods 51 through 62 are eye-region practice.

Periods   Eye Region Practice
51   Wrinkle forehead
52   Frown
53   Relax only
54   Close eyelids tightly
55   Look left with lids closed
56   Relax only
57   Look right with lids closed
58   Look up
59   Relax only
60   Look down with lids closed
61   Look forward with lids closed
62   Relax only

This progressive relaxation can continue into visualization practice, speech-region practice, and practice in other positions, such as sitting, and in "activities of daily living" as explained in Jacobson's *Self-Operations Control*.[23]

Another variation of Jacobson's progressive relaxation is a tool that has been used for years called the "Relaxation Lesson." The instructions given to the patient are as follows:

> Begin with diaphragmatic breathing; then do some combination breathing with the chest and diaphragm. Settle into a nice rhythmic breathing pattern, with the abdominal muscles relaxed, and the diaphragm doing all the work. Do this lying on your back with the proper supports so that you relax best. Coordinate the following exercises with the breathing rhythm. All exercises should be done with minimal effort; the relaxation period is most important. Concentrate so that you may establish new habits for your muscles.

—Bend fingers, wrist, and elbow (flexion pattern). Relax.
—Straighten fingers, pull back wrist and stiffen elbow (extension). Let go.
—Roll arm inward (inward rotation). Let go.
—Roll arm outward (outward rotation). Relax.

—Bend hip, knee, push foot down, curl toes (flexion). Let go.

—Pull toes and foot up, stiffen knee, push straight leg into bed (extension). Relax.

—Roll leg inward (rotation). Relax.

—Roll leg outward (outward rotation). Let go.

—Check breathing pattern and rhythm, thinking back to each arm and each leg. They should feel heavy and relaxed. As a muscle relaxes, it softens and lengthens. Concentrate; the exercise is not more important than the rest period.

—Squeeze buttocks together (attempt to use gluteals and spincters). Relax.

—Arch back. (erector spinae group). Let go.

—Pinch shoulder blades back toward spine (rhomboids). Let go.

—Pull shoulders forward (pectorals). Relax.

—Pull shoulders to ears (upper trapezius, etc.). Let go.

—Push shoulders toward knees (depressors). Relax.

—Pull abdominals in and relax. This alters breathing rhythm, so once again check your breathing. It should be belly breathing.

—Turn chin to right, left, and straight ahead. Release all the neck muscles.

—Push back of head into bed (neck extensors). Let go.

—Lift head (neck flexors). Relax.

—Pull corners of mouth downward. Let go. (Platysma Fish breathing).

—Raise eyebrows and wiggle scalp. Let go.

—Frown. Relax.

—Squeeze eyelids tightly together. Let go.

—With eyes lightly closed and without moving head, turn eyes right, left, up, down and straight ahead. Relax.

—Squeeze jaws together. Relax jaw muscles so mouth drops almost open.

—Push tongue against roof of mouth. Relax tongue.

—Swallow. Relax.

—Review mentally. Concentrate on feeling relaxed.

Minimum practice on this lesson is 1 hour per day—two 30-minute periods, six 10-minute periods, four 15-minute periods, or three 20-minute periods. Check your breathing hourly and practice diaphragmatic breathing 5 minutes out of every hour. You must establish new habits to break the pain-tension cycle.

The two control-relax tools explained above are slight variations of methods of teaching relaxation. The important point is to determine, after evaluating the patient, which method of practice will best suit the patient so that he may learn to relax his muscles. As the patient progresses in his ability to relax, the method will also certainly change and progress. Sometimes isolation of contract-relax is effective. With adhesive capsulitis, learning to relax the rotator cuff muscles can be effective. Learning to extend the neck can relieve tension headaches. Relaxation of the finger and wrists extensors is valuable in treating tennis elbow problems.

The patient must develop some understanding of what relaxation is, which means that those of us doing the teaching must have a greater understanding of the muscle relaxation process. However, the key to success is practice and repetition on the part of the patient. Since muscle relaxation is learned, the patient must practice. As mentioned before, 60 minutes is the recommended time period for daily practice. Frequently, the patient is so tense that he finds it extremely difficult to practice 60 continuous minutes, and shorter periods must be used. In very difficult cases, 5 minutes of practice out of each waking hour can be done. With contract-relax methods the emphasis must always be on the "letting go" phase. Patients will tend to emphasize the contraction phase of the exercises. You must carefully explain and repeat and re-emphasize that the "going negative" or "power off" phase is what is important. It is often helpful to tell the patient that even if he does every movement correctly but does not spend time "letting go" after the movement, the program will not be worth the paper it is printed on. On the other hand, even if half the movements are incorrect, but the patient really relaxes those muscles following the contraction, then muscle relaxation will be achieved.

Biofeedback

A comment about biofeedback or electromyography (EMG) equipment is appropriate at this time. As noted in Jacobson's *Progressive Relaxation*, these methods have been used for years. EMG equipment can reveal baseline data regarding the amount of muscle tension initially present and can indicate progress at a later date. Biofeedback equipment used a few times can help the patient to understand through sight and sound what muscle relaxation is. However, like muscle relaxant medications that do not seem to have solved tension conditions, biofeedback appears to be just another crutch for the patient if used as the relaxation method. The key to relaxation appears to be learning and practice on the part of the patient. The patient must accept the major responsibility in combating neuromuscular hypertension problems. The therapist is present to help, to teach, to clarify, to encourage, and to explain.

Practical Application

Learning to sense muscle relaxation is only the first step in the progressive relaxation process, just as in reading, learning the alphabet and the phonetic sounds are the basic steps. The learning is valuable when the letters and sounds are put into words—words with meaning. The same applies to relaxation. Until we begin to adapt our ability to relax to our daily lives, we have nothing more than a tool of no practical value. Practicality comes with continuing periods of awareness of what our muscles are doing throughout the waking hours. By checking ourselves for muscle tension during various activities (*e.g.*, working, driving, walking, eating, participating in recreational activities) we begin to realize how much we contract muscles excessively. Thus, we can begin to let go. Over time, the relaxation of muscle rather than the contraction becomes the habit pattern; relaxation acquires practical value in our lives. Reminders to help us become aware of muscle habits can be helpful. For example, we might use time to develop a mental connotation with relaxation. Every time we look at our watch, or the radio mentions the time, or someone says it is time for lunch or asks what time it is, we can check ourselves. However, reminders must be changed every few days, or the mental connotation will itself become a habit, and the needed awareness of muscle activity will not develop.

AUTOGENIC TRAINING

Autogenic training was developed by Schultz, a German neurologist, from investigations of hypnosis begun around 1900.[34,42] Two basic mental exercises are used: (1) the standard exercises and (2) the meditative exercises. The six standard exercises are physiologically oriented. The verbal content of the standard formula is focused on the neuromuscular system (heaviness of the limbs), the vasomotor system (warmth of the limbs and coolness of the forehead), the cardiovascular system, and respiratory mechanism. These exercises are practiced several times a day until the patient is able to shift to a less stressful state or the trophotropic state described by Hess.

A reduction of afferent stimuli requires observation of the following points:

—The exercises should take place in a quiet room with moderate temperature and reduced illumination.
—Restrictive clothing should be loosened or removed.
—The body should be as relaxed as possible, and the eyes closed. Three distinctive postures have been found adequate—a horizontal posture; a reclining arm-chair posture; and a simple, relaxed, sitting posture.
—The subject's attitude toward the exercises should not be tense or compulsive but of a "let it happen" nature, referred to as *passive concentration.*

The first exercise of the autogenic standard series aims at muscular relaxation. Right-handed individuals should start out with passive concentration on the right arm and heaviness, for example, "My right arm is comfortably heavy." Once the patient achieves the feeling of heaviness in the right arm, and the feeling spreads to the other extremities regularly, the formula is extended to include the other limbs (left arm, both arms, right leg, left leg, both legs, arms and legs). Concentration on heaviness continues until heaviness can be experienced more or less regularly in all four extremities. This may be achieved in 2 to 8 weeks.

Subsequently, passive concentration on warmth is added, starting with the right arm and warmth—"My right arm is comfortably warm." The warmth formula follows the same progressive procedures used for heaviness until all the extremities become regularly heavy and warm. This training on peripheral vasodilation may require another period of 2 to 8 weeks.

After having learned to establish the feeling of heaviness and warmth, the trainee continues with passive concentration on cardiac activity by using the formula "Heartbeat calm and regular," or just passively observing the heart beat. This is followed by the respiration formula "Respiration regular—It breathes me," or passively observing the breathing rhythm.

The last two, or final, exercises of the physiologically oriented standard exercises concern the abdominal region ("Solar plexus comfortably warm") and the cranial region, which should be cooler than the rest of the body ("My forehead is cool" or "Forehead pleasantly cool").

After the standard formulas have been repeated four to seven times in the sequence described, the altered state of consciousness is ended in a manner similar to awakening from a deep sleep by stretching, inhaling, or yawning, and gradually opening the eyes. Activation phrases are used, such as "I feel life and energy flowing through my legs, hips, solar plexus, chest, and arms. The energy makes me feel light and alive."

As training progresses, and after all six formulas have been added successively and mastered, they may be shortened. The time needed to establish these exercises effectively may require several months (4 to 6 months according to Schultz). In modern practice, however, Schultz or Luthe's Autogenic Training techniques have been modified to reduce training to a minimum of 6 weeks and so that a whole "round" can be practiced in 1 hour.[6] After several months of practice, the subject should be able to achieve the induced altered state of consciousness by simply thinking "Heaviness—Warmth—Heart beat and respiration—Solar plexus—Forehead."

The meditative exercises are reserved for the trainee who has mastered the standard exercises. They focus primarily on certain mental functions, single-focus mental concentration (as in yogic meditation), and finally meditation on abstract qualities of universal consciousness, much as in yogic or Zen meditation. The standard series of exercises and the single-focus meditation are primarily used in medical or psychological treatment.

Certainly, the autogenic standard exercises concentrate upon somatic attention and have a similar effect as progressive relaxation. According to Benson the first five standard exercises have been found to be the most effective in producing the relaxation response.[5] The meditative exercises that give an important role to single-focus concentration or to imagery are more cognitive in nature. They elicit subjective and physiological changes that are different from those that follow the practice of somatic procedures.

Clinical Application

The clinical usefulness of autogenic training in the treatment of muscular disorders according to Luthe and Schultz is largely based on the following factors: [34]

—Muscular relaxation
—Improved local circulation
—Decreased stimulation of pain
—Reduction of unfavorable reactivity to emotional stress
—Possible favorable effects on deviation of certain metabolic and endocrine functions
—Reduction or elimination of relevant pharmaceuticals
—Promotion of the patient's active participation in treatment

Regular practice of autogenic training has been found particularly helpful in relieving complaints associated with arthritis and related disorders (rheumatoid arthritis, osteoarthritis), nonarticular rheumatism (fibromyositis, myalgia), and cervical-root and low-back syndromes (particularly when associated with nerve-root pressure, such as lumbago-sciatic syndrome).

When musculoskeletal disorders involve the spine in conditions such as ankylosing spondylitis, degenerative joint disease, or herniation of a vertebral disc, autogenic training may prove to be very helpful when used in combination with other forms of treatment. These patients should be encouraged to learn all the standard exercises, with particular emphasis on the heavy and warm formulae. In addition, topographically adapted special formulae are used. Topographically specific heaviness and warmth formulae may cover the entire length of the spine or may be used with passive concentration on a particular area (*e.g.*, "The lower part of my spine is heavy" or "My pelvis is warm"). When used to cover the entire length of the spine, dynamic mental contact has a better effect. This implies that the mental contact does not remain fixed on a given topographic area but shifts progressively over different sections of the spine starting with the cervical section and moving to the coccygeal area, while the mental process of passive concentration (*e.g.*, "My spine is very warm") continues. The mental control travels repeatedly down the spine and is followed by concentration on the arms and legs.

Similarly, in musculoskeletal disorders affecting the joints of the extremities the emphasis is on frequent practice of the first two standard exercises (heavy and warm formulae) with relatively prolonged passive concentration on the affected area (*e.g.*, "My right knee is warm" or "My right shoulder is warm").

VARIATIONS OF AUTOGENIC TRAINING

Benson and Wallace have devised a simplified method incorporating a modification of the standard autogenic exercises and single focus attention.[5] Deep relaxation of the muscles, concentrating on heaviness and warmth, begins with the feet and works up progressively: feet, calves, thighs, back, neck, arms, shoulders. They use *one* as a mantra while breathing in and out for 10 to 20 minutes during the program. They suggest that there is not a single method that is unique in eliciting the relaxation response, and that any one of the age-old or newly developed techniques may produce the same physiological results, regardless of the mental device used.

Jencks has designed an interesting variation of autogenic training for children. Her variation includes all aspects of Schultz's standard formula but works through imagery instead of Schultz's precise meditative exercises.[26] Sensory awareness is aroused through images, for which suggestions are made in the form of Erickson's therapeutic double binds.[13] She refers to this approach as the "Autogenic Rag Doll."

Autogenic training has been found to be a useful adjunct to massage. Frances M. Tappin, a physical therapist and foremost authority on massage, states, "Since one purpose of massage is relaxation and relief of stress, it will be doubly effective if the one doing the massage can provide autogenic phrases to increase the effectiveness of massage."[49] She feels this is particularly true in situations where tension is a major part of the patient's problem. She suggests a series of autogenic phrases developed by Alyce and Elmer Green of the Menninger Clinic, that tend to bring the patient closer to the alpha brain rhythm, which is associated with feelings of calm.[17]

Alpha waves (slow brain-waves) increase during the practice of relaxation but are not commonly found in sleep. We still do not know the significance of alpha waves, but as presently noted, we do know that they are present when people feel relaxed.[5,6]

AN INTEGRATED RELAXATION APPROACH

Many physical therapists now use a combination of techniques or an integrated system using a sequential approach. Such an approach is best exemplified in a train-

ing program developed by Budzynski, Director of the Biofeedback Institute in Denver.[7,8] A gross awareness of muscle tension is acquired by moving from one form of relaxation to another in order of difficulty. The trainee progresses only after he has mastered a less difficult technique. His training program consists of three major components: progressive relaxation, autogenic training, and finally, a form of stress management combining autogenic training with systematic desensitization. There are six exercise elements that build upon each other to produce simultaneous mind-body relaxation. The approach may be used independently or as an adjunct to biofeedback or related clinical procedures.

The first set of exercises are used to develop a gross awareness of muscle tension using a modified variation of progressive relaxation. Once the trainee can perform the exercises to the therapist's satisfaction, he moves on to differential relaxation (also developed by Jacobson). This allows the trainee to integrate his ability to relax into everyday living situations.[25] Along with practice twice a day, the client is encouraged to become aware of specific tension areas in his body throughout the day.

The third set of exercises uses the autogenic formulae designed to develop further "muscle sense" with useful cognitive responses. The emphasis is on limb heaviness.

The fourth set moves on to limb heaviness and warmth, and the fifth to the forehead and the face. This fifth set attempts to put it all together.

The final set employs systematic desensitization, a behavioral therapy approach combined with the relaxation techniques. The therapist typically assists the client in developing a series of scenes or visualizations. These are then listed on a hierarchial order, based on their fear-evoking quality. The client begins by visualizing the scene that has the fewest anxious or fear-provoking properties. This scene is repeated until the trainee can visualize it while remaining relaxed. He then moves to the next scene.

GUIDELINES FOR ADMINISTERING RELAXATION TECHNIQUES IN MUSCULOSKELETAL DISORDERS

EVALUATION

The most obvious candidates for relaxation techniques that physical therapists see are patients with chronic back and neck problems. These conditions are often the result of many varying factors. The role of our urbanized, overstressed, under-exercised life in the etiology of premorbid states—of which neck and back pain are often the first symptoms—needs special consideration. Today, the initial attack of back pain is frequently precipitated by emotional problems, tension, or unaccustomed work or athletic activities. These causes are often masked by or combined with true mechanical factors, but rarely are they entirely missing. Therefore, when taking the case history, do not overlook physical signs of emotional stress and muscle tension. We need to emphasize the overall picture of the patient rather than concentrate on the local mechanical problems only.

Subjective Examination for Tension

An examination should always be conducted following lines similar to those described in Chapter 4, Assessment of Musculoskeletal Disorders, for the extremities, and for mechanical problems of the spine, which have been discussed and described by authors such as Cyriax, Grieve, and Maitland, among others.[10,18,36] In addition, we may need to further develop the history as it relates to tension and stress factors. The results of stress are often expressed as secondary manifestations, such as irregular sleeping habits, gastrointestinal problems, headaches, and so forth. People under stress experience a wide variety of physical responses, anxiety or restlessness, and emotional symptoms.

The nature of the patient's work, the way he works, and the manner in which he performs the predominant activities of his life are important clues to whether the patient is under tension. The following are some areas that may need to be explored:

Nature of his work Does he like his work, superiors, and co-workers? Is his job competitive and stressful?

Way the work is performed Do his daily activities require repetitive movements of the body? Does his activity allow free movement, or does he maintain a fixed position for prolonged periods?

Whether daily activity involves driving Commuting for long periods of time is often a source of tension not only from the standpoint of maintaining a fixed position, but also as a source of constant daily irritation from heavy traffic.

Physical activities Does his work give him much exercise? If not, what is he doing, if anything, to compensate for lack of exercise? What is the nature of such activity, and how frequently is it performed?

Home and family Is there illness in the family? If married, is the marriage relationship satisfactory? Are there children? The home situation is often an important source of tension.

People under stress may experience a wide variety of physical symptoms. These may include:

Cardiovascular and respiratory symptoms Does the patient experience chest pain, a rapid or racing heart beat, difficult breathing, or shortness of breath? Does he have a problem with high blood pressure?

ENT (eye, ear, nose, and throat) symptoms, headaches or head pain A special cause or starting point of neck pain may be related to grinding and clenching of the teeth. Does he frequently experience nasal stuffiness, hoarseness, or difficulty swallowing? Does he have frequent migraine or tension headaches? Does he experience transient somatic effects such as dizziness or fainting?

Digestive disorders Does the patient experience frequent stomach problems, a peptic ulcer syndrome, or a "nervous" stomach? Is he frequently bothered by indigestion, constipation, or nausea?

Endocrine imbalances The most frequent disorders causing muscle pain are hypothyroidism and estrogen deficiency.[29] Does the patient tire easily, require a lot of sleep, or have a weight problem? Is there increased or decreased perspiration? Are there problems with dysmenorrhea, or an irregular menstrual cycle?

Muscle-tension pain Patients often describe only the leading, most severe symptoms and forget a multitude of others that momentarily seem unimportant. Has he noticed excessive muscle tension or pain in other parts of his body (jaw, forehead, legs, shoulders)? Has he been bothered by stiff, sore, or cramping muscles? If so, where?

There must be close observation of whether the pain is primary or secondary. For example, did pain cause the stress or *vice versa*?

Stress is often accompanied by symptoms of anxiety or restlessness. Inquiry or observation during the interview may be useful in determining if some of the following manifestations are present:

—Chewing the lips, grinding and clenching the teeth, and nail biting
—Pacing
—Increased eating, smoking, or drinking
—Difficulty falling asleep, waking up feeling exhausted, and being keyed up and jittery during the day.

Stress is also accompanied by a variety of emotions. Possibly the most important question concerns the emotional stability of the patient. This aspect is often hard to obtain by direct questioning, but is frequently revealed in the course of the interview and treatment program. The patient's medical chart is also a useful source of information.

And finally, we will want to know

—In what type of situation does the patient become aware of unwanted tension? What is the environment, and what is he doing at the time and how?
—Is there any signal to warn him when tension may be coming on? Any thoughts or behaviors that are an indication of tension?
—When does he experience the most tension during a 24-hour day?
—What does he experience? When a patient states that he feels "nervous," what does he actually mean?
—How does he deal with anxiety or unwanted tension?
—What does he feel is the source of his tension?

Closer inquiry in these areas and others may pinpoint the source of tension and thereby make it possible to influence it.

Many times the history will indicate that tension is a factor, especially under the following circumstances:

—When symptoms have an insidious onset, with a number of general symptoms of a vague and aching quality
—If symptoms are related to a specific injury or particular activity and have taken a long time to improve or have actually become worse
—The patient tires easily and has general symptoms of fatigue
—When there is morning pain and stiffness, aggravated by activity—at times only a minor amount of activity—and

relieved by rest. (These patients many times have difficulty sleeping. They may tell you, "I never have been able to relax.")

—Particular problems have become recurrent. For example, the patient may have experienced a third or fourth episode of shoulder pain, or problems in the other shoulder as well. When muscle tension is involved, problems tend to recur.

—When questioned about medications, the patient indicates he has taken muscle relaxants in the past.

—The patient has gone from doctor to doctor without a specific diagnosis, or has been told he has a "functional illness."

—Many times it is a more specific condition, for example, adhesive capsulitis of the shoulder or various types of tendinitis with a very strong related factor of muscle tension.

—There are general health problems related to tension and fatigue.

A useful form for measuring the client's stress profile is the Symptoms of Stress Checklist, a questionnaire that measures the ways people respond to stressful situations.[31] Sets of questions dealing with physical, psychological, or behavioral responses are included. The questionnaire is filled out by the patient during the first week, or it may be filled out prior to the examination. Many other such evaluation forms are now available. They are not only a useful source of information, but many can also be used to assess the patient's progress during the training session and at its end.

Physical Examination for Tension

The physical part of evaluation will reveal many signs that point to tension. The first time you see the patient you will see that he is not resting or is constantly moving. For instance, the patient may prefer to stand rather than sit in the waiting room.

Once you begin the examination you may observe constant shifting of position in the chair, shifting and movement of arms or legs, use of arms in talking, constant movement of eyes, actual tremors, restlessness, rapid and short breathing patterns or constant sighing, diminished concentration, irritability, and other apparent overactivity of the skeletal muscles.

Inspection can be a relevant part of the examination for tension problems. Bony structure and alignment may be unremarkable, although subcutaneous soft tissues and the skin are affected (i.e., hard, stringy muscle fiber, and adherent skin). You may determine this during palpation. Atrophy from tension-fatigue, muscles that are well defined because of contraction in the muscle tissue, or poor general posture may be observed on inspection.

Selective tissue tension tests may elicit some positive signs as well. The patient may hesitate to move actively. There may be hypersensitivity to pain or general anxiety. Or he may move quickly rather than in the requested slow and deliberate pattern.

Passive testing is a key test for tension-related conditions, since it may be impossible to do a pure passive motion—the patient will actually assist you in moving the part. Even after you carefully explain to the patient that you would like him to completely let go, he will continue to assist. Patients often state that they are not aware of using their muscles. It thus becomes important in the remaining examination and treatment to stop frequently to point out that you want the patient to let go, and to explain relaxation. The patient quickly learns that by stopping movement or touching a particular muscle you can feel assistance or resistance, and therefore, he must "let go."

Be aware that although assistance is the most prevalent sign with passive movements, tense patients may actually resist movements. A hypersensitivity to pain and a muscle spasm or muscle tension end-feel will occur. Apparent involvement of joint play movements are more apt to be encountered because of resistance on the part of the patient. There will be involuntary, hyperactive muscle contractions that tend to prohibit testing of various joint play movements. Many joint play movements will appear painful, again because of the hyperactive muscle activity. Resistive testing will demonstrate a quick contraction on the part of the patient, and there will usually be several areas that have a pain response, rather than one or two specific movements. A general weakness may be prevalent. Neuromuscular tests may demonstrate hypersensitive responses to various stimuli, and will usually produce hyperactive responses when deep-tendon reflexes are tested.

Palpation will elicit distinct signs when tension is present. The skin is often tender and dry, has an elevated temperature, and is adherent to underlying tissue. Palpation of subcutaneous tissue, in particular muscle, is a key test. The muscle will feel hard and stringy and will be tender to palpation. It is difficult to distinguish between muscle tissue that is tense and that which is in spasm. Both are hard, but it is safe to assume that if several muscle groups are hard and tender, as well as numerous anatomical areas, there is a tension factor involved rather than pure protective spasm. Muscle tissue in a relaxed state is soft, pliable, not tender to palpation, and the various fibers are elongated. With tension (muscle is the only tissue in the body that contracts) there is just the opposite effect of the relaxed state, and this can be readily palpated.

Clearly, before initiating a program of relaxation training, the therapist must decide if it is realistic to expect that increasing relaxation skills will be a significant factor in alleviating the patient's problems. If the tension occurs in response to a serious problem in the patient's life, it must be dealt with differently (even though relaxation can be beneficial here as well). However, relaxation training can be helpful as a means of eliminating or reducing physical complaints, such as a headache or low-back pain, for which there are no strictly organic bases for the complaint that can be treated more directly by other means.

MANAGEMENT

A thorough knowledge of and experience with relaxation procedures, as well as the use of other clinical skills, are essential to effective relaxation training. Relaxation techniques are seldom used alone, since in most cases the patient's problem is combined with true mechanical factors, muscle imbalances and pain, emotional or behavioral problems, and so on. Relaxation training is an integral part of many behavioral procedures. Principles of behavioristic psychology, behavior modification, and biofeedback are often employed in conjunction with relaxation training but are beyond the scope of this chapter. These methods are discussed and described in many excellent books and articles in the current literature.

The first session of relaxation training is perhaps the most important. The therapist should

1. Explain and justify the procedures so that the patient can understand and accept the rationale underlying relaxation training
2. Instill a feeling of confidence in the technique as well as enthusiasm for carrying out necessary "home work." Success at learning relaxation skills requires regular practice once they have been learned in the training session.
3. Explain and set up long-term and short-term goals. An intermediate goal is for the patient to be able to relax at any time using any or all of the tech-

niques that work best for him. The ultimate goal is to produce relaxation independent of conditioned responses.

The Physical Setting

A suitable setting for training should be provided. Eliminate all sources of extraneous stimulation. Relaxation should take place in a quiet, dimly lit, attractive room. An important consideration is the chair or couch that the patient uses during relaxation training. Recliner chairs are considered ideal. A treatment table may be used as long as the basic requirement of complete support and comfort are met.

The client should wear loose fitting, comfortable clothing. Glasses, contact lenses, watches, and shoes should be removed to reduce extraneous stimulation and to allow free movement.

The therapist must be aware of self, touch, and tone of voice. The voice should be used as instrument to facilitate the relaxation process. How the therapist speaks is just as important as what is actually said. You should speak softly, and the pace of speech should gradually be reduced as the session progresses.

Directing the Procedure

The therapist directs the sequence of events, which will vary with the training technique employed. The clinical training should generally be continued until the therapist is convinced that the patient is performing a set of exercises corrrectly and that deep relaxation has in fact been achieved. This can usually be determined through questioning after the session and by nonverbal clues that are observed during the treatment session (*e.g.*, fidgeting in the chair).

Postrelaxation questioning should follow each session in order to determine if problems exist, and whether an alternative strategy should be employed. The patient's report usually is a sufficiently reliable guide to his ability to relax and is most helpful as an aid in modifying the approach to that patient. Ask the patient to describe in his own words what relaxation feels like, as well as more specific questions regarding any problems that occurred during the session. It is important to ask if anything that was said or done during the session made it more difficult for him to relax, and what statements or techniques seem to facilitate his relaxation so that they can either be eliminated or emphasized in subsequent sessions.

Assigned Home Programs

A home program of relaxation may be started from the very beginning or as soon as the therapist is convinced that the patient is performing a set of exercises correctly. Self-administered relaxation is ideally suited for problems in which tension is a major component and easily lends itself for use in "homework" assignments between therapy sessions. In general, self-administered relaxation can provide benefits as a treatment in itself, or it can be used in conjunction with additional therapeutic techniques.

The importance of practicing cannot be over emphasized to the patient. Relaxation is a skill that improves with practice. The trainee is usually required to practice once or twice a day (varying with the training technique employed, *e.g.*, anywhere from two 10-minute sessions to a single 1-hour session). In many cases, you will find that frequent, shorter sessions will be more effective for some patients. Caution the patient to practice at times when he is under minimal or no pressure. For example, just before bedtime is often recommended. He will usually discover for himself the best times for exercise. It is not advisable to practice on a full stomach.

As the patient becomes more and more proficient in his relaxation skill, the number of daily practice sessions as well as the time spent can gradually be reduced.

Gradually the patient should be weaned away from both therapist and any instrumentation used. He must be taught to rely upon his learned awareness and control, along with other self-generating aids, so that he can reduce tension at any time in day to day stressful situations.

Devices may be used to foster home practice and to incorporate these habits into routine activities of daily living. Some clinicians have used small parking-meter timers that can be set to buzz at hourly intervals to remind the patient to practice for anywhere from 30 seconds to 3 minutes. Patel uses an interesting reminder system, instructing patient to use everyday sounds such as ringing telephones or church bells.[39] Others use visual reminders such as stop lights, so that each time the patient comes to a lengthy stop in traffic, he practices his techniques. Others have patients replace their coffee breaks at work with relaxation breaks. Obviously, it is best if the patient will also allot long periods every day for serious practice in a conducive environment.

Standard relaxation tapes made from Jacobson's and Schultz and Luthe's relaxation techniques, which have been modified to reduce training time, are readily available commercially and are often used in home practice. Budzynski's relaxation approach described earlier is also available on tape. Tape practice, according to Brown, should be used with a bit of caution, however, and should be considered on an individual patient basis. Recent research indicates that recorded relaxation instruction may actually result in increased EMG tension levels in some patients.[6] Tape recorders offer far more flexibility than prerecorded tapes. Each relaxation session can be recorded during the clinical session on a tape recorder provided by the patient, which he can then take home for practice between sessions. This has several advantages. The relaxation technique can be modified to meet the patient's own needs and can become progressively shorter as the patient becomes more skilled in his learning techniques.

Tapes used for home practice have also been found to be useful for patients who have difficulty relaxing in the presence of a therapist. Patients may be started on relaxation learning in this way, and then at a later date start clinical practice with the therapist.

It is usually advisable for patients to do other homework as well. Patients may be requested to chart their painful activities during the day or to record situations that make them tense. This type of record keeping is useful in documenting the patient's progress as well as in helping to pinpoint sources of tension. Encourage the patient to make frequent body checks for muscle tension during the day in order to become more aware of the environment and what makes him tense.

Invariably, the patient will need "activity of daily living" (ADL) training. He needs to work on gait, posture, body mechanics, ways of conserving energy, and reducing tension. The most difficult step of all is transferring this learning to the patient's day to day living.

ASSESSING THE PATIENT'S PROGRESS

To assess the success of relaxation training, the therapist can employ several kinds of information—clinical observation, the subjective report of the patient with the help of a subjective stress profile or anxiety scale evaluation, and objective indicators of relaxation. Important indicators of progress that may be gained by observing the patient during the clinical session would include physical signs, such as less observable movement, a reduction in the breathing pattern during the course of the session, and a peaceful, relaxed appearance. (a relaxed open jaw or a sleepy-eyed appearance following successful relaxation). The patient's ability to gain deep relaxation in shorter and shorter periods of time is also an indicator.

There should be signs of symptomatic improvement. Furthermore, stimuli that once called forth muscle-tension or "fibrositis" pain (backache) no longer do so under the same condition. By deconditioning the muscle-tension habit or anxiety response that has been partly responsible for his problem, he brings about a proportionate reduction of the symptoms.

Secondary manifestations should decline. Stress-dependent reactions, whether migraines, intestinal cramps, grinding and clenching the teeth, or difficulty falling asleep, can also be used as measures of improvement. A reduction or termination of drugs to reduce pain or encourage muscle relaxation is also a useful indicator of improvement.

It is often an advantage to have objective indicators of relaxation. Jacobson has used EMG.[20] Recently, more convenient equipment, such as EMG biofeedback, have become available. They can be used as methods of evaluation, and as treatment to facilitate relaxation by that translating muscle potential into auditory or visual signal feedback to the patient. Other physiological measurements might include cardiovascular measurements (heart rate, blood pressure, skin temperature) and the use of brain wave biofeedback (electroencephalogram). Fortunately, the patient's report usually serve as a sufficiently reliable guide that relaxation skills have been a significant factor in alleviating his problems.

RESEARCH

Research in the area of relaxation and related techniques is poor up to this date. A bit of caution needs to be taken into consideration since there may be possible side effects. Symptoms ranging from insomnia to hallucinatory behavior and withdrawal have been reported when relaxation techniques have been practiced for long periods or to excess.[54] Clearly additional research is needed to test and clarify the numerous hypothesis presented in the current literature. We can help by documenting the claims made for relaxation and for specific treatment strategies that seem to be most effective. And, finally, we need to review the current studies involving relaxation for possible areas of clinical research as they apply to physical therapy and musculoskeletal disorders.

Relaxation has been found to be a successful alternative for drugs and numerous types of back surgery. A major advantage is it's cost effectiveness and that the patient's contribution. Relaxation is not a "magic bullet" and will not cure joint dysfunction or other musculoskeletal disorders. It is, however, a key to reducing muscle tension, anxiety, nervousness, and stress, that may lead to a variety of physical and psychological disabilities.

REFERENCES

1. Alexander FM: The Use of Self. London, Re-Education Publications, 1910
2. Barlow W: The Alexander Technique. New York, Alfred A Knopf, 1973
3. Beard G, Wood EC: Massage: Principles and Techniques. Philadelphia, W B Saunders, 1964
4. Benjamin BE: Are You Tense? The Benjamin System of Muscular Therapy: Tension Relief Through Deep Massage and Body Care. New York, Pantheon Books, 1978
5. Benson H: The Relaxation Response. New York, Avon Books, 1976
6. Brown BB: Stress and the Art of Biofeedback. New York, Harper & Row, 1977
7. Budzynski TH: Relaxation Training Program. New York, Bio Monitoring Audio Cassette Publications, 1977
8. Budzynski TH, Stoya J, Adler C: Feedback induced muscle re-education: Application to tension headaches. Journal of Behavioral Therapy and Experimental Psychiatry 1:205–211, 1970
9. Clynes M: Toward a View of Man. In Clynes M, Milsum J (eds): Biomedical Engineering Systems. New York, McGraw-Hill, 1970

10. Cyriax J: Textbook of Orthopedic Medicine, Vol I. Baltimore, Williams & Wilkins, 1972

11. Davidson RJ, Goleman DJ: Attentional and affective concomitant of meditation: A cross-sectional study. J Abnorm Psychol (in press)

12. Devi I: Yoga for Americans. Englewood Cliffs, NJ, Prentice-Hall, Inc, 1959

13. Erickson MH, Ross EL: Varieties of double bind. Am J Clin Hypn 17:143–157, 1975

14. Feldenkrais M: Awareness Through Movement. New York, Harper & Row, 1972

15. Feldenkrais M: Body and Mature Behavior. New York, International University Press, 1949

16. Gellhorn E: Principles of Autonomic-Somatic Interactions. Minneapolis, University of Minnesota Press, 1967

17. Green E, Green A: The ins and outs of mind body energy. In Science Year 1974: World Book Science Annual. Chicago, Field Enterprises Corporation, 1973

18. Grieves CP: Mobilisation of the Spine, 3rd ed. New York, Churchill Livingstone, 1979

19. Hess WR: Functional Organization of Diencephalon. New York, Grune & Stratton, 1957

20. Jacobson E: Anxiety and Tension Control. Philadelphia, J B Lippincott, 1964

21. Jacobson E: Progressive Relaxation. Chicago, University of Chicago Press, 1929

22. Jacobson E: Progressive Relaxation, 4th ed. Chicago, University of Chicago Press, 1962

23. Jacobson E: Self-Operations Control Manual. Chicago, National Foundation for Progressive Relaxation, 1964

24. Jacobson E: Tension in Medicine. Springfield, IL, Charles C Thomas, 1967

25. Jacobson E: You Must Relax. New York, McGraw-Hill, 1970

26. Jencks B: Respiration for Relaxation, Invigoration, and Special Accomplishment. Salt Lake City, Jencks, 1974

27. Jencks B: Your Body: Biofeedback at Its Best. Chicago, Nelson Hall, 1977

28. Kopell HR, Thompson AL: Peripheral Entrapment Neuropathies. Baltimore, Williams & Wilkins, 1963

29. Kraus H: Clinical Treatment of Back and Neck Pain. New York, McGraw-Hill, 1970

30. Kruger H: Other Healers, Other Cures. New York, Bobbs-Merrill, 1974

31. Leckie M, Thompson E: Symptoms of Stress Checklist. Seattle, University of Washington, 1977

32. Lowen A: Breathing, Movement and Feeling. New York, Institute for Bioenergetics Analysis, 1965

33. Lowen A: Physical Dynamics of Character Structure. New York, Grune & Stratton, 1958

34. Luthe W (ed): Autogenic Therapy, Vols I–VI. New York, Grune & Stratton, 1969–1972

35. Maharishi MY: The Science of Being and Art of Living. London, International SRM Publications, 1966

36. Maitland GD: Vertebral Manipulations, 3rd ed. London, Butterworth, 1972

37. Mason JW: A re-evaluation of the concept of nonspecificity in stress theory. Psychol Res 8:323–333, 1971

38. Mines S: The Conquest of Pain. New York, Grosset & Dunlap, 1974

39. Patel C: Randomized controlled trial of yoga and biofeedback in management of hypertension. Lancet 2: 93–95, 1975

40. Pierce F: Mobolizing the Midbrain. New York, G P Putnam's Sons, 1924

41. Ruch, TC: The nervous system: Sensory function. In Fulton JF (ed): Textbook of Physiology. Philadelphia, W B Saunders, 1955

42. Schultz JH, Luthe W: Autogenic Training: A Psychophysiologic Approach in Psychotherapy. New York, Grune & Stratton, 1959

43. Selye H: The Stress of Life. New York, McGraw-Hill, 1956

44. Selye H: Stress Without Distress. Philadelphia, JB Lippincott, 1974

45. Sinclair JD: Exercise in pulmonary disease. In Basmajian (ed): Therapeutic Exercise, 3rd ed. Baltimore, Williams & Wilkins, 1976

46. Sternbach RA: Psychophysiological bases of psychosomatic phenomena. Psychosomatics 7:81–84, 1966

47. Sternbach RA: Strategies and tactics in the treatment of patients with pain. In Crue BL (ed): Pain and Suffering: Selected Aspects. Springfield, IL, Charles C Thomas, 1970

48. Stewart E: To lesson pain: Relaxation and

rhythmic breathing. Am J Nurs 76:958–959, 1976

49. Tappin FM: Healing Massage Techniques: A Study of Eastern and Western Methods. Reston, VA, Reston Publishing, 1978

50. Vishnudevahada S: The Complete Illustrated Book of Yoga. New York, Julian Press, 1960

51. Wallace RK: Physiological effects of transcendental meditation. Science 167:1751–1754, 1970

52. Wallace RK, Benson H: The physiology of meditation. Sci Am 226:84–90, 1972

53. Whatmore GB, Kohli DR: Dysponesis: A neurophysiologic factor in functional disorders. Behav Sci 13:102–124, 1968

54. White J, Fadiman J (eds): Relax: How You Can Feel Better, Reduce Stress and Overcome Tension. The Confucion Press, 1976

55. Wolpe J: The Practice of Behavior Therapy, 2nd ed. New York, Pergamon Press, 1973

56. Wolpe J: Psychotherapy by Reciprocal Inhibition. Stanford, Stanford University Press, 1958

RECOMMENDED READINGS

STRESS THEORY-MANIFESTATION OF STRESS AND PSYCHOPHYSIOLOGY

Bakal DA: Headache: A biophysical perspective. Psychol Bull 32:369–382, 1975

Benson H, Beary JF, Carol MP: The relaxation response. Psychiatry 37:37–44, 1974

Benson H, Kotch JB, Crassweler KD: The relaxation response: A bridge between psychiatry and medicine. Med Clin North Am 61:929–938, 1977

Coleman JC: Life stress and maladaptive behavior. American Journal of Occupational Therapy 27(4):169–179, 1973

Dixon HH, O'Hara M, Peterson RD: Fatigue contracture of skeletal muscle. Northwest Medicine 66:813–816, 1967

DiCara L: Learning in the autonomic nervous system. Sci Am 222:30–39, 1970

Gellhorn E: Autonomic Imbalances and the Hypothalamus. Minneapolis, University of Minnesota Press, 1957

Kahn RL: Some propositions toward a researchable conceptualization of stress. In McGrath JE (ed): Social and Psychological Factors in Stress. New York, Holt, Rinehart & Winston, 1970

Kiely WF: From the symbolic stimulus to the pathophysiological response: Neurophysiological mechanisms. Int J Psychiatry Med 5(4):515–529, 1974

Lazarus RS: Psychological stress and coping in adaptation and illness. Int J Psychiatry Med 5(4):321–333, 1974

Lazarus RS: Psychological Stress and the Coping Process. New York, McGraw-Hill, 1966

Levi L (ed): Emotions: Their Parameters and Measurement. New York, Raven Press, 1975

Lipoloski ZJ, Lipsitt D, Whybrow PC (eds): Psychosomatic Medicine. New York, Oxford University Press, 1977

McGarth J (ed): Social and Psychological Factors in Stress. New York, Holt, Rinehart & Winston, 1970

Moss GE: Illness, Immunity and Social Interaction. New York, John Wiley & Sons, 1973

Rinehart RE: Evaluation of Behavior. In Tension Control. Chicago, Physical Biological Sciences, Ltd, 1975

Rinehart RE: Modern concepts in rheumatology. Northwest Medicine 56:578–581, 1957

Rinehart RE, Dixon HH: Muscular dysfunction. Northwest Medicine 60:707, 1961

Rubin R: Mind-brain-body interaction: Elucidation of psychosomatic intervening variables, pp 73–85. In Pasnau RO (ed): Consultation-Liaison Psychiatry. New York, Grune & Stratton, 1975

Selye H: Forth years of stress research: Principal remaining problems and misconceptions. Can Med Assoc J 115:53–56, 1976

Stein M, Schiavi RE, Canerino M: Influence of brain and behavior on the immune system. Science 191:435–440, 1976

Stoyva J, Budzynski TH: Cultivated low arousal—An antistress response? In Dicra LV (ed): Recent Advances in Limbic and Autonomic System Research. New York, Plenum, 1978

Tinbergen M: Ethology and stress disease. Science 185:20–27, 1974

RELAXATION AND RELATED TECHNIQUES

Benson H, Beary JF, Carol MP: The relaxation. response. Psychiatry 37:37–45, 1974

Brena S: Yoga and Medicine. New York, Penguin Books, 1972

French AP, Tupin JP: Therapeutic application of a simple relaxation method. Am J Psychother 28:282– 287, 1974

Frownfelter DL: Relaxation principles and techniques. In Frownfelter DL (ed): Chest Physical Therapy and Pulmonary Rehabilitation. Chicago, Year Book Medical Publishers, 1978

Goleman DJ, Schwartz GE: Meditation as an intervention in stress reactivity. J Consult Clin Psychol 44(3):456– 466, 1976

Grzesiak RC: Relaxation techniques in treatment of chronic pain. Arch Phys Med Rehabil 58:270– 272, 1977

LeShan L: How to Meditate. New York, Bantam, 1974

Lysebeth AV: Yoga Self-Taught. New York, Barnes & Noble, 1973

Morse DR, Martin JS, Furst ML, Dublin LL: A physiological and subjective evaluation of meditation, hypnosis and relaxation. Psychosom Med 39(5):304– 324, 1977

Rathbone JL: Relaxation. Philadelphia, Lea & Febiger, 1969

Roccia L, Rogora GA: Agopuntura e rilassamento. Minerva Med 67:1918– 1920, 1976

Showers M: Physical therapy and muscle re-education. In Tension Control. Chicago, Physical Biological Sciences, Ltd, 1975

Wallace RK, Benson H: The physiology of meditation. Sci Am, 1972

White J: What Is Meditation? New York, Doubleday & Co, 1974

Yorkston JF, Sergeant JD: Simple method of relaxation. Lancet 2:1319– 1321, 1960

MANAGEMENT OF STRESS

Beach CW, Marshall MG: Tension Control at Michigan State University. East Lansing, MI, American Association of Tension Control, 1974

Bonica J, Fordyce WE: Operant Conditioning for Chronic Pain. Springfield, IL, Charles C Thomas, 1974

Goldfried MR, Merbaum M: Behavior Change Through Self-Control. New York, Holt, Rinehart & Winston, 1973

Holzman PS: On learning and seeing oneself. J Nerv Ment Dis 148:198– 209, 1969

Hutchings D, Reinbing R: Tension headaches: What form of therapy is most effective? Biofeedback Self Regul 1:183– 190, 1976

Kanter FH: Self management methods. In Kanter FH, Goldstein AP (eds): Helping People Change. New York, Pergamon Press, 1975

Meichenbaum D: Toward a cognitive theory of self-control. In Schwartz GE, Shapiro D (eds): New York, Plenum Press, 1976

Miller NE: Visceral learning and other additional factors potentially applicable to psychotherapy. International Psychiatry Clinic 6:294– 312, 1968

Schwartz GE: Self-regulation of response patterning: Implications for psychophysiological research and therapy. Biofeedback Self Regul 1:7– 30, 1976

Schwartz GE, Shapiro D (eds): Consciousness and Self-Regulation. New York, Plenum Press, 1976

Whatmore G, Kohli K: The Physiopathology and Treatment of Functional Disorders, Including Anxiety States and Depression and the Role of Biofeedback Training. New York, Grune & Stratton, 1974

Wickramasekera I: Temperature feedback for the control of migraine. Journal of Behavior Therapy and Experimental Psychiatry 4:343– 345, 1973

BIOFEEDBACK TECHNIQUES

Blanchard E, Young L: Clinical applications of biofeedback training: A review of evidence. Arch Gen Psychiatry 30:573– 588, 1974

Budzynski T: Biofeedback procedures in the clinic. Seminars in Psychiatry 5(4):537– 547, 1973

Budzynski T, Stoyva J, Adler CS, Mullaney DJ: EMG biofeedback and tension headache: A controlled outcome study. Psychosom Med 35:484– 496, 1973

Gaarder K, Montgomery P: Clinical Biofeedback: A Procedural Manual. Baltimore, Williams & Wilkins, 1977

Lynch JJ: Biofeedback: Some reflections on modern behavioral science. Seminars in Psychiatry 5(4):551– 562, 1972

Miller N: Biofeedback: Evaluation of new technique. N Engl J Med 290:685, 1974

Miller N: Learning of visceral and glandular responses. Science 163:434– 454, 1969

Peck C, Kraft G: Electromyographic biofeedback for pain related to muscle tension: A study of tension headache, back and jaw pain. Arch Surg 112:889– 895, 1977

Schwartz GE, Shapiro D: Biofeedback and essential hypertension: Current findings and theoretical concerns. Seminars in Psychiatry 5:591– 603, 1973

Shapiro D, Schwartz GE: Biofeedback and visceral learning: Clinical applications. Seminars in Psychiatry 4:171– 184, 1972

Sterman L: Clinical biofeedback. Am J Nurs 75:2006– 2009, 1975

Stoyva J: Self-regulation: A context for biofeedback. Biofeedback Self Regul 1:1– 6, 1976

Turin A, Johnson W: Biofeedback therapy for migraine headaches. Arch Gen Psychiatry 33:517– 519, 1976

Venables PH, Martin I (eds): Manual of Psychophysiological Methods. Amsterdam, North Holland Publishing, 1966

Part Three
CLINICAL APPLICATIONS

Part Two

11 *The Temporomandibular Joint*

Darlene Hertling

TEMPOROMANDIBULAR JOINT AND THE STOMATOGNATHIC SYSTEM

Disease and dysfunction of the temporomandibular joints and the adjacent structures affect a large number of people. It is estimated that over 20% of the average population at one time or another has symptoms relating to the temporomandibular joint.[30] Practitioners of dentistry and medicine have long been aware that the temporomandibular joints are among the few joints in the body that, like the vertebral joints, function as a unit in a sliding–gliding action because of the mandible, which links the two condyles together. However, the many intricacies of the temporomandibular joint are just beginning to be appreciated.

In referring to the temporomandibular joints, the masticatory system, its component structures, and all the tissues related to it, the term *stomatognathic system* is used. This designation includes a number of systematically related organs and tissues that function as a whole. The components of this system include

—Bones of the skull, mandible, maxilla, hyoid, clavicle, sternum
—Temporomandibular and dentoalveolar joints
—Muscles and soft tissues of the head and neck, and the muscles of the cheeks, lips, and tongue
—Vascular, lymphatic, and nerve supply systems
—Teeth

The stomatognathic system functions almost continuously, not only in mastication and swallowing, but also in respiration and speech. It also directs the intricate postural relationships of the head, neck, tongue, and hyoid bone, as well as movements of the mandible. It must be constantly kept in mind that the entire system governs the movements of the mandible. Impaired physiological function results in breakdown not only of an individual tissue but also of the interdependent structures and eventual function of the other parts, thus setting up a chain reaction.

The relationship of the head and neck must be considered. Postural maintenance must consider the shoulder girdle, clavicle, sternum, and scapulae as the fixed base of operation. The head may be said virtually to teeter on the atlanto-occipital joint. Since the center of gravity of the head lies in front of the occipital condyles, it follows that a balance force must be applied to hold the head erect. That force is provided by the large posterior muscles of the neck. Normal balance of the head and neck unit requires normal balance of the anterior and posterior muscles, mandible and cranial relationship, and occlusion of the teeth. If one is off balance, the normal relationship is broken, leading to eventual dysfunction. Therefore, we must evaluate and treat the entire system.

A faulty relationship of the mandible and maxilla may result in faulty posture of the cranium upon the first and second cervical vertebrae, or an imbalance between these vertebrae may result in symptoms referable to the mouth, ear, face, or even the thoracic cavity. Furthermore,

233

faulty curvature of the cervical spine, along with the strains it produces, often is responsible for pain and dysfunction of the head, temporomandibular joints, shoulders, upper extremities, and chest.[3]

Management of the stomatognathic system is not limited to the discipline of any one particular field but encompasses in part nearly every specialty within dentistry and medicine. Treatment involves a team approach that may include physical, myofunctional, and speech therapists, the general dentist, oral-maxillofacial surgeon, orthodontist, otolaryngologist, psychologist, neurologist, allergist, and others.

FUNCTIONAL ANATOMY

OSTEOLOGY

The mandible, the largest and strongest bone of the face, articulates with the two temporal bones and accommodates the lower teeth. It is composed of a horizontal portion, the body, and two perpendicular portions, the rami, which unite with ends of the body nearly at right angles (Fig. 11-1).

The external surface of the body is marked by a midline, the mental protuberance, bilateral mental foramina (for passage of the mental artery and nerve), and the oblique line. Muscle attachments include the platysma, depressor anguli oris, depressor labii inferioris, mentalis, and buccinator. The internal surface is concave from side to side. The superior or alveolar border, wider posteriorly than anteriorly, consists of the dentoalveolar cavities for reception of the teeth. Extending upwards and backwards on either side of the internal surface is the mylohyoid line, to which the mylohyoid muscle attaches (Fig. 11-1). Other muscle attachments include the digastric and medial pterygoid muscles.

The ramus, which is quadrilateral in shape, has two processes, the coronoid process and the condylar process. The coronoid process serves as an insertion for the temporalis and masseter muscles. The triangular eminence varies in shape and size; its anterior border is convex, and its posterior border concave. The condylar process consists of two portions, the neck and the condyle. The condyle, which is convex in shape, articulates with the meniscus of the temporomandibular joint. The mandibular condyle is approximately 15 mm to 20 mm long and 8 mm to 10 mm thick, and resembles a little cylinder laid on its side. Its long axis is directed medially and slightly backward. An imaginary line drawn through the axis to the middle line would meet a line from the opposite condyle near the anterior margin of the foramen magnum (Fig. 11-2).* The lateral pterygoid inserts into a depression on the anterior portion of the neck of the condyle.

THE JOINT PROPER AND ITS LIGAMENTOUS STRUCTURES

The temporomandibular joint is located between the mandibular fossa (glenoid fossa) on the inferior surface of the temporal bone and the condylar process of the mandibular bone. Just posterior to the joint is the external ear canal. The temporal portion consists of the mandibular fossa, which is concave, and an anteriorly placed articular eminence, which is convex. After the mid-twenties, there is no fibrocartilage in the posterior portion of the mandibular fossa.†

From a functional point of view, the concave fossa serves as a receptacle for the condyles when the jaws are approximated and as a functional component in lateral

---

* This relationship is an important consideration in the application of mobilization techniques.

† Moffett BC: Personal communication, 1979

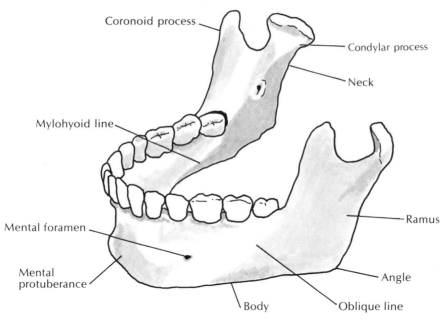

Fig. 11-1. Lateral and frontal aspects of the mandible

Fig. 11-2. Schematic representation illustrates how extensions of the long axis of the condyles meet near the anterior margin of the foramen magnum.

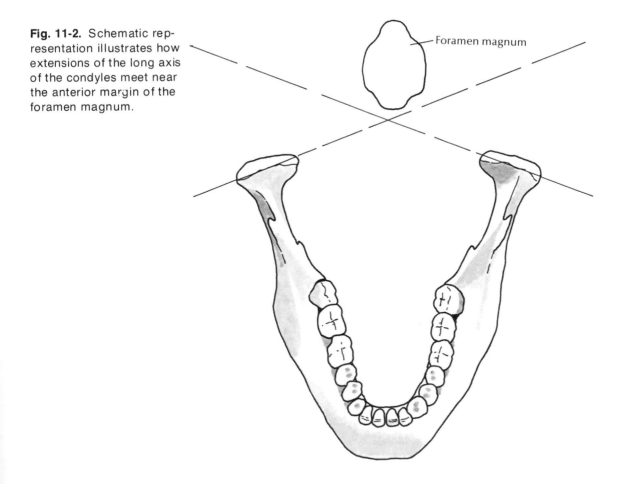

movements of the jaw. During opening, closing, protrusion, and retrusion, the convex surface of the condylar head must move across the convex surface of the articular eminence. The existence of the meniscus (interarticular disk) compensates functionally for the incongruity of the two opposing convex bony surfaces. In addition, the meniscus divides the joint into two portions, sometimes referred to as the upper and lower joints. The meniscus is concavoconvex on its superior surface to accommodate the form of the mandibular fossa and the articular tubercle. The inferior surface is concave over the condyle. In function both the condylar head and articular eminence of the temporal bone are not in contact with each other but with the opposing surfaces of the meniscus. The upper cavity is the larger of the two. The outer edges of the meniscus are connected to the capsule. Synovial

membranes line the two cavities above and below the meniscus (Fig. 11-3).

An excellent comprehensive study by Rees provides a more detailed analysis of the function and structure of the temporomandibular joint.[38]

Ligamentous Structures

The ligamentous structures around the temporomandibular joint include

—Articular capsule (capsular ligament)
—Lateral ligament (temporomandibular ligament)
—Sphenomandibular ligament (internal lateral ligament)
—Stylomandibular ligament

The capsular ligament is attached to the circumference of the mandibular fossa and the articular tubercle superiorly and

Fig. 11-3. Articular structures of the temporomandibular joint in the closed position

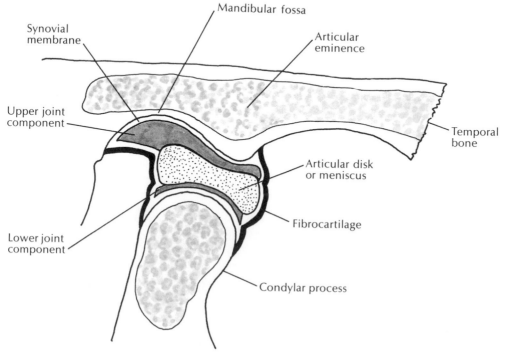

to the neck of the mandibular condyle inferiorly. It is a sleeve of thin, loose, fibrous connective tissue. The capsule is especially lax anteriorly in the superior cavity but very taut in the inferior cavity between the head and disk. Therefore, when the condyle moves forward, the disk follows (Fig. 11-4).

The temporomandibular ligament, a thickening of the joint capsule, is attached superiorly to the lateral surface of the zygomatic arch and articular eminence; inferiorly it attaches to the lateral surface and the posterior border of the neck of the mandible. The ligament prevents extensive forward, backward, and lateral movements and is the main suspensory ligament of the mandible during moderate opening movements (Fig. 11-4).

The sphenomandibular ligament, an accessory ligament, originates from the spine of the sphenoid and attaches to the lingula of the mandible at the mandibular foramen. It serves as a suspensory ligament of the mandible during wide opening. Following moderate opening, the temporomandibular ligament relaxes, and the sphenomandibular ligament becomes taut (Fig. 11-5). The medial pterygoid is associated with its medial surface.

The stylomandibular ligament is also considered an accessory ligament. It runs from the styloid process of the temporal bone to the posterior portion of the ramus of the mandible, and separates the masseter and medial pterygoid muscles. It acts as a stop for the mandible during extreme opening, preventing excessive anterior movement (Fig. 11-5).

The mandibular-malleolar ligament has been demonstrated by Pinto and others.[35] This ligamentous structure was found connecting the neck and anterior process of the malleus to the medioposterior part of the joint capsule, the meniscus, and the sphenomandibular ligament. According to Ermshar this anatomical association of the joint and middle ear may well explain many of the middle ear complaints associated with temporomandibular dysfunction.[11]

MANDIBULAR MUSCULATURE

The three major closing muscles of the mandible are the medial pterygoid, the masseter, and the temporalis. The superior head of the lateral pterygoid is also actively involved in mandibular closure.[24,28]

The *temporalis* muscle, which is fan shaped, arises from the temporal fossa and deep surface of the temporal fascia. The anterior fibers of the muscle are vertical, the middle are oblique, and the posterior are nearly horizontal. The fibers converge as they descend, becoming tendinous, and insert into the medial and anterior aspects of the coronoid process of the ramus. The temporalis muscle functions primarily as an elevator of the mandible, moving the jaw vertically and diagonally upwards. The posterior fibers also retract the mandible and maintain the condyles posteriorly (Fig. 11-6).

The *masseter* is a thick quadrilateral muscle composed of two bellies, the deep and superficial. The superficial portion arises from the lower border of the zygomatic arch and maxillary process; it extends down and back, and inserts into the angle and the inferior half of the lateral surface of the ramus. The muscle itself is formed by an intricate arrangement of tendinous and fleshy bundles that make it extremely powerful (Fig. 11-7,*A*). The smaller, deeper portion is fused anteriorly to the superficial portion but is separated from it posteriorly. It arises from the entire length of the zygomatic arch and passes anteriorly and inferiorly, inserting in the lateral surface of the coronoid process and superior half of the ramus (Figure 11-7, *B*). The masseter functions primarily as an elevator of the manible. The superficial fibers also protrude the jaw a little, and the deep portion acts as a retractor as well.

The *medial pterygoid* is located on the

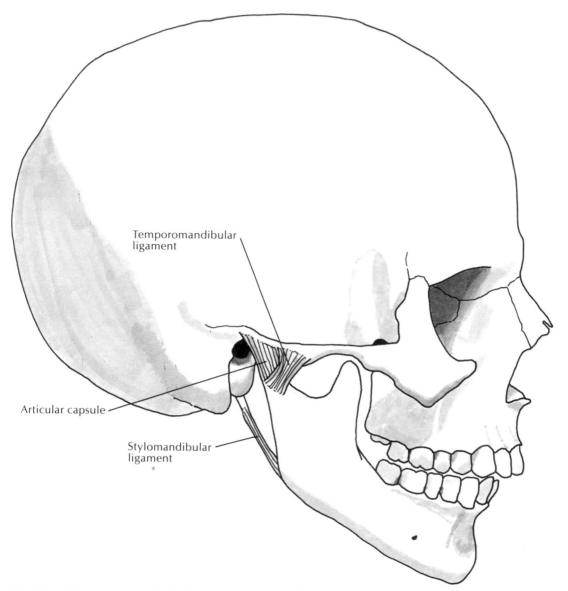

Fig. 11-4. Temporomandibular ligament and capsule

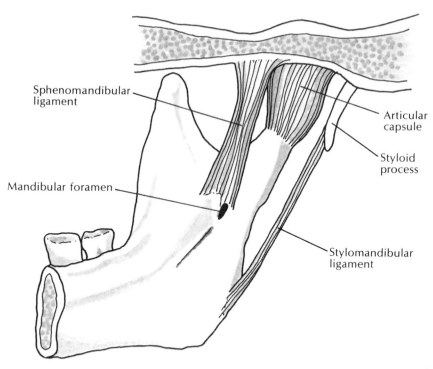

Sphenomandibular ligament

Mandibular foramen

Articular capsule

Styloid process

Stylomandibular ligament

Fig. 11-5. Sphenomandibular and stylomandibular ligaments as viewed from medial aspect of mandible

medial aspect of the ramus. Although less powerful than the masseter, its construction is similar to the masseter in that it is characterized by an alternation of fleshy and tendinous parts. The medial pterygoid, which is quadrilateral in shape, arises from the medial surface of the lateral pterygoid plate and pyramidal process of the palatine bone. The fibers pass laterally, posteriorly, and inferiorly, and insert onto the medial surface of the ramus and angle of mandible. Its primary function is closing and elevation of the mandible. It also protrudes and laterally deviates the jaw (Fig. 11-8).

The major muscles that depress the mandible are the lateral pterygoids and the anterior strap muscles, the suprahyoid and infrahyoid groups. The suprahyoid muscles are the digastric, stylohyoid, mylohyoid, and geniohyoid. They are all either opposed or assisted synergically by the infrahyoid muscles.

The *lateral pterygoid* is a thick conical muscle and consists of two bellies. The superior head arises from the infratemporal crest of the greater wing of the sphenoid bone. The inferior head arises from the lateral surface of the pterygoid plate. The two heads form a tendinous insertion in front of the temporomandibular joint. The lower fibers run horizontally and insert on the neck of the condyle, with some fibers attaching to the medial portion of the condyle as well. Fibers from the superior head are attached to the articular disk and capsule as well as to the condylar head (Fig. 11-8).[28,36] The attachment of the lateral pterygoid to the condyle and disk is significant in stabilizing the temporomandibular joint during bilateral protrusion, retrusion, and closing of the mandible. Lateral movement of the mandible is achieved by the action of the lateral and medial pterygoid on one side and the contralateral temporalis muscle. The

(*Text continues on page 244*)

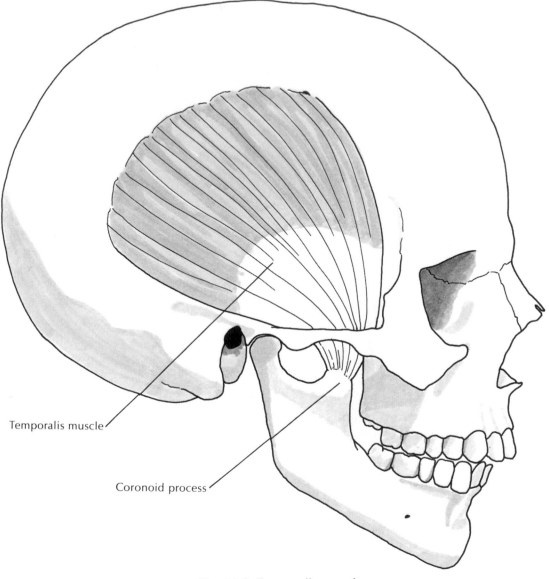

Temporalis muscle

Coronoid process

Fig. 11-6. Temporalis muscle

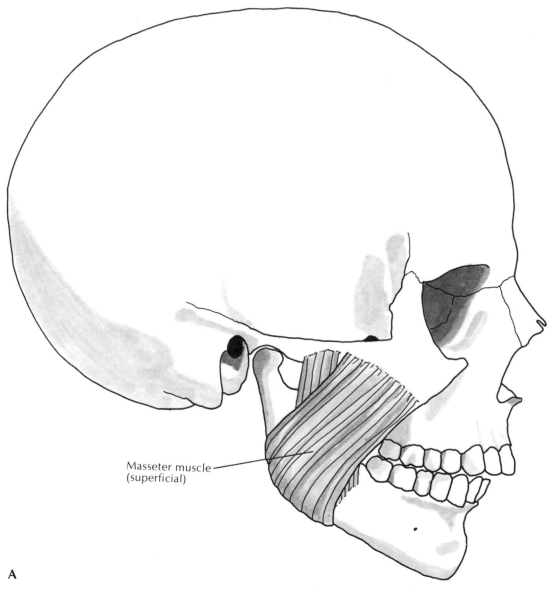

Masseter muscle
(superficial)

A

Fig. 11-7. (*A*) Superficial layer of masseter muscle

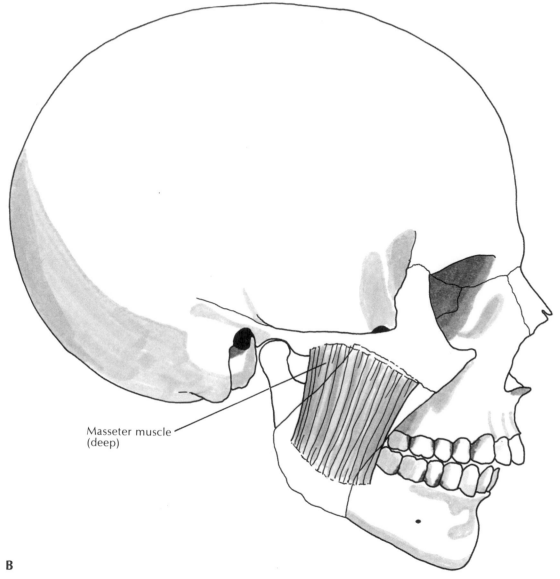

Masseter muscle
(deep)

B

Fig. 11-7. (*Continued*) (*B*) Deep layer of masseter muscle

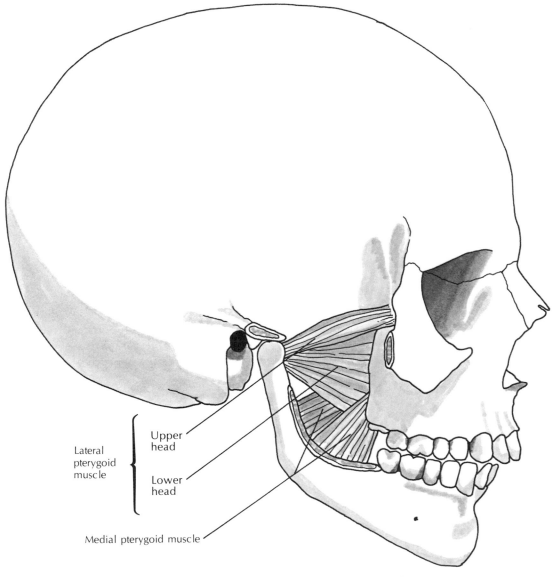

Lateral
pterygoid
muscle

Upper
head

Lower
head

Medial pterygoid muscle

Fig. 11-8. Medial and lateral pterygoid muscles

lateral pterygoid, especially its inferior head, is also the primary muscle used in opening the mouth, and in protrusion of the mandible. The superior head is thought to play an important role in stabilizing the condylar head and disk against the articular eminence during closing movement of the mandible.[28] This muscle is particularly important in cases of temporomandibular joint dysfunction and is the muscle most frequently involved.

The *digastric* consists of an anterior and posterior belly connected by a strong round tendon. The anterior belly arises from the lower border of the mandible close to the symphysis. The posterior belly, which is considerably longer than the anterior one, arises from the mastoid process of the temporal bone. Both bellies descend toward the hyoid bone and are united by the intermediate tendon, which is connected to the hyoid bone by a loop of fibrous tissue (Fig. 11-9). The function of the digastric is to pull the mandible back and down. The digastric, assisted by the suprahyoids, plays a dominant role in forced opening of the mandible when the hyoid bone is fixed by the infrahyoid muscle group. It also aids in retraction of the jaw and elevation of the hyoid bone.

The *stylohyoid* muscle arises from the styloid process of the temporal bone and inserts on the hyoid bone. Along with the geniohyoid it determines the length of the floor of the mouth. It also acts in initiating and assisting jaw opening and draws the hyoid bone upwards and backwards when the mandible is fixed (Fig. 11-9).

The *geniohyoid* is a narrow muscle, wider posteriorly than anteriorly, that lies adjacent to the midline of the floor of the mouth and above the mylohyoid muscle. It arises from the symphysis of the mandible and inserts onto the anterior surface of the hyoid bone. Like the digastric, it acts to pull the mandible down and back when the hyoid bone is fixed and assists in elevation of the hyoid bone. (Fig. 11-10).

The *mylohyoid* arises from the whole length of the medial surface of the mandible, from the symphysis to the last molar teeth, and makes up the floor of the mouth. The fibers pass downward with some meeting in the median raphe and some attaching directly to the hyoid bone. The mylohyoid elevates the floor of the mouth. It also assists in depression of the mandible when the hyoid is fixed and elevation of the hyoid bone when the mandible is fixed (Fig. 11-10).

The *infrahyoid* muscles (sternohyoid, thyrohyoid, and omohyoid) act together to steady the hyoid bone or depress it and therefore allow the suprahyoids to act on the mandible (Fig. 11-9).

Muscle Group Action

Mandibular movements are complicated, owing to the wide range of positions that the mandible can potentially assume. Briefly, group action might be summarized as follows:

Mandibular Elevators. The mandibular elevators include the coordinated action of the masseter, temporalis (for retrusion), superior head of the lateral pterygoid (for stabilization), and the medial pterygoid (for protrusion).

Mandibular Opening. The inferior head of the lateral pterygoid and the anterior head of the digastric are considered the primary muscles used in opening the mandible. The inferior head of the lateral pterygoid acts synergistically with the suprahyoid muscle group in the translation of the condylar head downward, inferiorly and contralaterally during opening movements. Opening is assisted by the other suprahyoid muscles which also act in initiating motion when the hyoid bone is fixed by the infrahyoid muscles. The masseter and the medial pterygoid muscles also help draw the jaw slightly forward.

Retrusion of the Mandible. The posterior fibers of the temporalis draw the condyles backward during retrusion and are assisted by the digastric and suprahyoids.

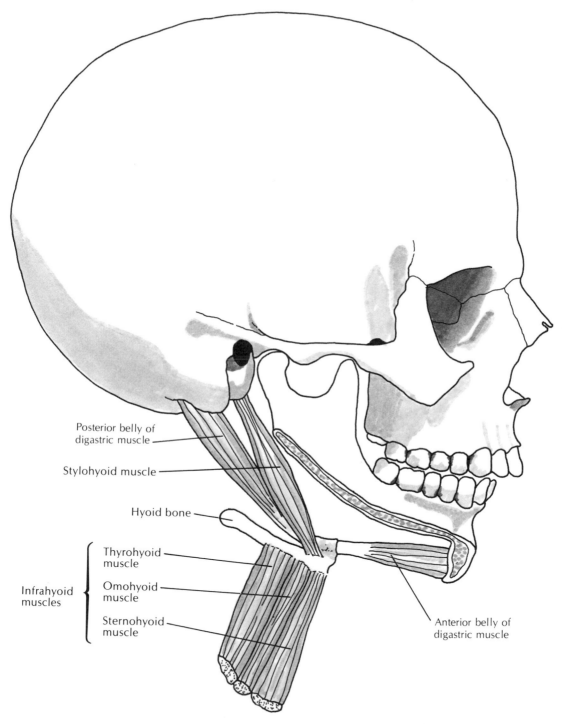

Posterior belly of
digastric muscle

Stylohyoid muscle

Hyoid bone

Thyrohyoid
muscle

Infrahyoid
muscles

Omohyoid
muscle

Sternohyoid
muscle

Anterior belly of
digastric muscle

Fig. 11-9. Digastric, stylohyoid, and infrahyoid muscles

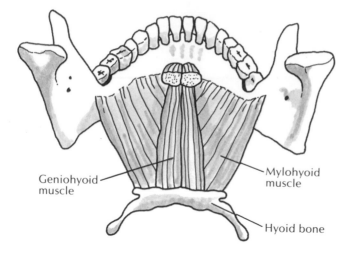

Geniohyoid muscle

Mylohyoid muscle

Hyoid bone

Fig. 11-10. Mylohyoid and geniohyoid muscles viewed from above and behind the floor of the mouth

Protrusion of the Mandible. Protrusion is performed by the masseter and medial and lateral pterygoids.

Lateral Movements. Action is achieved primarily by the lateral and medial pterygoids on one side and the temporalis muscle on the contralateral side. When the mandible moves to the right side, the left lateral pterygoid and medial pterygoid moves the chin across the midline toward the right side. The digastric, geniohyoid, and mylohyoid also are actively involved.

DYNAMICS OF THE MANDIBLE AND TEMPOROMANDIBULAR JOINTS

Before evaluating the dynamics of the various mandibular movements, certain physiological positions of the jaw should be defined. These are the rest position, occlusal positions, hinge position, and centric position. The terminology of some of these positions is confusing and controversal. No basic terminology has been universally adopted, and each investigator has had to establish his own.

The rest position of the mandible is considered the position the jaw assumes when there is minimal muscle-action potential. It usually implies that the head is also in its normal rest position when the individual is in an upright posture. The mandibu-

lar rest position is considered to be an equilibrium between the tonus of the gravity, or jaw opening, muscles and that of the antigravity, or jaw closing, muscles. The residual tension of the muscles at rest is termed *resting tonus*. In this position there is no occlusal contact between the maxillary and mandibular teeth. The space between the upper and lower teeth is called the *free-way space* or *interocclusal clearance*. It normally measures from 2 mm to 5 mm between incisors.

The importance of the rest position lies in the fact that it permits the tissues of the stomatognathic system to rest and thus repair themselves. If the vertical dimension is abnormally decreased—eliminating the interocclusal space—the teeth will be in constant contact. This eliminates the rest position and creates constant muscular tension and stress on the supporting structures and teeth. Factors that influence muscle tonus and the rest position are function, sleep, pathologic conditions, and the normal aging process.

Occlusal positions are functional positions in which contact between some or all of the teeth occur. One occlusal position, termed *median occlusal position* by Sicher and DuBrul, is highly significant.[45] This is the position in which the jaws are closed so that all upper and lower teeth meet, resulting in full occlusion with a balanced intercuspation of the upper and lower dental arches. From the median occlusal position, the mandible can move forward into protrusive occlusal positions, laterally, and backward to a limited extent in all normal jaws. Absent or abnormally positioned teeth can displace the mandible from the normal median occlusal position, disturbing the complete balance between the teeth, temporomandibular joints, and the musculature.

The hinge position is the position of the mandible from which a pure hinge opening and closing of the jaw can be made.[45] In the hinge position, the condyles are in the most retruded position that the muscles of the jaw can accomplish; it is determined by the length of the temporomandibular ligaments. The position is considered a retruded position or "strained relationship" that the mandible can assume actively or passively. Determination of this position is useful for some clinical procedures.

Centric position, or centric relation occlusion, denotes a concept of normal mandibular posture. Centric position implies the most retruded, unstrained position of the mandible from which lateral movements are possible and the components of the oral apparatus are in balance. Normal centric position is slightly forward of the most posterior position that the mandibular musculature can actually achieve. Ideally, median occlusal position should coincide with centric position.

Mandibular movements are complicated owing to the wide range of positions that the mandible can assume. Involved and integrated in mandibular movements are the shape of the fossae, the degree of tension of the associated ligaments, the menisci, the neuromuscular system, and the guiding incline of the teeth.

Kinematically, the mandible may be considered a free body that can rotate in any angular direction. It has, therefore, three degrees of freedom; each of these de-grees of freedom of motion is associated with a separate axis of rotation.[48] The two basic movements required for functional motion are rotation and translation. The mandible is capable of affecting these movements in three planes—sagittal, horizontal, and frontal. The joint has three functional motions—opening and closing, protrusion and retrusion, and lateral motions. A considerable degree of rotation is also possible.

When the mouth is opened, the condyles first rotate around a horizontal axis. This motion is then combined with gliding of the condyles forward and downward with the lower surface of the meniscus at the same time as the meniscus slides forward and downward on the temporal bone. This movement results from the attachment of the meniscus to the medial and lateral poles of the head of the mandible and from the contraction of the lateral pterygoid which carries the condyle with the meniscus onto the articular eminence. The forward sliding of the meniscus ceases when the fibroelastic tissue attaching to the temporal bone posteriorly has been stretched to the limits. Thereafter, there is some further hinging and gliding forward of the condyle until it articulates with the most anterior part of the meniscus and the mouth is fully opened. The condyles essentially rotate on an axis in the horizontal plane and translate against the posterior slope of the articular eminence in the sagittal plane.

Opening movements of the mandible are caused by the synergistic action of the lateral pterygoid muscles and the depressors of the mandible. Although the lateral pterygoid pulls the condylar head and meniscus forward, the digastric and geniohyoid muscles pull the mandible downward and backward, affecting rotation. This blending of muscle action makes possible the rotatory and translatory movements of jaw opening. This motion affects all the other muscles anchored to the mandible. The elevators of the mandible must lengthen to ensure smoothness of performance, and the muscles of the cranium and hyoid bone must act as holders to establish a fixed position (Fig. 11-11).

In mandibular closure, the movements are reversed. In the first phase of the movement, the condyles glide backward and then hinge on the menisci, which are held forward by the lateral pterygoids. The backward glide of the mandible results from interaction between the retracting portions of the masseter and temporal muscles and the retracting portions of the depressors. During the second phase, the inferior head of the lateral pterygoids relaxes while the upper head allows the menisci to glide backward and upward on the temporal bone along with the condyles.[24] The second phase begins with the contraction of the masseter, the medial pterygoid, and temporalis muscles; it ends with intercuspation of the teeth. The onset of superior head, or lateral pterygoid function is usually concurrent with that of the elevator musculature.[28]

In protrusion, the teeth are retained throughout in the occlusal position, so far as possible, and the lower teeth are drawn forward over the upper teeth by both lateral pterygoids. In contrast to opening movements, the condyles and menisci move downward and forward along the articular eminences without rotation of the condyles around a transverse axis. To prevent the mandible from falling, the elevating muscles exhibit some degree of contraction. They must make the necessary adjustment with the balancing depressor–retractors as they lengthen to allow the mandible to slide forward just free of the interlocking dentition.

In retraction, the mandible is drawn backward by the deep portion of the masseter muscles and by the posterior fibers of the temporalis muscles to the rest position. At the same time, the geniohyoid and the digastric muscles and the elevators synergistically balance each other to maintain the mandible in the horizontal position.

In lateral movements of the mandible, asymmetrical muscular patterns develop on both sides. In this movement, one condyle and meniscus slides downward and forward in the sagittal plane and medially in the horizontal plane along the articular

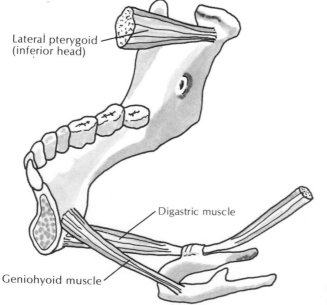

Lateral pterygoid
(inferior head)

Digastric muscle

Geniohyoid muscle

Fig. 11-11. Mandibular muscles involved in opening

eminence. At the same time, the other condyle rotates laterally on a sagittal plane around a shifting vertical axis and translates medially in the horizontal plane while remaining in the fossa. The condylar translation in the horizontal plane is known as the Bennett movement.[45,48,49] If one views the mandible from above, it will be seen that the medial pole of the condyle juts far medially from the plane of the jaw, while the coronoid process leans laterally. The lateral pterygoid muscle, inserted on the medial pole of the condyle, pulls inward and forward in the horizontal plane, while the horizontal fibers of the temporal muscle, inserted on the coronoid process, pull outward and backward (Fig. 11-12). These muscles, operating as a force-couple, contribute to the torque of rotating the condyle which is necessary to effect chewing on this side. The condyle is known as the working-side condyle. Therefore, in lateral deviation to the left, the lateral pterygoid on the right, together with the right and left anterior bellies of the digastric and geniohyoid, contract. This causes the right condyle to move downward, forward, and medially while the actions of the left temporal and the lateral pterygoid rotate the left condyle in the fossa and displace the mandible to the left. This is described as left lateral excursion with a Bennett shift to the left. The left condyle is called the *working side condyle* and the right condyle is the *nonworking condyle*, or balancing condyle. Basic types of working condylar motions include[49]

1. Rotation with no lateral shift (Fig. 11-13,*A*)
2. Rotation with movement backward, upward, and/or laterally (Fig. 11-13,*B*)
3. Rotation with movement downward, forward, and laterally (Fig. 11-13,*C*)
4. Rotation with a lateral shift (Fig. 11-13,*D*)
5. Rotation with movement downward, backward, and laterally (Fig. 11-13,*E*)

It is apparent that the right lateral pterygoid has also entered into the force-couple system. In the closing stroke, the force-couple changes in direction and components. Thus, in the rotatory movements of grinding or chewing, these alternating movements swing the mandible from side to side.

Although masticatory movements are highly complex, they become automatic in each individual as a result of the integration of the proprioceptive mechanism and muscular action. All of the muscles of mastication are involved in the act of chewing because it involves all four movements of the mandible—elevation, depression, protrusion, and retrusion.

APPLIED ANATOMY

Dislocation of the Jaw

Dislocation may result from actual trauma to the chin during opening of the mouth or may occur without actual trauma, for example, with a sudden muscular spasm during a yawn. This dislocation is always anterior and may be unilateral or bilateral, resulting in displacement of one or both condyles forward into the infratemporal fossa anterior to the articular eminences.[43] In bilateral dislocations, the chin is displaced forward so that the patient shows some degree of prognathia with an open bite. In unilateral dislocation the mandible is displaced toward the noninjured side.

Reduction is accomplished unilaterally by depressing the mandible with the thumb placed on the last molar teeth and at the same time elevating the chin. The downward pressure overcomes the spasm of the elevating muscles, and elevating the chin repositions the condyles backward behind the articular eminences. Reduction is usually followed by several days of rest.[41]

Habitual dislocations, subluxations, or self-reducing dislocations are not especially rare. According to Dufourmentel and Axhausen, there are two kinds of habitual subluxation that patients themselves may learn to adjust either by a spe-

(*Text continues on page 252*)

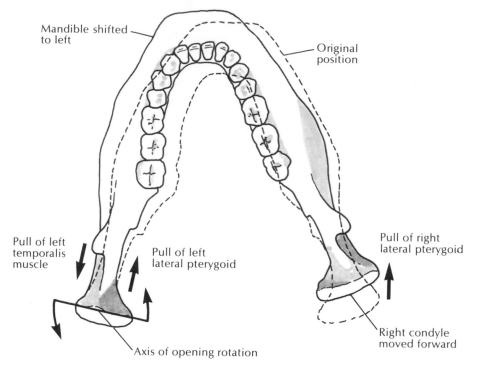

Mandible shifted to left

Original position

Pull of left temporalis muscle

Pull of left lateral pterygoid

Pull of right lateral pterygoid

Right condyle moved forward

Axis of opening rotation

Fig. 11-12. Mandibular muscles involved in lateral movement of the mandible to the left. The suprahyoid muscles are not shown.

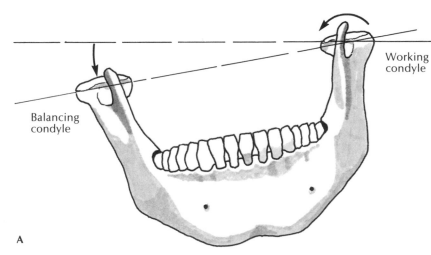

Working condyle

Balancing condyle

A

Fig. 11-13. The basic types of working condylar motions are (A) rotation with no lateral shift; (B) rotation with movement backward, upward and/or laterally; (C) rotation with movement downward, forward, and laterally; (D) rotation with a lateral shift; and (E) rotation with movement downward, backward, and laterally. (After Weinberg LA: J Prosthet Dent 13:622–644, 1963)

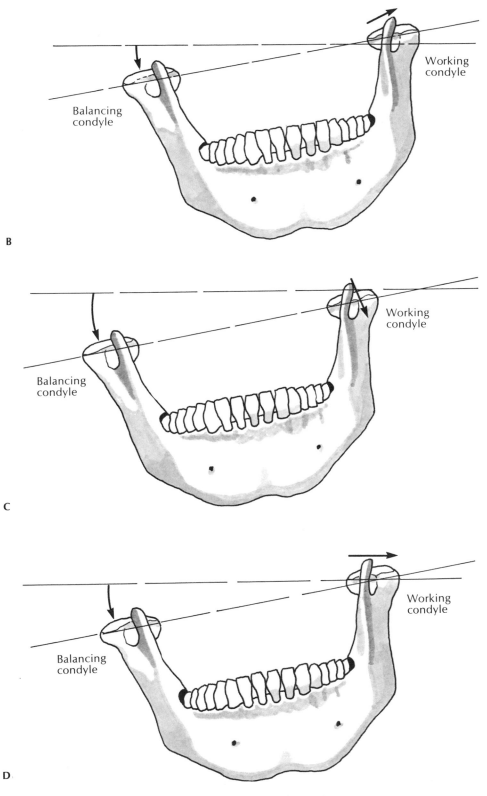

Fig. 11-13. (*Continued*)

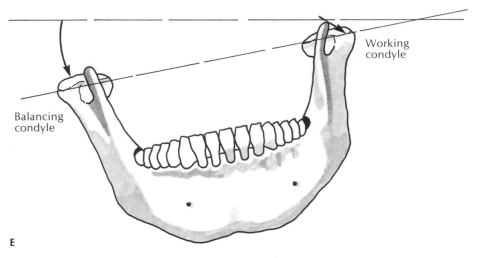

E

Fig. 11-13. (*Continued*)

cial jaw movement or with the hand. These are luxation in the upper cavity (meniscotemporal) and luxation in the lower cavity (meniscocondylar).[1,10]

Derangement of the Meniscus

Trauma, overclosure of the mouth with backward displacement of the condyle, or malocclusion may cause derangement of the meniscus. Trauma to the meniscus can vary from an inflammatory condition to a complete or partial tearing of the meniscus from its capsular attachment. If the meniscus remains attached to the anterior capsule and the external pterygoid, an anterior dislocation of the meniscus occurs. It may be manifested by displacement of the mandible toward the affected side and possible blockage of mandibular opening and closing.[43] If the meniscus remains attached to the posterior capsule, a painful blockage in closing the mandible results.[43]

The most widely accepted view is that clicking is the result of derangement of the meniscus. However, many investigators have reported various other theories of its etiology in addition to derangement of the meniscus. Among these are incoordinate contraction of the two bodies of the lateral pterygoid, so that the disk snaps over the condyle rather than following its movement smoothly and coordinately when the mouth is open; deterioration of the disk and cartilaginous surfaces; and stretching of the joint ligaments by frequent subluxation.[44]

Clicking may occur as one or more clicks in one joint, or clicking may occur in both joints; it may or may not be associated with pain. Various types of clicking noises have been observed during sagittal opening, including an opening click, an intermediate click during the opening phase, and a full opening click. Each of these clicks appears to be associated with various pathologic occlusions.

An opening click is felt to be due to an anterior displacement of the meniscus, with the condyle displaced posteriorly and superiorly. As the mandible opens, the condyle must pass over the posterior surface of the meniscus.[44]

Clicking during various parts of the opening of the mandible is thought to result from incoordinate movements of the upper and lower heads of the external pterygoid, so that the condyle cannot remain in its normal relationship with the meniscus.[44] A more likely cause is possible anteroposterior displacement of the disk, or ruptures or rents of the disk.[54]

A final click occuring in the full opening phase may be caused by the condyle passing over the anterior portion of the meniscus, or by the meniscus being pulled forward of the condyle, or by both the meniscus or condyle passing over the articular eminence.[44]

In addition to clicks produced during mandibular opening, clicks may be produced by eccentric movements. Again these may be largely due to structural changes in the disks or incoordinate functioning of the parts of the joint.[44]

Crepitus has been associated with perforation in the disk. Moffett and co-workers demonstrated that perforation of the disk is usually followed by osteoarthritic change on the condylar surface, which is in turn followed by similar bony alterations on the opposing surface of the fossa.[29]

COMMON LESIONS

TEMPOROMANDIBULAR JOINT DYSFUNCTION SYNDROME

A common temporomandibular joint disorder found clinically is temporomandibular (TMJ) joint dysfunction syndrome, also referred to as mandibular pain–dysfunction syndrome, arthrosis temporomandibularis,[44] temporomandibular joint arthrosis, and myofascial pain syndrome.

TMJ dysfunction syndrome cannot be considered a disease of aging or senility, since it commonly occurs in patients between the ages of 20 and 40 years.[41] It is most frequently found among women. The early incoordination phase associated with clicking, subluxation, and recurrent dislocation is most commonly found among women in the third to fourth decade of life, and in men during the third decade. The later limitation phase occurs most frequently in women in the fourth to fifth decade.[42]

Signs and symptoms of the early incoordination phase are usually unilateral but may be bilateral. They may include muscular tenderness, limited motion, and a dull aching pain in the periarticular area often radiating to the ear, face, head, neck, and shoulders and aggravated by function. Usually, the syndrome first manifests itself in the form of functional incoordination of the mandibular muscles with symptoms of clicking in the temporomandibular joint, which is otherwise asymptomatic, and subluxation or recurrent dislocation. Additionally, clinical examination often reveals hypermobility of the joints or a tendency to protrude the mandible or both during the initial opening movement.[46] These symptoms are followed in many cases by spasms of the masticatory muscles characterized by pain on movement of the joint, especially during mastication. Gradually, the pain becomes worse and is accompanied by decreased mobility. Pain and mobility tend to be worse in the morning. In unilateral conditions, the mandible deviates to the symptomatic side, resulting in compensation of the contralateral joint by hypermobility, subluxation, and irregular mandibular opening and closing movements. Mandibular "catching" or "locking" in certain positions may also occur on opening. Often pain may accompany movement of the hypermobile joint and may require treatment as well.

The temporomandibular joint dysfunction syndrome is usually reversible, but its perpetuation may and often does result in organic changes. When spontaneous recovery does not occur and when spasm is not relieved by treatment, such spasm may set up a sustaining cycle. If dysfunction is of a long duration, contracture of the masticatory muscles with limited painless mandibular movement may occur. This is referred to as the *limitation phase*. At this stage, pathologic changes are noted and are mainly degenerative. They are located in the fibrous covering of the articular eminence, in the condylar head, and in the fibrous articular meniscus. There is, however, little evidence to support the view that there is a relationship between degenerative changes within the joint and symptoms of TMJ dysfunction.[41] Marked changes are often seen without symptoms, and frequently, marked symptoms are seen without radiographic evidence of changes in structure. When arthrosis of the temporomandibular joint shows extreme changes in the structure of the joint or joints, the disease is sometimes referred to as *arthrosis temporomandibularis deformans*.[44]

It is generally accepted that TMJ dysfunction–pain syndrome is a neuromuscular or joint dysfunction and that the etiology of pain is multicausal. The five major causes of pain may be (1) neurologic, (2) vascular, (3) the TMJ joint itself, (4) muscular, or (5) hysterical conversion.[52] Pain that originates from the joints themselves can be caused by infection, disk derangement, condylar displacement, microtrauma, and traumatic injury.[50] Many patients, particularly those with painful limited mandibular movements, complain of sudden onset of symptoms upon awaking, after rapid or extensive mandibular opening (*e.g.*, yawning or following a long dental appointment), or when changes are made in occlusion (*e.g.*, through restoration, grinding, or the use of a dental appliance).

Many authors point out that many conditions called TMJ disorders are not in the strict sense of the word disorders of the joint at all, but simply dysfunction of the masticatory muscles. The presence of painful areas within the muscles and signs of mandibular dysfunction were Schwartz's most constant finding.[41] Such painful areas and accompanying dysfunction have been given various names such as *myalgia, myositis, fibrositis,* and *myofascial pain syndromes*. The precipitating factor is held to be motion that stretches the muscle, setting off a self-sustaining cycle of pain, spasm, and pain. The muscles that are commonly involved are the masseter, medial and lateral pterygoids, temporals, suprahyoids, infrahyoids, sternocleidomastoids, scaleni, and rhomboids. The muscles most frequently involved are the lateral pterygoids.

Emotional tension may also play a predominant role. With stress, the tension of the skeletal muscles increases, often with clenching of the teeth or bruxism resulting in local disharmony of the masticatory apparatus. When hypertonicity occurs in the masticatory muscles for a long period of time, we may observe pain–dysfunction syndrome, occlusal wear, and tooth mobility. Once the pattern is established, it appears to be self-perpetuating. Other habit manifestations seen in these patients that cause pathologic occlusal contact are numerous and include unilateral mastication, abnormal swallowing, and "tooth doodling" during the waking hours.[14,46] What the patient does to his occlusion in reaction to stress seems to be more important than any existing malocclusion. Certainly malocclusion, by mechanically increasing the amount of force or altering its direction, can make the chance of injury more likely. More important than the type of malocclusion, however, may be the amount and kind of muscular activity and the reaction of the individual to such activity. In some individuals, change in proprioception, no matter how slight, seems to be more important than a longstanding malocclusion, no matter how irregular.

Diagnostic procedures to establish the presence of TMJ dysfunction and a definitive diagnosis include

—An accurate history
—Determination of the patient's emotional state and daily habits
—Examination of mandibular movements
—Measurement of mandibular opening, lateral deviation, and protrusion
—Palpation of the temporomandibular joint and muscles of mastication
—Dental and oral examination
—Occlusal analysis
—Radiographs

—Electromyography
—Physical examination of related structures (cervical spine)
—Neurological testing

The primary methods of therapy revolve around the correction of occlusal disharmonies and tension habits, as well as physical therapy to eliminate spasm and increase range of motion through therapeutic exercise and mobilization techniques.

DEGENERATIVE JOINT DISEASE—OSTEOARTHRITIS

Although osteoarthritis may occur at any age, it is considered primarily a disease of middle or old age. It is estimated that it may be found in 80% to 90% of the population over 60 years of age.[30]

The etiology is generally felt to be the result of normal wear and tear associated with aging and function, as well as the result of repeated minor trauma. It is speculated that damage consists primarily of degeneration of the chondroitin-collagen-protein complex.[17] Radiographic examination may reveal narrowing of the tempomandibular joint space with condensation of bone in the region of the articular cortex, spur formation, and marginal lipping at the articular margins of the condylar head.[17] In some cases there is considerable thickening of the synovial membrane due to chronic synovitis. There may be perforation of the disc without bony changes. Erosion of the condylar head, articular eminence and fossa may be noted.

Symptoms do not seem to be related to the extent of articular damage. Osteoarthritis may be asymptomatic even in the presence of extensive articular damage, while on the other hand, articular findings may be completely absent in patients with acute symptoms. The onset is generally insidious with mild symptoms. Pain, which is usually a dull aching in or around the joint, is usually not constant. Typically, painful stiffness of the jaw muscles is noted in the morning or following periods of rest. With use, the symptoms may disappear and then reappear with fatigue at the end of the day. Pain may be precipitated on opening or during mastication. Crepitation, crackling, or clicking may occur in one or both joints. Subluxation and locking of one or both joints during certain movements are common complaints. The patient may also complain of symptoms of the ear, impaired hearing, frequent headaches, and dizziness. At the onset, symptoms are usually short-lived, but as degeneration progresses they occur more frequently and last longer. Crepitation and limited motion are the most constant findings.

Diagnostic procedures to establish the presence of osteoarthritis can be difficult but again depend on an accurate history, the determination of the patient's emotional state, physical examination, and radiographs. Physical examination may or may not reveal discrete painful areas in the musculature; minimal emotional tension may be noted.

The primary method of therapy is directed at symptoms and may involve correcting the occlusion of the teeth or prosthesis, drug therapy, and physical therapy. During the painful phase, the application of hot packs may help to reduce muscle spasm and pain. Active range of motion exercises (often in conjunction with ultrasound), passive range of motion exercises, mobilization techniques (preceded by deep frictions to the capsule[7]), and stretching may be used during the chronic phase. Graded exercises involving a few simple movements performed frequently during the day are frequently prescribed as a home treatment. Advanced bony changes within the joint may necessitate arthroplasty with joint debridement.

RHEUMATOID ARTHRITIS

There is little agreement regarding the incidence of patients with rheumatoid arthritis who also develop the disease in the temporomandibular joints; estimates vary from 20% to 51%.[17] Women are affected more often than men.

There are three groups of symptoms— transitory, acute, and chronic. Transitory symptoms include limitation of motion and referred pain. Acute symptoms consist of transitory symptoms plus joint pain, swelling, and warmth lasting 6 to 10 wks. Chronic symptoms are characterized by severe pain and limitation of motion. The joint and muscle symptoms are severest in the morning and diminish with the day's activity. Inflammatory changes are noted in the synovial membrane and periarticular structures by atrophy and rarefraction of bone. A serious sequela of ankylosis may restrict or even eliminate movement. If symptoms are not relieved by conservative management, surgical intervention may be indicated.

The primary method of therapy is directed at symptoms and may involve drug therapy, if indicated by specific signs and symptoms, and physical therapy. In the acute phase, immobilization is contraindicated, but rest in the form of a soft or liquid diet is advocated. After inflammation has subsided, treatment is directed at reducing muscle spasm and restoring mandibular movements by correction exercises.

Surgical procedures such as condylectomies and condylotomies frequently used in the past are now felt to be obsolete for the most part but are occasionally performed.[40] Following surgery, corrective exercises and exercises of mandibular excursions, using mouth props to insure that range of motion is not compromised, should be performed several times a day.[25]

TRAUMA AND DISORDERS OF LIMITATION

One of the most frequent cause of TMJ dysfunction is a direct or indirect blow to the area, including resultant fracture in the region of the condyle. When there is no fracture, injuries may result in edema and possible soft-tissue damage, such as tearing of the capsular ligaments or meniscus and simple dislocations and subluxations. Other causes of limitation include postoperative trismus following tooth extraction and whiplash injuries.

There is adequate proof that whiplash injuries are responsible for many TMJ dysfunctions. Whiplash can be explained as a deceleration effect on the mandible and thus on the temporomandibular joint either through direct injury or through neurologic involvement. When the head is snapped back abruptly, the mouth flies open, evoking a stretch reflex of the masseter. The capsule, ligaments, and interarticular mensicus act as a restraining ligament; tearing or stretching these tissues may result. Immediately following, the jaw snaps shut; this may strain the attachment of the meniscus if malocclusion is present. Cervical traction, commonly used in the management of the cervical spine, may also produce TMJ dysfunction or the primary TMJ dysfunction may be aggravated.

Treatment and management of such injuries will depend on the structures involved, the extent of displacement, the effect on function, and the degree of pain. During the acute phase, soft and liquid diets, head bandages or intermaxillary immobilization, and splints may be used to rest the joint. Surgical procedures, open and closed reduction, and manipulations may be necessary.

Physical therapy may consist of heat and other methods to reduce pain and muscle spasm; early mobility exercises postsurgically or following immobilization to ensure range of motion is not compromised; and muscle re-education and corrective exercises. Stretching and mobilization techniques may be necessary to treat contracture of the musculature or capsules. When cervical traction is considered necessary in the treatment of the neck and whiplash injuries, the temporomandibular joint should be protected with bite plates or soft splints and the proper use of traction.[53]

OTHER CONDITIONS

Other conditions that may cause TMJ dysfunction include a variety of neurologic and muscular disorders, bone disease, tumors, infections, psychogenic disorder, growth and developmental disorders, diseases causing disturbance of the occlusion of the teeth or supporting structures, faulty habits of the jaw, improper swallowing, oral-facial imbalance, and others.

PHYSICAL THERAPY MANAGEMENT

TMJ dysfunction, arthritic conditions, ankylosing diseases, traumatic injuries, and postsurgical entities may be a few of the causes that bring a patient to the physical therapist.

When degenerative disease, bony or fibrous ankylosis, fractures, occlusal disharmony, and other conditions necessitate surgery, follow-up physical therapy may become necessary to maintain or regain motion, as well as regain normal mandibular osteokinematics. In the majority of postsurgical cases, muscle tonus remains good, except after long-term ankylosis or degenerative joint disease. In these cases there is greater possibility that the muscles have atrophied, making rehabilitation more difficult and necessitating a more extensive program of therapeutic exercises to increase the physiological elasticity and strength of the muscles.

Following condylectomy, we must keep in mind that the lateral pterygoid's attachment to the condyle has been severed, and that the jaw will increasingly deviate ipsilaterally. Postoperative rehabilitation for the lost function should encourage the similarly functioning muscles of the masseter, temporalis, and suprahyoid muscles on the healthy side to perform with increased strength. At least partial use of the lateral pterygoid muscle should be stressed so that it is able to contribute to contralateral mandibular excursion and to prevent posterior drifting of the ramus in its tonic state.

Signs and symptoms of the TMJ syndrome vary, but generally include a cluster of symptoms.

—Pain and tenderness of the masticatory muscles
—Limited or altered mandibular function (*i.e.*, hypermobility or a tendency to protrude the mandible in the initial opening phase)
— Crepitation or clicking
— Deviation of the mandible on opening
— Disturbed chewing patterns
— Locking of the jaw
—Vague, remote subjective complaints.

The means of treatment of TMJ syndrome is basically like that for other myofascial pain syndromes—anesthetics, exercise, and physical and pharmacologic agents. There are, however, additional considerations. There are two traditional concepts of the etiology of TMJ dysfunction. Some clinicians stress malocclusion as the causal factor. They advocate treatment involving mainly mechanical factors, such as equilibration of the occlusion.[7,19] Others emphasize that psychological factors, especially response to stress, and harmful habits of the jaw may influence both the onset and course of symptoms. They advocate patient education, the elimination of habitual protrusion or other harmful habits, and muscular relaxation.

The effective management of TMJ disorders requires first of all a diagnosis based on a complete history, thorough physical examination, and when indicated, adjuncts such as a detailed study of the patient's occlusion, radiography, and electromyography.

TREATMENT OF LIMITATION DISORDERS

STRETCHING TECHNIQUES

For the purpose of increasing limited mandibular movements, a variety of exercises involving the muscles of mastication may be employed. They are used, on one hand, to help break up the muscle spasm, and on the other, to maintain and increase limited jaw movement to full physiologic function.

Active Stretch — Opening

This exercise consists of having the patient actively open his mouth as wide as possible several times following a series of warming up exercises.[42] By having the patient repeat a gentle, rhythmic, hingelike movement a number of times before active stretch, muscle spasm can be physiologically diminished or eliminated. With the patient in a comfortable, relaxed, reclining position or in a recliner chair, have him place his tongue in contact with the hard palate as posteriorly as possible, while keeping the mandible in a retruded position. In this position with the tongue on the hard palate, the patient's articular movements are mainly rotatory, and early protrusion is avoided. It is helpful to have the patient palpate the condyles so that he can feel the movement. If glide occurs too early, with little or no rotatory motion, there is an early protrusion problem. Instruct the patient to open his mouth slowly and rhythmically within this limited range 10 times or so in succession. He then performs active stretch by opening his mouth as wide as possible within the pain-free limit, as slowly as he can two or three times. The opening position should be held for 5 seconds, followed by relaxation in the rest position for 5 seconds. Ultrasound may be effective during this active stretch.

REFLEX RELAXATION — HOLD-RELAX

A variety of neuromuscular facilitation exercises may be used when range of motion is limited by shortening, contracture, or spasm.[22,41,53] One of the most frequently used methods is hold-relax to make stretching of the masticatory muscles more effective. This technique implies a contraction of the antagonist against maximal resistance followed by relaxation and then active or assistive stretch of the agonist. For example, to increase mandibular opening, the patient is asked to close his mouth tightly as resistance is applied gently and slowly to the mandible. This is followed by a relaxation and then by active or passive motion. Isometric contraction of the mouth elevator muscles facilitates their relaxation. The resultant stimulation of the jaw opening muscles permits increased active or passive stretch. You might use the following commands:

1. "Just hold your jaw closed and don't let me move it." Apply resistance gently and slowly to the mandible.
2. "Let go." Maintain gentle support of the mandible and wait for relaxation to occur.
3. "Open your mouth." Have the patient move the mandible actively with or without resistance.

Unresisted reversing movements may also be used as a follow up procedure by either active or assistive stretch.

A variety of similar techniques, such as maximal resistance superimposed upon an isotonic or isometric conraction, slow-reversal-hold, and contract-relax, may be used.[22,41,53] Such exercises may also be used for increasing range of protrusion, retrusion, and lateral deviation. The therapist provides resistance, or the patient may be asked to do so with his own hand.[41] By using resistance, the patient effects an increased relaxation of the antagonist muscles. This sets up a reflex mechanism called reciprocal inhibition.

PASSIVE AND ASSISTIVE STRETCH

Mechanical Methods — Mouth-opening

A simple method of mechanical stretch is to use a mouth prop with padded ends to protect the teeth. (A surgical mouth prop with a rachet or spring may be used for prolonged or static stretching, or the rachet may be removed for brief assistive or passive stretching.)

In static or prolonged stretching the patient is made as comfortable as possible in the reclining position. Moist heat may be applied to the cervical spine and both temporomandibular joints for 15 to 20 min. Place the side-action mouth prop between the molar teeth on one side, with the patient's mouth at a tolerable position of maximal opening.[53] Change the mouth prop from side to side during the course of the treatment to help distribute even pressure.

A somewhat more effective approach is to use a series of tongue blades. These are built up, one on top of the other, and placed between the front teeth to maintain a position of maximal tolerable opening. As the jaw begins to relax, additional tongue blades may be added. Contract-relax procedures and transverse pressure mobilization techniques may be administered with the mouth open at its maximum.[26]

In assistive and passive stretching the patient assumes a sitting position. The therapist, who stands behind the patient, uses one hand to place the prop between the patient's teeth and the other hand to support the mandible under the chin.[41] The patient then actively opens his mouth as wide as possible as he is assisted by the force of the separating arms of the prop. To provide passive stretch, the patient is first asked to bite down on the prop and then to relax as he is assisted into further mandibular opening. This contract opening reflex method helps the elevators to relax more readily.

A mouth prop can also be used for home treatment, both as a static stretch and for briefer periods of active and passive strain. A mouth prop, however, must be used with caution since too vigorous application may cause injury. Shore recommended the use of a tapered cork.[44] The cork, which is approximately 15 mm at its narrow end and 30 mm at its widest end, is gradually inserted—small end first—into the patient's mouth until the jaws are separated. Once the jaw begins to relax, the cork can be placed further into the mouth, thus progressively opening the jaw wider and wider. Shore recommends using this technique as a home treatment for 30-second periods, every 2 hours.

Direct Methods

Again with the patient sitting, the therapist stands behind and places both thumbs over the patient's lower teeth and his index fingers over the upper teeth. A sterile gauze or a cloth may be placed over the lower teeth. The patient is instructed to support the mandible with one hand under the chin. The mandible is then opened with gentle but maximal effort. If a less vigorous stretch is indicated, use one hand, with the index finger and thumb in the same position, and support the patient's mandible with the opposite hand.[41]

The patient may be taught to use this method as self-treatment, using the thumb and index finger in a reverse position and supporting the mandible with one or two hands.[41]

All of these exercises should emphasize movement without pain or undue force. Stretching should be done slowly and can be done actively—with or without resistance to the mandible—or passively.

Reflex relaxation of the elevator muscles followed by active stretch, as used for the opening movement, as well as passive and assistive stretch may also be applied to lateral, protrusive, and retrusive movements. With instruction, the patient can carry out many of these exercises by himself.

MOBILIZATION TECHNIQUES

Mobilization techniques in the treatment of temporomandibular joint disorders are aimed at restoring normal joint mechanics in order to allow full, pain-free osteokinematics of the mandible to occur. The techniques described are based on courses presented by M. Rocabado and the works of Kaltenborn.[21,37] They are restricted to a description of manual techniques, which are best learned and practiced under supervision in a postgraduate course or in physical therapy schools.

Temporomandibular Joint

1. *Caudal Traction*

P—Lies supine on a semi-reclining table or in dental chair that supports the head and trunk.

O—Stands at patient's side and faces left side of her head. Right hand and forearm are placed around patient's head, fixating head against the table. A stabilizing belt across the forehead may be used instead. Left hand holds with thumb in the mouth over the left inferior molars and with the fingers outside around the patient's jaw.

M—Ask patient to swallow. While maintaining the forearm in a straight line (hand and forearm act as a unit) apply traction caudally (Fig. 11-14). Reverse for the opposite side.

Comments: Caudal traction may be combined with ventral and dorsal glide (protraction and retraction). The mandible is first distracted caudally and while traction is maintained, the mandible is glided ventrally, then dorsally, followed by a gradual release of caudal traction.

2. *Protrusion*—ventral glide

P—Lies supine on a semi-reclining table or in dental chair that supports the head and trunk.

Note: For the sake of simplicity, the operator will be referred to as male, and the patient as female. (P—patient; O—operator; M—movement; X—fixation)

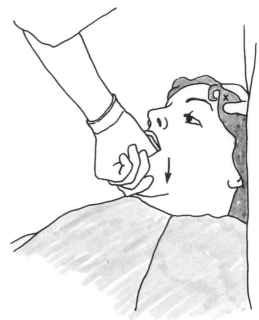

Fig. 11-14. Caudal traction

O—Stands at patient's side and faces left side of her head. Right hand and forearm are placed around the patient's head, fixating against the operator's body. Left hand holds onto the angle of the ramus with index and third finger. The rest of the hand contacts the patient's jaw.

M—Ask patient to swallow. While maintaining the forearm in a straight line, glide the mandible ventrally into protrusion (Fig. 11-15). Reverse for opposite side.

Comments: An alternate hand hold would be to place the thumb in the mouth on the right inferior molars and the fingers outside around the right side of patient's jaw. This same handhold can be used for retrusion (dorsal glide).

Gliding movements ventrally may be combined with a little rotation. The right mandible is first glided forward, as described, and then rotated to the left by rotation of operator's body.

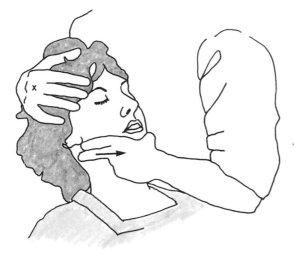

Fig. 11-15. Protrusion (ventral glide)

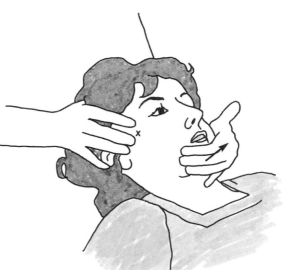

Fig. 11-16. Medial-lateral glide

3. *Medial-Lateral Glide*
  a. Rotation of the left joint and forward glide of the right joint
    P—Lies supine on a semi-reclining table or dental chair that supports the head and trunk
    O—Stands behind patient. Right hand holds around her head, fixating head against table. Left hand is positioned so that the hypothenar eminence is placed just caudal to the left temporomandibular joint with the fingers wrapped around the patient's jaw.
    M—Ask patient to swallow. The hypothenar eminence acts as a pivot point as the mandible is glided forward and medially to the left (Fig. 11-16). Reverse for opposite side.
  b. Alternate technique
    P—Lies supine on a semi-reclining table or in dental chair that supports the head and neck.
    O—Stands at patient's side and faces left side of her head. Right hand is placed around patient's head, fixating head against table. Left hand holds with thumb in mouth on medial aspect of

body of mandible near the right inferior molars, with the fingers (outside) wrapped around the jaw.
    M—Ask patient to swallow. With the thumb acting as a pivot point, move the wrist ulnarly so that the right condyle moves outward, forward, and laterally as the mandible is moved medially to the left (Fig. 11-17). Reverse for opposite side.

Many of the semi-reclining techniques described above may be carried out in a sitting position. The patient's head may be stabilized against the operator's body and supported with the free hand. However, the semi-reclining or supine position is preferred since the head and mandible are in a better position for fixation. Furthermore, if a stabilizing belt is used, the operator's other hand is free to assist the mobilizing hand or to palpate the joint to determine if correct motion is obtained. Mobilization techniques using pressures against the head of the mandible, which have been developed by Maitland are particularly useful (Fig. 11-18).[23] One of the greatest difficulties encountered when

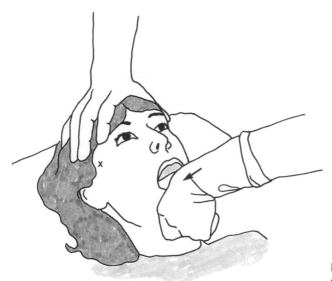

Fig. 11-17. Medial-lateral glide (alternate technique)

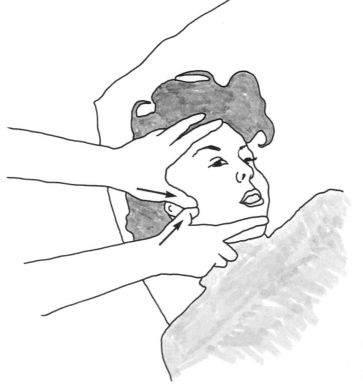

Fig. 11-18. Mobilization techniques (here a medial glide) may be applied directly to the condyle.

mobilizing the jaw is the patient's inability to relax the jaw completely. By mobilizing the condyle directly rather than through the mandible (which involves large movements), the patient is able to relax more readily, and treatment is often times more successful. Also, overstretching of the upper joint compartment is avoided. Medial glide is particularly useful in restoring rotation (lower joint compartment).

TREATMENT OF DISK DERANGEMENT AND CONDYLAR DISPLACEMENT

Signs and symptoms of early TMJ dysfunction include primarily muscular hyperactivity and pain, disturbed chewing habits, clicking, "catching" or "locking" of the jaw (recurrent sublaxations), and limited motion or hypermobility of the joints. Palliative therapy is directed at reducing muscle spasm (the pain-spasm-pain cycle) and relieving intrajoint symptoms caused by trauma, inflammation, condylar displacement, or disk derangement.[52] Treatment may include drug therapy, injections, application of various forms of heat or cold, disengagement of the occlusion by prostheses or voluntarily, and alterations in dietary and oral habits.

Causative therapy procedures may include manipulations and joint mobilization techniques to restore normal joint mechanics; correction of condylar displacements with the use of occlusal repositioning splints or occlusal equilibration; and correction of disk derangement by mandibular manipulations or repositioning appliances.[23,26,33,44,52] Occasionally, surgical correction may be necessary.

Adjunctive therapy may include the use of ultrasound, electrical stimulation, patient education, relaxation techniques, psychotherapy, biofeedback, and exercises. According to Somers, treatment directed towards patient education, the elimination of poor oral habits, and the acquisition of muscle relaxation, is often all that is required to relieve the patient's symptoms.[46]

PATIENT EDUCATION

A most important step is to educate the patient regarding the functioning of his joints, the reason for his symptoms, and the means of removing his symptoms. Advice should include reassurance, which is often simply gained by understanding the anatomy of the joint and the physiological mechanisms at work.

Using a skull, the patient's radiograms, or simple diagrams will help you to explain the structure and function of the temporomandibular joints and the rationale for the various procedures that must be undertaken. Your instructions should emphasize diet and careful use of the jaw.[44] The harmful effects of wide opening, yawning, biting off large mouthfuls of hard food, habitual protrusion, diurnal clenching or nocturnal bruxism should be explained. Because an emotional overlay is often present, counseling on how emotional conflicts are translated into muscle tension and pain is usually an important consideration. Point out that methods to achieve muscle relaxation and abolish well-established patterns of inappropriate muscular activity and methods to acquire new ones are important means of removing symptoms.

RELAXATION TRAINING

In addition to patient education, relaxation training for jaw and facial muscles is often considered, although it may be difficult to achieve. Muscle tension is one of the most frequent single contributing causes of muscular derangements of the temporomandibular joint, whether or not the derangement occurred through trauma. A report by Heiberg, Heloe, and Krogstad indicates that of a group of patients with a diagnosis of TMJ syndrome, almost all exhibited tense muscles in the neck and back as well, indicating that muscular tension is not confined to the masticatory muscles alone. Increased muscular tension, especially in the erector trunci, was present in 95% of these patients.[20] Typically these patients present with a tightly closed jaw, stiffened neck and back, elevated shoulders and a forward head. Faulty respiration patterns are also a common finding.

Relaxation of the whole body or body regions is frequently indicated in the treatment of these overly tense patients. More often than not, general relaxation techniques will have to precede training for local relaxation. (See Chapter 10, Relaxation.) Relaxation exercises such as those modified from Jacobsen, autogenic training, and reflex relaxation exercises, may all be used.

You can show the patient the presence of unnecessary muscular contraction at the end of the initial physical examination or during the first treatment session. Most patients are unable to relax the jaw muscles so that the mandible can be moved freely by the therapist. They are unable to let the head loll back when the shoulders are supported since the neck muscles remain rigid. They cannot permit their elevated arm to fall limply to the treatment table when requested by the examiner.

Perhaps one of the hardest of all relaxation procedures to achieve is elimination of overcontraction of the jaw muscles. An example of a local technique using a modification of Jacobson's approach follows:

— Clench the jaw firmly and concentrate on feeling the sense of tightness in the temples as well as the jaw itself.
— Switch off and let the jaw fall open
— Push the jaw open against the pressure of an assistant's hand
— Relax completely
— Move the jaw sideways to the left as far as possible with or without resistance and experience the sensation this gives to the jaw and temples before relaxing
— Repeat the same exercise to the left
— Complete the sequence by clenching the jaw firmly again, and let the jaw drop open loosely.

Somers suggests that total relaxation cannot be assumed until the assistant can take the patient's chin between the thumb and forefinger and tap the teeth together rapidly without any opposition from the jaw muscles.[46] It is often most helpful for the patient to adapt this method for use from time to time to assess the degree of tension and his progress in attempting to achieve relaxation. Autosuggestion techniques to guard against clenching and tooth contact are also helpful. He may be told to repeat the following after each meal: "Lips together, teeth apart." He should also be instructed to make frequent checks during the day for jaw clenching and to attempt to maintain the rest position of the mandible in which only the lips touch while the teeth are held apart. These methods of treatment are often considered the first line of defense against clenching and nocturnal bruxism.[44]

The use of biofeedback methods to guide the patient in controlling muscle activity and promoting relaxation has increased in recent years.[19,34,47] Feedback from electromyogram (EMG) of the frontal, temporal, and masseter muscles have been the most popular methods.

In addition, the therapist must spend time instructing the patient in good body mechanics, postural control and correct body positioning for maximum relaxation of the cervical spine and masticatory muscles. Cervical traction, exercises, and mobilization may also be indicated when associated cervical symptoms or pathology coexist. Occlusal splints may be indicated to create relaxation of the elevator muscles and disorientation of an acquired noxious occlusal sensory input. Splints may also be used to disorient the sensory input in patients who clench by changing the quality of afferent touch information.[23,44] Occlusal analysis and equilibration, if indicated, are usually best deferred until relaxation has been achieved.

EXERCISE THERAPY

The use of retraining exercises to overcome spasm and incoordination of the mandibular musculature, to promote harmonious coordinated mechanism, to reduce momentary luxation of the disk and to increase muscle strength have long been advocated; however, they are now considered controversial.[2,7,33,41,42]

Cyraix feels that clicking of the jaw due to momentary luxation of the intra-articular meniscus can usually be relieved by strengthening the muscles of mastication. Opening, protrusion, and lateral resistive movements are performed. It is usually not necessary, he feels, to develop the closing muscles since most patients usually maintain normal strength of these muscles by chewing.[7]

Schwartz and Bertoft recommend a training program of exercises against resistance to promote reflex relaxation of the antagonistic muscles. This stimulates the maximum number of motor units within the lateral pterygoids during opening and lateral mandibular movements.[2,41,42]

Paris feels that major derangements should be treated in the same manner as subluxations by mobilization techniques. Minor derangements, however, are best treated by isometrics to the lateral pterygoids (i.e., protrusion and lateral movements).[33] Regardless of the type of exercises used, they should always be carried out without clicking and pain.

Such strengthening-resistive exercises, according to Weinberg, are not indicated in the TMJ pain–dysfunction syndrome because the neuromuscular mechanism involved is associated with overfunction rather than underfunction.[52] Such exercises do not seem to have a rational basis as an effective therapy. Strengthening and re-education exercises may be indicated when true muscle weakness is found (as in the limitation phase) or when habits such as deviant swallowing or habitual protrusion reverses normal muscle function and contributes to the TMJ pain–dysfunction syndrome.[46,52]

TREATMENT OF ORAL-FACIAL IMBALANCES

Muscles of the entire stomatognathic system and the oral-facial complex play a major role in proper balance and function of the temporomandibular joint. It should be kept in mind that the oral-facial muscles are under stress 24 hours a day. Swallowing takes place 2000 times a day as a reflexive act. Forces during eating, drinking, speech, and the rest position of the tongue must be taken into consideration. If there is an imbalance of forces, there will be a tremendous amount of pressure against normal balance of forces of the temporomandibular joint that can cause malfunction of the joint apparatus.

Protrusion of the mandible resulting in an abnormal palatal swallow may be caused by ankylotic tongue, shortened frenulum, or abnormal use of facial muscles, particularly the mentalis.[13,16] Abnormal use or position of the tongue at rest, muscle imbalance of the masseter, decreased strength of the orbicularis oris, neuromuscular problems, post-traumatic and surgical conditions (e.g., unilateral condylectomies), pain conditions of the head, face or cervical spine, and other pathologies can result in malfunction of the temporomandibular joint.

In many of these conditions, real or apparent reduction in muscle strength of one or more muscles may be disclosed during examination. This may point to lack of use (e.g., in unilateral function), atrophy of muscle fibers, muscular fibrositis, and other pathologic conditions localized in or near the muscle and its tendon, causing pain on contraction. Although strengthening-resistive exercises are usually not indicated in muscles that are already refusing to relax, they do need to be considered in the proper balance and function of the temporomandibular joint complex when weakness exists, from whatever cause.

FACILITORY EXERCISES

There is a wide variety of well-known facilitory and strengthening-resistive exercises that are at the therapist's disposal.[12,13,22,41,42,55] Exercises employing postural reflexes, brushing, vibration, synergistic muscles, surrounding facial and cervical muscles, and activities of daily living may be used as facilitory techniques. Stimuli—consisting of stretch, maximal resistance, pressures, stroking, or tapping—may be given manually. Popping or clucking of the tongue on the hard palate may be used to strengthen the muscle of the tongue and encourage greater range of motion of the jaw. Gargling after each brushing helps facilitate mandibular depressors. Resistive tongue exercises may be used to facilitate the three major jaw muscles. Resisted neck motion may facilitate tongue motions as well as mandibular motions. In general, facial and mandibular motions that require depression or downward motions are facilitated by neck flexion; conversely, facial and mandibular motions that require elevation and upward motions are facilitated by neck extension. Neck rotation reinforces motion on the side of the face or the mandible toward which the head is turned.

Early protrusion of the mandible during opening that is due to an imbalance of the synergistic action of the suprahyoids and lateral pterygoids is often revealed during examination. A translatory rather than a rotatory movement is occurring; its abolition should be a major step in manage-

ment. An excellent, initial exercise requires the patient to place his tongue as posteriorly as possible in contact with the hard palate, to effect retrusion. By assuming this position, protrusion of the lower jaw is eliminated, since the patient's articular movements are mainly rotatory and limited by the constraints of the internal pterygoids. By limiting the movement to the interocclusal clearance, any subsequent translatory movement is eliminated. Instruct the patient to open his mouth slowly and rhythmically within the pain limits several times in succession. He should practice this simple exercise frequently during the day.

The next step is to instruct the patient to repeat this exercise with the addition of one critical modification, voluntary resistance. The patient should grasp the chin firmly or position a closed first under the mandible to resist the motion of pressing the jaw down and back.

Both of these exercises rely upon synergistic action of the suprahyoids and lower bodies of the lateral pterygoids. In normal opening, all of these muscle pairs contract strongly. However, when the lateral pterygoids contract more strongly than the suprahyoids, the mandible will protrude. These exercises are felt to help train the suprahyoids to contract more forcefully than the lateral pterygoids.

Another useful exercise for the development of the suprahyoids, described by Shore, consists of teaching the patient to perform isometric contraction of these muscles in front of a mirror.[44] The patient is taught to contract these muscles with the mouth closed and the teeth in light contact. He then makes a conscious effort to retrude the jaw and depress the floor of the mouth without actually moving it. Once acute spasms have subsided, the patient repeats the exercise with the mouth slightly open. Each day he can gradually increase the extent of mouth opening until coordinated mandibular muscular action is achieved.

Once the patient has mastered rotation during limited opening without forward condylar movement, the range of opening is gradually increased. While the patient is looking in a mirror, he is asked to place his index finger over each condylar head or his palms over the sides of the face to monitor and correct any abnormal protrusion of the condylar head during opening and closing. He should also note any irregular movements such as one condylar head preceding movement of the other. Keeping the hands in place, the patient is instructed to carry out slow rhythmic full opening and closing within the pain-free range, avoiding any clicking, abnormal protrusion, or lateral deviation of the jaw. If abnormal deviation or protrusion does occur, he is taught to guide the motion with his thumb or forefinger positioned on his chin so that the mandible moves smoothly in a coordinated hingelike fashion without protrusion.[41] Initially, this exercise should be performed with the therapist, who assists by guiding the motion of the mandible as the patient actively opens and closes his mouth.

Of particular interest is the rehabilitation of unilateral condylar fractures following immobilization. Residual mandibular kinesiopathy often persists and is referred to as *postfracture condylar syndrome*. It consists of deviation of the mandible on depression and inadequate mandibular excursion toward the contralateral side. Begin management by first explaining to the patient the difference between a hinge joint and a gliding joint, and how he must develop a gliding joint to masticate with the contralateral side. He is then given a lateral tongue exercise to facilitate using the mylohyoid muscle to assist the weakened lateral pterygoid muscle in accomplishing lateral mandibular excursion. To perform this exercise, described by Gerry, the patient works before a mirror; places the tip of his tongue on the palatal surface of the contralateral maxillary molars and presses as hard as he can while elevating and depressing his mandible.[15] It is suggested that this exercise be performed for 5 minutes hourly. As lateral excursions develop, periarticular fibrosis of the injured joint resolves, and normal lateral pterygoid function tends to return.

TEMPOROMANDIBULAR EVALUATION

I. **History.** The general format of the initial evaluation should follow the same lines of questioning as set out in Chapter 4. Information on when the problem started and how it occurred as well as previous management and the results obtained by them is helpful. If the problem was caused by injury or surgical procedure, you will need to know what was done by the attending personnel and physicians. A most important aspect of taking the history is the attempt to clarify any emotional factors in the patient's background that may provoke habitual protrusion or muscular tension.

The history may be handwritten from answers to your verbal questions. Perhaps a more complete history can be obtained, however, by using a personal history form, which is completed by the patient. After reviewing the form, all pertinent facts may be reviewed in detail with the patient. The work of Day, Shore, and Morgan and Rosen, provides excellent detailed outlines and the rationale for obtaining such information as a means of compiling a complete history relating specifically to TMJ disorders.[9,31,44] Such forms have been designed to include most of the information that will be found useful in treating TMJ disorders and related oral–facial problems. Certainly no specific set of questions is adequate, and more detailed questioning will usually be necessary. It is also unlikely that you will obtain all relevant information at the initial evaluation. A few pertinent questions that apply particularly to TMJ disorders include

1. Does the joint grate, click, pop, snap, or lock?
2. Do you have difficulty opening and closing your mouth?
3. Do you have frequent headaches? What area of the head? How long do they last?
4. Have you ever had a severe blow to the head or a whiplash injury?
5. Are your jaws clenched or your teeth sore when you awaken from sleep?

Perhaps one of the most common complaints of head pain is what is generally termed *tension headache*. Berry has studied 100 patients with mandibular dysfunction pain and reports that over 50% of his patients had headaches and pain in the neck, back, and shoulders.[4] This condition may be the result of structural cervical disease, may be associated with vascular pain syndrome, or may occur as a separate entity.[3,9]

II. **Physical Examination.**
  A. *Observation.* Record significant findings. The physical examination in a sense occurs simultaneously when you take the history. The appearance, general posture, and characteristics of bodily movements are often revealing. Physically the typical patient with TMJ pain–dysfunction, with an emotional overlay, have a posture of elevated shoulders, forward head, stiff neck and back, and have shallow, restricted breathing.[20] Also observe facial expression and habits of the jaw (*i.e.,* clenching or grinding the teeth, biting the fingers, or twitching the masseter).
  B. *Inspection of the head, face, and neck.* Record significant findings.
    1. *Skin.* Examine the face for blem-ishes, moles, pigmentations, scars, and texture.
    2. *Soft tissue.* Note any swelling. Swelling of the joint must be moderate or marked before it is apparent on inspection. If swelling is detectable, it appears as a rounded bulge just anterior to the external meatus. The face should be further examined for atrophies and hypertrophies. Asking the patient to clench his jaws together may help to disclose asymmetry.
    3. *Bony structure and alignment.* Record significant findings.
        Viewing the profile of the face in both the frontal and sagittal plane will reveal the relative development of the skull, face, and mandible. The size of the mandible should be compared with that of the skull, and abnormal positions or asymmetry of the jaw noted. Asymmetry may be indicative of a growth or developmental problem or unusual muscular activity. Take particular note of the occlusal and rest positions of the jaw. An abnormal protrusive position may be associated with tongue thrust (deviate swallowing) or habitual protrusion.
        The examiner should briefly inspect the upper spine, shoulder girdles, and arms for obvious muscle atrophy or deformities.
  C. *Selective tissue tension tests.* Record significant findings.
    1. *Active movements* (with passive over pressure). Observe the general patterns of active movements (depression, elevation, lateral deviation, protraction, retraction) for freedom of movement, range, and symmetry. Ascertain if any pain ac-

companies active movements and in what part of the range it occurs and where. Pain may be felt in the area of the joint and about the ear, but many times it is also felt diffusely through the face, teeth, jaws, and mouth. Masticatory pain is typically not well localized. (During the palpation portion of the examination, actual sites of tenderness can be established.)

Abnormal movements such as "jumps" or "facet slips" should be noted. In particular ask the patient to open his mouth to a limited extent (about 1 cm) while you observe whether the mandible is making an initial rotation or translatory movement. Forward movement will be revealed by a reduction in incisal overjet and by excessive prominence of the condylar heads.

Record the restriction of movement, deviations to one side, and asynchronous patterns of movement; measure the maximum opening the patient can achieve without pain. Lateral movements to the left and right, using the bite position as the control as well as protrusion–retrusion, again using normal bite as control, should be recorded when restricted. Lateral motion may be lost earlier and to a greater degree than vertical motions.

Note whether pain is provoked when the jaws are in firm occlusion and when the patient is asked to bite against a tongue blade on one side. Such tests help distinguish muscle spasms from discitis and retrodiscitis (3).

2. *Passive movements* (anatomical ranges). With passive movements, in addition to seeing how easily the jaw can be moved and making a comparison with active range of motion, note the type of end feel as well as the presence of pain and spasms. To determine the nature of the end feel, have the patient open his mouth and then apply additional pressure with the thumbs and index fingers on the edge of the upper and lower teeth, noting the type of end feel present. Passive movements should routinely include depression, elevation, protraction, retraction, and lateral movements.

3. *Resisted movement* (static tests). Determine the strength and presence of pain by applying resistance to mandibular opening, protrusion, and lateral deviations. Pain arising in the pterygoid muscles may be provoked by resisted deviation to the painful side as well as clenching the teeth. Weakness of the muscles that close the mouth is rather uncommon, since strength is usually maintained by mastication.

4. *Passive joint play movements.* Routinely include accessory posterior–anterior, transverse movements, and longitudinal movements (cephalad and caudal to the heads of the condyle) with and without compression.[26,47] Note stability—mobility, presence of pain, guarding, spasm, and behavior.

D. *Palpation*
1. *Skin.* Palpate for warmth, tenderness, temperature, moisture, and mobility.
2. *Muscles.* Palpate for consistency, mobility, continuity, tenderness, pain, and signs of

spasm. Palpation of the muscles of mastication should routinely include the origin and insertion of the masseter, temporalis, internal pterygoid, and the origin of the external pterygoid.[41]

When indicated, all the muscles of the maxillofacial region should be palpated, including the facial muscles, sublingual and suprahyoids, and the cervical muscles, especially the sternocleidomastoid and trapezius. Various structural or functional cervical diseases may result in spasms of the masticatory muscles. A comprehensive thesis on the musculature and differential diagnosis of oral-facial pain is described by Bell.[3]

3. *Temporomandibular joint.* First, palpate the condylar heads laterally with the mouth closed; then palpate the distal aspect with the jaw apart for tenderness. Determine if any such tenderness is definitely accentuated when the mandible is moved contralaterally. This maneuver brings the condyle more firmly under the palpating finger. The posterior aspect can be palpated through the external auditory meatus with the palpating finger. Pain and tenderness on palpation suggests a capsulitis, particularly if tenderness is found posteriorly. Abnormal capsular thickening, warmth, and swelling should also be noted. Moderate degrees of swelling in the joint prevent the fingertip from entering the depressed area overlying the joint. Swelling of a marked degree may be palpable as a rounded, often fluctuant mass overlying the joint.

The range and dynamics of condylar motion can also be ascertained by means of palpation. From a position behind the patient, place your forefingers on the lateral aspects of the condylar heads as the patient actively opens his mouth. Inability to feel protrusion of the condylar head suggests a lack of forward movement.

You can determine the presence and the amount of rotation by placing the fingertips in the ear. Palpation should be done bilaterally so that a comparison of both joints can be made and any asymmetrical movements ascertained. Palpable snapping, clicking, or jumps should also be noted.

Bony palpation should include palpation of the zygomatic arch, the hyoid bone, and the upper cervical spine.

4. *Auscultation.* Palpation of the temporomandibular movements often reveals the presence of clicking or crepitus. However, such sounds can be more accurately evaluated with the bell of a stethoscope placed over the condylar head as the patient actively opens his mouth. Note the type of sound associated with the movements and particular phase of movement in which it occurs. All movements—opening, closing, lateral deviation, protrusion, and retrusion—should be assessed.

E. *Dental and oral examination.* Make a general survey of the oral cavity, since both facial pain as well as TMJ disorders may have their origin in dental or oral lesions. The examination of the teeth and their supporting structures, other oral structures, and mucosa is important.

By having the patient open his mouth maximally, the examiner is able to observe the oropharynx, tonsillar areas, and surfaces of the palate and tongue. Note any alteration in the color and texture of the lingual tissues. Include palpations.

Cavities and restored and missing teeth should be noted. Wear of biting edges and chewing surfaces that appears excessive for the patient's age often points to tensional oral habits such as bruxing. Also note the occlusion of the teeth, premature contact, overclosure of the vertical dimension, and the degree of overjet.[6] Detailed occlusal analysis should always be deferred until muscle relaxation has been achieved.

F. *Sensory and motor response.* Masticatory and oral-facial functioning and the neurologic system that integrates it are complex. Involvement of the muscles innervated by the fifth to twelfth cranial nerve and at least the upper three cervical spinal nerves may be reflected in masticatory malfunctioning or pain.[3] Not only the chief masticatory and secondary muscles, but also the muscles of the lips, cheeks, tongue, floor of the mouth, neck, palate, and pharynx may be involved. Sensory as well as motor function testing may be indicated.

G. *Other tests.* A cervical-upper extremity scan exam is frequently indicated in the evaluation of TMJ disorders. It should be noted that the upper cervical spinal nerves are more likely sources of pain that refer or spread to the masticatory region than are the lower cervical nerves. Passive movements (physiological) and passive joint play movements of the upper cervical spine should be included.[26,47]

Adjuncts, such as radiography and electromyography may be indicated. Only electromyography can reveal how a muscle acts at any point during mandibular movements and postures; it is felt by some researchers to be more reliable diagnostically than radiographs of the temporomandibular joints.[5,26,30]

Analgesic blocking of tender muscles of the joint proper may be needed to confirm the source of pain as well as to help identify secondary pain effects.[3]

Examination of the ear, nose and throat may be necessary to exclude a variety of diagnosable and treatable conditions that may be confused with temporomandibular joint pathology. In addition to the history and clinical examination, further procedures are often necessary to evaluate tinnitus, hearing loss and vertigo to establish or rule out otological or neurological cause for these symptoms.

REFERENCES

1. Axhausen G: Pathology and therapy of the temporomandibular joint. Fortschritte der Zahnaerz 6:177–201, 1930; 7:199–215, 1931; 8:201–215, 1932
2. Bertoft G: The effect of physical training on temporomandibular joint clicking. Odontologisk Revy 23:297–304, 1972
3. Bell WE: Orofacial Pains—Differential Diagnosis. Dallas, Denedco of Dallas, 1973
4. Berry DC: Mandibular dysfunction pain and chronic minor illness. Br Dent J 127:170–175, 1969
5. Bessette RW, Mohl ND, DiCosimo CJ: Comparison of results of electromyographic and radiographic examinations in patients with myofascial pain-dysfunction syndrome. J Am Dent Assoc 89:1358–1364, 1974
6. Curnutte DC: The role of occlusion in diagnosis and treatment. In Morgan DH, Hall WP, Vamvas SV (eds): Disease of the Temporomandibular Apparatus: A Multidisci-

plinary Approach. St Louis, CV Mosby, 1977

7. Cyriax J: Textbook of Orthopedic Medicine, Vol I: Diagnosis of Soft Tissue Lesions, 7th ed. London, Balliere Tindell, 1978

8. Dachi SF: Diagnosis and management of temporomandibular dysfunction syndrome. J Prosthet Dent 20(1):53–61, 1968

9. Day LD: History taking. In Morgan DH, Hall WP, Vamvas SV (eds): Disease of the Temporomandibular Apparatus: A Multidisciplinary Approach. St Louis, CV Mosby, 1977

10. Dufourmentel L: Chirurgie de l'articulation temporo-maxillaire. Paris, Masson, 1920

11. Ermshar CB: Anatomy and neuroanatomy. In Morgan DH, Hall WP, Vamvas SV (eds): Disease of the Temporomandibular Apparatus: A Multidisciplinary Approach. St Louis, CV Mosby, 1977

12. Farber SD: Sensorimotor Evaluation and Treatment Procedures, 2nd ed. Bloomington, Indiana University Press, 1974

13. Garliner D: Myofunctional Therapy. Philadelphia, WB Saunders, 1976

14. Gelb H: The craniomandibular syndrome. In Garliner D: Myofunctional Therapy. Philadelphia, WB Saunders, 1976

15. Gerry RG: Condylar fractures. In Schwartz L: Disorders of the Temporomandibular Joint. Philadelphia, WB Saunders, 1959

16. Greene BJ: Myofunctional Therapy. In Morgan DH, Hall WB, Vamvas SJ (eds): Disease of the Temporomandibular Apparatus: A Multidisciplinary Approach. St Louis, CV Mosby, 1977

17. Grokoest A: Osteoarthritis. In Schwartz L: Disorders of the Temporomandibular Joint. Philadelphia, WB Saunders, 1959

18. Grokoest A, Chayes CM: Rheumatic disease. In Schwartz L, Chayes CM: Facial Pain and Mandibular Dysfunction. Philadelphia, WB Saunders, 1968

19. Grossan M: Biofeedback. In Morgan DH, Hall, WP, Vamvas SV (eds): Disease of the Temporomandibular Apparatus: A Multidisciplinary Approach. St Louis, CV Mosby, 1977

20. Heiberg AN, Heloe B, Krogstad BS: The myofascial pain dysfunction: Dental symptoms and psychological and muscular function: An overview. Psychother Psychosom 30:81–97, 1978

21. Kaltenborn F: Manual Therapy for the Extremity Joints. Oslo, Olaf Norlis Bokhandel, 1974

22. Knott M, Voss DE: Proprioceptive Neuromuscular Facilitation. New York, Harper & Row, 1962

23. Krogh-Poulsen WG, Olsson A: Management of the occlusion of the teeth. In Schwartz L, Chayes CM: Facial Pain and Mandibular Dysfunction. Philadelphia, WB Saunders, 1968

24. Luschei ES, Goodwin GM: Patterns of mandibular movement and muscle activity during mastication in the monkey. J Neurophysiol 35(5):954–966, 1974

25. Mahan PE, Kreutziger KL: Diagnosis and management of temporomandibular joint pain. In Alling C, Mahan P (eds): Facial Pain. Philadelphia, Lea and Febiger, 1977

26. Maitland GD: Peripheral Manipulations, 2nd ed. Boston, Butterworth, 1977

27. McNamara DC: Examination, diagnosis and treatment of occlusal pain-dysfunction. Aust Dent J 23(1):50–55, 1978

28. McNamara JA: The independent function of the two heads of the lateral pterygoid muscle. Am J Anat, 138:197–205, 1973

29. Moffett BC, Johnson LC, McCabe JB, Askew HC: Articular remodeling in the adult human temporomandibular joint. Am J Anat 115:110–130, 1964

30. Morgan DH, Hall WP, Vamvas SJ (eds): Disease of the Temporomandibular Apparatus: A Multidisciplinary Approach. St Louis, CV Mosby, 1977

31. Morgan DH, Rosen LM: Interpretation of radiograph. In Morgan DH, Hall WP, Vamvas SJ (eds): Disease of the Temporomandibular Apparatus: A Multidisciplinary Approach, St Louis, CV Mosby, 1977

32. Munro RR: Electromyography of the masseter and anterior temporalis muscle in the open-close-clench cycle in the temporomandibular joint dysfunction. Monogr Oral Sci 4:117–125, 1975

33. Paris SV: The Spinal Lesion. Christchurch, New Zealand, Pegasus Press, 1965

34. Peck C, Kraft G: Electromyographic biofeedback for pain related to muscle tension: A study of tension headache, back and jaw pain. Arch Surg 112:889–895, 1977

35. Pinto OF: A new structure related to the temporomandibular joint and the middle ear. J Prosthet Dent 12(1):95–103, 1962

36. Porter MR: The attachment of the lateral pterygoid muscle of the meniscus. J Prosthet Dent 24:555–562, 1970

37. Rocabado M: Management of the temporomandibular joint. Presented at a course on physical therapy in dentistry. Vail, January 1978

38. Rees LA: The structure and function of the temporomandibular joint. Br Dent J 96:125–133, 1954

39. Rood M: Neurophysiological reactions as a basis for physical therapy. Physical Therapy Review 34:444–449, 1954

40. Scheman P: Surgery of the temporomandibular articulation. In Gelb H (ed): Clinical Management of Head, Neck and TMJ Pain and Dysfunction: A Multidisciplinary Approach to Diagnosis and Treatment. Philadelphia, WB Saunders, 1977

41. Schwartz L (ed): Disorders of the Temporomandibular Joint. Philadelphia, WB Saunders, 1959

42. Schwartz L, Chayes CM (eds): Facial Pain and Mandibular Dysfunction. Philadelphia, WB Saunders, 1968

43. Shira RB, Alling CC: Traumatic injuries involving the temporomandibular joint articulation. In Schwartz L, Chayes CM (eds): Facial Pain and Muscular Dysfunction. Philadelphia, WB Saunders, 1968

44. Shore MA: Temporomandibular Joint Dysfunction and Occlusal Equilibration. Philadelphia, JB Lippincott, 1976

45. Sicher H, Du Brul EL: Oral Anatomy, 5th ed. St Louis, CV Mosby, 1970

46. Somers N: An approach to the management of temporomandibular joint dysfunction. Aust Dent J 23(1):37–41, 1978

47. Trott PH, Goss AN: Physiotherapy in diagnosis and treatment of the myofascial dysfunction syndrome. Int J Oral Surg 7(4):360–365, 1978

48. Viener AE: Oral surgery. In Garliner D (ed): Myofunctional Therapy. Philadelphia, WB Saunders, 1976

49. Weinberg LA: An evaluation of basic articulators and their concepts, Part I, Basic concepts. J Prosthet Dent 13:622–644, 1963

50. Weinberg LA: The etiology, diagnosis, and treatment of TMJ dysfunction-pain syndrome, Part I: Etiology. J Prosthet Dent 42(6):654–664, 1979

51. Weinberg LA: The etiology, diagnosis and treatment of TMJ dysfunction-pain syndrome, Part II: Differential diagnosis. J Prosthet Dent 43(1):58–70, 1980

52. Weinberg LA: The etiology and treatment of TMJ dysfunction-pain syndrome, Part III: Treatment. J Prosthet Dent 43(2):186–196, 1980

53. Wetzler G: Physical therapy. In Morgan DH, Hall WP, Vamvas SV (eds): Disease of the Temporomandibular Apparatus: A Multidisciplinary Approach. St Louis, CV Mosby, 1977

54. Whinery JG: Examination of patients with facial pain. In Alling C, Mahan P (eds): Facial Pain. Philadelphia, Lea and Febiger, 1977

12 The Shoulder

Randolph M. Kessler

REVIEW OF FUNCTION ANATOMY

OSTEOLOGY

The Glenohumeral Joint (Fig. 12-1)

The *humeral head*, in the anatomical position, faces medially, slightly posteriorly, and superiorly. The head forms almost half a sphere, with an angular value of about 150°. It forms an angle of about 45° with the humeral shaft.

The glenoid cavity faces laterally, forward, and superiorly. It has an angular value of only 75°. This incongruity between the humeral head and the glenoid cavity is partially compensated for by the fibrous or fibrocartilaginous glenoid labrum which serves to deepen the glenoid cavity. The glenoid is pear shaped—narrow superiorly, and wider inferiorly.

The Acromioclavicular Joint (Fig. 12-2,A)

The clavicle is S shaped, the lateral third being concave anteriorly. This provides for extra motion during elevation of the arm (see under the section, Biomechanics). The lateral end of the clavicle is a convex articular surface. This articular surface faces medially and somewhat anteriorly and superiorly. These surfaces are oriented in such a way that a strong compression force tends to cause the clavicle to override the acromion. This is what occurs in an acromioclavicular separation,

usually caused by a fall on the tip of the acromion.

The Sternoclavicular Joint

The sternal end of the clavicle is somewhat bulbous, and is convex in the frontal plane while having a slight concavity anteroposteriorly. It articulates with the upper lateral edge of the manubrium, as well as with the superior surface of the medial aspect of the cartilage of the first rib. It tends to extend above the superior surface of the manubrium by as much as one half its width.

The Scapulothoracic Joint (Fig. 12-2,A)

The scapula, viewed from above at rest, makes an angle of about 30° with the frontal plane. It makes and angle of about 60° with the clavicle, viewed from above.

The medial portion of the scapular spine usually lies level with the T3 spinous process, while the inferior angle lies level with the T7 or T8 spinous process. The medial border lies about 6 cm lateral to the thoracic spinous processes.

LIGAMENTS

Glenohumeral Joint (Fig. 12-3)

The articular capsule is quite thin and lax with redundant folds situated anteroinferiorly when the arm is at rest. This allows a full range of elevation. Because of the laxity of the joint capsule, the head of the humerus can be distracted laterally about 2 cm in the cadaver, with the arm in a position of slight abduction. With the arm at the side, the superior joint capsule remains taut, whereas the remainder of

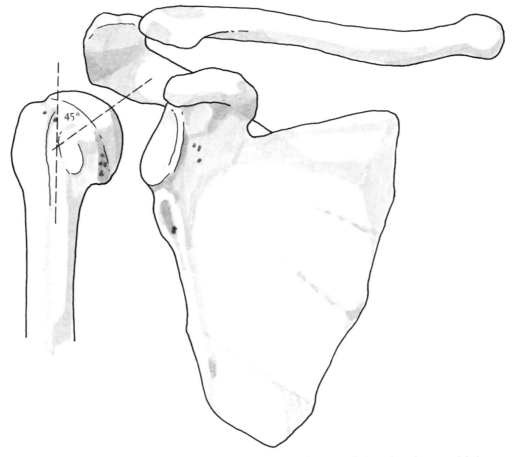

Fig. 12-1. Anterior view of the relationship of the bones of the glenohumeral joint

the capsule assumes a forward and medial twist. The tendons of the supraspinatus, infraspinatus, teres minor, and subscapularis blend with the fibers of the joint capsule.

The glenohumeral ligaments provide some reinforcement to the capsule anteriorly; helping to check external rotation.

The coracohumeral ligament strengthens the superior capsule. From the root of the coracoid process, it passes laterally and downward to the greater tubercle, blending with the supraspinatus tendon. Running somewhat anteriorly to the vertical axis about which rotation occurs, it also checks external rotation, and perhaps extension.

The transverse humeral ligament traverses the intertubercular (bicipetal) groove, acting as a retinaculum for the tendon of the long head of the biceps.

Acromioclavicular Joint

The acromioclavicular ligament appears to be quadrilateral when viewed from above. It strengthens the superior joint capsule.

Coracoclavicular Ligaments

Although situated away from the joint, these ligaments are of most importance in providing acromioclavicular joint stability.

The trapezoid ligament lies almost

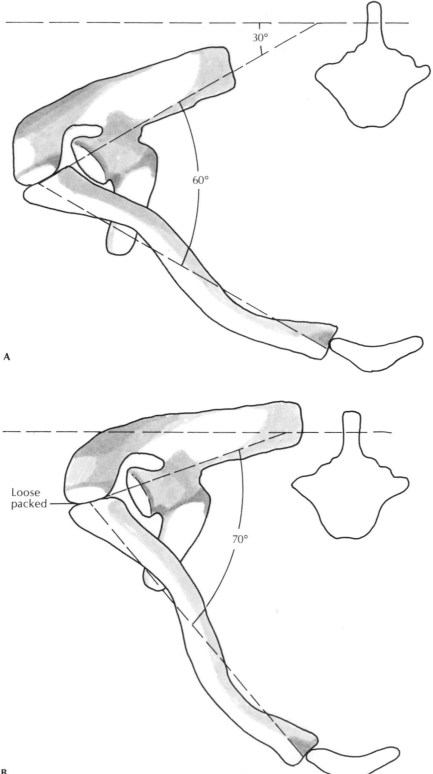

A

B

Loose
packed

30°

60°

70°

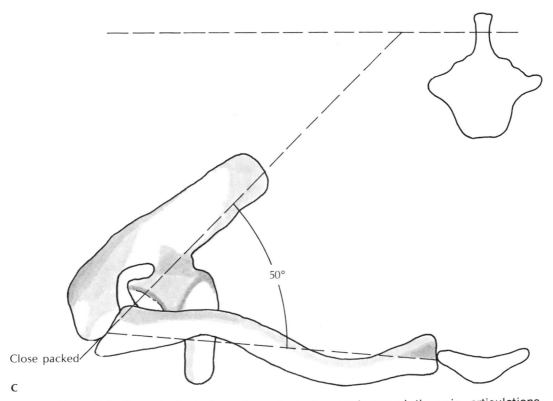

50°

Close packed

C

Fig. 12-2. Acromioclavicular, sternoclavicular, and scapulothoracic articulations shown (A) at rest, (B) in retraction, and (C) in protraction

horizontally in the frontal plane and is positioned such that it can check overriding, or lateral, movement of the clavicle on the acromion. It also helps prevent excessive narrowing of the angle between acromion and clavicle (viewed from above), as occurs with protraction.

The conoid ligament is oriented vertically, medial to the trapezoid ligament, and is twisted upon itself. It primarily checks superior movement of the clavicle on the acromion; it also prevents excessive widening of the scapuloclavicular angle, viewed from above. Note that as the arm is abducted, the scapula rotates in such a way that the inferior angle swings laterally and superiorly. This movement increases the distance between the clavicle and the coracoid process, pulling the conoid ligament taut. This tightening causes a backward axial rotation of the clavicle, bringing the acromioclavicular joint back

into apposition (because of the "s" shape of the clavicle). It is necessary for full elevation of the arm (see under the section, Biomechanics).

The Sternoclavicular Joint (Fig. 12-4)

The relatively lax joint capsule is reinforced anteriorly by the anterior sternoclavicular ligament, posteriorly by the posterior sternoclavicular ligaments, and superiorly by the interclavicular ligament. The costoclavicular ligament lies just lateral to the joint. Its anterior fibers run superiorly and laterally, and check elevation and lateral movement of the clavicle. The posterior fibers run superiorly and medially from the first rib, and check elevation and medial movement of the clavicle.

An intra-articular disk is attached above to the clavicle and below to the first costal

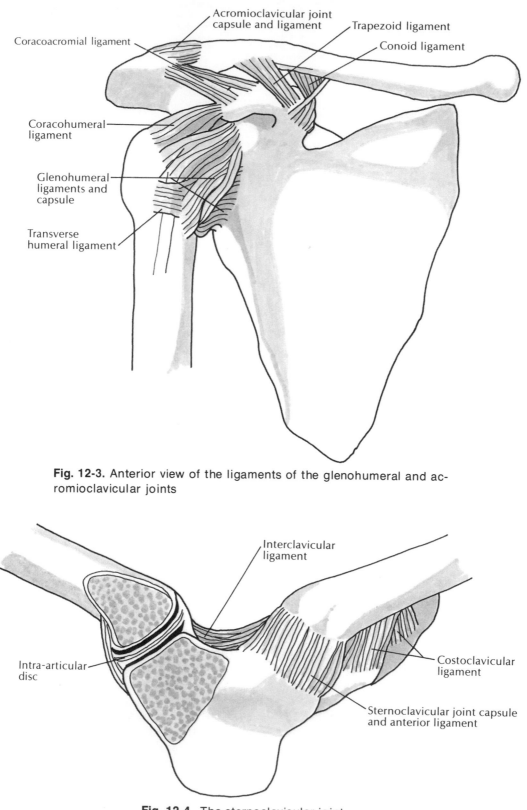

Coracoacromial ligament

Acromioclavicular joint capsule and ligament

Trapezoid ligament

Conoid ligament

Coracohumeral ligament

Glenohumeral ligaments and capsule

Transverse humeral ligament

Fig. 12-3. Anterior view of the ligaments of the glenohumeral and acromioclavicular joints

Interclavicular ligament

Intra-articular disc

Costoclavicular ligament

Sternoclavicular joint capsule and anterior ligament

Fig. 12-4. The sternoclavicular joint

cartilage and the sternum. It is especially important in helping to prevent medial dislocation of the clavicle, which can occur with a fall on the outstretched arm or on the point of the shoulder. Invariably the clavicle will break or the acromio-clavicular joint will dislocate before the sternoclavicular joint dislocates medially. This is true in spite of the fact that the medial sloping of the joint surfaces and the superior overlap of the clavicle on the sternum would seem to make the joint susceptible to medial dislocation.

The Scapula

The coracoacromial ligament does not serve to restrict movement, but forms a "roof" over the underlying glenohumeral joints. It thus protects structures beneath it and prevents upward displacement of the humeral head. It can be the site of impingement of the greater tubercle, supraspinatus tendon, or subdeltoid bursa in cases of abnormal joint mechanics.

BURSAE

There are usually considered to be eight or nine bursae about the shoulder joint. Practically speaking, only two are worth considering here, because of their clinical significance.

The Subacromial or Subdeltoid Bursa

This bursa extends over the supraspinatus tendon and distal muscle belly beneath the acromion and deltoid muscle. At times it extends beneath the coracoid process (Fig. 12-5,*A*). It is attached above to the acromial arch and below to the rotator cuff tendons and greater tubercle. It does not normally communicate with the joint capsule but may in the case of a rotator cuff tear. This is seen on arthrogram as dye leaking over the top of the supraspinatus tendon. The bursa is susceptible to impingement beneath the acromial arch, especially if it is inflamed and swollen (Fig.

12-5,*B*). Inflammation of the bursa is often attributed to rupture of a supraspinatus calcium deposit superiorly into the underside of the bursa.

The Subscapular Bursa

This bursa overlies the anterior joint capsule and lies beneath the subscapularis muscle. It communicates with the joint capsule and fills with dye on arthrography. Articular effusion may be manifested clinically by an anterior swelling due to distension of the bursa (Fig. 12-6).

VASCULAR ANATOMY OF THE ROTATOR CUFF TENDONS

The tendons of the rotator cuff include the supraspinatus, infraspinatus, teres minor, and subscapularis. As implied by the term *rotator cuff*, they do not exist as discrete tendons but blend to form a continuous cuff surrounding the posterior, superior, and anterior aspects of the humeral head. The fibers of the tendinous cuff attach to the articular capsule of the glenohumeral joint by blending with it. This allows the cuff to provide dynamic stabilization of the joint.

The rotator cuff is a frequent site of pathology—usually of a degenerative nature—in response to fatigue stresses. Lesions usually affect the supraspinatus, and to a lesser extent, the infraspinatus portions of the cuff. Since such degeneration often occurs with normal activity levels, the nutritional status of this frequently involved area of the cuff is of particular interest. Most fatigue or degenerative lesions occur either from increased stress levels or from a nutritional deficit.

The primary blood supply to the rotator cuff tendons is derived from six arteries, three of which contribute in virtually all individuals, and three of which are sometimes absent (Fig. 12-7).[18] The posterior humeral circumflex and the suprascapular arteries are usually present; they sup-

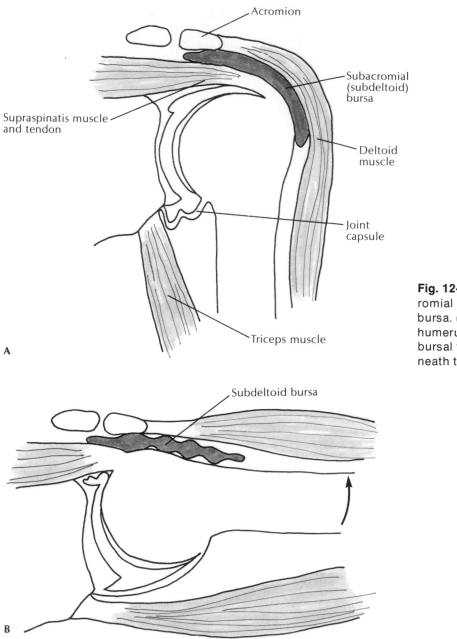

Fig. 12-5. (*A*) The subacromial (subdeltoid) bursa. (*B*) As the humerus elevates, the bursal tissue gathers beneath the acromion.

ply primarily the infraspinatus and teres minor areas of the cuff. The subscapularis is supplied by the anterior humeral circumflex artery, which is usually present; the thoracoacromial artery, which is occasionally absent; and the suprahumeral and subscapular arteries, which are often absent. The supraspinatus region receives its supply primarily from the thoracoacromial artery which, as mentioned, is sometimes absent. This artery anastomoses with the two circumflex arteries, which also contribute some to the supraspinatus region.

The most significant feature of the blood supply to the rotator cuff is that the su-

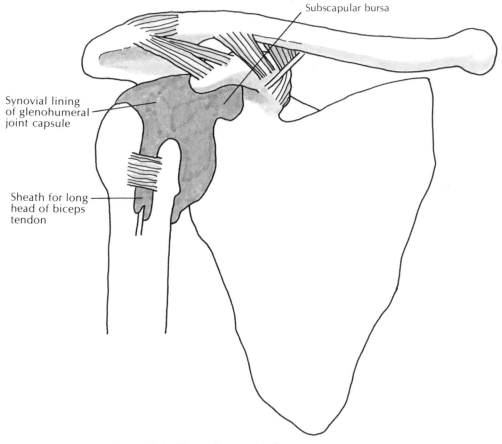

Subscapular bursa

Synovial lining
of glenohumeral
joint capsule

Sheath for long
head of biceps
tendon

Fig. 12-6. The subscapular bursa

praspinatus and, to a lesser extent, the infraspinatus regions of the cuff are areas that are often considerably hypovascular with respect to the rest of the tendinous cuff. This has been confirmed by injection studies as well as by histologic sections. In Rothman and Parke's investigation, it was found that, regardless of age, the supraspinatus region was hypovascular in 63% of 72 specimens, and that the infraspinatus region was hypovascular in 37%. It was further noted that when the infraspinatus was undervascularized, so was the supraspinatus. Hypovascularity was demonstrated in the subscapularis region in only 7% of the specimens.

Clinically, the relative incidence of tendinitis in these tendons correlates well with the above relative incidences of hypovascularity. Also, the incidence of shoulder tendinitis tends to increase with advancing age, which is consistent with the findings that tendon hypovacularity, in general, progresses with age.[18]

It is proposed that the hypovascularity in the supraspinatus region is at least partly the result of pressure applied to the underside of the tendon by the superior aspect of the humeral head as the tendon passes around and over its insertion on the greater tubercle of the humerus.[14]

BIOMECHANICS

JOINT STABILIZATION

As indicated in the discussion of functional anatomy, the glenohumeral joint capsule

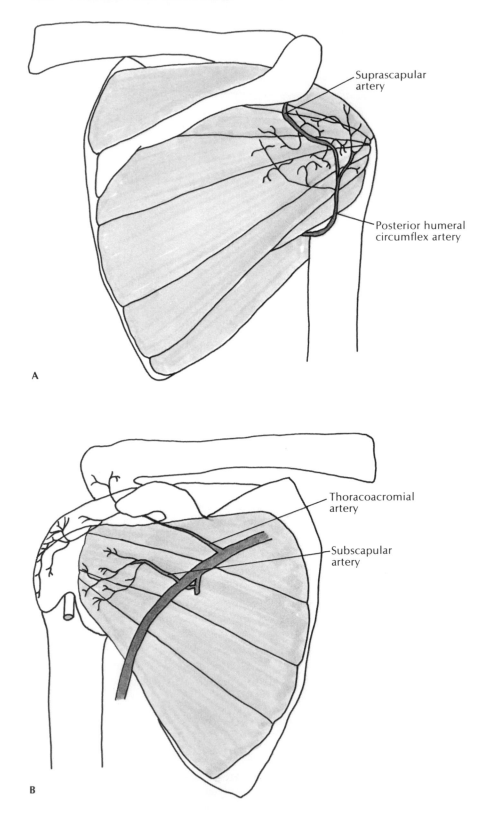

Suprascapular artery

Posterior humeral circumflex artery

A

Thoracoacromial artery

Subscapular artery

B

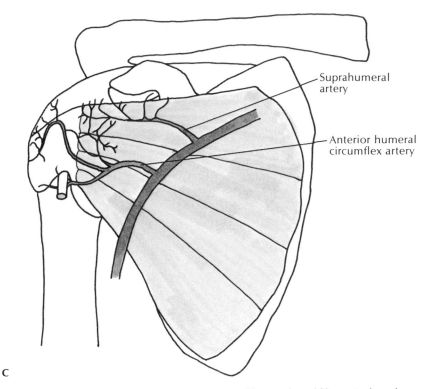

C

Fig. 12-7. Vascular supply of the rotator cuff muscles: (*A*) posterior view; (*B*) anterior view, showing the thoracoacromial and subscapular arteries; and (*C*) anterior view, showing the suprahumeral and anterior humeral circumflex arteries

is relatively lax. This is somewhat unique, since most joints rely primarily upon their capsules and ligaments to maintain proper orientation of joint surfaces during movement and in response to external forces. The shoulder joint capsule does provide some stabilization of the joint when the arm is at the side, and it does help to guide movement of the joint. At the shoulder, however, the muscles also play an essential role in these functions. The shoulder, then, relies on active and passive stabilizing components to maintain joint integrity. This is necessary at the glenohumeral joint because the incongruent bony constituents confer little intrinsic stability, such as is present at the hip joint.

When the arm hangs freely to the side, the superior joint capsule and coracohumeral ligament are normally taut, and the plane of the glenoid cavity faces somewhat upward. A vertical force produced by the weight of the hanging arm is met by a reactive tensile force to the superior joint capsule. The result of these two forces is a force that tends to pull the head of the humerus in against the upward-facing glenoid cavity (Fig. 12-8). In this way the tightness of the superior joint capsule and the orientation of the glenoid stabilize the humerus when the arm hangs freely at the side. Little or no muscle contraction by the deltoid or the rotator cuff muscles is necessary in order to prevent inferior subluxation of the humerus, even when some weight is held in the hanging hand.[1,3]

Once the arm is elevated from the side in any plane, tension is lost in the superior joint capsule so that it can no longer con-

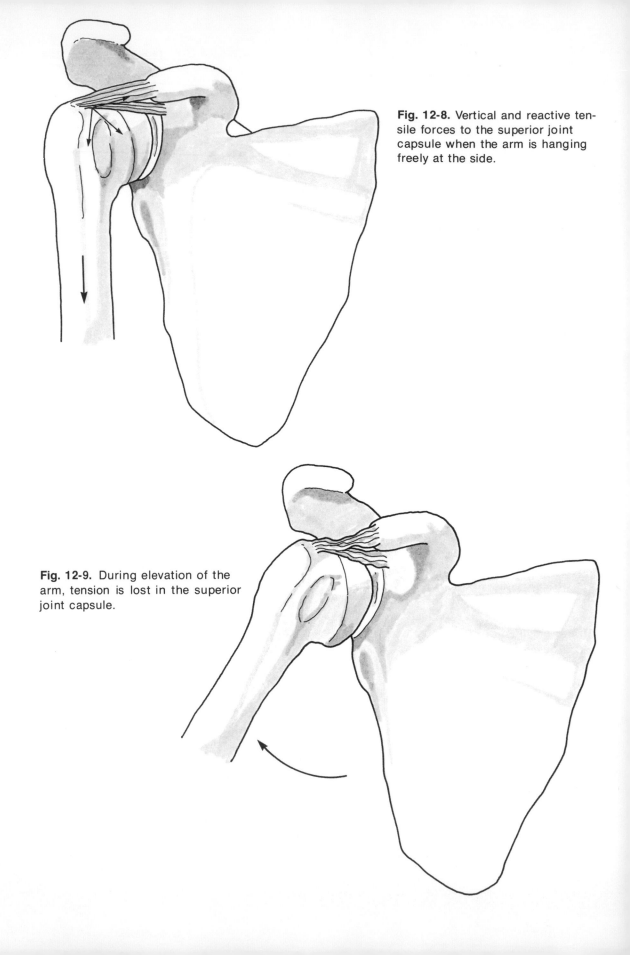

Fig. 12-8. Vertical and reactive tensile forces to the superior joint capsule when the arm is hanging freely at the side.

Fig. 12-9. During elevation of the arm, tension is lost in the superior joint capsule.

tribute to the maintenance of joint interity (Fig. 12-9). Now the rotator cuff muscles, supraspinatus, subscapularis, and teres minor must contract to hold the humerus in a proper orientation with respect to the glenoid cavity during movement of the arm (Fig. 12-10). In this way, the rotator cuff tendons, which blend with the joint capsule, provide for stabilization of the glenohumeral joint when the arm is held away from the side.[1,2,3,10]

Clinically there are some common conditions in which these normal stabilizing mechanisms are compromised. The two common causes are (*1*) alterations in the normal structural alignment of the bony constituents of the shoulder girdle and (*2*) rotator cuff muscle weakness. In a person with a thoracic kyphosis, the scapula fol-

lows the contour of the thorax and assumes a downward rotated position; the glenoid cavity no longer faces upward. Also, in this position the freely hanging humerus assumes a position of relative abduction with respect to the scapula, and tension is lost in the superior joint capsule (Fig. 12-11). In this situation, the rotator cuff muscles must contract to maintain joint integrity with the arm at the side, thus preventing inferior subluxation of the humerus. Therefore, the person with a thoracic kyphotic deformity must maintain increased tone in his rotator cuff muscles to compensate for the loss of capsular stabilization. It is possible that thoracic kyphosis is an etiologic factor in some cases of frozen shoulder. The increased tone of the rotator cuff muscles results in

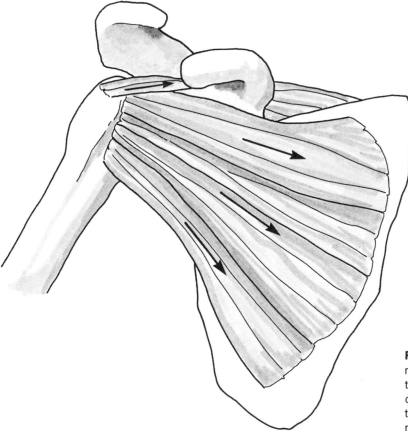

Fig. 12-10. Rotator cuff muscles contract to hold the humerus in proper orientation with respect to the glenoid during movement of the arm.

increased tensile stresses to the joint capsule, with which the rotator cuff tendons blend (Fig. 12-12). The increased stress to the capsule stimulates an increase in collagen production, which leads to a gradual loss of extensibility of the capsule, in other words, capsular fibrosis.

In the patient with shoulder girdle muscle paresis, a similar situation may exist; the weakness of the scapular muscles allows the scapula to assume a downward rotated position on the chest wall (Fig. 12-13,A). The common condition in which this occurs is hemiplegia following a stroke. In these individuals, rotator cuff muscle activity may also be reduced, and the arm is predisposed to inferior subluxation because of the loss of active and passive stabilizing components (Fig. 12-13,B).

INFLUENCE OF THE GLENOHUMERAL JOINT CAPSULE ON MOVEMENT

The orientation and configuration of the shoulder joint capsule play a major role in determining the degree and type of movement that occur at the joint. When the arm hangs freely to the side the fibers of the joint capsule are oriented in a forward and medial twist (Fig. 12-14).[11] Because the plane of the scapula is oriented midway between the frontal and sagittal planes, this capsular twist is increased with abduction (elevation in the frontal plane) and decreased with flexion (elevation in the sagittal plane) (Fig. 12-15). Thus, as the arm swings into abduction, the increasing twist in the joint capsule begins to pull the head of the humerus in

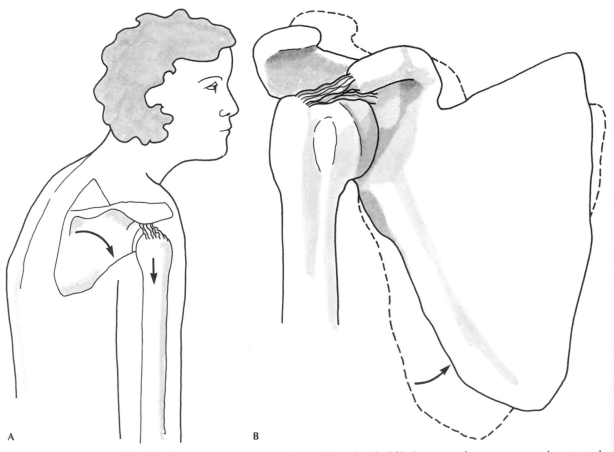

A   B

Fig. 12-11. In a person with thoracic kyphosis (A) the scapula assumes a downward, rotated position so that the glenoid fossa no longer faces upward. (B) The freely hanging humerus assumes a position of relative abduction with loss of tension in the superior joint capsule.

tightly against the glenoid cavity, and the tension in the capsular fibers gradually increases as the twisting continues. The tension eventually causes the capsule to pull the humerus around into external rotation (Fig. 12-16). This external rotation untwists the joint capsule and allows further movement to occur. If the humerus were not to rotate externally, the joint would lock at the midrange of abduction from the combined effects of abnormal compression of joint surfaces and excessive tension on the capsular fibers. The external rotation that occurs also causes the greater tubercle to clear the acromiocoracoid arch during abduction.[4,10,13] In this way, the external rotation of the humerus that takes place during abduction is a passive phenomenon occurring as a result of the twisted configuration of the glenohumeral joint capsule, and because abduction involves movement out of the plane of the scapula in a direction that tends to increase the twist. If lateral rotation does not occur, full movement is restricted because the joint locks and the greater tubercle impinges on the acromial arch (Fig. 12-17).

A common condition in which external rotation of the humerus becomes restricted is frozen shoulder. With capsular fibrosis at the shoulder, the anterior joint capsule becomes especially tight. The capsule adheres to the anterior aspect of the humeral head while the redundant folds of the capsule situated anteroinferiorly adhere to one another.[17] It is important for the clinician to realize that in the presence

(*Text continues on page 290*)

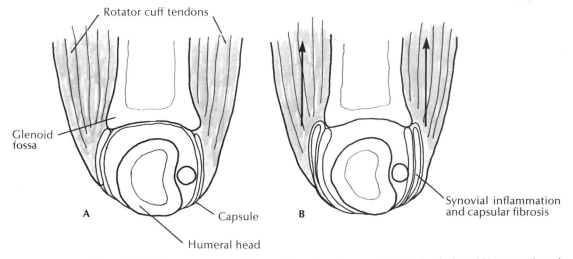

Fig. 12-12. Transverse section of the glenohumeral joint depicting (*A*) normal and (*B*) increased cuff tension

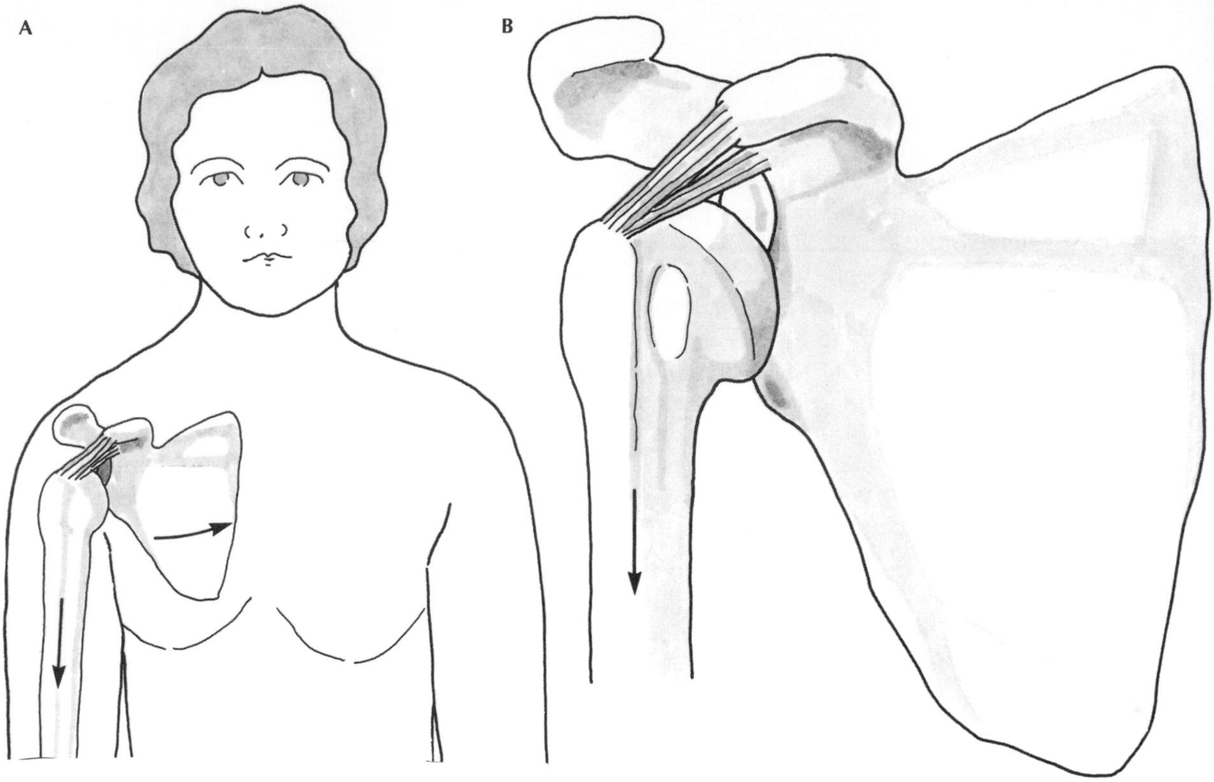

Fig. 12-13. In the person with shoulder-girdle muscle paresis (*A*) the scapula assumes a downward, rotated position on the chest wall. (*B*) Reduced rotator-cuff tension predisposes to inferior subluxation.

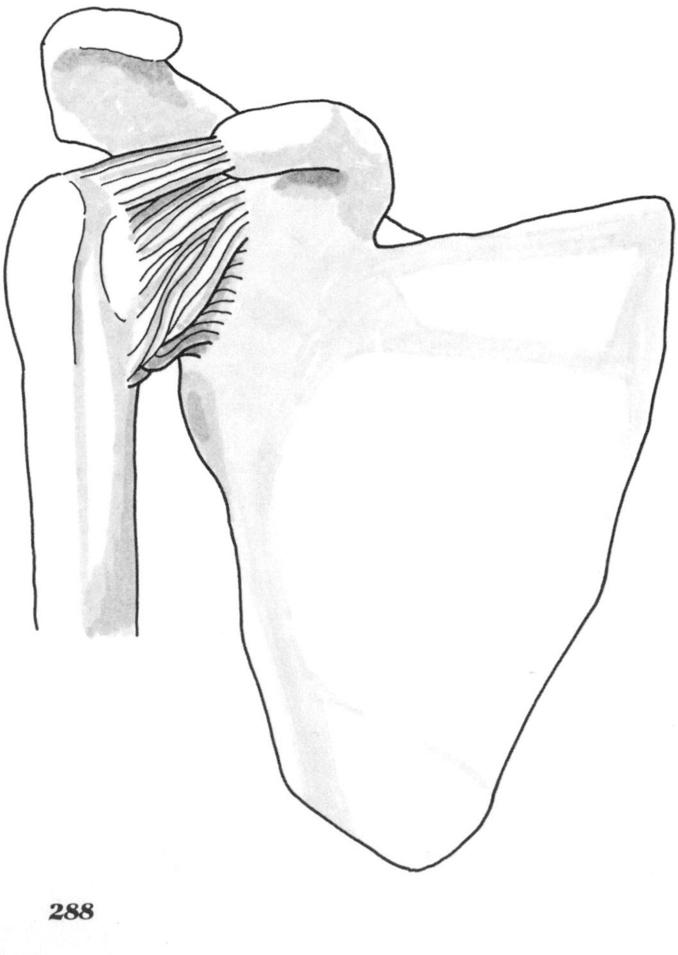

Fig. 12-14. Anterior view of the orientation of the fibers of the joint capsule when the arm hangs freely at the side

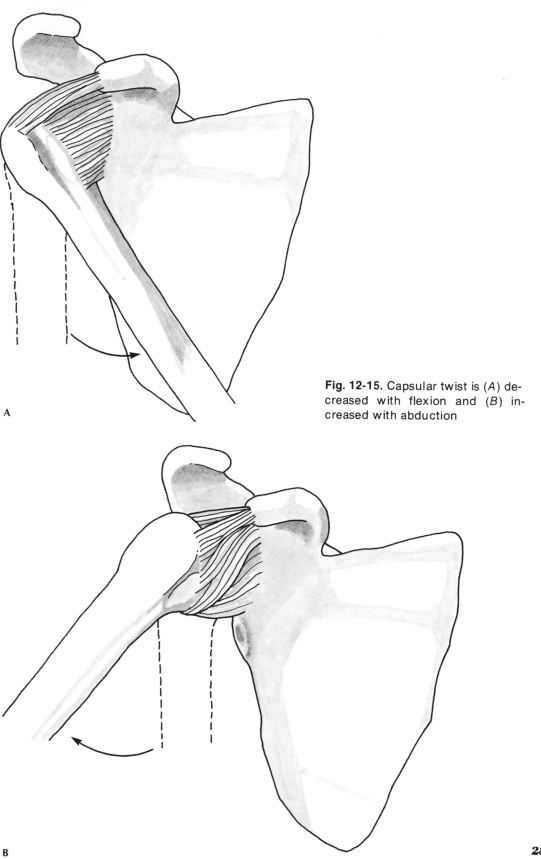

Fig. 12-15. Capsular twist is (*A*) decreased with flexion and (*B*) increased with abduction

A

B

of capsular tightness at the shoulder, abduction is restricted by locking and impingement. This movement should not be forced until external rotation is gained.

MUSCULAR FORCE-COUPLE

The rotator cuff muscles act with the deltoid muscle in a force-couple mechanism during elevation to guide the humerus in its movement on the glenoid cavity.[6,10,13,19] If only the deltoid alone were to contract to elevate the arm from the side, the head of the humerus would jam superiorly into the overlying acromial arch (Fig. 12-18). This is because with the arm at the side, the fibers of the deltoid pass across the axis of movement, and there would be no moment arm by which to rotate the humerus about the axis of abduction (Fig. 12-19,A). Once the arm is elevated somewhat from the side, the orientation of the deltoid is such that a moment arm is created. This allows the deltoid to abduct on its own, although the rotator cuff muscles do remain active during this phase (Fig. 12-19,B). Thus, at the initiation of abduction, contraction of the rotator cuff muscles is necessary in order for the arm to be swung from the side (Fig. 12-20). Acting as part of a force-couple with the deltoid, these muscles maintain depression of the head of the humerus during abduction.

The long head of the biceps also aids in humeral head depression because of the way the tendon acts as a pulley around the superior aspect of the humerus.[10,13] If the arm is externally rotated so that the bicipital groove faces laterally, the long head of the biceps works as a pulley to assist in abduction of the arm (Fig. 12-21).

Clinically, a large rotator cuff tear, involving most of the supraspinatus tendon region, will usually result in the inability to actively abduct the arm from the side. The patient often attempts to swing the arm up passively to a point at which the deltoid can take hold and complete the movement of elevation. On the other hand, a person with loss of deltoid function from, for example, an axillary nerve lesion, may very well be able to abduct the arm using the rotator cuff and long head of the biceps. A person with a biceps tendon rupture will usually not have a functional deficit, but may be predisposed to subacromial impingement because of inadequate depression of the humeral head during elevation. The same may hold true for someone with mild to moderate rotator cuff weakness. Chronic subacromial impingement tends to cause irritation to the subdeltoid bursa or supraspinatus tendon attachment.

The clinician who deals with stroke patients, or any patient with diffuse paralysis of the shoulder musculature, must be aware of the importance of the rotator cuff muscles in guiding glenohumeral movement. If passive range of motion of the shoulder is performed in such cases, the head of the humerus must be guided into inferior glide (depression) passively during flexion and abduction. If it is not, the subacromial tissues may be subjected to repeated trauma. This may explain the onset of shoulder pain in many of these patients as sensation to the shoulder returns. It also emphasizes that "routine" range of motion be performed by a skilled professional.[16]

ANALYSIS OF SHOULDER ABDUCTION

When we consider function at the shoulder, we must be concerned with the contribution of several joints in addition to the glenohumeral articulation. These include the acromioclavicular joint, the sternoclavicular joint, the articulation between the scapula and the thorax, the joints of the lower cervical and upper thoracic spines, and the articulation between the coracoacromial arch and the subacromial tissues. An analysis of the functioning of each of these during abduction of the arm emphasizes the importance

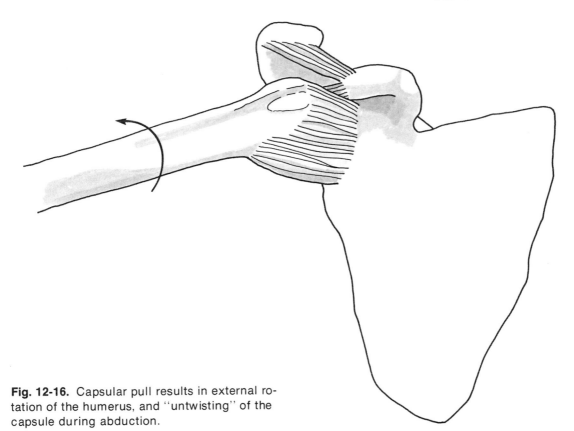

Fig. 12-16. Capsular pull results in external rotation of the humerus, and "untwisting" of the capsule during abduction.

of a normal interplay between each of the components of the shoulder complex.

During the first 15° to 30° of abduction, much of the movement occurs at the glenohumeral joint, although this varies among individual.[7,10,12] During this early phase, the muscles controlling the scapula contract to stabilize the scapula against the chest wall, preparing it for subsequent movement. Because the glenohumeral joint capsule is twisted forward and medially at the starting position, and because abduction is a movement of the humerus out of the plane of the scapula, the medial twist of the capsule begins to increase as abduction proceeds.*[11]

---

* The increasing medial twist is a result of medial conjunct rotation from movement of the humerus around the medial axis as defined at the beginning of movement. This occurs because abduction is an impure swing in which the humerus moves out of the plane of the scapula.

Beginning at 15° to 30° of abduction, the scapula begins to move to contribute to elevation of the arm. In doing so, it moves around forward, elevates, and rotates upward on the chest wall. Much of this movement of the scapula can occur because of movement at the sternoclavicular joint; the clavicle protracts about 30°, elevates about 30°, and rotates backward around its long axis about 50°.[5,10,13] The acromioclavicular joint contributes much less to scapular movement because its planar joint surfaces do not allow much angular movement. The scapula does rotate some at the acromioclavicular joint at the beginning of scapular movement. Viewed from above, the angle between the scapula and clavicle narrows as the scapula slides around and forward on the chest wall (Fig. 12-2,C). The rotation which the scapula undergoes in the frontal

(*Text continues on page 294*)

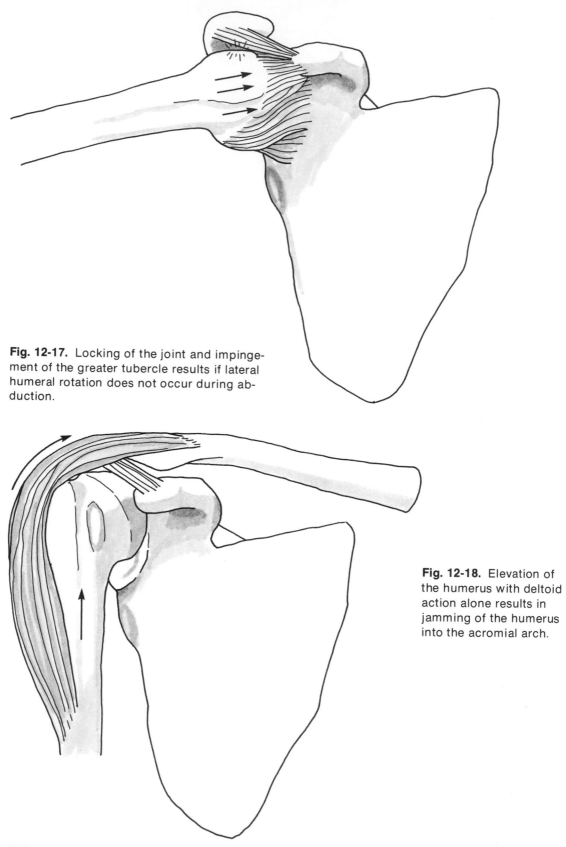

Fig. 12-17. Locking of the joint and impingement of the greater tubercle results if lateral humeral rotation does not occur during abduction.

Fig. 12-18. Elevation of the humerus with deltoid action alone results in jamming of the humerus into the acromial arch.

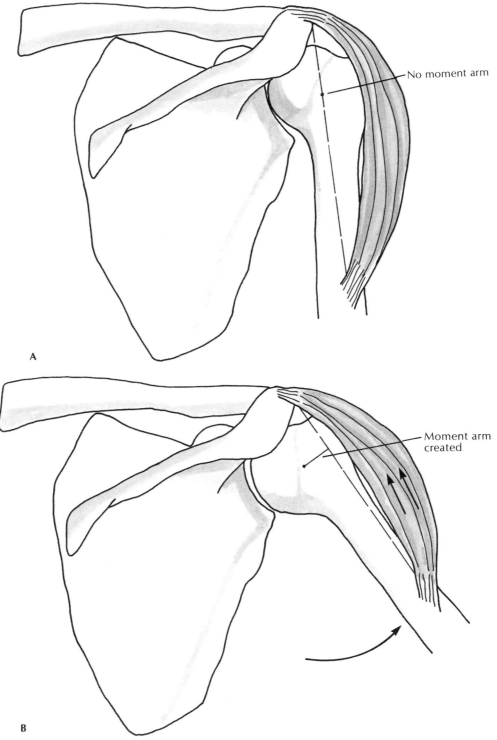

Fig. 12-19. Muscular force couple mechanism: (*A*) no-moment arm with the arm at the side; (*B*) moment arm created during humeral elevation

plane, with respect to the clavicle, causes the conoid ligament to tighten. Since this ligament attaches to the backside of the clavicle, as it pulls tight, it pulls the clavicle into a backward axial rotation. As the angle between the scapula and clavicle narrows (viewed from above), the joint close-packs quite early. However, because the clavicle rotates axially and because it is S shaped, the joint surfaces maintain a more constant relationship than they would otherwise. Furthermore, less movement is required of the acromioclavicular joint because of this axial rotation and the shape of the clavicle. Thus, out of the total of the approximately 60° that scapular movement contributes to elevation of the arm, about 30° occurs at the sternoclavicular joint, and the remaining 30° occurs from the combined effects of clavicular rotation, which cause the

clavicular joint surface to face upward, and the movement that occurs at the acromioclavicular joint.

From 15° or 30° of abduction the humerus continues to elevate with respect to the scapula through a total of 90° to 110°.[7,10,12,13] The humerus contributes about 15° of movement for every 10° contributed by scapular motion. As the humerus elevates, the greater tubercle begins to approximate the coracoacromial arch, and the capsular fibers continue to twist medially. Once a certain amount of tension develops in the joint capsule, the capsule pulls the humerus around into a lateral axial rotation, causing the greater tubercle to be directed behind and beneath the acromion. As this occurs the subdeltoid bursal tissue is gathered proximally beneath the acromion (Fig. 12-5). If the bursa is distended, or if the tubercle

Fig. 12-20. Rotator-cuff mechanism acts as part of the muscular-force couple during humeral elevation.

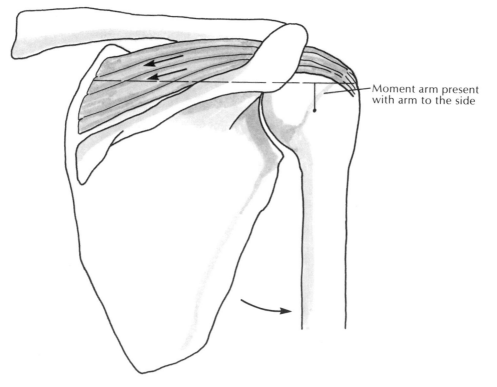

Moment arm present with arm to the side

rides too high or does not rotate laterally, subacromial impingement will occur with either loss of movement or chronic trauma to the subacromial tissues, or both.

The combined glenohumeral and scapular movements contribute about 160° to the full range of abduction. The remaining movement occurs as a result of movement at the lower cervical and upper thoracic spines. If both arms are raised simultaneously, extension occurs at these regions. If unilateral abduction is performed, the spine bends away from the side of arm movement. The contribution of spinal movement to the full 180° elevation of the arm is often overlooked. The person with a fixed spinal deformity, such as a thoracic kyphosis, cannot be expected to demonstrate full elevation of the arm.

EVALUATION OF THE SHOULDER

A general approach to evaluation of soft-tissue lesions is discussed in Chapter 4; the concepts it presents all apply to evaluation of the shoulder. However, there are concepts and techniques specific to evaluation of the shoulder region.

We must realize that the shoulder and the arm are common sites of referred pain from other areas, such as the myocardium, cervical region, and diaphragm. Usually the history will suggest the origin of pain. If not, a scan exam consisting of active motion of the neck and all major upper-extremity joints, with passive over-pressure at the extremes of each motion, may be useful in reproducing the pain and suggesting the site of the lesion. In discussing examination of the shoulder itself, we assume that the physician's examination, the history, or the scan examination has localized the lesion to the shoulder region. The physical therapist's in-depth examination clarifies the nature and extent of the lesion so that he may safely and effectively apply prescribed

treatment modalities and may quantify physical findings by which to set a baseline for judging progress.

I. **History**
   A. *Specific questions* for shoulder lesions include the following:
      1. Does the pain ever spread to below the elbow?
      2. Can you lie on the shoulder at night time?
      3. Are you able to comb your hair with the arm?
      4. Can you reach into your hip pocket/fasten a bra behind you?
      5. Can you eat comfortably with the arm?
      6. Does it hurt to put on or remove a shirt or jacket?
      7. Is it difficult to perform activities that require reaching above shoulder level?

   Comments relative to common lesions that affect the shoulder deal with the location, nature, and onset of pain.
   B. *Site of pain*—Except in acromioclavicular joint sprains, pain is seldom felt at the shoulder itself but rather over the lateral brachial region. It may spread to all or any part of, from which the glenohumeral joint structures are primarily derived, usually the C5 segment or C4 in the case of acromioclavicular problems.
   C. *Nature of pain*—Common lesions at the shoulder tend to be aggravated by use and relieved by rest. Patients with capsular lesions give a history of painful limitation, especially with movements into external rotation and abduction. Patients with noncapsular lesions often present with painful "twinges" during various func-

(*Text continues on page 298*)

Fig. 12-21. Long head of biceps acts in the muscular-force couple to create (*A*) vertical and reactive tensile forces and (*B*) moment arm during humeral elevation.

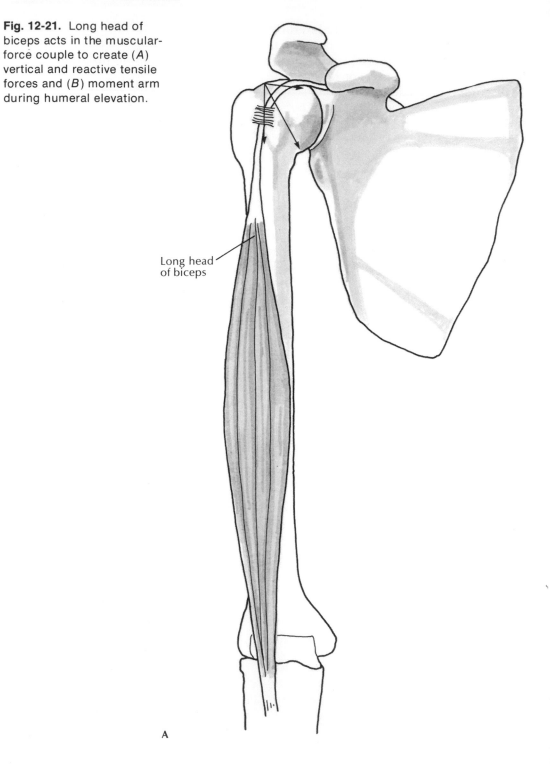

Long head
of biceps

A

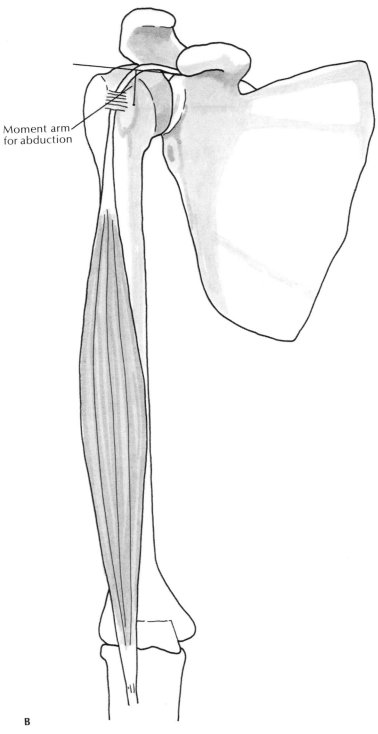

Moment arm
for abduction

B

Fig. 12-21. (*Continued*)

tions, such as donning a jacket or reaching above shoulder level.

In the case of acute bursitis, which is relatively rare, the pain may become quite intense and is often felt even at rest.

    D. *Onset of pain*—Except in athletic settings, a history of trauma does not accompany most common shoulder lesions. More often, the onset is insidious, as is the case in tendinitis or capsular tightening. In these, the onset is very gradual, whereas in acute bursitis, the patient notes a rapid buildup of pain over 12 to 72 hours.

II. Physical Examination

    A. *Observation* (*record findings*)
      1. Posture of the arm and shoulder girdle
        a. does the patient hold arm close to side or across chest?
        b. does the patient tend to support arm?
      2. Function, particularly dressing, and general willingness to use arm
    B. *Inspection* (*record findings*)
      1. Structure. Observe the patient in relaxed standing position for
        a. upper spinal curvatures
        b. shoulder heights
        c. bony relationships—acromioclavicular joint; acromion-to-greater tubercle distance; sternoclavicular joint
        d. position of scapulae
        e. rotary position of humerus hanging freely at the side, as judged by the orientation of the epicondyles and antecubital space
      2. Soft tissues. With patient in sitting position, observe for
        a. atrophy—especially over the shoulder girdles
        b. swelling

        i. anteriorly for joint effusion
        ii. laterally for bursal swelling
        iii. entire extremity for edema, as from reflex sympathetic dystrophy
        c. general contours—note asymmetries
      3. Skin (entire extremity and shoulder girdle)
        a. color
        b. moisture
        c. texture
        d. scars and blemishes
    C. *Selective tissue tension tests*
      1. Active movements (sitting)
        a. observe
        i. flexion and extension
        ii. abduction—determine whether a painful arc exists
        iii. horizontal adduction
        iv. hand to neck
        v. hand behind back—note which spinous process can be reached with the thumb
        b. Apply slight passive overpressure at the limits of each active movement.
        c. Record for each movement
        i. range of motion
        ii. presence of pain
        iii. nature of end-feel
        iv. presence of crepitus
      2. Passive movements (supine)
        a. perform
        i. flexion and extension
        ii. internal-external rotation (with elbow bent and arm at 45° abduction)
        iii. abduction—note painful arc
        iv. horizontal adduction
        b. record
        i. range of motion

ii. pain

iii. end-feel

iv. crepitus

3. Resisted movements (supine)

   a. strong isometric contractions with the arm close to the side (parentheses indicate tendons most commonly involved if test is positive)

     i. internal rotation (subscapularis)

     ii. external rotation with arm close to side (infraspinatus)

     iii. external rotation with arm at 75° abduction (teres minor)

     iv. abduction with arm close to side (supraspinatus)

     v. elbow flexion (long head of biceps)

     vi. forearm supination (biceps)

     vii. others as necessary for differentiation

   b. Record whether strong or weak, painful or painless

4. Joint play movements (supine)

   a. tests

     i. inferior glide

     ii. lateral glide

     iii. anterior glide

     iv. posterior glide

     v. backward glide

     vi. backward and downward glide

     vii. backward and outward glide

     viii. scapular rotations

   b. Compare to other arm and record

     i. amplitude of joint play (normal, restricted, hypermobile)

     ii. presence of pain or muscle guarding

D. *Neuromuscular tests.* These tests may be performed if neurologic involvement is suspected, such as that following anterior humeral dislocation, or that accompanying a cervical nerve root impingement. (See Chapter 4, Assessment of Muskuloskeletal Disorders.)

—Included might be upper extremity muscle testing, sensory testing, and reflex testing (see Table 4-1, Chapter 4).

E. *Palpation (record findings)*

1. Skin

   a. temperature, over joint regions and entire extremity

   b. moisture, especially distally

   c. mobility of skin over subcutaneous tissues

   d. tenderness, especially if neurologic involvement is suspected

   e. texture

2. Soft tissues

   a. consistency, tone, and mobility of shoulder girdles and brachial region

   b. swelling. Joint effusion may be palpable anteriorly; bursal effusion may be noted laterally

   c. pulse. Radial pulse tests (*e.g.,* Adson's maneuver) may be carried out if thoracic outlet syndrome is suspected. Be sure to compare to the opposite side.

   d. tenderness. Referred tenderness over the lateral brachial region accompanies most common shoulder lesions. Don't be mislead.

3. Bones and soft tissue attachments

   a. bony relationships

     i. acromioclavicular joint

     ii. sternoclavicular joint

   iii. acromion-to-greater-
      tuberosity distance
   b. tenderness
      i. tenoperiosteal junctions
         of the supraspinatus, in-
         fraspinatus, subscapu-
         laris, teres minor, and
         biceps
      ii. acromioclavicular joint
      iii. sternoclavicular joint
   c. bony contours
F. *Other*. It is important to determine
   during the history what studies
   have been done and to gain access
   to the results of any radiographs,
   blood tests, or arthrograms which
   may have been taken. This information is often important in developing the treatment program
   but is usually not communicated
   in the routine referral.

COMMON LESIONS

TENDINITIS

Tendinitis at the shoulder is a very common disorder. It occurs in young active
individuals as well as in older persons,
and about equally in males and females.
In the case of a younger person it may be
caused by activities such as tennis, racquetball, or baseball, which increase the
stress levels to the rotator cuff tendons. In
the older person it is more likely to be a
degenerative lesion. Because of the relatively poor blood supply near the insertion
of the supraspinatus, nutrition to the area
may not meet the metabolic demands of
the tendon tissue. The resultant focal cell
death sets up an inflammatory response,
probably due to the release of irritating
enzymes and dead tissue acting as a for-
eign body.[6,14] The body may react by laying down scar tissue or calcific deposits.
Such calcific deposits may be visible on
radiographs; however, they are often seen
in the absence of symptoms and, conversely, they are not always present in
known cases of tendinitis. Superficial migration of these deposits with rupture into
the underside of the subdeltoid bursa is
thought to be a major cause of acute bursitis at the shoulder.[15] Because of the poor
blood supply to the region, adequate repair may not take place, and the lesion
may develop into an actual tear in the
tendon.

The degenerative lesions tend to be
persistent, with little tendency toward
spontaneous resolution. The combined
effects of poor blood flow and continued
stress to the tendon do not allow for
adequate maturation of the healing
tissue. It is not unusual for a patient to
describe a history of several years of constant or intermittent problems with the
shoulder. This should by no means suggest that such patients cannot be helped,
since they do respond well, and often
dramatically, to the program outlined
below. Transverse friction massage is an
essential component of the treatment program in chronic cases. The beneficial effects of friction massage in such cases are
not well understood. However, it is proposed that an increase in the mobility of
the developing, or developed, scar tissue
takes place without stressing the tendon
longitudinally (see Chapter 9, Friction
Massage). This prevents the healing tissue
from being continually retorn during
daily activities.

A factor that may contribute to chronicity and recurrence is weakening of the
rotator cuff muscles from reflex inhibition
or from actual disuse. Such weakening
would predispose to subacromial impingement during elevation of the arm and
further mechanical irritation to the site of
the lesion. Rotator cuff strengthening is,
therefore, an important part of the treatment program. However, if recent or repeated steroid injections of the tendon
have been performed, you must proceed

gradually with the strengthening program. While local steroids do relieve the pain through inhibiting the inflammatory response, they have an antianabolic effect on connective tissue, which may result in structural weakening of the injected tendon.[22]

I. **History**
   A. *Site of pain*—Lateral brachial region, possibly referred below to the elbow in the C5 or C6 sclerotome
   B. *Nature of pain*—Sharp twinges felt on various movements, such as abduction, putting on jacket, or reaching above shoulder level
   C. *Onset of pain*—Usually gradual with no known trauma. May be related to occupational or recreational overuse. May have been present for many months, or even years.
II. **Physical Examination**
   A. *Active movements*—Relatively full range of motion. Often a painful arc is present at midrange of abduction. There is usually slight limitation and pain at full elevation due to pinching of the lesion between the greater tubercle and the posterior rim of the glenoid cavity.
   B. *Passive movements*
      1. Essentially full range of motion
      2. Pain at full elevation, but full range of motion is usually present
      3. May be a painful arc on rotation and abduction
      4. May be pain on stretch of the involved tendon (*e.g.,* on full internal rotation in the case of supraspinatus or infraspinatus tendinitis)
   C. *Resisted movements*—This is the key test
      1. Maximal isometric contraction of the relevant muscle will reproduce the pain.
      2. In the case of simple tendinitis, the contraction will be fairly strong; if an actual tear exists, it will be weak.
      3. The supraspinatus is the most commonly involved tendon.
      4. Others (biceps, subscapularis, teres minor) are rarely involved.
   D. *Palpation*
      1. Tenderness usually over the involved tendon, near its insertion
      2. Usually referred tenderness over the lateral brachial region. *Don't be mislead.*
   E. *Inspection*
      1. Usually negative
      2. Some atrophy may be noted if a chronic tear exists.
III. **Management.** The presence or absence of a calcific deposit, as demonstrated by radiographs, should not affect the treatment plan.
   A. *Ultrasound*
      1. Resolution of inflammatory exudates
      2. Increased blood flow to assist the healing process
      3. May provide some pain relief although persistent pain is usually not a problem
   B. *Friction massage*—This is a key component of the treatment program
      1. To form mobile scar
      2. The hyperemia induced by the massage may enhance blood flow to the area to assist the healing response.
   C. *Instruction in appropriate use of the arm*
      1. Strict avoidance of activities that may cause impingement or tension stress at the site of

involvement while formation of painless scar takes place

2. Gradual return to normal use as healing ensues

D. *Restrengthening* of involved muscles and other measures to restore normal joint mechanics

E. *General comments*

In most of cases of tendinitis at the shoulder, perhaps the only dispensable component of the above program is the use of ultrasound. In the authors' experience, failure to appropriately institute any of the remaining measures will increase the likelihood that treatment will be unsuccessful or that the patient will suffer a recurrence. The younger person whose primary complaint is pain during recreational activities such as baseball or racquetball must be advised that temporary abstinence from certain activities is an essential remedial measure. However, restricting activities to "resting" the part is usually not sufficient in itself to effect a resolution of the pathology, although the reduction in pain experienced may often suggest this. Usually, resumption of activities will be accompanied by a recurrence of the previous symptoms because simply resting the part does not insure the development of a mature, mobile cicatrix. This is also true for the older person, who may experience pain during normal daily activities. Although appropriate control of activities is usually necessary for resolution of the problem, it alone is usually not adequate. The use of friction massage and especially restrengthening exercises should not be excluded.

The therapist must, through a complete history, become aware of the patient's habitual daily activities. This is important because the patient often engages in activities that may contribute to the problem without actually realizing it. Such "fatigue" pathologies typically result from the cumulation of otherwise asymptomatic stresses. Activities that particularly need to be avoided are those involving repetitive elevation of the arm to shoulder level or above.

The importance of strengthening exercises can be appreciated by understanding the key role the muscles play in the normal functioning of the shoulder joint. As pointed out in the section on biomechanics, the supraspinatus is largely responsible for maintaining adequate depression of the humeral head during abduction. In the presence of a weak supraspinatus, the head of the humerus will tend to ride high in the glenoid during elevation of the arm due to the disproportionate contraction of the deltoid. This would predispose to impingement of the greater tubercle, along with its tendinous attachments, against the coracoacromial arch. Thus, in cases of tendinitis there is a tendency toward muscle atrophy from reflex inhibition or disuse that may often be a factor in prolonging the pathology. Remedial strengthening exercises are best performed with the arm close to the side to prevent the possibility of impingement and reflex inhibition during performance of the exercises.

The successful use of friction massage requires precision with respect to the site of application and the intensity or depth of application. (See Chapter 9, Friction Massage.) If for some reason it is not practical for the patient to present for treatment, you should consider instruction to a family member in the technique of application or instructions to the patient in self-administration. However, application by a skilled and experienced practitioner is preferred, when feasible, in order to assure that the appropriate technique is used and to accurately monitor and document results. As athletic activities or activities involving repetitive elevation of the arm are resumed, instructing the patient in self-administered friction massage prior to engaging in the particular function may be an important preventative measure.

ADHESIVE CAPSULITIS — FROZEN SHOULDER

Capsular tightening at the shoulder is also a common disorder, usually referred to as *frozen shoulder* or *adhesive capsulitis.* The majority of cases seen by physical therapists are those in which no specific cause can be determined for the stiffening. It affects women more often than men, and middle-aged and older persons more often than younger persons. It is probable that some of the so-called idiopathic cases of frozen shoulder come about from an alteration in scapulohumeral alignment, as occurs with thoracic kyphosis. This is consistent with the fact that women are more frequently affected, since women are also more predisposed to developing thoracic kyphosis than men. (See section on biomechanics.) Some believe this problem to be a progression of rotator cuff lesions, in which the inflammatory/degenerative process spreads to include the entire joint capsule, resulting in capsular fibrosis.[6,15,16] While this may be so in some cases, there are two major contradictions to this proposal: (*1*) rotator cuff tendinitis affects men and women fairly equally, whereas frozen shoulder is much more common in women; (*2*) persons with a frozen shoulder rarely present with coexistent tendinitis, as evidenced by the absence of pain on resisted movement.

It is commonly said that these people stop using the arm because for some reason it is painful, and motion is therefore lost from disuse. In our experience, this is rarely the case. Instead, the loss of motion is responsible for the pain. The patient continues to use the arm until the restriction of motion progresses to the extent that it interferes with daily activities. It is not until this point that the patient feels much pain or is aware of a problem with the arm. The woman first notices that it is difficult to comb her hair and fasten a bra. She may also be awakened at night when rolling onto the affected side. The man notes difficulty reaching into the hip pocket and combing his hair, and may be similarly awakened at night. Because much shoulder motion can be lost before interfering with daily activities of persons in this age group, these patients invariably do not seek medical help until the shoulder has lost about 90° of abduction, 60° of flexion, 60° of external rotation, and 45° of internal rotation. In fact, it is somewhat rare to see a patient present with significantly more, or significantly less, than this amount of movement. Of course, there are some cases of capsular tightening at the shoulder that are associated with particular disease states or conditions. Conditions that might result in capsular tightness at the glenohumeral joint include

—Degenerative joint disease—This is rare at the shoulder and, if present, is relatively symptomless.
—Rheumatoid arthritis—The smaller joints of the hand and feet are usually affected first.
—Immobilization—For example, following fracture of the arm, forearm, or wrist, or perhaps following dislocation of the shoulder.

—Reflex sympathetic dystrophy (see Chapter 14, The Wrist)—This condition may follow certain visceral disorders such as a myocardial infarction, or it may follow some trauma, such as a Colles' fracture. Capsular stiffening of the joints of the hand, wrist, and shoulder is a common component of this syndrome. A frozen shoulder occurring in conjunction with a reflex sympathetic dystrophy is usually more refractory to treatment, probably because of the abnormal pain state that tends to accompany the disorder.

I. **History**
   A. *Site of pain*—Lateral brachial region, possibly referred distally into the C5 or C6 segment
   B. *Nature of pain*—Varying from a constant dull ache to pain felt only on activities involving movement into the restricted ranges. The patient is often awakened at night when rolling onto the painful shoulder.
   C. *Onset of pain*—Very gradual. May be related to minor trauma, immobilization, chest surgery, or myocardial infarction. More commonly, no cause can be cited.

II. **Physical Examination**
   A. *Active movements*—Limitation of motion in a capsular pattern: little glenohumeral movement on abduction, much difficulty and substitution getting the hand behind the neck. Some limitation when flexing the arm or trying to put the hand behind the back
   B. *Passive movements*—Limitation in a capsular pattern: external rotation is markedly restricted, abduction moderately restricted, flexion and internal rotation are somewhat limited.

1. May be limited by pain with a muscle-guarding end-feel (acute)
2. May be limited by stiffness with a capsular end-feel (chronic)
   C. *Joint play*—Restriction of most joint play movements, especially inferior glide
   D. *Resisted movements*—Strong and painless, unless a tendinitis coexists
   E. *Palpation*—Often referred tenderness over the lateral brachial region. Often a feeling of increased muscle tone, with induration over the lateral brachial region.
   F. *Inspection*—Often negative. Observe for a surgical scar.

III. **Acute vs. Chronic**
   A. *Acute*
      1. Pain radiates to below the elbow.
      2. The patient is awakened by pain at night.
      3. On passive movement, limitation is due to pain and muscle guarding, rather than stiffness *per se.*
   B. *Chronic*
      1. Pain is localized to the lateral brachial region.
      2. The patient is not awakened by pain at night.
      3. On passive movement, limitation is due to capsular stiffness, and pain is felt only when the capsule is stretched.
   C. *Subacute*—Some combination of the above findings

IV. **Management**
   A. *Acute stage*—See above criteria for acute vs. chronic
      1. Relief of pain and muscle guarding to allow early, gentle mobilization
         a. ice or superficial heat
         b. grade I or II joint play oscillations

2. Maintenance of existing range of motion and efforts to gently begin increasing range of motion
   a. grade I or II joint play mobilization. At this stage it is often best to perform these with the patient lying prone and the arm hanging freely at the side of the plinth. Inferior glide is particularly comfortable for most patients and is usually most helpful in relieving muscle spasm. This is an important movement to perform since the spasm, which is usually present in the acute stage, causes the humerus to assume a superior position in the glenoid cavity, further interfering with normal joint mechanics.
   b. Initiation of active assisted range of motion exercises at home, such as wand and pendulum exercises
3. Instruction in isometric strengthening exercises, especially for the rotator cuff muscles. The movement associated with isotonic exercises will usually cause pain and reflex inhibition, thus reducing their effectiveness.
4. Prevention of excessive kyphosis and shoulder girdle protraction. When appropriate instruction in postural awareness for the upper trunk and shoulder girdles such that the patient learns to differentiate proprioceptively between a kyphotic, protracted posture and a relatively upright, retracted position. A system of regular "postural checks" should be incorporated into the patient's daily activities.
5. Gradual progression of the above program as the condition becomes more chronic (see below).
B. *Chronic stage*—Increase the extensibility of the joint capsule, with special attention to the anteroinferior aspect of the capsule.
   1. Ultrasound preceding or accompanying stretching procedures.
   2. Specific joint mobilizations with emphasis on the anteroinferior capsular stretch (see Chapter 7, Joint Mobilization Techniques).

When using specific joint mobilization techniques in the presence of a chronically tight joint, the primary objective is to stretch the joint capsule. In order to do so the more vigorous, grade IV, techniques must be used. It is usually best, however, to commence with the use of grade I or II oscillations in preparation for more intensive stretching. The lower grades of oscillations promote reduced muscle spasm and pain, probably by increasing large-fiber, sensory input. Perhaps the best technique to use at the initiation of glenohumeral mobilization is *inferior glide* with the arm to the side, since this technique, especially, seems to induce relaxation. For this reason, this is also a good technique for relieving the "cramping" sensation a patient may experience during more vigorous movements.

Prior to or during capsular stretching procedures, you may use ultrasound to help increase the extensibility of the tissue. For example, you may perform the anteroinferior capsular stretch while an assistant directs ultrasound to the anteroinferior aspect of the joint. Specific joint mobilization techniques are most effective when used in conjunction with the motions they are intended to restore, such as inferior glide simultaneous with abduction or flexion, posterior capsular stretch with internal rotation, and anterior capsular stretch with external rotation.

You may combine passive stretching with appropriate accessory movements, for example, flexion with inferior glide or abduction with inferior glide.

Instruct the patient in home range of motion exercises. These are necessary to maintain gains made in treatment and to use as a measure to help increase movement.

General Comments

A major goal of the treatment program is to promote independence in mobilization procedures. Once approximately 120° of abduction, 140° of flexion, and 60° of external rotation are achieved, many patients will continue to make satisfactory improvement in range of motion by continuing on a supervised home exercise program. From the outset, though, it is difficult for most patients to make substantial gains in range of motion with home exercises alone; skillfully applied passive movement will significantly accelerate improvement in the early phases of treatment. The probable reason for this is that in the relatively acute stage, the reflex muscle spasm that accompanies active movement of the joint prevents the patient from exerting an effective stretch to the joint capsule—he simply fights against his own muscles. The therapist skilled in the use of passive joint mobilization procedures is able to localize the stretch to specific portions of the joint capsule and carefully graduate the intensity of the stretch to avoid eliciting protective muscle contraction. Also, the therapist can combine joint play movements with certain movements of the arm to reduce cartilaginous or bony impingement at the extremes of movement. For example, while

moving the arm into abduction, the therapist can passively move the head of the humerus inferiorly to prevent impingement of the greater tubercle against the acromial arch, which would tend to occur from the loss of external rotation and from a loss of inferior glide of the joint. By doing so, muscle spasm is reduced and a more effective stretch to the inferior capsule is affected. In fact, until significant gains in external rotation are made, the patient should not be instructed to stretch into abduction on his own, since attempting to do so will tend to traumatize the subacromial tissues more so than stretching the inferior aspect of the joint capsule.

It must be emphasized that the primary goal of treatment is restoration of painless functional range of movement and that regaining full movement of the arm is not always realistic. This is especially true for individuals with some degree of increased thoracic kyphosis since full elevation of the arm involves extension of the upper thoracic spine. For these patients "normal" elevation is usually about 150° to 160°. Range of motion of the uninvolved shoulder should serve as a guide for setting treatment goals.

In the more acute cases of frozen shoulder, the patient's major complaint is often the inability to get a good night's sleep. Each time the patient rolls onto the involved side, he is awakened by pain. The resultant fatigue adds to the patient's general debilitation. Fortunately, with appropriate management this is usually the first aspect of the problem to resolve. In fact, subjective improvement, in the form of significant reduction in night pain, will usually precede any evidence of objective improvement, such as increased range of motion. It has been our experience that one or two sessions of gentle joint play oscillations, especially into inferior glide, preceded by superficial heat or ice, will frequently be sufficient to alleviate nocturnal symptoms. This leads us to speculate whether perhaps the night pain is due more to the fact that the joint is compressed in a position in which the humerus is held into a cephalad malalignment by muscle spasm, rather than being the result of compression of an inflamed joint capsule. At any rate, it seems that relaxation of the associated muscle spasm is one of the more important measures in reducing pain in the acute phase.

In the chronic stage, pain is primarily the result of repeated tensile stresses to the tight joint capsule during daily activities. Treatment should be directed primarily toward increasing range of motion, although some restriction of activities may be warranted. For the most part, however, in the chronic stage, encourage the patient to use the arm as much as tolerable to minimize habitual disuse, which can be a factor in perpetuating the disorder.

Some sources in the literature claim that adhesive capsulitis is a self-limiting disorder, and that spontaneous resolution can be expected in about 12 months' time. This has not been consistent with our clinical experience. Even if it were the case, this should not be used as a reason for not instituting active treatment since, with appropriate therapy, satisfactory results can be expected within 3 to 4 months, usually sooner. The only frequent exception is when a frozen shoulder results as part of a sympathetic reflex dystrophy. These cases are often quite refractory to conservative management and may require supplementary measures such as sympathetic blocks or manipulation under anesthesia.

Although in most cases of frozen shoulder the prognosis for functional recovery is good, the time frame of recovery is rarely linear. Improvement tends to be characterized by spurts and plateaus. Both the therapist and the patient should be cognizant of this to avoid undue frustration during periods of limited progress.

ACUTE BURSITIS

This condition is relatively rare and is thought by many to occur secondary to a calcific tendinitis, in which the deposit migrates superficially into the floor of the subdeltoid bursa.[16]

I. **History**
   A. *Site of pain*—Lateral brachial region, possibly referred distally
   B. *Nature of pain*—Intense, constant, dull, sometimes throbbing pain. The patient may present with the arm in a sling, or supporting the arm at the elbow with the uninvolved hand. During this acute period, very little relief is found in any position. All movements are reported to be painful.
   C. *Onset of pain*—May be a history suggestive of a chronic tendinitis. The acute pain, however, usually arises over a period of 12 to 72 hours, with a gradual buildup of pain over this period.

II. **Physical Examination**
   A. *Active movements*—Marked restriction in all planes with evidence of rather severe pain on attempts to elevate the arm
   B. *Passive movements*—Restricted by pain in a noncapsular pattern with an "empty" end-feel; no resistance is felt to movement, but the patient insists that movement be ceased because of intense pain. Rotation with the arm at the side may be fairly free, but abduction past 60° or flexion past 90° is usually not permitted because of complaints of severe pain.
   C. *Resisted movements*—There may be some hesitance to perform a maximal contraction, with perhaps some pain on resisted abduction, owing to squeezing of the inflamed bursa. When carefully

tested, however, most contractions are strong and painless.

D. *Palpation*—Possibly some warmth and swelling noted over the region overlying the subdeltoid bursa. There is usually considerable tenderness in this area.

E. *Inspection*—Often unremarkable. Possibly some visable swelling laterally at the site of the bursa

III. **Management**

A. *Early stages*

1. Resolution of the acute inflammatory process
   a. Ice or superficial heat
   b. Support of the arm with a sling to reduce postural tone in the muscles adjacent to the bursa, thereby relieving pressure to the inflamed area.

2. Maintaining range of motion— Gentle active-assisted exercises such as wand and pendulum exercises

B. *Chronic stage*

With the above measures, it is rare for the condition to remain "acute" for longer than a few days. Resolution of the acute stage is characterized by the absence of pain at rest, and localization of pain to the lateral brachial region. The patient is able to actively elevate the arm to at least 90° of flexion or of abduction.

1. Resolution of chronic inflammatory process. Bursitis at the shoulder and of the trochanteric bursa are, in our experience, the two conditions in which the use of ultrasound to provide relief of symptoms, in the presence of a subacute or chronic inflammation, will often have an unequivically beneficial effect. The increased blood flow induced by the local heat apparently aids in a more rapid resolution of inflammatory irritants and debri.

Unlike tendinitis or frozen shoulder, acute bursitis at the shoulder tends to be self-limiting over a period of several weeks. With appropriate therapy few patients have significant pain or disability after 2 weeks from the time of the onset of acute symptoms. However, because calcific rotator cuff tendinitis is often a pre-existing condition, as the acute phase of the bursitis resolves you should take care to test for the presence of tendinitis, the clinical signs of which may be obscured by the acute symptoms of bursitis. If tendinitis does exist, appropriate treatment measures should be instituted. (See previous discussion on tendinitis.)

2. Restoration of full range of motion, joint play, and strength
   a. instruction in home range of motion procedures
   b. specific joint mobilization (automobilization or passive movements) if warranted
   c. instruction in home strengthening exercises

OTHER LESIONS

There are, of course, other more serious lesions that commonly affect the shoulder, such as anterior dislocation and acromioclavicular joint separation. These are usually not seen by a physical therapist until they have been treated by the physician with prolonged immobilization, or perhaps surgery followed by immobilization. At this point, the therapist no longer deals with the original injury so much as with the effects of immobilization. As a result, the goals and techniques of management in such cases are often essentially the same as those for a patient with capsular tightness. There are, however, some special considerations with which one should be familiar, depending upon the original problem. For example, surgery for recurrent anterior dislocation may be performed with the specific intent to limit external rotation to some degree to help provide some anterior stabilization.[15,21] Or, following an anterior dislocation, it may be desirable for the sake of preventing recurrence to allow the anterior capsule to heal in a tightened state. In both cases emphasis on regaining external rotation will be less than what it might be in other cases of capsular tightness. Certain surgical fixations for acromioclavicular separation, such as those involving insertion of a screw from the clavicle to the coracoid, may permanently restrict normal clavicular axial rotation. So long as such a screw is still in place, full elevation of the arm should not be expected; it can only occur if the screw should break.

Since it is not within the scope of this book to discuss them at length, the therapist must be familiar with these injuries, the current surgical procedures, and such special considerations as discussed above.

REFERENCES

1. Basmajian JV: Factors preventing downward dislocation of the abducted shoulder joint. J Bone Joint Surg 414(A):1182– 1186, 1959
2. Basmajian JV: Surgical anatomy and function of the arm–trunk mechanism. Surg Clin North Am 43:1471– 1482, 1963
3. Basmajian JV: Weight bearing by ligaments and muscles. Can J Surg 4:166– 170, 1961
4. Codman EA: The Shoulder. Boston, Thomas Todd, 1934
5. DePalma AF: Surgical anatomy and function of the acromioclavicular and sternoclavicular joints. Surg Clin North Am 43:1541– 1550, 1963
6. DePalma AF: Surgical anatomy of the rotator cuff and natural history of degenerative periarthritis. Surg Clin North Amer 43:1507– 1521, 1963
7. Fisk GH: Some observations of motion at the shoulder joint. Can Med Assoc J 50:213– 216, 1944
8. Freedman L, Munro R: Abduction of the arm in the scapular plane: Scapular and glenohumeral movements. J Bone Joint Surg 48(A):1503– 1510, 1966
9. Heppenstall RB: Fractures of the proximal humerus. Orthop Clin North Am 9(2):467– 75, 1975
10. Inman VT, Saunders JB, Abbott LC: Observations of the function of the shoulder joint. J Bone Joint Surg 26:1– 30, 1944
11. Johnston TB: The Movements of the shoulder joint, a plea for the use of the plane of the scapula as the plane of reference for movement at the humeroscapular joint. J Bone Joint Surg 25:232– 260, 1937
12. Lockhart RD: Movements of the normal shoulder joint. J Anat 64:288– 302, 1936
13. Lucas DB: Biomechanics of the shoulder joint. Arch Surg 107:425– 432, 1973
14. MacNab I: Local steroids in orthopaedic conditions. Scott Med J 17:176– 186, 1972
15. MacNab I: Rotator cuff tendinitis. Ann R Coll Surg Engl 53:271– 287, 1973
16. Moseley HF: The natural history and clinical syndromes produced by calcific deposits in the rotator cuff. Surg Clin North Amer 43:1489– 1492, 1963
17. Najenson T, Yacibovich E, Pikielni S: Rotator cuff injury in shoulder joints of hemiplegic patients. Scan J Rehabil Med 3:131– 137, 1971
18. Neviaser JS: Adhesive capsulitis of the shoulder: A study of pathological findings in periarthritis of the shoulder. J Bone Joint Surg 27:211– 222, 1945

19. Rothman RH, Parke WW: The vascular anatomy of the rotator cuff. Clin Orthop 41:176, 1965

20. Rothman RH, Marvel JP, Heppenstall RB: Anatomical considerations in the glenohumeral joint. Orthop Clin North Am 6(2):341, 1975

21. Turek SL: Orthopaedics: Principles and Their Application, 3rd ed. Philadelphia, JB Lippincott, 1977

13 The Elbow

Randolph M. Kessler

REVIEW OF FUNCTIONAL ANATOMY

OSTEOLOGY

Looking anteriorly at the distal end of the humerus, we see two articular surfaces: the trochlea which is pulley-shaped, somewhat like an hour glass or spool lying on its side, and the capitellum, which forms most of a sphere mediolaterally and half of a sphere anteroposteriorly. The lateral epicondyle extends laterally above the capitellum for attachment of the extensor muscles. The medial epicondyle is the site of attachment of the flexor–pronator group. The coronoid fossa lies immediately above the trochlea, and the radial fossa immediately above the capitellum. They receive the coronoid process and the anterior rim of the radial head, respectively, on full elbow flexion (Fig. 13-1).

Looking laterally, or medially, the distal humerus angulates anteriorly such that the longitudinal axis of the trochlea is directed anteriorly, 45° to the shaft of the humerus. As implied above, the hemisphere of the capitellum faces anteriorly, the articular surface having an angular value of about 180° (Fig. 13-2).

Looking posteriorly (Fig. 13-3) the large, deep olecranon fossa accepts the olecranon process on full elbow extension. At times it communicates with the coronoid fossa. The trochlear articular surface, with its median groove, extends posteriorly. The groove usually runs obliquely, distally, and laterally; the medial half of the trochlea extends farther distally than the lateral half does. The asymmetry of the trochlea causes the ulna to angulate laterally on the humerus when the elbow extends. This abduction of the forearm on full extension is referred to as the *carrying angle* of the elbow.

The radial head is concave on its superior surface for articulation with the convex capitellum. Viewed from above, the radial head is slightly oval, being longer anteroposteriorly, so that with pronation it is displaced slightly laterally (Fig. 13-4).

The proximal ulna consists of the olecranon and the coronoid process, between which is the trochlear notch. With the elbow extended, the trochlear notch faces anteriorly and superiorly, corresponding to the 45° angulation of the distal humerus (Fig. 13-2,A). Lying inferiorly and medially to the trochlear notch is the radial notch, which faces laterally for articulation with the radial head (Fig. 13-1).

The angulation of the distal humerus and trochlear notch of the proximal ulna allow about 160° of elbow flexion and 180° of extension. The angulation is necessary in order to provide room for the anterior muscle groups of the arm and forearm, which approximate on elbow flexion (Fig. 13-5). Any bony malalignment that interferes with these critical angles (*e.g.,* following a supracondylar fracture) will make normal movement impossible.

LIGAMENTS

The capsule of the elbow is reinforced by medial and lateral collateral ligaments. These serve to restrict medial or lateral
(*Text continues on page 314*)

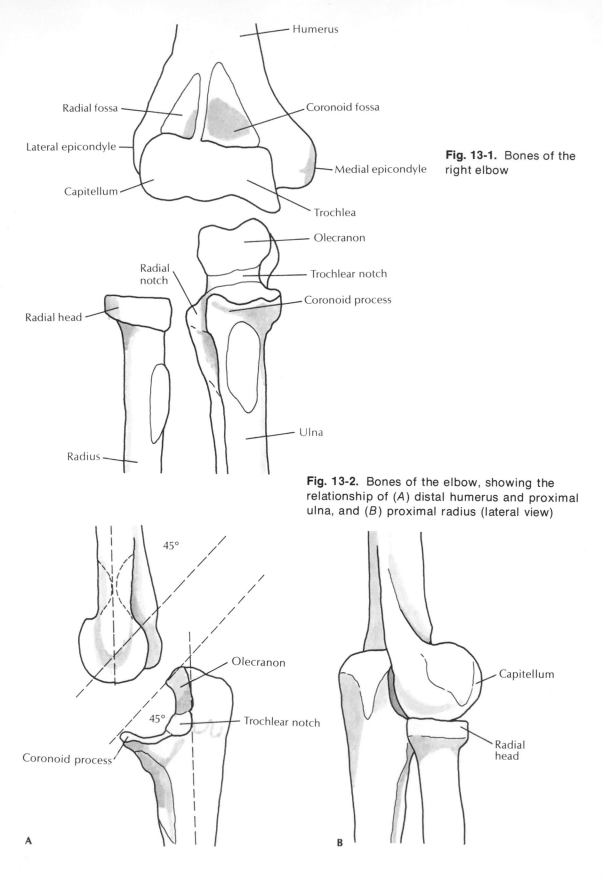

Radial fossa

Lateral epicondyle

Capitellum

Radial head

Radius

Radial notch

Humerus

Coronoid fossa

Medial epicondyle

Trochlea

Olecranon

Trochlear notch

Coronoid process

Ulna

Fig. 13-1. Bones of the right elbow

Fig. 13-2. Bones of the elbow, showing the relationship of (A) distal humerus and proximal ulna, and (B) proximal radius (lateral view)

45°

Olecranon

45°

Trochlear notch

Coronoid process

Capitellum

Radial head

A

B

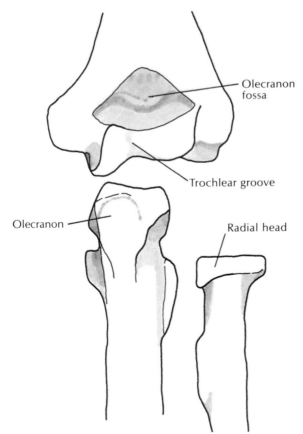

Fig. 13-3. Posterior view of bones of the elbow

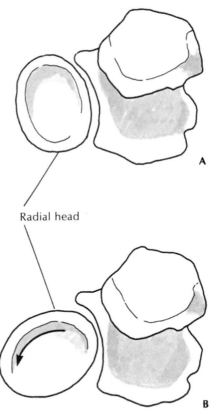

Fig. 13-4. Relationship of proximal radius and ulna in (A) supination and (B) pronation, as viewed from above

Fig. 13-5. Elbow in flexion

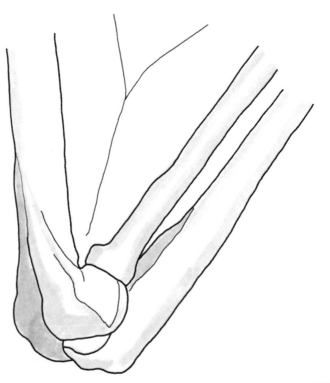

angulation of the ulna on the humerus. They also help prevent dislocation of the ulna from the trochlea. Each collateral ligament consists of anterior, intermediate, and posterior fibers. The anterior fibers of both help reinforce the annular ligament of the radioulnar articulation (Fig. 13-6). The capsule is strengthened anteriorly by an anterior oblique ligament (Fig. 13-7).

The annular ligament runs from the anterior margin of the radial notch of the ulna around the radial head to the posterior margin of the radial notch. It is lined with articular cartilage so that with pro-

nation and supination, the radial head articulates with the capitellum of the humerus and the radial notch of the ulna, as well as with the annular ligament (Figs. 13-6 and 13-7).

The joint capsule of the elbow encloses the humeroulnar joint, the radiohumeral joint, and the proximal radioulnar joint (Figs. 13-6, 13-7, and 13-8).

BURSAE

The olecranon bursa overlies the olecranon posteriorly, lying between the su-

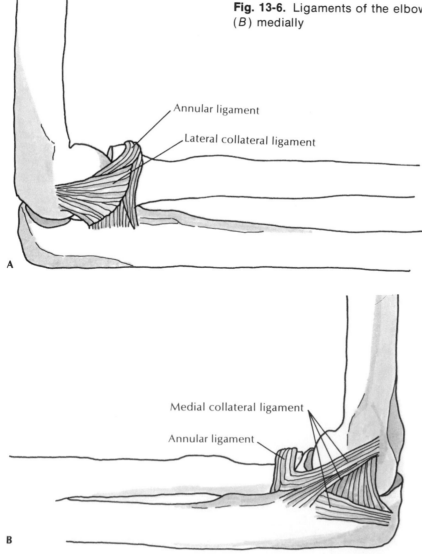

Fig. 13-6. Ligaments of the elbow viewed (*A*) laterally and (*B*) medially

Annular ligament

Lateral collateral ligament

A

Medial collateral ligament

Annular ligament

B

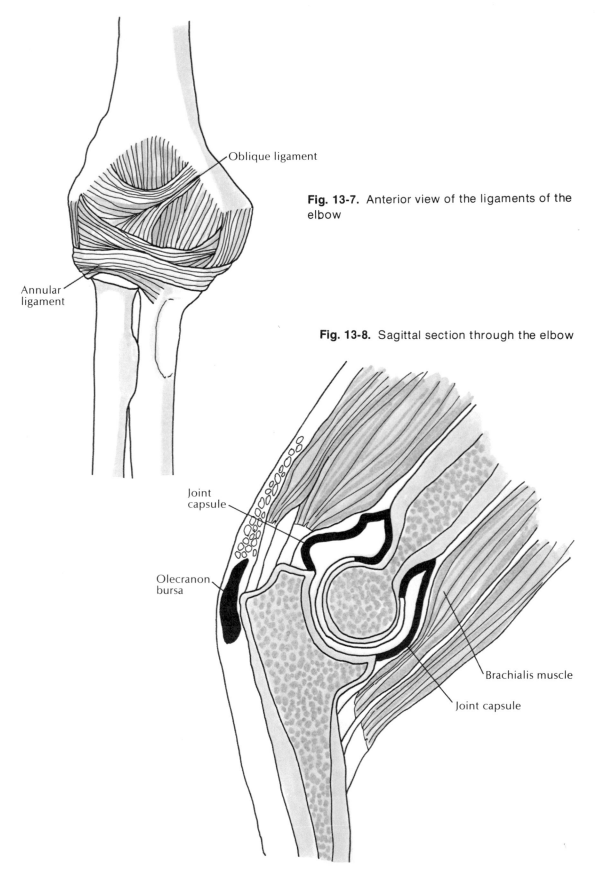

Oblique ligament

Fig. 13-7. Anterior view of the ligaments of the elbow

Annular ligament

Fig. 13-8. Sagittal section through the elbow

Joint capsule

Olecranon bursa

Brachialis muscle

Joint capsule

perior olecranon and the skin. It may become inflamed from trauma, prolonged pressure ("Student's elbow"), or other inflammatory afflictions such as infection and gout (Fig. 13-8).

TENDINOUS ORIGINS

The flexor–pronator muscles of the wrist have their tendinous origins at a common aponeurosis that originates at the medial epicondyle of the humerus. The wrist extensor group has its common aponeurotic origin at the lateral epicondyle. From superior to inferior on the humerus, the brachioradialis inserts first, followed by the extensor carpi radialis longus, the extensor carpi radialis brevis, and the remaining extensor muscles (Fig. 13-9). The extensor carpi radialis brevis is the upper-

Fig. 13-9. Lateral view of the tendinous origin of the forearm muscles

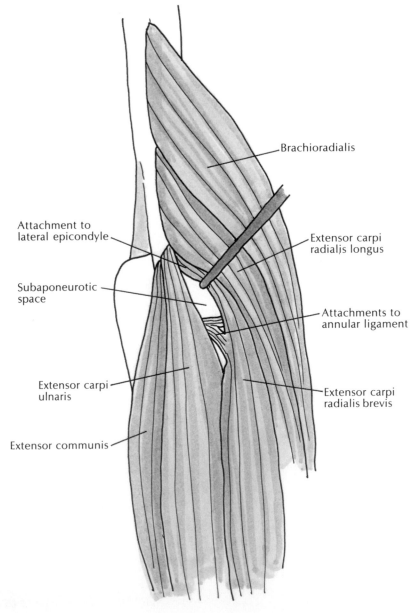

most muscle to attach to the common extensor tendon. The extensor carpi radialis longus and the brachioradialis do not contribute to the common tendon, but rather attach above the epicondyle.

The extensor carpi radialis brevis is important clinically since its tendon is most frequently involved in cases of tennis elbow.

Although it originates in part from the common extensor tendon, the extensor brevis also has proximal attachments to the lateral collateral ligament of the elbow, and often to the annular ligament (Fig. 13-9).

Deep to the tendon of the extensor brevis, and just distal to its insertion at the lateral epicondyle, there is a small space normally filled with loose, areolar connective tissue. This is termed the *subaponeurotic space*.[6] This space is bordered on the ulnar side by the extensor digitorum tendon and distally by the attachment of the brevis to the annular ligament (Fig. 13-9). Surgical findings commonly reveal granulation tissue in this space in cases of tennis elbow. Histologic studies show hypervascularization and the ingrowth of numerous free nerve endings into this space with granulation.[3,6] The granulation probably represents the reactions of adjacent tissues to chronic irritation of the extensor brevis origin resulting from tension stresses.[6,7]

On full forearm pronation, with the elbow extended, the orientation of the extensor carpi radialis brevis becomes such that proximally it is stretched over the prominence of the radial head (Fig. 13-4). This fulcrum effect from the radial head adds to the normal tensile forces transmitted to the origin of this muscle when stretched during combined wrist flexion, forearm pronation, and elbow extension.[7] This may in part explain the susceptibility of this tendon to chronic inflammation at or near its attachment.

EVALUATION OF THE ELBOW

HISTORY

Routine questions to be pursued during evaluation of patients with common musculoskeletal disorders are discussed in Chapter 4. However, the following questions are of particular concern when evaluating patients with elbow disorders:

1. What activities (*e.g.*, athletic or occupational) do you engage in that involve vigorous or repetitive use of the arm? (Except for the arthritides, the majority of elbow conditions seen are traumatic conditions or degenerative conditions, such as tennis elbow, that become active with certain activities.)
2. Are any other joints involved? (Except for the degenerative or traumatic lesions, rheumatoid arthritis is one of the few remaining causes of elbow pain of local origin.)

The elbow is largely derived from C6 and C7 and may, therefore, be the site of referred pain from other structures of the same segmental derivation; it may also itself refer pain to other structures in these segments.

PHYSICAL EXAMINATION

I. **Observation**
   A. Posture and attitude in which the arm is held
   B. Functional use of the arm during gait, dressing, and other activities
II. **Inspection** (include the entire extremity)
   A. *Structure*—Observed in a relaxed, standing position
     1. Shoulder height
     2. Elbow carrying angle (valgus–varus angle)

3. Elbow flexion–extension angle
4. Positions of medial and lateral epicondyles, radial head, and olecranon
B. *Soft tissue*
  1. Atrophy—Observe and measure the girth of arm or forearm
  2. Swelling
     a. Marked posterior swelling is usually bursal swelling.
     b. Articular effusion is often visible anteriorly as well as posteriorly.
  3. General contours
C. *Skin*
  1. Color
  2. Scars or blemishes
  3. Moisture
  4. Texture
III. **Selective Tissue Tension Tests**
A. *Active movements* (sitting)
  1. Observe
     a. elbow flexion–extension
     b. forearm pronation–supination (with elbow at 90°)
     c. wrist flexion–extension
  2. Apply slight overpressure. Assess effect on pain; assess end-feel; feel for crepitus.
  3. Record significant findings relating to range of motion, pain, end-feel, and crepitus.
B. *Passive movements* (supine for optimal stabilization)
  1. Tests
     a. elbow flexion–extension with the shoulder flexed, extended, and in neutral positions for constant-length phenomenon in case of muscular pain and tightness
     b. elbow pronation–supination
     c. wrist flexion with ulnar deviation; (The elbow is held extended and the forearm

pronated, stretching the common extensor tendon.
     d. wrist extension with the forearm supinated and elbow extended (common flexor–pronator tendon stretched)
  2. Record whether the resisted contraction is strong or weak, and whether it is painful or painless.
C. *Joint play movements*
  1. Tests (see Chapter 7, Joint Mobilization Techniques)
     a. Inferior glide of the ulna on the humerus
     b. Medial–lateral (valgus–varus) movement of ulna on humerus
     c. Superior–inferior glide of the radius
     d. Anterior–posterior movement of radial head
     e. Rotation of the radial head
     f. Anterior–posterior glide of distal radioulnar joint
  2. Record significant findings related to the degree of mobility and the presence of pain and muscle guarding.
IV. **Palpation**
A. *Skin*
  1. Temperature—Especially over brachialis and joint
  2. Moisture—Especially over the hand and forearm
  3. Texture
  4. Mobility of skin over subcutaneous tissues, especially after immobilization
  5. Tenderness—Primarily if neurologic involvement is suspected (*e.g.,* ulnar nerve lesion)
B. *Subcutaneous soft tissues*
  1. Consistency, tone, and mobility
  2. Swelling—Joint effusion is often palpable anteriorly by ballottement.

3. Tenderness
   a. common tendon insertions
   b. soft-tissue attachments
C. *Bones*
   1. Bony relationships—Especially the position of the radial head
   2. Tenderness—Tenoperiosteal junctions of common flexor and common extensor groups
   3. Bony contours
V. **Other**—Results of radiographs, lab tests, and electromyograms, if available

COMMON LESIONS

TENDINITIS

This is a very common disorder affecting the elbow. The tendon most commonly involved is the extensor carpi radialis brevis, at or near its insertion at the lateral epicondyle.[2–4,6,7] At times, other of the common extensor tendons will also be involved concurrently or, rarely, by themselves. Much less frequently, the common flexor tendon is involved at the tenoperiosteal junction near the medial humeral epicondyle. Involvement of the extensor tendon is usually referred to as *tennis elbow*, while involvement of the flexor tendon is called *golfer's elbow*. We will discuss both conditions together, since their history, objective signs, and management are similar.

Tendinitis affecting the elbow is rarely of acute traumatic origin. Except in sports medicine clinics, most patients presenting with tennis elbow do not relate the onset or aggravation of the problem to athletic endeavors such as tennis. Even when the chief complaint is the development of pain during some activity, the onset is usually gradual, and pain is felt most *after* the activity. This is because tennis elbow is usually a "degenerative" disorder; it represents tissue response to fatigue stresses. The inflammatory response, which char-acterizes the disorder, is an attempt to speed up the rate of tissue production to compensate for an increased rate of tissue microdamage (*e.g.*, collagen fiber fracturing). The increased microdamage rate occurs because of greater internal strain to the tendon fibers over time. This might come about from some increase in use of the tendon, for example, with carpentry, pruning shrubs, or tennis. It may also occur with normal activity levels if the capacity of the tendon to attenuate tensile loads is reduced. This typically occurs with aging, in which a loss of the mucopolysaccharide chondroitin sulfate makes the tendon less extensible; more of the energy of tensile loading must be absorbed as internal strain to collagen fibers rather than by deformation of the tissue. The explanation for the susceptibility of the extensor carpi radialis brevis to excessive strain is probably related to the added tensile load imposed on the tendon by the radial head when the tendon is stretched (*e.g.*, wrist flexion, elbow extension, and forearm pronation). In this position the tendon is further stretched over the prominence of the radial head.[7] Because the development of tennis elbow may be due to age-related tissue changes, most individuals presenting with this problem are 35 years old or older.[2,3,4]

Tennis elbow is classically a very persistent disorder that does not tend toward spontaneous resolution. If the individual with tennis elbow continues to perform activities that stress the tendon, the immature collagen that is produced in an attempt at repair continues to break down before it has the chance to adequately mature, and the chronic inflammatory process continues. If the part is completely immobilized, there may not be adequate stress to the new collagen to stimulate maturation, in which case the scar will again break down upon resumption of activities. In order for treatment to be successful, this dilemma must be resolved.

Examination and Management

I. History

  A. *Site of pain*

    1. Tennis elbow—Over the lateral humeral epicondyle, often referred into the C7 segment, down the posterior forearm into the dorsum of the hand, and perhaps into the ring and long fingers

    2. Golfer's elbow—Over the medial epicondyle, rarely referred into the ulnar aspect of the forearm

  B. *Onset of pain*—Usually gradual. May be related to wrist extension activities in tennis elbow, such as grasping, hitting a backhand at tennis, or pruning shrubs, or to wrist flexion and pronation activities in gollfer's elbow. The patient rarely recalls a sudden onset of pain during these activities, however. At times a direct blow to the epicondyle will initiate the problem.

  C. *Nature of pain*—Varies from a dull ache or no pain at rest to sharp twinges or straining sensation with activities as mentioned above. Tennis elbow is particularly aggravated by grasping activities because the wrist extensors must contract to stabilize the wrist during use of the finger flexors.

II. Physical Examination

  A. *Active movements*—These are usually fairly painless. In more severe cases of tennis elbow, there may be some pain with active wrist flexion with the elbow in extension from the stretch placed on the tendon. Active wrist extension does not usually produce enough tension to reproduce the pain. Similarly, there may be some pain with active wrist extension with the elbow extended in golfer's elbow, but usually not on active wrist flexion.

  B. *Passive movements*

    1. One of the key tests that should reproduce the pain in tennis elbow is full passive wrist flexion with ulnar deviation, forearm pronation, and elbow extension. Passive elbow movements alone are painless.

    2. Full wrist extension with supination and elbow extension reproduces the pain in golfer's elbow.

  C. *Resisted movements*—The other key test is resisted wrist extension (with the elbow extended) reproducing the pain in tennis elbow; resisted wrist flexion reproduces pain in golfer's elbow. At times, resisted pronation is painful in golfer's elbow.

  D. *Joint play movements*—These should be full and painless.

  E. *Palpation*

    1. Rather exquisite tenderness, usually over the epicondyle

    2. In tennis elbow, the tenderness may often extend down into the muscle belly. Less often, the tenderness is felt superior to the epicondyle at the insertion of the extensor carpi radialis longus.

    3. There may be some warmth noted over the respective epicondyle.

  F. *Inspection*—Usually no significant findings

III. Management

  A. *Goals*

    1. Restoration of normal, painless use of the involved extremity

    2. Prevention of recurrence

  B. *Objectives*

    1. Resolution of the chronic inflammatory process

    2. Maturation of the scar (healed area of the tendon). The new collagen must be sufficiently

"strong" and extensible to withstand the tensile stresses imposed by the patient's particular activity level; there must be an appropriate amount of tissue that is oriented to attenuate tensile stresses with a minimum of internal strain.

3. Restoration of strength and extensibility to the muscle–tendon complex

C. *Techniques*

1. *Acute cases* — Tennis elbow is, by nature, a chronic disorder, but as indicated in the criteria suggested in Chapter 4, some patients may present with acute symptoms and signs associated with tennis elbow; pain is referred into the entire forearm and perhaps the hand, and occasionally up the back of the arm. There may be some pain at rest, and some degree of muscle spasm is elicited when the tendon is stressed passively or by resisted movements.

   In such cases, the immediate goal is to promote progression to a more chronic state by assisting in the resolution of the acute inflammation.

   a. Instruct the patient to apply ice to the site of the lesion several times a day.

   b. Continued stress to the tendon must be prevented. If the patient presents with acute symptoms and signs as outlined above, this is best achieved by immobilization of the wrist, hand, and fingers (not the elbow) in a resting splint. In some cases a simple wrist cock-up splint will suffice, since this will obviate the need for the wrist extensors to contract when the finger flexors are used. Activities involving grasping, pinching, and fine finger movements must be restricted. This is often the most difficult component of the program to institute but at the same time the most important at this stage. The effectiveness of any other treatment measures will be compromised if the patient continues to engage in activities that stress the lesion site. This requires, for example, that the carpenter take some time off from work or temporarily change his duties, that the tennis player abstain from playing for a while, and that the person who enjoys knitting, sewing, or gardening temporarily alter his activities.

   c. A few times a day, the patient should remove the splint and actively move the wrist into flexion, the forearm into pronation, and the elbow into extension, simultaneously, to minimize loss of extensibility of the muscle and tendon. This should be done *gently*, avoiding significant discomfort, and very slowly to prevent high strain-rate loading of the tissue.

   If appropriate instructions are given and the patient faithfully follows the program outlined, progression to a more chronic status should occur over a period of a few (*i.e.*, 3 to 5) days.

2. *Chronic state* — If pain is fairly localized over the lateral elbow region and there is little or no pain at rest, the disorder

should be treated as chronic tendinitis.

a. Advise the patient explicitly as to the appropriate level and type of activity that may be performed. Strong, repetitive, grasping activities, such as hammering, and activities that particularly stress the tendon, such as tennis, must be restricted until there is very little pain on resisted isometric wrist extension, and little or no pain when the tendon is passively stretched (wrist flexion, forearm pronation, and elbow extension). Such activities must be resumed very gradually, with some protection of the part. Protection may be provided by an inelastic cuff made from a 2-in to 3-in wide piece of webbing worn firmly around the proximal forearm with a Velcro-type fastener. The fit of the cuff automatically tightens when the forearm pronates and the wrist flexes passively, providing additional afferent input to signal increasing stress to the wrist extensor group. This may reflexly enhance the action of the wrist extensors to contract in order to resist sudden passive tensile stress to the extensor tendons. Thus, a potentially high strain rate of loading is attenuated over time and transmitted to the tendon as a more gradually applied load, a type of load more easily absorbed by the viscoelastic tendon tissue. If the use of such a device is instituted, gradually wean the patient from it as strength, mobility, and painless function increase.

Also, as normal activities are resumed, certain adaptations may be implemented to minimize the stresses that may be imposed upon the wrist extensors. For example, the tennis player typically receives high strain-rate loading to the wrist extensor group when using a backhand stroke if the ball strikes the racquet above the center point of the strings. This produces a moment arm about which the force of the ball hitting the racquet can create a high pronatory torque. If the wrist extensors are somewhat weak, the wrist might also be forced into flexion. The combined effects of the active and passive tension created in the wrist extensor group result in high loading of the extensor tendons. The passive component can be minimized by hitting the ball on center and by having adequate wrist extensor strength to keep the wrist from flexing. The passive pronatory torque can also be reduced by increasing the diameter of the racquet handle. Other considerations would include the tension of the strings on the racquet head and the flexibility of the racquet shaft. High string tension and low racquet flexibility will result in reduced attenuation of forces by the racquet and, therefore, greater transmission of high strain rate forces to the arm. Also, the larger the head on the racquet, the greater the potential moment arm about which pronatory forces can act. Thus, a tennis player might benefit from taking lessons to improve the likelihood of hitting the ball on center, from reducing string tension, and from using a relatively flexible racquet with a handle of maximum tolerable diameter and a head of standard size. Each patient's activities should be similarly assessed for ways to reduce the loads imposed on the wrist extensor group.

b. Ultrasound and friction massage should be used to assist in the resolution of the chronic inflammatory process and to promote maturation at the site of healing.

Resolution of inflammatory exudates, such as lysosomal enzymes and other cellular "debri," may be enhanced by the increased blood flow stimulated by the heating effects of the ultrasound. Ultrasound must often be applied under water because of the irregular surface contour of the lateral elbow region.

Friction massage is an essential component of the treatment program. Its beneficial effects in cases of tendinitis are not well understood, but are probably related to the induced hyperemia and the mechanical influence it may have on tissue maturation (see

Chapter 9, Friction Massage). The hyperemic effects are of greatest importance in cases of tendinitis that may be related to hypovascularity, for instance, at the shoulder. Hyperemia does not seem to be a significant factor in the etiology of tennis elbow, however, and this may in part explain why friction massage is effective over a shorter period of time in cases of rotator cuff tendinitis than it is in cases of tennis elbow. The mechanical effects of the deep massage may promote orientation of immature collagen along the lines of stress. This would be an important factor in pathologies, such as tennis elbow, in which some type of mechanical stimulus is necessary for adequate tissue maturation. Use of deep transverse massage may assist in tissue maturation without imposing a longitudinal stress to the healing tendon tissue and, therefore, without continued rupturing of fibers at the site of the lesion. Thus, the defect heals with a maximum degree of tissue extensibility and is less likely to be overstressed as use of the part is resumed. This seems to be a solution to the dilemma mentioned above. If the patient continues to use the part, he perpetuates the problem by producing continued damage at the lesion site; if he completely immobilizes the part, there is no stimulus for tissue maturation and as soon as activity is resumed, the healed tissue begins to break down.

c. Strength and mobility must be restored. As symptoms and signs indicate improvement, the patient must resume activities gradually. Excessive internal strain to the tendon can be minimized during stressful activities by optimizing tissue extensibility. No vigorous activities should be allowed until you determine that the muscle–tendon complex has sufficient extensibility. Following the ultrasound and friction massage, gently and slowly stretch the tissue by holding the elbow extended, the forearm pronated, and the wrist ulnarly deviated, while flexing the wrist and fingers. Instruct the patient to perform this stretch at home, emphasizing that it must be performed slowly and gently. The patient should notice a stretching sensation but no pain. As the patient resumes vigorous activities such as tennis, carpentry, and gardening, teach him to administer friction massage for a few minutes prior to engaging in the activity.

Also, before a normal activity level is resumed, you must be sure that good wrist extensor strength has been restored. Wrist extensor strengthening exercises are always necessary, since the muscles will invariably undergo atrophy from disuse and reflex inhibition. Good extensor strength is necessary to protect the tendon from high strain-rate passive loading which may occur with many types of activities. A convenient method of wrist extensor strengthening is to have the patient tie a 3-ft rope to the center of a 1-in dowel and a weight to the end of the rope; the patient grasps both ends of the dowel and rotates it toward him until the entire rope becomes wrapped around the dowel. This can be repeated as appropriate; the weight may be varied as necessary.

d. Local anti-inflammatory therapy, such as infiltration with a steroid preparation, is commonly used in cases of tendinitis. It must be emphasized that although symptomatic improvement is often dramatic, such treatment has only temporary value. It has no lasting beneficial effect on the pathologic process and certainly does not influence etiologic factors. At best, it should be considered as an adjunct to management in the acute state. Too often other important components of the treatment program are ignored when an apparent "cure" is heralded by dramatic symptomatic improvement.

POSTIMMOBILIZATION CAPSULAR TIGHTNESS

Patients with restricted movement at the elbow from capsular tightness are often referred to physical therapists. Since capsular restriction from degenerative joint disease at the elbow is rare, the patients with capsular restriction who are seen by physical therapists are usually those whose elbows have been immobilized. The only other frequent cause of capsular restriction at this joint is inflammatory arthritis, usually rheumatoid arthritis but occasionally traumatic arthritis.

The common injuries for which management may involve elbow immobilization include fractures of the arm or forearm (humeral shaft fractures, supracondylar fractures, and Colles' fractures are the most common) and elbow dislocations (usually posterior dislocation of the ulna on the humerus).

I. **History**—Determine a time frame of events that indicates the date of injury, dates of subsequent surgeries (if any), duration of immobilization, and date of removal of supports or splints. Any suggestion of complications following the injury or immobilization, such as vascular dysfunction, should be noted. Determine whether there have been previous attempts at remobilization, and if so, what these entailed. Assess the patient's functional disability in terms of limitations on dressing or grooming and on occupational and recreational activities. These should be documented and used as a means by which to judge progress.

II. **Physical Examination**—The key sign is limitation of motion in a capsular pattern. However, take note of any complication that may have ensued.

A. *Reflex sympathetic dystrophy* (see Chapter 14, The Wrist)

1. Key signs include capsular restriction of all or most upper extremity joints, to varying degrees; generalized edema of the forearm and hand; trophic changes in skin and nails (glossy smooth skin, hyperhidrosis, hypohidrosis, cyanosis, brittle or ridged nails); dysesthesias, with pain hypersensitivity even to light tough.

Radiographs often reveal marked osteopenia, especially of the bones of the hand and wrist.

2. The exact cause of this disorder is not known. It is especially prevalent in persons who have sustained a Colles'-type fracture. It is thought to be related in some way to nerve trauma (such as trauma to the median nerve in Colles' fracture), the degree of edema, immobilization, and psychological factors. Preventive measures to be taken during the period of immobilization should include frequent active exercise of the free joints (usually shoulder and fingers) and regular periods of elevation of the involved extremity.

Development of a true reflex sympathetic dystrophy, often referred to as a shoulder–hand syndrome, can be a significant complicating factor in the rehabilitation program following immobilization. The marked articular restrictions and pain hypersensitivity make efforts at remobilization especially difficult.

B. *Malalignment of bony fragments*—This is occasionally seen following a supracondylar fracture at the elbow and invariably follows a Colles' fracture (see Chapter 14, The Wrist).

Elbow malalignment is easily detected by observing the carrying angle of the arm and by assessing structural alignment. With a supracondylar fracture, the distal fragment tends to displace posteriorly and medially with an angulation medially. Rotational displacement, medial or lateral displacements, and posterior or anterior displacements are not significant in the young person since these usually resolve with remodeling of the bone. Angular displacements, however, tend to persist. Typically, the malalignment following a supracondylar fracture presents as a decrease or reversal of the normal carrying angle. The medial epicondyle is positioned higher than the lateral epicondyle, and the olecranon becomes directed medially. Such malalignment usually does not result in a functional deficit, but may be cosmetically unacceptable.

C. *Brachialis contusion*—The displacement of bony parts that accompanies supracondylar elbow fractures and elbow dislocations may result in a contusion to the distal brachialis muscle belly, which overlies and is in close contact with the distal end of the humerus (Fig. 13-10). The consequence of such a contusion may be eventual metaplasia of the contused portion of this muscle into osseus tissue—a condition referred to as myositis ossificans.[1,5] Myositis ossificans usually results in permanent restriction of motion at the elbow; extension is restricted more than flexion.

It is questionable whether mobilization of the part—active, passive, prolonged, or otherwise—actually affects the eventual outcome. It is believed by some that the condition is often the result of over zealous attempts to remobilize the part. This may indeed be the case if the brachialis muscle is stretched. In cases of capsular restriction, however, in which the stretch is applied to the anterior capsule rather than the brachialis muscle, it is doubtful that any form of mobilization would predispose to development of myositis ossificans of the brachialis muscle. It is probable that the development of myositis ossificans, following injuries in which the brachialis muscle is traumatized, occurs as an inevitable event resulting from the original injury.

The therapist must protect himself medicolegally in the event that myositis ossificans should occur. This can be done by (*1*) recognizing the two common conditions (supracondylar fracture and posterior dislocation) that especially predispose to development of myositis ossificans, and (*2*) distinguishing between capsular and muscular restriction of motion at the elbow. Fortunately, fractures and dislocations at the elbow occur primarily in children. Because of this, remobilization is not a major problem, and passive mobilization is seldom required. However, if mobilization procedures are requested for a patient who has been immobilized following a supracondylar fracture or elbow dislocation, you must take certain precautions. First, determine the cause of the restriction. Limitation of extension more than flexion with an elastic end-feel is very suggestive of a muscular restriction. Use the constant length phenomenon to determine whether it is biceps or brachialis. Limitation of motion in a capsular pattern with a capsular end-feel suggests a capsular restriction. Stretching a tight elbow flexor muscle in such a case must not be done vigorously, except in cases of persistent restriction of elbow extension, and then only with agreement of the referring physician and with the patient's understanding.

Secondly, whether the restriction appears to be capsular or muscular, you must attempt to

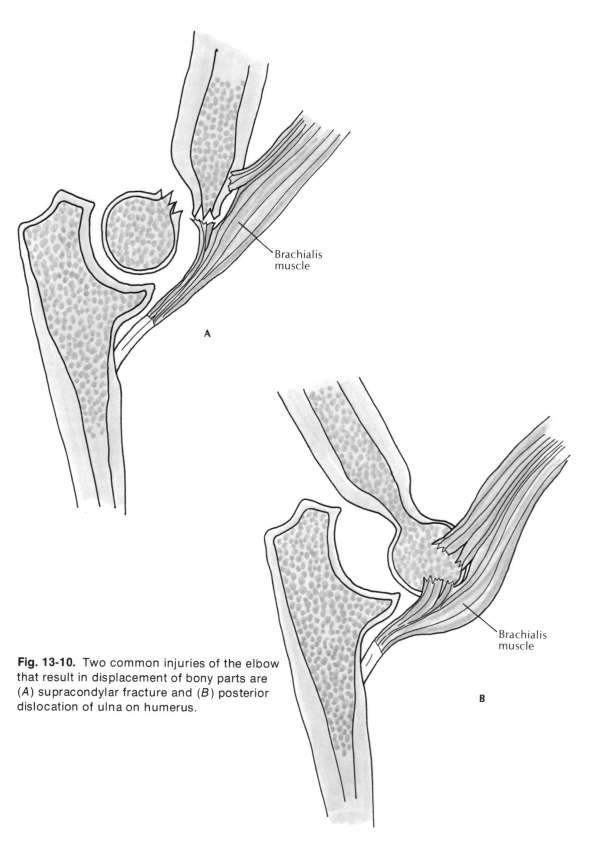

Fig. 13-10. Two common injuries of the elbow that result in displacement of bony parts are (*A*) supracondylar fracture and (*B*) posterior dislocation of ulna on humerus.

detect any signs of inflammation of the brachialis muscle. This is done by palpating for a hematoma or excessive tenderness over the distal brachialis muscle belly. Any suggestion of inflammation or hematoma of the distal brachialis muscle belly should preclude vigorous mobilization, barring the stipulations indicated above. Regardless of the intensity of the mobilization program, the therapist would do well to record thermistor readings over the distal brachialis region before and after each treatment session. A rise in temperature that persists over, for example, a 24-hour period might indicate that you should reduce the intensity of the program, especially if a muscular restriction is at fault.

III. **Management of Capsular Tightness**
  A. *Acute* (see criteria for acute *vs.* chronic in Chapter 5). Since most capsular elbow restrictions are those that follow immobilization after injury, you will rarely see them in an acute stage, since the acute inflammatory process subsides during the period of immobilization.
    1. Provide relief of pain and muscle guarding using ice, superficial heat, grade I and II joint play movement
    2. Maintain existing range of motion and increase movement as pain and guarding abate.
      a. gentle joint play movements, grades I and II
      b. initiation of an active-assisted home range of motion exercise program
    3. Progressive strengthening of muscles controlling the shoulder, elbow, forearm, and wrist as necessary. Use isometrics in acute stage, since joint move-

ment might cause reflex inhibition of the muscles to be strengthened.
  B. *Chronic*
    1. Ultrasound to tight capsular tissues along with or followed by capsular stretching, with joint play mobilization techniques (see Chapter 7). If treating a stiff elbow following a radial head resection, give special attention to preventing the development of a valgus contracture at the elbow by use of the "varus tilt" mobilization technique. The radius tends to migrate superiorly since the radial head no longer abuts the capitellum of the humerus. This may also result in problems at the distal radioulnar joint.
    2. Progression of home program to include prolonged stretch as tolerated and as indicated.
    3. Progression of home strengthening program.

REFERENCES

1. Ackerman LV: Extra-osseous localization non-neoplastic bone and cartilage formation. J Bone Joint Surg 40(A):279, 1958
2. Boyd HB: Tennis elbow. J Bone Joint Surg 55(A):1183–1187, 1973
3. Coonrad RW: Tennis elbow: Its course, natural history, conservative and surgical management. J Bone Joint Surg 55:1177, 1973
4. Cyriax J: *Textbook of Orthopaedic Medicine*, Vol I, pp 307–318. Baltimore, Williams & Wilkins, 1969
5. Gilmer WS, Anderson LD: Reaction of soft somatic tissue which may progress to bone formation: Circumscribed myositis ossificans. South Med J 52:1432, 1959
6. Goldie I: Epicondylitis lateralis humeri. Acta Chir Scand (Suppl) 339:3–119, 1964
7. Nirschl RD: Tennis elbow. Orthop Clin N Amer 4:787, 1973

14 *The Wrist*

Randolph M. Kessler

REVIEW OF FUNCTIONAL ANATOMY

OSTEOLOGY

Distal End of Radius

The radius flares distally and this end is much larger than the distal end of the ulna. It extends further distally than medially. The distal lateral extension of the radius is the radial styloid process. The radial styloid normally extends about 1 cm further distally than the ulnar styloid (Fig. 14-1).

The medial aspect of the distal radius is a concave surface anteroposteriorly. The medial concavity is the ulnar notch, which articulates with the head of the ulna, allowing pronation and supination to occur. The distal end of the radius is triangular in its transverse cross section. The distal articular surface of the radius is composed of two concave facets, one for articulation with the scaphoid and one for articulation with the lunate (Fig. 14-2). The distal articular surface of the radius faces slightly palmarly (average of 10°) and somewhat ulnarly (average of 20°) (Fig. 14-3).

Distal End of Ulna

The distal end of the ulna flares only mildly compared to the distal end of the radius. The ulnar styloid process is a small conical projection from the dorsomedial aspect of the distal end of the ulna. The radial aspect of the ulnar head is convex anteroposteriorly. It is cartilage-covered for articulation with the ulnar notch of the radius during pronation and supination (Figs. 14-1 and 14-2).

The distal end of the ulna is somewhat circular on transverse cross-section, except for the irregularity formed by the styloid process dorsomedially. The distal surface of the ulna is covered with articular cartilage for articulation with the articular disk (not with the carpals). There is movement between the ulna and disk primarily on pronation and supination, during which the disk must sweep across the distal end of the ulna.

Carpals

The proximal row of carpals consists of the triquetrum, pisiform, lunate, and scaphoid bones. The scaphoid has a biconvex articular surface proximally for articulation with the lateral facet of the distal end of the radius. The lunate is also convex proximally and articulates with the medial facet of the distal radius and with the articular disk in positions of radial deviation. The triquetrum has a small convex articular surface proximally. This surface is in contact with the ulnar collateral ligament when the wrist is in neutral position and articulates with the articular disk primarily in positions of ulnar deviation. The flexor carpi ulnaris tendon inserts onto the pisiform bone, which lies palmarly over the triquetrum.

The distal end of the scaphoid consists of two distal articular surfaces. The radial surface of the distal scaphoid is convex for articulation with the concave surface formed by the combined proximal ends of the trapezoid and trapezium. The ulnar

329

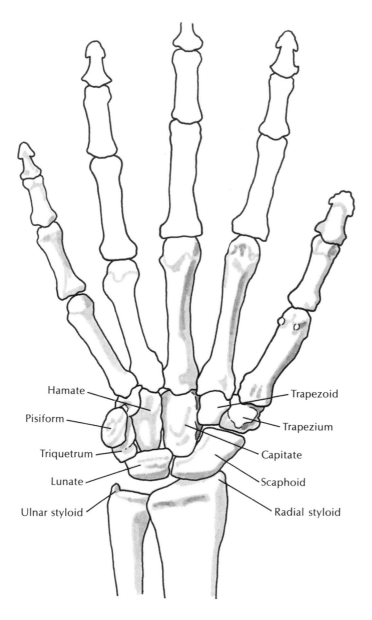

Fig. 14-1. Palmar aspect of the bones of the right wrist and hand

articulating surface of the distal scaphoid is concave and faces somewhat palmarly and ulnarly. It articulates with the proximal end of the capitate. The distal surface of the lunate is quite concave anteroposteriorly but less so mediolaterally. It grasps the convex proximal end of the capitate and also articulates, to a lesser extent, with the hamate. The distal surface of the triquetrum is concave for articulation with the hamate (Figs. 14-1 and 14-2).

There is some movement between the bones of the proximal row of carpals. For this reason each of the proximal carpals are lined with articular cartilage on their radial or ulnar surfaces, or both, to allow for such movement.

Ulnarly to radially, the distal carpals consist of the hamate, capitate, trapezoid, and trapezium (Fig. 14-1). As indicated above, the combined proximal surfaces of the hamate and capitate form a convex surface that articulates with the concave

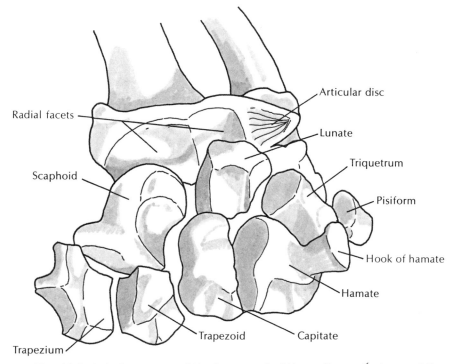

Radial facets

Scaphoid

Trapezium

Trapezoid

Capitate

Articular disc

Lunate

Triquetrum

Pisiform

Hook of hamate

Hamate

Fig. 14-2. Inferior aspect of the lower end of the radius and ulna and the carpal bones of the hand

surface formed by the combined distal surfaces of the triquetrum, lunate, and scaphoid (Fig. 14-2). The combined proximal surfaces of the trapezoid and trapezium form a concave surface for articulation with the convex distal articular surface of the scaphoid. The distal end of the trapezium is a sellar surface that articulates with the correspondingly sellar surface of the proximal aspect of the first metacarpal. The trapezoid articulates distally with the second metacarpal, the capitate with the third metacarpal, and the hamate with the fourth and fifth metacarpals (Fig. 14-1).

Because there is a small amount of movement between adjacent bones of the distal row, these are also lined with articular cartilage radially and ulnarly to allow for such intercarpal movement.

The carpals, taken together, form an arch in the transverse plane that is concave palmarly. This arch deepens with wrist flexion and flattens on wrist exten-

sion. The "hook" of the hamate, a rather large prominence on the palmar aspect of the hamate, and the pisiform bone, situated on the palmar aspect of the triquetrum, form the ulnar side of this arch. The trapezium, which tends to be oriented about 45° from the plane of the palm, and the radial aspect of the scaphoid, which curves palmarly, form the radial side of the arch. The flexor retinaculum, or transverse carpal ligament, traverses this arch (Fig. 14-4). The flexor ulnaris tendon inserts onto the pisiform. When this muscle contracts it pulls on the pisiform, causing tightening of the flexor retinaculum. This tightening deepens the transverse carpal arch.

LIGAMENTS, CAPSULES, SYNOVIA,
AND DISK

The articular cavity of the distal radioulnar joint is usually distinct from the articular cavity of the radiocarpal joint,

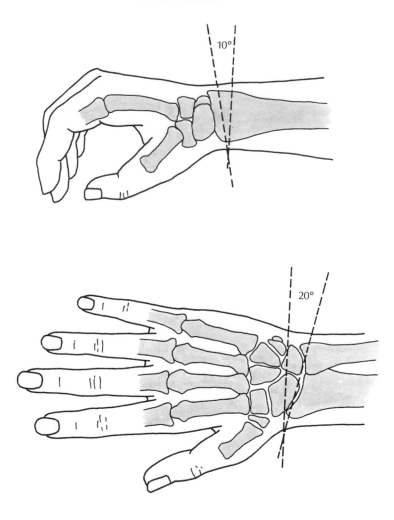

Fig. 14-3. Normal wrist alignment

which is also separate from that of the midcarpal joint. The carpometacarpal joints often share a common joint cavity which, in some cases, communicates with the midcarpal joint (Fig. 14-5).

The distal radioulnar joint is bordered proximally by the lax "sacciform recess" in the capsule, which loops proximally between the radius and ulna. Distally this joint is bordered by the triangular articular disk. This fibrocartilagenous disk attaches ulnarly to the ulnar styloid process and radially to the ulnar margin of the distal radial articular surface. It is what separates the distal radioulnar joint from the radiocarpal joint. Anteriorly and pos-

teriorly the margins of the disk attach to the joint capsule. The superior aspect of the disk is a cartilage-lined concave surface for articulation with the distal end of the ulna. As implied above, the disk moves with the radius on pronation and supination and must therefore sweep across the distal end of the ulna on these movements. During flexion and extension of the wrist the disk remains stationary relative to the ulna. With this movement the lunate or triquetrum, or both, articulates with the distal surface of the disk, which is also concave and cartilage-covered. The disk, then, provides two articular surfaces for the ulna and carpals, respectively, sepa-

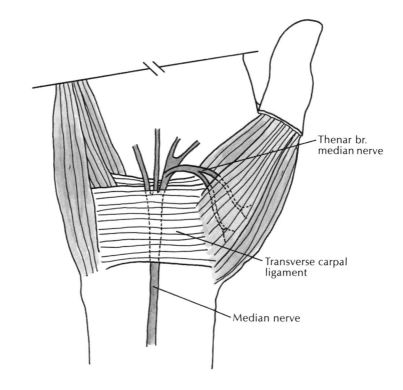

Fig. 14-4. Transverse carpal
ligament and median nerve

rates the adjacent joint cavities, and binds together the distal ends of the ulna and radius (Fig. 14-5).

The *radiocarpal joint* is bordered proximally by the radius and the articular disk. Distally it is bordered by the three proximal carpals and their respective interosseus ligaments, which are flush with the continuous convex articular surface formed by the proximal carpals. Medially and laterally the joint is bordered by the strong ulnar and radial collateral ligaments. Both collateral ligaments attach proximally to the styloid processes. Distally, the ulnar ligament attaches to the triquetrum and pisiform; the radial ligament attaches to the scaphoid and trapezium. Palmarly and dorsally, the capsule of this joint is reinforced by the palmar radiocarpal ligament and the dorsal radiocarpal ligament (Fig. 14-6). Palmarly, there is also an ulnocarpal ligament. These ligaments assure that the carpals follow the radius during pronation and supination. Synovium lines the cap-

suloligamentous structures mentioned, as well as the interosseus ligaments between triquetrum and lunate and between scaphoid and lunate.

The articulations between the proximal and distal carpal bones are enclosed in a common joint cavity. Anatomically, we can refer to the *midcarpal joint* as being the compound joint between the two rows of carpals. However, functionally, as explained under Biomechanics, the distinction is not so simple. Proximally, the midcarpal joint is bordered by the scaphoid, lunate, and triquetrum and their interosseus ligaments, which as mentioned intervene between the proximal ends of these bones. In this way the intercarpal articulations between the proximal carpals are enclosed within the midcarpal joint cavity. Distally, the midcarpal joint is bordered by the distal carpals and their interosseus ligaments, which intervene about midway, or further distally, between the distal carpals. Occasionally an interosseus ligament intervenes between

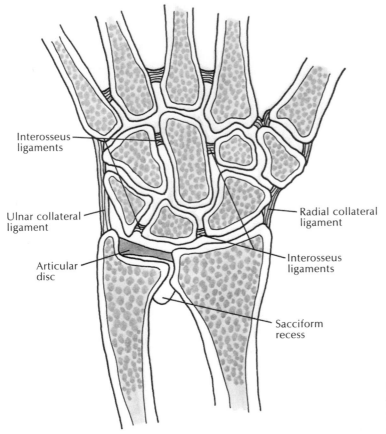

Interosseus ligaments

Ulnar collateral ligament

Articular disc

Radial collateral ligament

Interosseus ligaments

Sacciform recess

Fig. 14-5. Cross-section through the articulations of the wrist, showing the synovial cavities

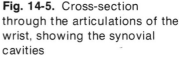

capitate and scaphoid, dividing the mid-carpal joint into medial and lateral cavities. Since an interosseus ligament is often missing between trapezoid and trapezium, the midcarpal joint often communicates with the common joint cavity of the carpometacarpal joints (Fig. 14-5). Medially and laterally, extensions of the ulnar and radial collateral ligaments connect the triquetrum to the hamate and the scaphoid to the trapezium. There are also dorsal and palmar intercarpal ligaments between the bones of the two rows. Palmarly these intercarpal ligaments are often referred to as the *radiate ligament* as they tend to radiate outward from the capitate (Fig. 14-6).

Palmar and dorsal intercarpal ligaments also connect the carpals within a row. The pisohamate ligament (from the pisiform to the hook of the hamate) and the pisometacarpal ligament (to the base of the fifth metacarpal) are thought to be continuations of the flexor carpi ulnaris tendon that attaches to the pisiform (Fig. 14-6). The joint between the pisiform and triquetrum is usually distinct from the other joints mentioned, having its own joint capsule and synovial lined cavity.

TENDONS, NERVES, AND ARTERIES

We will not discuss these structures in detail here. The reader will benefit from studying cross-sectional diagrams that depict anatomical relationships of these structures (Fig. 14-7). The relationships described below are of most importance clinically.

As mentioned, the transverse carpal lig-

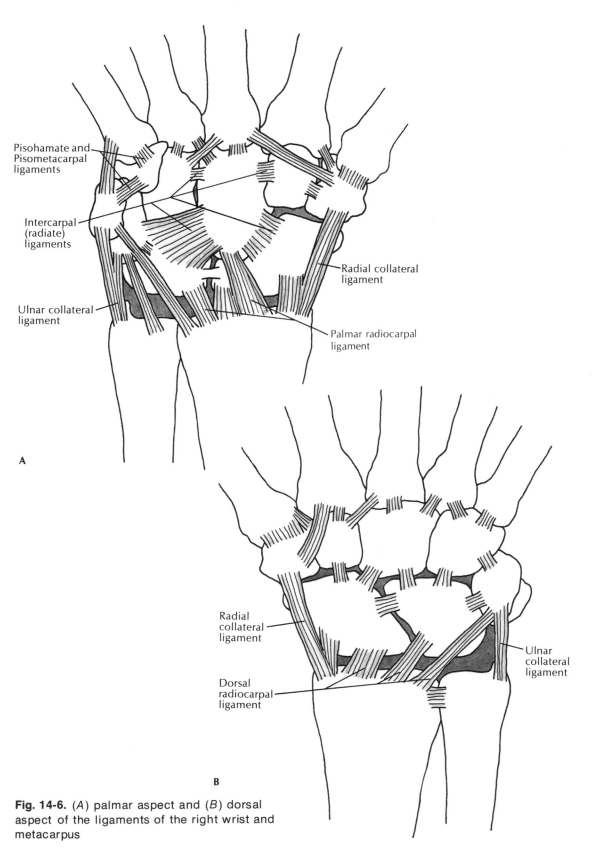

Fig. 14-6. (*A*) palmar aspect and (*B*) dorsal aspect of the ligaments of the right wrist and metacarpus

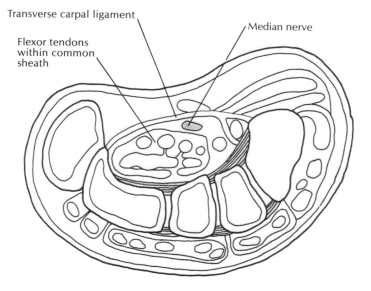

Transverse carpal ligament

Flexor tendons within common sheath

Median nerve

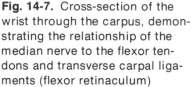

Fig. 14-7. Cross-section of the wrist through the carpus, demonstrating the relationship of the median nerve to the flexor tendons and transverse carpal ligaments (flexor retinaculum)

ament (flexor retinaculum) forms a roof over the palmar arch of the carpal bones (Figs. 14-4 and 14-7). Through the resulting tunnel pass the tendons of the flexor digitorum profundus and flexor digitorum superficialis. These tendons are all enclosed in a common synovial sheath. The flexor carpi radialis tendon and the flexor pollicis longus tendon also pass through the "carpal tunnel," each enclosed in a separate sheath. Superficial to the common flexor tendon sheath and deep to the flexor retinaculum passes the median nerve. At the distal end of the tunnel the nerve divides into several digital branches, one of which turns rather sharply around the distal border of the flexor retinaculum to innervate the thenar muscle (Fig. 14-4). "Carpal tunnel syndrome" is the result of compression of the median nerve within the tunnel, or occasionally, of just the thenar branch of the nerve as it turns around the distal border of the retinaculum. The palmaris longus tendon and the ulnar nerve and artery pass superficially to the flexor retinaculum. The nerve and artery travel beneath the flexor carpi ulnaris tendon, then radially to the pisiform bone before dividing to enter the hand.

The tendons of the extensor pollicis brevis and the abductor pollicis longus are enclosed in a common sheath as they pass across the lateral aspect of the distal radius. Inflammation of this sheath, or of the tendons within the sheath, is a fairly common disorder, referred to as *de Quervain's disease*, or tenosynovitis. These tendons form the radial side of the "anatomical snuff box." The extensor pollicis longus tendon passes around Lister's tubercle on the dorsal aspect of the distal radius in a pulleylike fashion. It turns obliquely toward the thumb to form the ulnar side of the "snuff box." The radial artery travels laterally to the flexor carpi radialis tendon before turning deep beneath the abductor polfor longus and extensor pollicis brevis tendons. It becomes superficial dorsally and can be palpated in the anatomical snuff box.

SURFACE ANATOMY

Because the wrist consists of many small structures in close proximity, the clinician must pay special attention to identification of these structures. There are some guidelines that can be followed to help identify the clinically significant structures about the wrist. The following exercise may be performed on yourself.

The distal end of the radius is easily palpated. Notice how it flares distally. Palpate along its radial border to the styloid process; note the gap between the radial styloid and the carpals when the wrist and thumb are relaxed. Extend the thumb and notice how the abductor pollicis longus and extensor pollicis brevis tendons bridge this gap. The prominence on the dorsal aspect of the distal radius, Lister's tubercle, is easily palpated. Again, extend the thumb and follow the extensor pollicis longus tendon from this tubercle, about which it curves, down to the thumb.

With the thumb extended and the wrist slightly dorsiflexed, once again locate the abductor pollicis longus tendon. Now palpate ulnarly on the palmar aspect of the wrist, level with the radial styloid. The next prominent tendon is the flexor carpi radialis tendon. Palpate the radial pulse just radial to this tendon. Once again palpate in an ulnar direction. The next tendon, just ulnar to the flexor carpi radialis, is the palmaris longus tendon. The median nerve lies deep to this tendon, beneath the flexor retinaculum.

The distal end of the ulna is also easily palpated. Feel the interval between it and the distal radius. Notice how much smaller the distal ulna is compared to the radius. The ulnar styloid process is quite prominent on the dorsoulnar aspect of the distal ulna. Palpate to the end of the ulnar styloid and notice the gap between it and the carpals, which opens with radial deviation and closes with ulnar deviation. With the wrist in radial deviation, the ulnar collateral ligament can be felt bridging this gap.

From the ulnar styloid dorsoulnarly, palpate distally to the next large prominence—the dorsal aspect of the triquetrum. From the dorsal aspect of the triquetrum, palpate around palmarly to the prominent pisiform situated in the palmoulnar corner of the palm. Grasp the pisiform with two fingers and notice how it can be wriggled back and forth with the wrist in flexion, but not with the wrist in extension. This is because of the increased tension on the flexor carpi ulnaris tendon that attaches to the pisiform. Palpate the flexor carpi ulnaris tendon proximal to the pisiform. Feel the pulse from the ulnar artery just radial to this tendon. The ulnar nerve is situated just deep to and between the ulnar artery and the flexor carpi ulnaris tendon. Once again, locate the dorsal aspect of the triquetrum, the large prominence just distal to the prominent ulnar styloid. Slide your palpating finger distally over the dorsal aspect of the triquetrum. Feel the small interval or "joint line" between it and the hamate. With the index finger over the dorsal aspect of the hamate, bring the thumb around palmarly at the same level. With the thumb palpate the prominent "hook" of the hamate deep in the hypothenar eminence; it is usually slightly tender to palpation. Between the hook of the hamate and the pisiform, beneath the pisohamate ligament, is the "tunnel of Guyon." The ulnar nerve and artery pass through this tunnel.

Now image a line running dorsally from the base of the middle finger to Lister's tubercle. At the midpoint of this line, or just radial to it, the base of the third metacarpal can be felt as a prominence. The capitate lies just proximally to this prominence. With the wrist in neutral position, the dorsal concavity of the capitate can be palpated as a depression at the dorsum of the wrist. Just proximal to this depression is the lunate. If you place a palpating finger over the lunate and capitate while passively flexing and extending the wrist, the distal end of the lunate can be felt to slide into the depression in the capitate on extension and out on flexion.

In the deepest portion of the anatomical snuff box the dorsoradial aspect of the scaphoid bone can be palpated. It is most easily felt with the wrist in ulnar deviation. Just distal to the scaphoid you can feel the trapezium. You should be able to identify the traperzium–first metacarpal articulation. The trapezoid is easily palpated as a prominence at the base of the second metacarpal.

BIOMECHANICS

We speak of the wrist as being composed, anatomically, of three joints: the distal radioulnar joint, the radiocarpal joint, and the midcarpal joint. With this description it is understood that the radiocarpal joint includes the articulation between the disk and the carpals, since the disk acts as an ulnar extension of the distal radial joint surface. From a functional standpoint, however, it is best to speak of an ulnomenicotriquetral joint in addition to the three joints listed above. In this way we are in a better position to consider the movements of the ulna in relation to the disk, and the carpals in relation to the disk. (Refer to the Appendix for a description of the movements that occur at these joints and the arthrokinematic motions that accompany these movements.)

Movements among the many bones of the wrist are, indeed, complex. The clinician must have a basic knowledge of the major interarticular movements if he is to be successful in evaluating painful conditions affecting the wrist and in restoring movement when it is lost. The important features of movement at the wrist, as a whole, will be reviewed here.

FLEXION – EXTENSION

The primary axis of movement for wrist flexion–extension passes through the capitate. The wrist close-packs in full dorsiflexion, since it must assume a state of maximal intrinsic stability in order to allow one to transmit pressure from the hand to the forearm. In functional activities such force transmission usually occurs with the wrist in dorsiflexion, for

example, when pushing a heavy object or walking on all fours. As with any synovial joint, the close-packed position at the wrist is achieved by a "screw home" movement—a movement involving a conjunct rotation (see Chapter 2). The carpus, on dorsiflexion, moves in a supinatory rotation. This is easily observed by watching your own wrist as it passes from neutral to full extension. The reason for this rotation is that the scaphoid moves in a manner that differs from the movement of other proximal carpal bones.[6] As the wrist moves from a position of flexion to neutral, the distal row of carpals remains relatively loose-packed with respect to the proximal row, and the proximal row remains loose-packed with respect to the radius and disk; movement occurs at both the radiocarpal joint and the mid-carpal joint. At about the neutral position, or just slightly beyond, as the wrist continues into dorsiflexion, the distal row of carpals becomes close-packed with the scaphoid but not with the other proximal carpals (lunate and triquetrum). Because of this close-packing, the scaphoid moves with the distal row of carpals as the wrist moves into full dorsiflexion. During this final stage of dorsiflexion, then, movement must occur between the scaphoid and lunate as the distal row continues to dorsiflex against the lunate and triquetrum. Looking at it another way, the scaphoid moves more with respect to the radius than do the lunate and triquetrum. This asymmetry of movement results in a supinatory twisting within the carpus that twists capsules and ligaments to closepack the remaining joints at full dorsiflexion (Fig. 14-8).

As with any joint, the bones forming the wrist are most susceptible to fracture or dislocation when in the close-packed position. Most frequently fractured are the scaphoid and the distal end of the radius. The most common dislocation is a palmar dislocation of the lunate relative to the radius and remaining carpals, or a dorsal

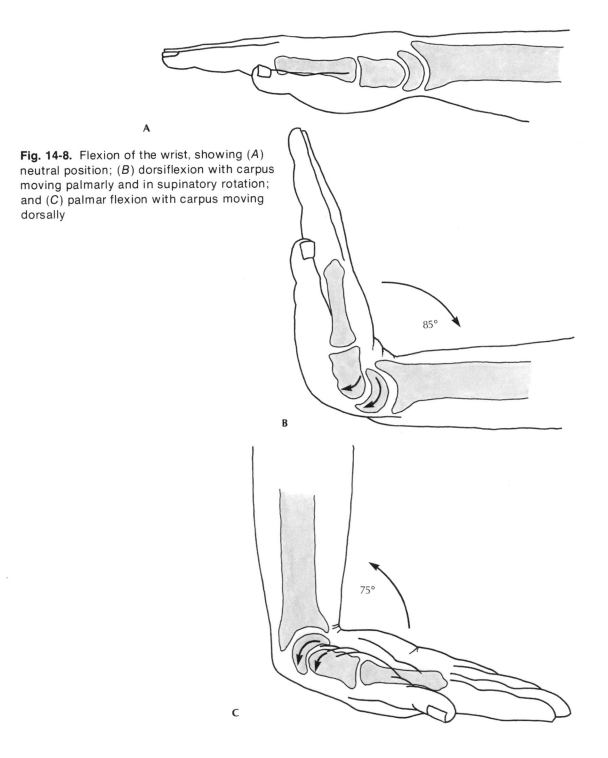

Fig. 14-8. Flexion of the wrist, showing (A) neutral position; (B) dorsiflexion with carpus moving palmarly and in supinatory rotation; and (C) palmar flexion with carpus moving dorsally

A

85°

B

75°

C

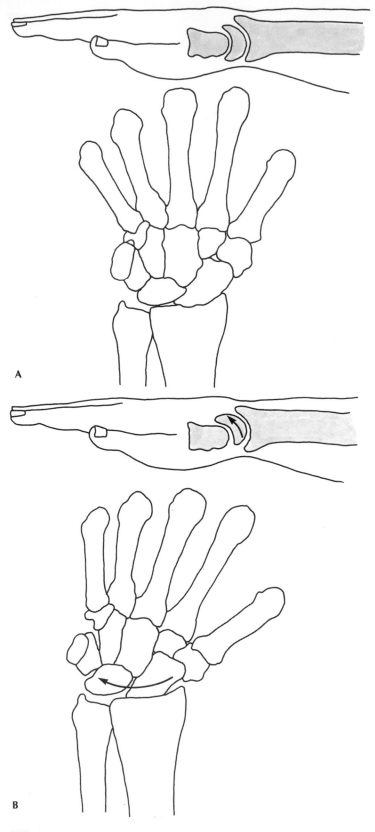

Fig. 14-9. Radial deviation of the wrist. The wrist is shown (*A*) in neutral position. (*B*) With radial deviation, the proximal row of carpal moves into dorsal and ulnar glide.

A

B

Fig. 14-10. Ulnar deviation of the wrist. The proximal row of carpals moves into palmar and radial glide.

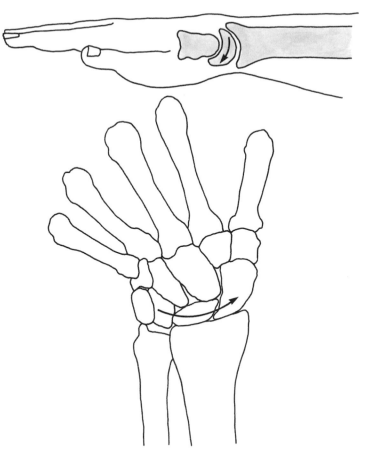

dislocation of the carpals with respect to the lunate and the radius. The common mechanism of injury for all the above injuries, as would be expected, is a fall on the dorsiflexed hand.

RADIAL—ULNAR DEVIATION

The axis of movement for radial-ulnar deviation also passes through the capitate. Ulnar deviation occurs over a much greater range of movement than radial deviation. This is because radial deviation is limited by contact of the scaphoid tubercle against the radial styloid, whereas the triquetrum easily clears the ulnar styloid, which is situated more dorsally and is less prominent than the radial styloid. Both radial and ulnar deviation involve movements at the radiocarpal and midcarpal joints. The associated arthrokinematic movements are not pure, but rather involve rotary movements between proximal row and radius, and between distal row and proximal row. As described by Kapandji, the proximal row tends to move into pronation, flexion, and ulnar glide during radial deviation with respect to the radius and disk (Fig. 14-9). At the same time, the distal row moves into supination, extension, and ulnar glide with respect to the proximal row. The opposite movements occur during ulnar deviation (Fig. 14-10). This can be easily observed on a cadaver, and seems to be due entirely to the shapes of the joint surfaces rather than from capsuloligamentous influences. Radial deviation involves close-packing of primarily the midcarpal joint.

EXAMINATION

The wrist structures are innervated primarily from C6–C8. Lesions affecting structures of similar segmental derivation may refer pain to the wrist, and conversely, lesions at or about the wrist may refer pain into the relevant segments. Since the wrist is located distally, and pain is more commonly referred in a proximal to distal direction than in a retrograde direction, pain from lesions at or about the wrist are fairly well localized. Symptoms experienced at the wrist or hand, however, must always be suspected as possibly having a more proximal origin. Common lesions that often refer pain to this region include lower cervical pathology (spondylosis, disc disease, etc.), tendinitis or capsulitis at the shoulder, thoracic outlet syndrome, and tennis elbow. If subjective findings do not seem to implicate a local problem, a scan exam of the neck and entire extremity may be warranted before proceeding with an in depth evaluation of the wrist (see Chapter 15, The Cervical–Upper Extremity Scan Examination).

HISTORY

A structured line of questioning should be pursued as set out in Chapter 4, Assessment of Musculoskeletal Disorders.

Common lesions at or about the wrist vary in onset from insidious (carpal tunnel syndrome, de Quervain's tenosynovitis, rheumatoid arthritis) to those in which an incident of trauma is definitely recalled (Colles' fracture, scaphoid fracture, lunate dislocation, or capsuloligamentous sprains). Again, be prepared to direct the line of questioning to elicit information concerning more proximal regions, especially if the onset is insidious. If a traumatic event is sited, the examination should attempt to determine the exact mechanism of injury. Since rheumatoid arthritis is not uncommon at

the wrist, one might inquire about possible bilateral problems and problems with the metacarpophalangeal joints and joints of the feet.

PHYSICAL EXAMINATION

I. **Observation**
    A. *General appearance and body build*
    B. *Functional activities.* Observe the way the person shakes hands, noting the firmness of grasp, temperature and moisture of the hand. Note during dressing activities whether one hand tends to be favored. Observe for fumbling with fasteners or small objects—a problem typical of carpal tunnel syndrome or neurologic dysfunction of more proximal origin. Note whether the patient willingly puts pressure through the wrist, as when standing up from a chair.
    C. *General posture and positioning of body parts.* Note how the arm and hand are carried and especially whether they swing naturally when walking. The person with a sympathetic reflex dystrophy, not an infrequent complication following healing of a Colles' fracture, invariably walks in with the elbow flexed and the forearm held across the upper abdomen.

II. **Inspection**
    A. *Bony structure and alignment.* This is especially important following a fracture of the distal radius. The most common complication following a Colles' fracture is healing of the fragments in a malaligned position, resulting in a "dinner fork" deformity (Figs. 14-11 and 14-12). In such a deformity the distal end of the radius is displaced and angulated dorsally, foreshortened, and often rotated into supination. Such a deformity must be considered when deter-

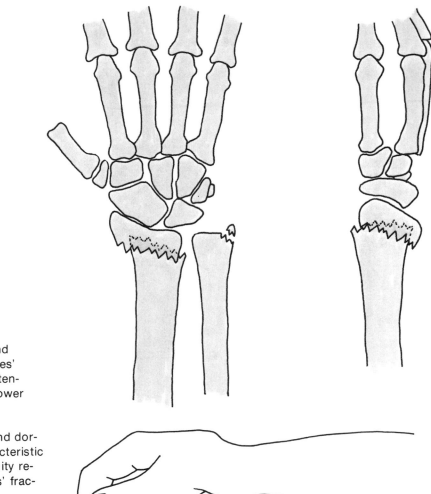

Fig. 14-11. Dorsal and lateral view of a Colles' fracture, showing extension fracture of the lower end of radius

Fig. 14-12. Lateral and dorsal view of the characteristic "dinner fork" deformity resulting from a Colles' fracture

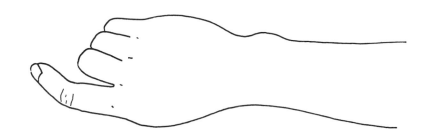

mining treatment goals, since normal range of motion can never be obtained in such cases.

1. Note structural alignment of head, neck, shoulder, girdle, arm, and forearm.
2. Note carefully the structural alignment and relationships of the distal end of the radius and ulna, the carpals, and metacarpals (see section on surface anatomy).
3. Note any structural deformities of the hands and fingers such as boutonnière or swan-neck deformities, ulnar drift, claw hand, or ape hand.

B. *Soft tissue*
1. Muscle contours
   a. Note especially any atrophy of the thenar muscles (this may accompany carpal tunnel syndrome), the hypothenar muscles (suggestive of an ulnar nerve lesion), and intrinsics.
   b. Note any generalized atrophy of the arm or forearm (this invariably occurs with immobilization, but may be masked by edema).
   c. Note any localized atrophy about the shoulder girdles and rest of limb, which may suggest neuromuscular involvement of related segments.
2. Joint regions
   a. Inspect for effusion of any upper extremity joints.
   b. Notice other periarticular swellings: Herberden's nodes about the distal interphalangeal joints, characteristic of osteoarthrosis of those joints.
   c. Small pea-sized ganglia are commonly found on the dorsal or palmar aspect of the wrist and are usually of little significance.
   d. Large nodules about the wrist, extensor surface of the forearm, and elbow are characteristic of rheumatoid arthritis.
3. General soft tissue inspection
   a. Generalized edema of the distal extremity is invariably present following immobilization in all but younger patients.
   b. Localized edema over the dorsum of the hand suggests an infection involving any part of the hand.
   c. If swelling or edema is present, volumetric measurements and girth measurements should be taken for documentation of a baseline.

C. *Skin*
1. Color
   a. redness with inflammation
   b. often cyanotic in reflex sympathetic dystrophy
   c. colorless with severe neurological deficit
2. Texture (see under palpation)
3. Moisture (see under palpation)
4. Scars, blemishes

D. *Nails*
1. Splitting, ridging (typical in reflex sympathetic dystrophy)
2. Clubbing (may suggest cardiopulmonary disorder)
3. Hollowing

III. **Selective Tissue Tension Tests**
A. *Active movements.* Record range of motion, pain, crepitus
1. Wrist flexion—extension and radioulnar deviation. Forearm pronation and supination. Active radial and ulnar deviation performed with the thumb held in a fist under the other fingers may be helpful in dis-

tinguishing de Quervain's tenosynovitis from osteoarthrosis of the trapezium–first metacarpal joint (both of which are common lesions).

2. Include shoulder and elbow movements, especially after immobilization and when reflex sympathetic dystrophy is suspected.

B. *Passive movements.* Record range of motion, pain, crepitus, end-feel

1. Same movements as above
2. Also ask patient to place the hand flat on table with wrist dorsiflexed, elbow extended, and to lean forward so as to transmit body weight through forearm and wrist.

C. *Resisted movements.* Record strong or weak, painful or painless

1. Resist all wrist, forearm, finger, and thumb movements.
2. If referred pain from more proximal regions is suspected, include resisted elbow and shoulder movements.

D. *Joint play movements.* Record mobility and irritability (pain or muscle guarding)

1. See Chapter 7, Joint Mobilization Techniques, for joint play movements at wrist and hand
2. Special intercarpal movements should be performed if an intercarpal ligament sprain is suspected. The therapist may use his knowledge of surface anatomy to move any of the carpal bones against its neighbors.

IV. Neuromuscular Tests (see Chapter 4 for relevant tests)

A. Strength, sensation, reflex, and coordination testing should be performed at this point if neuromuscular involvement is suggested by findings thus far in the exam.

B. A useful test for median nerve pressure at the carpal tunnel is to ask the patient to strongly flex the wrist while maintaining a strong three-jaw-chuck grasp. This position should be held for 1 minute. The onset of paresthesias into the first three or four fingers during this test is suggestive of a carpal tunnel syndrome.

C. If carpal tunnel syndrome is suspected, percuss the median nerve where it passes through the carpal tunnel. Reproduction of paresthesias suggests nerve involvement at this level (Tinel's sign).

V. Palpation

A. *Skin*

1. Moisture
2. Texture
3. Temperature
4. Mobility
5. Tenderness. Dysesthesias, such as burning on light palpation, suggests nerve root or peripheral nerve pathology, for example, pressure.
6. A common condition following immobilization (especially after a Colles' fracture) is the development of a reflex sympathetic dystrophy. The exact cause is unknown. Many believe it to be related to the development of edema during immobilization. Some feel it results from trauma to a nerve from the original injury, for example, contusion of the median nerve from the displaced distal fragment in a Colles' fracture. Others believe psychological factors also play an important role. In early phases of the development of this disorder the skin may be dry, rough and warm from decreased sympathetic activity. Later, increased sympathetic

activity, with hyperhidrosis and vasoconstriction, seem to predominate. Skin palpation reveals several findings in this disorder.

   a. Hyperhidrosis

   b. Smooth, glossy skin

   c. Decreased temperature (cold, clammy hands)

   d. Hypersensitivity to normally non-noxious sensory stimuli; even light touch may be painful

   e. Loss of mobility of the skin in relation to subcutaneous tissues from interstitial fibrosis accompanying tissue edema

B. *Soft tissues*

   1. Tenderness (Palpate tendons and ligaments, especially for local tenderness.)

   2. Mobility, consistency (Soft tissues feel indurated and adherent in reflex sympathetic dystrophy from interstitial fibrosis, as well as atrophied, fibrotic muscle.)

   3. Edema and swelling (Common with reflex sympathetic dystrophy)

   4. Pulse, radial and ulnar arteries. This may be performed in conjunction with various maneuvers of the arm (hyperabduction), shoulder girdle (depression, elevation, and retraction), and neck rotation, if thoracic outlet syndrome is suspected.

C. Bones

   1. Tenderness. The radial styloid is often the site of referred tenderness from more proximal lesions within usually the C5 or C6 segment. It is usually also tender in de Quervain's tenosynovitis

   2. Relationships. Palpate for structural alignment and positioning of the various bony components of the wrist as discussed in Inspection and Surface Anatomy.

COMMON LESIONS

CARPAL TUNNEL SYNDROME

This is a very common condition. Women present with this problem more commonly than do men. It rarely affects the young people. The cause is variable. In certain instances it is due to some known disorder involving increased pressure within the carpal tunnel. Such situations include a displaced fracture of the distal radius, a lunar or perilunar dislocation, and swelling of the common flexor tendon sheath. In most cases, the cause is not readily determined. Some believe it to be a vascular deficiency of the median nerve at the carpal tunnel, while others believe direct pressure to the nerve to be the cause. Symptoms and signs accompanying this disorder are more suggestive of a pressure phenomenon.[2]

  I. **History**

    A. *Onset of symptoms.* Usually insidious unless, of course, following trauma resulting in fracture, dislocation, or swelling of the wrist

    B. *Nature of symptoms.* The complaint is most often that of paresthesias (pins and needles) felt into the first three or four fingers of the hand. The patient is most troubled by being awakened at night, usually in the early hours of the morning, from paresthesias in the hand. Onset of paresthesias often occurs with activities involving prolonged use of the finger flexors such as writing and sewing. Often the patient complains of clumsiness on activities requiring fine finger movements. At times a burning sensation is felt in the median nerve distribution of the hand as well. Subjective complaints of actual weakness are rare. The problem can be unilateral or bilateral. **Note:** C6 or C7 nerve root involvement and thoracic outlet syndrome often present with paresthesias in a similar distribution as that of carpal tunnel syndrome. In the case of nerve root involvement, however, the patient is rarely awakened by paresthesias, and use of the hand does not bring on symptoms. Differentiation from thoracic outlet syndrome, based on subjective findings, is more difficult, since these patients are usually awakened at night with paresthesias, and paresthesias may come on with certain activities involving use of the upper extremity. In thoracic outlet syndrome, paresthesias are more likely to involve the entire hand (though often the patient is not sure in just how many fingers paresthesias are felt) or perhaps just the more ulnar side of the hand from lower cord involvement only. The objective exam will help differentiate in any case.

II. Physical Examination
  A. *Observation.* Perhaps some clumsiness with activities requiring fine finger movements, such as handling buttons or other fasteners
  B. *Inspection.* Some thenar atrophy may be noticed, but usually in chronic cases only.
  C. *Selective tissue tensions tests.* Noncontributory, except perhaps some subtle weakness or resisted thumb movements
  D. *Neuromuscular tests.* Only in severe, chronic cases can true

thumb or lumbricals weakness be noticed. Substitution, overlapping innervation, or subtle involvement make motor testing unreliable.
  1. Careful sensory testing may reveal some deficit in the tips or dorsal ends of the first three or four fingers (usually the second or third). However, mild cases or early cases sufficient to cause significant symptoms may not present with a detectable sensory deficit.
  2. The special test mentioned under Examination will usually reproduce the paresthesias.
  3. Tinel's sign (reproduction of paresthesias by tapping the median nerve at the wrist) may be positive.
  4. Nerve condition studies of the median nerve is the most reliable objective test, but often unnecessary diagnostically.
  E. *Palpation.* Usually noncontributory.

III. Management
These patients often do remarkably well simply by wearing a night resting-splint for the wrist. The reason why this helps is not entirely clear, except that it maintains the wrist in a neutral position, the position of least pressure within the carpal tunnel. (For this reason it seems more likely that this disorder is a pressure phenomenon rather than a release phenomenon.)

Show the patient how to don the splint without impairing venous return from fastening straps or wraps too tightly. The splint may or may not include the fingers. It is usually not necessary to wear the splint during the day. However, if night use does not provide relief of symptoms, a several-day trial of continuous use of the splint followed by gradual wean-ing should be instituted. Whether the splint is worn continuously or at night only, after a week or two of relief from symptoms, use of the splint can gradually be decreased and eventually discontinued.

Only in persistent cases is surgery required to divide the flexor retinaculum and relieve the pressure.

LIGAMENTOUS SPRAINS

These are also quite common and often lead to chronic wrist pain unless treated appropriately. Most commonly involved, in our experience, are the lunate–capitate ligament, dorsally, and the radiocarpal ligament, palmarly. However, any other of the several ligaments about the wrist may conceivably be sprained.

I. History

  A. *Onset of pain*. Ligamentous lesions are invariably of traumatic rather than degenerative onset. The patient usually recalls the traumatic event. A fall on the outstretched hand may rupture one or more of several ligaments about the wrist, but often one of the ligaments attached to the lunate is sprained. This is because of the tendency toward a lunar or perilunar dislocation with such an injury. In fact, at this point in the exam, such a dislocation cannot be ruled out. Because a fall on the outstretched hand tends to force the wrist into hyperextension, the palmar radiolunate and palmar lunocapitate ligaments tend to be sprained. However, if the lunate partially dislocates palmarly with spontaneous reduction, the dorsal radiolunate ligaments may also be sprained (Fig. 14–13).

  Occasionally the fall is such that the person strikes the dorsum of the hand, forcing the wrist into extreme palmar flexion. This usually results in a sprain of one of the ligaments attached dorsally to the capitate. The ulnar collateral ligament is often sprained with a Colles' fracture.

  B. *Site of pain*. The pain is usually well localized to a small area that corresponds well to the site of the lesion.

  C. *Nature of pain*. The pain is felt with use of the wrist. Often a particular activity is cited as being most aggravating; the activity stresses the involved ligament. In the case of a dorsal radiocarpal sprain, often the activity that tends to reproduce the pain puts pressure down through the hand (as when doing pushups).

II. Physical Examination

  A. *Observation*. Usually noncontributory

  B. *Inspection*. Usually noncontributory. Localized swelling following an injury to the wrist almost never accompanies a ligamentous injury only. Fracture or dislocation should be suspected.

  C. *Selective tissue tension tests*
    1. Active movements. Possibly (but not necessarily) some pain on the extreme of a movement that stresses the ligament
    2. Passive movements
      a. It is quite possible for a ligamentous lesion to exist that is not stressed at the extreme of any passive anatomical movement.
      b. Often the only maneuver that reproduces the pain, other than some specific joint play movement test, is having the patient lean forward, transmitting the body weight through the arm, forearm, extended wrist, and hand. This is

most likely to reproduce pain from a lesion of the palmar radiolunate or dorsal lunocapitate ligaments.

c. Also note that the dorsal radiocarpal ligament may be stressed on full passive pronation (applying the force through the hand and wrist to the forearm), and the palmar radiocarpal ligament may be stressed on full passive supination.

3. Resisted movements. Strong and painless. **Note:** Resist pronation and supination at the distal forearm, not at the hand, to avoid stressing the radiocarpal ligaments.

4. Joint play movements

a. The specific intra-articular movement that stresses the involved ligament is likely to reproduce the pain, but again, joint play movement in itself may not be sufficient to reproduce the pain.

b. The most important movements to perform are dorsal–palmar glide of the capitate on lunate and lunate on radius.

c. Some hypermobility of the lunate may be detected fol-

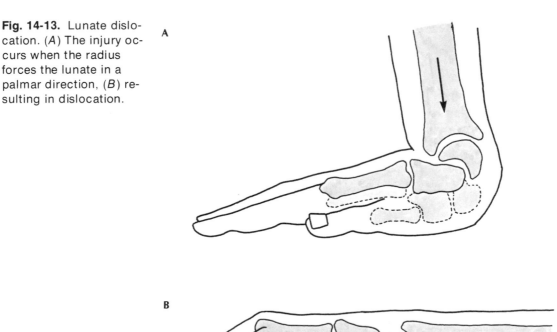

Fig. 14-13. Lunate dislocation. (A) The injury occurs when the radius forces the lunate in a palmar direction, (B) resulting in dislocation.

A

B

lowing partial dislocation and spontaneous reduction of the lunate with a fall on the dorsiflexed hand.

d. Some hypermobility of the capitate may be detected following a fall on the palmarly flexed hand in which a lunocapitate or capitate–third metacarpal ligament may be ruptured

D. *Neuromuscular tests.* Noncontributory

E. *Palpation.* Localized tenderness that usually corresponds well with the site of the lesion

III. **Management**

A. Temporary restriction of activities that tend to stress the involved ligament

B. Friction massage to the site of the lesion to increase mobility of the collagen fibers without longitudinally stressing the ligament. As an adjunct you may use ultrasound to assist in the resolution of chronic inflammatory exudates.

POST-COLLES' FRACTURE

In most out-patient settings, patients who have sustained a Colles' fracture comprise the largest proportion of those with wrist disorders. The term *Colles' fracture* is usually used now to refer to fractures of the distal end of the radius, with or without an associated fracture at the distal ulna. This is one of the most common of all fractures. It affects primarily older people, women more often than men. This is because of the prevalence of osteoporosis, especially in older women. Physical therapists are often referred these patients following the period of immobilization because of complications resulting in residual loss of function. The most common complications following these injuries are (*1*) malunion (*not* nonunion) of bony fragments and (*2*) development of a reflex sympathetic dystrophy. Pain and residual loss of movement are the major factors limiting function following immobilization of a Colles' fracture.

Mechanism and Nature of Injury

A Colles' fracture invariably results from a fall on the outstretched hand in an older individual. The patient lands with the wrist in dorsiflexion and the forearm in pronation. The lunate acts as a wedge to shear the distal 2 cm, or so, of the radius off in a dorsal direction. The momentum of the body weight causes the distal fragment to displace radially and rotate in a supinatory direction with respect to the proximal bone end (Fig. 14-11). Because this metaphyseal area of bone is typically osteoporotic, the compression force often results in comminution and impaction of the distal fragment. The major fracture line runs transversely across the distal radius, usually about 2 cm proximal to the radiocarpal joint. The momentum that results in radial displacement may also cause a sprain of the ulnar collateral ligament and an avulsion fracture of the ulnar styloid.[3]

The characteristic "dinner fork" deformity results from the wrist and hand being displaced dorsally with respect to the forearm (Fig. 14-12). Often included in the deformity is radial displacement of the wrist and hand.

Physician's Management

Closed manipulative reduction is usually carried out in an effort to bring the fragments back into anatomical alignment. Reduction is usually not so much of a problem as is maintenance of reduction. In unstable, comminuted fractures there is a tendency for the distal fragment to slip back into its post-injury position of dorsal, radial, and supinatory displacement. In an attempt to maintain anatomical reduction, the wrist is usually splinted in a position of flexion and ulnar deviation, with pronation. In some cases external fixation with a Roger Anderson device may be used. The elbow is usually left free. Note that since the elbow is left free, splinting in a position of excessive pronation may result in a force tending to pull the distal fragment into radial displacement and supination from tension on the brachioradialis with elbow extension. This would defeat the original purpose of positioning the part in pronation and ulnar deviation.

The plaster splint is left on for at least 4 weeks. Nonunion is rare since this facture occurs in highly vascularized, metaphyseal bone.

Complications

Malunion. It is rare for a Colles' fracture to heal without some residual malalignment. The radius invariably ends up foreshortened such that the radial styloid no longer extends beyond the ulnar styloid. The distal end of the radius also tends to be angulated and displaced dorsally; the distal radial articulation surface no longer faces 10° to 15° in a palmar direction. It should be realized that the malalignment described above will result in a permanent loss of full wrist flexion and ulnar deviation. In addition, there may be some residual malalignment of the distal fragment toward supination, resulting in a permanent loss of pronation. The distal fragment may also heal when displaced radially, but this would have little effect on motion.

Reflex Sympathetic Dystrophy. This condition is not uncommon following a Colles' fracture. In fact, in our experience this condition develops more often following a Colles' fracture than after any other injury. Also, according to our experience, the majority of patients sent to physical therapy following immobilization of a Colles' fracture have this condition to some degree (otherwise they probably would not require ongoing physical therapy management).[1,4,7–10]

The pathophysiology of this condition is not well understood nor agreed upon. It is generally agreed, however, that a sympathetic dysfunction occurs as part of a viscious cycle initiated reflexly by some alteration in afferent input from the periphery. Several different proposals have been offered as to the precipitating factor in this condition, including direct trauma to a peripheral nerve, edema from prolonged immobilization, pain, and psychological predisposition. The characteristic features of the disorder are hyperalgesia, edema, and capsular tightness of the joints of the hand, wrist, and often the shoulder (it is often referred to as shoulder–hand syndrome, although the shoulder is not always involved). The elbow occasionally stiffens, as well. As mentioned in other than the early phases of this condition, there is usually increased sympathetic activity involving the distal part of the extremity, with vasoconstriction and hyperhidrosis. The vasoconstriction causes a cyanotic appearance and atrophy of the musculoskeletal tissues; the skin becomes glossy and thin, the nails brittle, and the bones, osteoporotic. (Early osteopenia, seen on radiography, is often marked. This early bone atrophy is thought to be a result of hyperemia that is often present in the earlier stages; excessive blood flow to bone causes increased resorption).

Carpal Tunnel Syndrome. The median nerve may be traumatized at the time of injury. Prolonged pressure to the nerve may come about from malalignment of bony fragments, persistent edema involving the carpal tunnel, or both. (See section on carpal tunnel syndrome for discussion of symptoms and signs.)

Late Rupture of the Extensor Pollicis Longus Tendon. This tendon normally takes quite a sharp turn around Lister's tubercle at the dorsum of the distal radius on its way to inserting at the thumb. Malalignment of bony parts following a Colles' fracture may cause excessive friction to this tendon which may result in fraying to the tendon and eventual rupture. Pain on active and passive thumb flexion or apposition along with pain on resisted thumb extension are suggestive of such a problem before actual rupture. Painless weakness of thumb extension, some time after injury, is characteristic of rupture of the tendon.

I. History

A. Determine the date of initial injury, subsequent treatment, the length of time the part was immobilized, and the dates of removal of splints. Inquire as to whether exercise and elevation activities were performed while immobilized. Of course, the patient sent to you who had been immobilized for 8 weeks with no instruction in shoulder exercises and elevation activities, and who has not used the part since removal of the splint 2 weeks ago, will be expected to present with more dysfunction and disability than the patient who has just come out of the splint after having been immobilized for 6 weeks, during which time range of motion for the shoulder was carried out along with intermittent periods of elevation and active finger movements.

B. The standard questions, as discussed in Chapter 4, Assessment of Musculoskeletal Disorders, relating to the patients pain should be asked. Any acute inflammatory process, initiated at the time of injury, should have resolved during the period of immobilization. Considering this, you would expect any residual pain to be due primarily to stiffness and to be associated with use of the part. Complaints of pain at rest, pain that awakens the patient at night, and inability to use the part because of pain, are suggestive of reflex sympathetic dystrophy in this case. Take note of any complaints of shoulder pain because of the possibility of stiffening of the shoulder from immobilization, and perhaps "shoulder–hand syndrome." Pain on use of the thumb may be suggestive of involvement of the extensor pollicis longus tendon as described above. Complaints of burning pain or paresthesias into the median nerve distribution of the hand should alert you to the possibility of a carpal tunnel syndrome.

C. Determine and document the patient's present functional status.
 1. What specific daily activities cannot be performed with the involved hand, that could be performed before the injury?
 2. What activities can be performed but with some difficulty or pain?
 3. Consider, especially, eating, grooming, dressing, household chores, occupational activities, and recreational activities.

II. Physical Examination

A. *Observation.* Typically these patients walk in holding the hand and forearm out in front of them, across the chest or abdomen.
 1. Is the arm used when rising from a chair?
 2. Does the arm hang normally to the side and swing freely and normally when walking?
 3. Does the patient use the hand and arm during dressing activities, or does he guard it carefully?
 4. Observe the facies for wincing during movement of the part.

B. *Inspection*
 1. Skin and nails. Note especially trophic changes that are sug-

gestive of a reflex sympathetic dystrophy: brittle, split nails; smooth, glossy skin; cyanotic appearance to skin in the distal part of extremity.

2. Subcutaneous soft tissue. Atrophy of the forearm musculature is invariably found, but perhaps somewhat masked by edema, which is usually noticed most in the hand and forearm.

3. Bony structure and alignment. Some degree of malalignment is likely to be present. In the classic "dinner fork" deformity, the wrist and hand are offset dorsally with respect to the forearm. There is usually some displacement radially also. The radial styloid process may no longer extend further distally than the ulnar styloid, as it should, because of impaction of the distal fragment.

C. *Selective tissue tension tests*

1. Active and passive range of motion

   a. The interphalangeal (IP) and metacarpalphalangeal (MCP) joints of the hand are usually restricted in a capsular pattern, the MCPs being especially restricted in flexion, the IPs especially restricted in extension.

   b. Wrist and forearm movements are restricted in all planes. Flexion, ulnar deviation, and pronation are likely to be restricted from bony malalignment; check for "bony end-feel." Extension, radial deviation, and supination are likely to be limited because the hand is usually immobilized in a position opposite each of these movements (see above).

   c. All movements are likely to be painful at the extremes, especially in the presence of a reflex sympathetic dystrophy.

   d. Be sure to check shoulder range of motion for possible capsular tightening.

2. Resisted movements

   a. Pain on resisted thumb extension may suggest some involvement of the extensor pollicis longus tendon secondary to bony malalignment.

   b. Otherwise, resisted movements should be strong and painless.

3. Joint play movements. Considerable restriction of all joint play movements of the wrist and hand is likely to be found.

D. *Neuromuscular tests.* Here you should be concerned primarily with the function of the median nerve. The special test mentioned under carpal tunnel syndrome should be performed.

E. *Palpation*

1. Skin

   a. The skin is likely to feel cool, moist, smooth, and tight, especially in the presence of a reflex sympathetic dystrophy.

   b. Tenderness to light palpation of the skin is characteristic of a reflex sympathetic dystrophy.

2. Subcutaneous soft tissue
   Pitting-type edema is very often present distally. The tissues may feel "tight" and bound down in the hand and forearm because of the fibrosis accompanying prolonged edema.

3. Bones. Careful bony palpation will reveal the extent of residual malalignment.

F. *Other.* A radiologist's report should be ordered so that the therapist can determine the degree of bony malalignment. This is helpful in setting treatment goals. Also, marked osteoporosis usually accompanies a reflex sympathetic dystrophy. It is often said that as much as 40% of bone resorption may take place before osteopenia shows on radiographs. If radiographs suggest considerable osteoporosis, techniques to regain range of motion must not be performed using forces applied over a long lever-arm.

Management

Functional use of the part is lost or restricted primarily due to pain and loss of motion. As with any joint in which motion is lost from capsular tightening, much of the patient's pain may be due to joint stiffness; the joint capsule is stretched excessively during use of the part. However, these patients often complain of pain that is out of proportion to the extent of the dysfunction. Such an abnormal pain state is characteristic of a reflex sympathetic dystrophy. In such situations the patient may complain of severe pain to light touch or other normally non-noxious stimulation. Needless to say, this may act as a considerable barrier to efforts to regain joint motion.

Pain Management. If such an abnormal pain state is apparent, take special care not to reinforce the patient's pain behavior, and do not allow such reinforcement by family members, so as to avoid development of an operant pain problem. You cannot, on the other hand, ignore totally the patient's very real pain problem. The patient must be advised that, while in no way is their pain imagined, the pain is not in this case serving a useful function by signaling potential harm to tissues.

Unless the problem is carefully explained to the patient, he cannot be expected to carry out home instructions that may well ask the patient to perform exercises and other activities that may be somewhat painful. He will also have doubts of your professional judgement if you should use certain techniques that cause considerable discomfort unless you carefully explain your rationale.

In addition to discussing the problem with the patient, take some measures to try to make the treatment sessions as painless as possible. This is one disorder in which some modality or procedure might be used solely for its effect to reduce the patient's pain, so as to allow one to carry out other treatment procedures, such as joint mobilization. A whirlpool during, or just before, mobilization procedures may act as a counterirritant, as well as increasing blood flow to the part. The part may be kept in the water for application of ultrasound in preparation for mobilization procedures.

Restoration of Joint Motion. These patients require an intensive mobilization program. All the joints of the extremity, with the possible exception of the elbow, are likely to be restricted in the case of reflex sympathetic dystrophy. It is usually desirable to have the patient come in for treatment at least three times a week for passive mobilization. Treatment should include ultrasound to help increase the extensibility of capsular tissue, followed by specific joint mobilization techniques. Such techniques are especially indicated because they are performed with forces applied over very short lever-arms.

A home program of active and active-assisted range of motion exercises should be instituted. Take care to show the patient exercises that do not involve forces applied over long lever-arms, especially when working on finger flexion and extension. These patients usually have some degree of tissue edema that contributes to the restriction in range of motion. Frequent elevation of the part with activation of the muscle pump should be included in the home program. Encourage use of the part for dressing, grooming, and light activities.

Simple strengthening exercise for finger, wrist, and shoulder muscles should be instituted. Strengthening the rotator cuff is especially important because of the important role these muscles play biomechanically. Exercises should be kept simple, and the number of exercises should be kept at a minimum. The patient who becomes confused or exhausted with a home program is likely to abandon the program completely. This is an important consideration here because these patients need to perform range of motion exercises for most of the upper-extremity joints, in addition to strengthening exercises and elevation activities. Whenever possible, design exercises that incorporate strengthening range of motion and elevation so as to keep the program simple and concise.

In cases in which a marked or persistent reflex sympathetic dystrophy presents a major obstruction to rehabilitation, the patient may undergo a series of sympathetic blocks. In such a program the patient may be admitted to the hospital or to short-procedure surgery. The stellate ganglion is injected with an anesthetic in an attempt to reduce sympathetic activity to the part and to break up the cycle. Typically, a series of five injections are given on a daily basis. Such a program in no way precludes continuation of the normal physical therapy program. In fact, the ideal situation is for the patient to be seen in physical therapy each day following the block for mobilization procedures. Obviously, close communication and cooperation among orthopaedics, anesthesiology, and physical therapy is an important factor here.

In our experience, the active phase of a reflex sympathetic dystrophy following a Colles' fracture tends to resolve over a period of several months. However, a patient may be left with some residual disability. Some residual loss of motion is not unlikely because of the often extensive fibrosis of joint capsules as well as extra-articular structures. Goals, in these cases, should be set toward restoration of *functional* motion, not necessarily *physiological* motion. In older people, the two are less likely to coincide. Of more significance, however, is the tendency toward development of a chronic pain state. Operant management at this point may be indicated over, or in addition to, continued physical treatment. The possibility of psychological consultation should be discussed with the physician.

All too often these patients continue to come in for treatment over a prolonged period of time without demonstrable improvement in function. While vigorous treatment is indicated in the early phase after immobilization, once improvement plateaus for, say, a 2-week or 3-week period, treatment should gradually be discontinued in favor of a progressive home program. Keep in mind, however, that improvement is rarely linear in such cases, and some fluctuation between spurts of improvement and periods of plateauing can be expected. Until satisfactory, functional use of the part is regained, intermittent follow-up visits should be arranged for reassessment and progression of the home program. As usual, improvement should be based primarily upon objective findings and subjective reports of increased function (not on subjective reports of decreased pain).

DE QUERVAIN'S TENOSYNOVITIS

This is a relatively common condition. It is generally believed to be an inflammation and swelling of the synovial lining of the common sheath of the abductor pollicis longus and the extensor pollicis brevis tendons where they pass along the distal, radial aspect of the radius.

I. **History.** Pain is felt over the distal, radial aspect of the radius, perhaps radiating distalling into the thumb or even proximally up the forearm. The onset is usually insidious. The patient notes pain primarily with activities involving thumb movements, such as wringing or grasping activities.

II. **Physical Examination.** This condition must be differentiated from osteoarthrosis of the trapezium–first metacarpal joint, which is also a fairly common disorder. In osteoarthrosis, *A.* and *B.* below are negative, and joint play movements at the trapezium–first metacarpal joint will be restricted and painful.

  A. Pain on resisted thumb extension and abduction

  B. Pain on ulnar deviation of the wrist with the thumb held fixed in flexion. On this movement the tendons and the sheath are placed on a stretch.

  C. Tenderness to palpation over the tendon sheath in the region of the radial styloid.

III. **Management**

  A. The physician may elect to inject the sheath with a steroid preparation or a local anesthetic. Surgical incision of the sheath is occasionally performed.

  B. If injection is not contemplated or if it is unsuccessful, a trial of ultrasound and friction massage over a 1-week or 2-week period on a basis of three to five times per week is warranted. The rationale of this program is to maintain and increase mobility of the tendons within the sheath and to help resolve the chronic inflammatory process. In more severe or persistent cases, temporary restriction of thumb movements with a small opponens splint should be considered, to prevent continued irritation to the inflammed sheath.

SCAPHOID FRACTURE AND LUNATE DISLOCATION

In the older person, a fall on the outstretched hand results in a Colles' fracture, since the proximal carpals are jammed into the weak osteoporotic radius. However, in the younger person, in whom the radius is strong and healthy, the scaphoid may fracture on impact, or the radius may force the lunate palmarly, resulting in lunate dislocation in a palmar direction (see Fig. 14-13).

A lunate dislocation may be detected on a standard anteroposterior radiograph by the lunate's appearing triangular in shape rather than quadrangular, and in a lateral view by its abnormal position. In any event, always palpate for lunate positioning in patients sent to physical therapy after a fall on the outstretched hand.

A scaphoid fracture is not always so obvious. Many times a fracture here will not show on standard radiographs. A key clinical sign is localized bony tenderness in the anatomical snuff box on palpation. When this is found in a patient sent to you following a fall on the outstretched hand, suspect a scaphoid fracture and also consult the physician. A rather high incidence of avascular necrosis of the proximal fragment of the scaphoid occurs with this fracture because the blood supply to the scaphoid often enters only from the distal aspect of the bone. The fracture, then, cuts off the blood supply to proximal fragment. It is generally agreed that strict, prolonged immobilization of the wrist and thumb is necessary to minimize the possibility of avascular necrosis and nonunion.

REFERENCES

1. Caillet R: Reflex sympathetic referred pain. In Shoulder Pain, 2nd ed, pp 108–124. Philadelphia, FA Davis, 1981
2. Cyriax J: Textbook of Orthopaedic Medicine, 5th ed, Vol 2, pp 333–338. Baltimore, Williams & Wilkins, 1969

3. De Palma F: The Management of Fractures and Dislocations; an Atlas, 2nd ed. Philadelphia, WB Saunders, 1970

4. deTakas G: Nature of painful vasodilatation in causalgic states. Arch Neur Psychiat 50:318, 1943

5. Kapandji IA: The Physiology of the Joints, Vol I, Upper Limb. New York, Churchill Livingstone, 1970

6. MacConaill MA: Mechanical anatomy of the carpus and its bearing on surgical problems. J. Anat 75:166– 175, 1941

7. Moberg E: Shoulder– hand– finger syndrome. Surg Clin North Am 40(2):367– 373, 1960

8. Steinbrocker O, Argyros TG: The shoulder– hand syndrome: Present status as a diagnostic and therapeutic entity. Med Clin North Am 42:1533, 1958

9. Steinbrocker O, Spitzer N, Friedman NH: The shoulder– hand syndrome in reflex dystrophy of the upper extremity. Ann Int Med 29:22– 52, 1948

10. Woolf D: Shoulder– hand syndrome. Practitioner, 213(1274):176– 183, 1974

11. Youm Y, McMurtry RY, Flatt AB, Gillespie TE: Kinematics of the wrist. I. An experimental study of radial-ulnar deviation and flexion-extension. J Bone Joint Surg 60(A)432– 431, 1978

15 The Cervical–Upper Extremity Scan Examination

Randolph M. Kessler

The extremities are derived from spinal segments; the myotomes, dermatomes, and sclerotomes corresponding to C4 through T1 extend into the arms, whereas those from L2 through S2 extend into the legs. The clinical significance of this is that symptoms and signs related to spinal pathology are often referred into the extremities, and, conversely, symptoms from common extremity lesions are often referred to the spine (or other parts of the involved extremity). In the case of deep somatic pathologies, referred symptoms and signs are the rule rather than the exception. This is most significant with respect to pain, since pain is the most frequent clinical manifestation of deep somatic pathology. Thus, the patient with a cervical problem is very likely to experience scapular, shoulder, or arm pain, perhaps even moreso than cervical pain. In addition, paresthesias, weakness, or sensory changes may affect the related segment in the arm or hand. Similarly, it is not unusual for patients with common extremity disorders to experience pain that is referred in a retrograde direction to the proximal aspect of the extremity or the related spinal region. Indeed, patients with carpal tunnel syndrome often experience pain up the forearm and arm into the scapular region and neck.

The clinical problem encountered when dealing with the common phenomenon of referred symptoms is that information elicited from the history does not always reliably narrow the source of the problem to a particular region. When this is the case, the clinician may have trouble knowing in which area to direct the physical, or objective, examination. The situation may be compounded by the fact that many individuals present with symptoms that occur as the result of summation of afferent input from two separate disorders affecting tissues innervated by the same segment. This is especially true for middle-aged and older people, since degenerative joint changes in the cervical spine are common by middle age and may cause "hyperexcitability" of the involved segments.

The purpose of performing a spinal–extremity scan examination is to help identify the major area of involvement so that you can direct the physical examination accordingly. It is most useful in cases in which the history or the referring diagnosis does not provide adequate information to indicate the area to be examined. It should be used with most middle-aged or older patients presenting with chronic musculoskeletal complaints because it will often reveal disorders, other than those identified by the referral or by the history, that are the primary pathology. For example, a scan exam often reveals that the patient who describes symptoms suggestive of a C6 radiculopathy actually has carpal tunnel syndrome, that the patient with carpal tunnel syndrome may have symptoms that are enhanced by lower cervical facet-joint tightness, that a person with some lower cervical problem is also developing a frozen shoulder, or that someone who describes what sounds like pain referred distally into the C7 segment from the neck actually has pain referred proximally from a tennis elbow condition. Such situations are surprisingly common and can be a frequent source of error in evaluation and treatment planning unless recognized.

The tests that make up the scan exam include those that can be considered *key tests* for the common musculoskeletal lesions affecting the cervical spine and upper extremity, or the lumbar spine and lower extremity. Listed below are the key tests and positive findings for the common disorders for which the scan exam is intended to be sensitive.

COMMON DISORDERS OF THE CERVICAL SPINE AND UPPER EXTREMITY

A. Localized cervical facet joint restriction
   1. Typical subjective complaints include
      a. Aching in the scapular region, perhaps into the arm, usually unilaterally; occasional headaches
      b. Gradual onset with perhaps a history of cervical trauma or intermittent acute episodes of neck pain
      c. Worse at the end of the day and during periods of prolonged muscular tension such as during emotional stress and long periods of holding the head against gravity (*e.g.*, typing or reading)
      d. The patient is usually 25 to 50 years old.
   2. Key objective findings
      a. Active cervical movements with passive overpressure
         i. Pain at the extremes of side bending and rotation to the involved side
         ii. Possible pain on extension
      b. Quadrant test (passive rotation, side bending, and extension to one side). Pain when performed toward the side of involvement
B. Generalized cervical degenerative changes with bilateral, multisegmental facet-joint capsular tightness.
   1. Typical subjective complaints include
      a. Gradual onset of neck stiffness with associated pain into shoulder girdles and perhaps the arms. Pain and stiffness may be bilateral, though usually worse on one side. Frequent headaches originating from the occiput and radiating to the frontal region.
      b. History of intermittent cervical problems over many years
      c. Stiffness and headaches noted in the morning, easing somewhat during midday, with increased neck and shoulder pain by evening
      d. The patient is usually 50 years old or older.
   2. Key objective findings. Active cervical movements with passive over-pressure.
      a. Marked restriction of extension, moderate restriction of side bending, mild to moderate restriction of rotations and flexion
      b. Pain at the extremes of some movements
C. Cervical nerve root impingements
   1. Typical subjective complaints include
      a. Gradual or sudden onset of unilateral neck, scapular or arm pain. Often paresthesias into fingers are described. Arm pain may be sharp or aching.
      b. Pain may be intense, relieved somewhat with recumbency, worse with weight bearing

c. The patient is usually 35 to 60 years old.

2. Key objective findings
   a. Quadrant test (foraminal compression). Reproduction of *arm* pain
   b. Upper extremity sensory, motor, and reflex tests. Neurological deficit confined to the involved segment.
      C5—Weak shoulder abduction or external rotation
         —Sensory changes over the radial aspect of the forearm
         —Diminished biceps or brachioradialis jerk
      C6—Weak elbow flexion or wrist extension
         —Sensory changes over the thumb or index finger
         —Diminished biceps or brachioradialis jerk
      C7—Weak elbow extension or wrist flexion
         —Sensory changes over the middle three fingers
         —Diminished triceps jerk
      C8—Weak thumb abduction, small finger abduction, or wrist ulnar deviation
         —Sensory changes over the small or ring fingers.

D. Frozen shoulder (adhesive capsulitis)
   1. Typical subjective complaints include
      a. Gradual onset of shoulder pain and stiffness, noted especially when combing hair, fastening buttons, bras, etc., behind the back, or reaching into the hip pocket
      b. Frequently there are problems with being awakened at night when rolling onto painful side.
      c. The patient is more often a woman, usually 40 years old or older.
   2. Key objective findings. Active

shoulder movements with passive overpressure
   a. Considerable loss of external rotation and abduction, mild to moderate loss of flexion and internal rotation
   b. Pain at the extremes of shoulder movements, especially external rotation and abduction, with a capsular or muscle-spasm end-feel.

E. Shoulder tendinitis (rotator cuff or biceps)
   1. Typical subjective complaints include
      a. Gradual onset of lateral brachial pain, occasionally radiating into arm and forearm
      b. The onset may be associated with increased use of the arm, such as athletics.
      c. Painful twinges are felt with specific movements, such as putting on jacket and reaching behind the back.
      d. The patient is likely to be 20 to 50 years old.
   2. Key objective findings. Resisted shoulder, elbow, and forearm movements. Pain on contraction of the involved muscle–tendon complex
      a. Supraspinatis: pain on resisted shoulder abduction
      b. Infraspinatis: pain on resisted external rotation
      c. Subscapularis: pain on resisted internal rotation
      d. Biceps (long head): pain on resisted elbow flexion or forearm supination

F. Shoulder tendon rupture (rotator cuff or biceps)
   1. Typical subjective complaints include
      a. Gradual onset of inability to use the arm normally, especially above shoulder level if a rotator

cuff tendon is involved. The onset may be sudden, especially in the case of a biceps rupture.

b. History of intermittent shoulder pain over many years

c. Possible history of repeated local steroid injections

d. Pain may or may not be a problem

e. The patient is usually 50 years old or older

2. Key objective findings

  a. Resisted movement tests

    i. Supraspinatis: resisted abduction weak and painless

    ii. Infraspinatis: resisted external rotation weak and painless

    iii. Biceps: resisted elbow flexion and forearm supination weak and painless

  b. Observable muscular atrophy

G. Acute subdeltoid bursitis

1. Typical subjective complaints include

  a. Gradual development of relatively intense, constant lateral brachial pain over a 48-hour to 72-hour period. Pain may radiate down the entire arm.

  b. Often a history of more minor, intermittent shoulder problems suggestive of preexisting tendinitis

  c. Difficulty sleeping or using the arm at all because of intense pain

  d. The patient is likely to 30 to 50 years old.

2. Key objective findings. Active shoulder movements with passive overpressure. Marked restriction of active flexion and abduction, with an empty end-feel to passive overpressure. Mild-to-moderate restriction of internal and external rotation with the arm to the side.

H. Elbow tendinitis

1. Typical subjective complaints include

  a. Gradual onset of medial or lateral elbow pain that may radiate into the ulnar aspect of the forearm (golfer's elbow) or into the dorsum of the forearm and hand and into the posterior brachial region (tennis elbow)

  b. Onset may be associated with some activity such as tennis, golf, or pruning shrubs

  c. Pain is aggravated by grasping activities such as hammering or carrying a suitcase and by prolonged fine finger activities such as knitting or sewing.

  d. The patient is usually 35 to 60 years old.

2. Key objective findings

  a. Resisted wrist movements, performed with elbow extended

    i. Tennis elbow (tendinitis at origin of extensor carpi radialis brevis): pain on resisted wrist extension

    ii. Golfer's elbow (tendinitis at common flexor–pronator origin): pain on resisted wrist flexion

  b. Active wrist movements with passive overpressure, performed with elbow extended

    i. Tennis elbow: pain on full wrist-flexion with the elbow extended and forearm pronated

    ii. Golfer's elbow: pain on full wrist-extension with the elbow extended and forearm supinated

I. Carpal tunnel syndrome (pressure on the median nerve in the carpal tunnel)

1. Typical subjective complaints include

  a. Gradual onset of paresthesias into any or all of the median nerve distribution of hand (thumb and middle three fingers). An aching sensation may be referred up the forearm and arm to the scapula and neck.

b. Symptoms often awaken the patient at night and are aggravated by activities involving the finger flexors, such as writing, sewing, or knitting.

c. Women are affected more often than men. The patient is usually 40 years old or older.

2. Key objective findings. Three-jaw-chuck pinch with wrist held in sustained flexion (modification of Phalen's test). Reproduction of paresthesias into median nerve distribution of the hand.

J. De Quervain's disease (tenosynovitis of the abductor pollicis longus and extensor pollicis brevis at the wrist)

1. Typical subjective complaints include

a. Gradual onset of pain over the radial aspect of the distal radius that may radiate distally into the thumb or proximally up the radial aspect of the forearm.

b. Pain is worse with activities involving thumb movements or wrist ulnar deviation.

c. The patient is usually 40 or older.

2. Key objective findings

a. Resisted finger movements. Pain over the radial styloid region on resisted thumb extension

b. Active wrist movements with passive overpressure. Pain over the radial styloid region on full ulnar deviation with thumb held in patient's clenched fist.

K. Carpal ligament sprain

1. Typical subjective complaints include

a. History of acute trauma, usually a fall on the dorsiflexed or palmarly flexed hand, followed by chronic wrist pain. The patient often has trouble localizing the pain to a particular aspect of the wrist.

b. Pain is often felt only with specific activities, such as those requiring repeated wrist movements or weight bearing through the hand and wrist.

c. The patient is usually a young or active individual.

2. Key objective findings

a. Active wrist movements with passive overpressure

i. Dorsal radiocarpal, dorsal lunocapitate, or capitate–third metacarpal ligament: pain on full wrist flexion

ii. Palmar radiocarpal or palmar lunocapitate ligament: pain on full wrist extension

b. Upper extremity weight bearing (through dorsiflexed wrist and straight arm). Pain with either dorsal or palmar ligament sprains

FORMAT OF THE CERVICAL–UPPER EXTREMITY SCAN EXAM

The patient sits at the edge of the plinth with the neck, arm, and shoulder girdles exposed. The examiner briefly inspects the upper spine, shoulder girdles, and arms for obvious muscular atrophy or deformity.

I. **Cervical Tests**

A. *Resisted cervical movements.* Place one hand on each side of the patient's head (without covering auditory meatus). The forearms and elbows rest over the patient's trapezial ridges to help stabilize against trunk movements. From this position the examiner resists cervical rotation and side bending to the left and right, without allowing movement of the head.

To resist cervical extension, place one hand over the back of the patient's head such that the wrist lies over the patient's cervical spine and the forearm rests against the thoracic spine. The other hand reaches across the front of the patient to grasp the opposite shoulder. Extension of the patient's head and neck are resisted without allowing movement.

Flexion is resisted by approaching the patient from behind, resting the elbows against the back of the patient's shoulders, and placing both hands over the patient's forehead.

1. Tests the integrity of the upper cervical myotomes
2. Tests for lesions of the cervical muscles

B. *Active cervical movements with passive overpressure.* Ask the patient to perform each of the six cervical movements, and gently apply some passive over-pressure at the extreme of each movement. Ask the patient if there is pain and observe for muscle guarding or other signs of discomfort. Also note restricted movement.

1. Tests for cervical joint restriction

C. *Quadrant test.* Position the patient's head in combined rotation, side bending and extension to one side. With the head in this position, apply a gentle axial compression through the neck by downward pressure to the top of the head.

1. Tests for localized capsular facet-joint tightness
2. Tests for interforaminal nerve root impingement

II. **Shoulder Tests**

A. *Active shoulder movements with passive overpressure.* Ask the pa-tient to perform flexion of the arm (in the sagittal plane), abduc-tion (in the frontal plane), hori-zontal adduction (reaching across to behind the opposite shoulder), to touch the palm to the back of the neck and retract the elbow, and to crawl the thumb up the back as far as possible. Apply gentle passive overpressure at the end point of each movement. Both arms are tested simulta-neously for comparison. Note the presence of pain, muscle spasm, or loss of movement.

1. Tests for shoulder tendinitis: Typically full range of motion with pain at the extremes of elevation and movements which stretch the involved tendon. A painful arc on ab-duction suggests rotator cuff tendinitis.
2. Tests for capsular restriction of the glenohumeral joint: Considerable pain and restric-tion on external rotation and abduction, moderate restric-tion of flexion and internal ro-tation.
3. Tests for acute bursitis: Marked pain and restriction of elevation of the arm in any plane.

B. *Resisted shoulder movements.* The patient sits with the elbows close to the sides, the elbows bent to 90°, and the fingers pointed for-ward. Resist abduction with the arms held at about 30° of abduc-tion. Resist external rotation and internal rotation with the elbows held tight against the sides, ap-plying counterpressure just prox-mal to the wrist. All movements are resisted bilaterally and simul-taneously for easy comparison of one side with the other and for most efficient stabilization against trunk movements. Maximal contractions should be encouraged. Attempt to prevent any joint movement. Note the presence of pain or weakness.

1. Tests for the presence of tendinitis: The contraction of the involved muscle and tendon will be strong and painful.
2. Tests for the presence of a tendon rupture: The contraction will be weak and painless.
3. Tests the integrity of the C5 and C6 myotomes

III. Elbow Tests

A. *Active movements with passive overpressure.* Ask the patient to fully flex and extend both elbows together. Apply passive overpressure at the extremes of each movement and observe for pain, spasm, or restricted movement. These tests may be performed with the shoulder extended, in neutral, or flexed to test for involvement of the long head of the biceps or triceps.

1. Tests for capsular restrictions: Flexion is limited to about 90° to 100°, extension is lacking by 20° to 30°.
2. Tests for extracapsular pain or restrictions
   a. Loose body—extension is restricted, flexion is relatively free. Often there are painful twinges or crepitus noted during movement.
   b. Brachialis tightness—extension is limited, flexion is free. Tightness is felt anteriorly by the patient on forced extension. The restriction is unaffected by the position of the shoulder.
   c. Biceps tendinitis—Pain may be reproduced with elbow extension performed

with the shoulder extended.

B. *Resisted movements.* Stabilize the trunk by placing a hand over the top of the patient's shoulder and resist isometric flexion and extension of the elbow. Pronation and supination are resisted with the elbow bent to 90°. Note pain or weakness.

1. Tests the integrity of the C6 and C7 myotomes
2. Tests for biceps tendinitis: Resisted elbow flexion and forearm supination will be strong and painful.
3. Tests for biceps tendon rupture: Flexion and supination will be weak and painless.

IV. Wrist Tests. The patient's elbow is maintained in extension. Turn away side to be examined. Hold the patient's arm snugly between your elbow and side and cradle the patient's forearm in your forearm and hand.

A. *Active movements with passive overpressure.*

1. With the forearm pronated, move the wrist into full flexion and ulnar deviation. Apply passive overpressure, once with the patient's fingers flexed, once with them relaxed. Note pain or restricted motion.
2. With the forearm supinated, the wrist is brought into full extension and radial deviation. Apply overpressure once with the fingers extended, once with them relaxed. Note pain or restricted motion.
   a. Tests for tennis elbow: Elbow pain is reproduced on full wrist flexion and ulnar deviation with the forearm pronated and the fingers flexed.

b. Tests for golfer's elbow: Elbow pain is reproduced with full wrist extension with the fingers extended and forearm supinated.

c. Tests for carpal ligament sprain: Pain on the movement that stretches the involved ligament

d. Tests for de Quervain's disease: Pain over the radial styloid region when the wrist is ulnarly deviated while the thumb is held flexed

e. Tests for capsular restriction of wrist movements: All wrist movements are limited.

B. *Resisted wrist movements.* With the patient's arm held as described above and the patient's fist clenched, resist wrist flexion, extension, ulnar deviation, and radial deviation. Note pain or weakness.

1. Tests the C6 (extension), C7 (flexion), and C8 (ulnar deviation) myotomes.

2. Tests for tennis elbow: Pain on resisted wrist extension

3. Tests for golfer's elbow: Pain on resisted wrist flexion

C. *Modified Phalen's test.* Instruct the patient to perform a "three-jaw-chuck" pinch with both hands and to maintain both wrists in extreme flexion by pressing the dorsum of the hands against one another. This position is held for 30 to 60 seconds. Note the production of pain or paresthesias.

1. Tests for carpal tunnel syndrome: Paresthesias into the thumb or middle three fingers are reproduced on the involved side.

2. Tests for dorsal carpal liga-ment sprain: Wrist pain is reproduced on full wrist flexion.

D. *Upper extremity weight bearing.*

1. While he is still sitting, ask the patient to place both hands to his side on the plinth and attempt to raise his body off the plinth by pressing down with the hands.

2. Tests for carpal ligament sprain: This is often the only maneuver that will reproduce the wrist pain.

V. Finger Tests

A. *Grasp–release.* Ask the patient to squeeze two of your fingers, simultaneously with both hands, as hard as possible, and then to open the hands as wide as possible. Note pain, weakness, or joint restriction.

1. Tests for the integrity of the T1 myotome: Weakness will be noted on grasp.

2. Tests for tennis elbow: Strong grasp may reproduce the elbow pain because the wrist extensors must contract to stabilize.

3. Tests for restriction of finger movement

B. *Resisted abduction–adduction.* The patient attempts to keep the fingers spread apart as you adduct the small finger and thumb simultaneously. Both hands are tested at the same time for comparison. Then interlace your fingers between the patient's extended fingers and ask the patient to adduct his fingers. Note pain or weakness.

1. Tests the C8 myotome (thumb and small finger abduction) and the T1 myotome (finger adduction)

2. Tests for de Quervain's disease: Pain is produced with resisted thumb abduction.

VI. Sensory Tests. The patient sits with the forearms resting on the thighs, palms facing upward. Using a sharp pin or pinwheel, assess sensation by applying the stimulus first to a small area on one extremity, and asking the patient if it feels sharp, then repeating the test on the same area on the opposite extremity. Then ask the patient if it feels the same on both sides. The key sensory areas in the hand are checked first, then various aspects of the forearms, arms, and shoulder girdles, using the procedure described above. Note asymmetries and reduction of sensation. For more subtle testing, a wisp of cotton or tuning fork may be used.

1. Tests the integrity of the C4 through T1 dermatomes: Rarely is a deficit noted proximal to the distal forearm in the case of nerve root lesions because of the extensive overlapping of dermatomes in all but the wrist and hand.
   C4—Trapezial ridge to tip of shoulder
   C5—Upper scapula, lateral brachial region, radial aspect of forearm
   C6—Upper scapula, lateral brachial region, radiovolar aspect of forearm, thumb and index finger
   C7—Midscapula, posterior brachial region, dorsum of forearm and hand, middle three fingers
   C8—Middle to lower scapula, ulnar aspect of forearm and outer two fingers
   T1—Ulnovolar aspect of forearm
2. Tests sensory integrity of upper extremity peripheral nerves

VII. Deep Tendon Reflex Tests. The patient sits with forearms resting on thighs.

A. *Biceps* (C5,C6). As the patient maintains relaxation of the arm, place your thumb firmly over the patient's biceps tendon at the antecubital fossa and strike the dorsum of his thumb with the reflex hammer to elicit the reflex. Feel for tensing of the tendon; observe for contraction of the muscle and slight flexion of the elbow. Note asymmetries in responses and clonic responses.

B. *Triceps* (C7): As the patient maintains relaxation of the arm, grasp the patient's wrists and, while supporting the forearm at 90° elbow flexion, strike the distal triceps tendon just above the olecranon. Observe for triceps contraction and feel for slight elbow extension. Note asymmetrical or clonic responses.

C. *Brachioradialis* (C5,C6): As the patient maintains relaxation of both arms, support both forearms at about 90° elbow flexion by grasping both of the patient's thumbs in one hand. Strike the brachioradialis tendon just above the radial styloid process, slightly volarly. Observe the brachioradialis muscle belly for contraction and feel for slight elbow flexion and forearm pronation. Note asymmetrical or clonic responses. Tests the integrity of the C5, C6, and C7 segments.

SUMMARY OF STEPS TO CERVICAL–UPPER EXTREMITY SCAN EXAM

In order for the scan exam to be of practical use, it must be performed within a very short period of time—5 minutes or less. Otherwise, one of its primary purposes, that of saving time in the clinic, is defeated. In order to perform the scan exam within a reasonable period of time, the clinician must sequence the tests so that they are performed as efficiently as possible. In doing so, take care to avoid undue haste, which might lead to poor evaluatory technique and inaccurate findings. The scan exam condenses a number of tests within a short time period; in order to avoid confusion or the possibility of omitting crucial steps, the clinician must drill himself on the sequencing of steps and the rationale for each step in order to be able to use the scan exam effectively in the clinic.

The following lists the steps to the scan exam in the order which they can be most efficiently performed:

1. Cervical resisted movements
2. Active cervical movements with passive overpressure
3. Quadrant test, left and right
4. Active shoulder movements with passive overpressure
   a. Flexion
   b. Abduction
   c. Hand to opposite shoulder
   d. Hand to back of neck, wing elbow back
   e. Hand behind and up back
5. Resisted shoulder movements
   a. Abduction
   b. Internal rotation
   c. External rotation
6. Active elbow movements with passive overpressure, resisted elbow movements
   a. Flexion: passive overpressure, resist flexion
   b. Neutral: resist extension, resist pronation and supination
   c. Extension: passive overpressure
7. Active forearm and wrist movements with passive overpressure
   a. Combined wrist flexion and ulnar deviation with the forearm pronated and elbow extended: passive overpressure with fingers flexed; passive overpressure with fingers relaxed
   b. Combined wrist extension and radial deviation with the forearm supinated and elbow extended: passive overpressure with fingers extended; passive overpressure with fingers relaxed
8. Resisted wrist movements
   a. Flexion
   b. Extension
   c. Radial deviation
   d. Ulnar deviation
9. Modified Phalen's test
10. Active and resisted finger movements
    a. Grasp–release
    b. Finger abduction
    c. Finger adduction
11. Upper extremity weight bearing
12. Sensory tests
    a. C4–T1
13. Reflex testing
    a. Biceps
    b. Triceps
    c. Brachioradialis

16 The Hip

Randolph M. Kessler

REVIEW OF FUNCTIONAL ANATOMY

OSTEOLOGY

The acetabulum is formed superiorly by the ilium, posteroinferiorly by the ischium, and anteroinferiorly by the pubis. The acetabulum faces laterally, anteriorly, and inferiorly (Fig. 16-1,*A*). It is deepened by the fibrocartilaginous acetabular labrum, allowing it to enclose slightly more than half a sphere. The bony, fibrocartilaginous labrum and cartilaginous constituents of the acetabulum are interrupted inferiorly by the acetabular notch (Fig. 16-1,*B*). This notch is traversed by the transverse ligament of the acetabulum (Fig. 16-1,*C*).

The head of the femur constitutes about two thirds of a sphere. Slightly below and behind the center of the articular surface of the head is a roughened indentation called the *fovea*, to which the ligament of the head of the femur attaches (Fig. 16-1,*B*). The neck of the femur connects the head and shaft of the femur. In the frontal plane, the angle formed by the neck and shaft of the femur is about 125° in the adult, but closer to 150° in the young child. This is often termed the *angle of inclination* (Fig. 16-2). In the transverse plane, the neck forms an angle of about 15° with the transverse axis of the femoral condyles, such that with the transverse axis of the condyles lying in the frontal plane, the neck of the femur is directed about 15° forward (Fig. 16-3). This is referred to as the *angle of torsion* or *angle of declination* of the hip. Note, then, that in the anatomical position, both the acetabulum and the neck of the femur are directed anteriorly. Because of this, in the normal standing position, a large area of the articular surface of the head of the femur is exposed anteriorly, and the effective weight-bearing surface of the head is confined to a relatively small area on the posterosuperior aspect of the head.

An increase in degrees of the normal inclination angle is referred to as *coxa valgum*; a decrease in the angle is called *coxa varum* (Fig. 16-2). When an increased torsion angle is present, we speak of an *anteverted hip*, whereas a hip in *retroversion* is one in which there is less than a normal torsion angle (Fig. 16-3). Clinically, it should be apparent that a patient with an anteverted hip will appear to lack external rotation, and a patient with a retroverted hip will appear to lack internal rotation. Also, the person with an anteverted hip will tend to walk with a toe-in gait; with retroversion, a toe-out gait is characteristic.

The greater trochanter is a prominence projecting laterally and superiorly from the junction of the neck and shaft of the femur. It serves as an area for attachment of many of the muscles controlling movement at the hip. Situated posteromedially to the junction of the neck and shaft is a smaller prominence, the lesser trochanter; it also provides an area of insertion for muscles controlling the hip (Fig. 16-1,*A*).

Trabeculae

The trabecular patterns of the upper femur reflect the normal stresses sustained by the hip; they correspond to the normal lines of force in this area (Fig. 16-4). The main system of trabeculae consists of two sets of trabeculae. The arcuate bundle resists a bending moment or a tendency for the weight of the body to shear the head and neck inferiorly with respect to the shaft of the femur; this bending moment is brought about by the lever arm created by the medially projecting neck of the femur. The vertical bundle resists vertical compressive forces through the head of the femur. The arcuate bundle runs from the lateral cortex of the shaft of the femur, just inferior to the greater trochanter, upward and medially to the middle and inferior cortical region of the head of the femur. The vertical bundle is contiguous with the medial cortex of the shaft of the femur, running straight upward to the superior cortex of the head.

Another trabecular system runs from the medial cortex at the base of the neck, upward laterally through the greater trochanter. These resist the tensile forces from the muscles attaching to the trochanter.

The areas where the vertical bundle and the trochanteric bundle intersect the arcuate bundle are areas of particular strength. The intervening region is an area of relative weakness, made weaker by osteoporosis in older people. This region is often the site of femoral neck fractures.

ARTICULAR CARTILAGE

The area of the acetabulum covered by articular cartilage is a horseshoe-shaped region. The area not covered by articular cartilage corresponds to the total sweep of the ligament of the head of the femur when the hip is moved through a full range of movement in all planes. This nonarticular portion is the acetabular fossa and is lined by a fat pad (Fig. 16-1,*B*). The entire head of the femur is covered by articular cartilage except for the small fovea where the ligament of the head attaches.

LIGAMENTS AND CAPSULE

The joint capsule of the hip joint is thick and strong and is reinforced by strong ligaments. Its fibers run longitudinally, parallel to the neck of the femur (Fig. 16-5). The capsule runs from the rim of the acetabulum and labrum to the intertrochanteric line anteriorly and to about 1 cm proximal to the *intertrochanteric crest* posteriorly. Much of the neck of the femur, then, is intracapsular. Some deep fibers of the joint capsule run circularly around the neck of the femur, forming the zona orbicularis.

The iliofemoral ligament is one of the strongest ligaments in the body. It is sometimes referred to as the *Y ligament of Bigelow*, since it resembles an inverted Y. It attaches proximally to the lower portion of the anteroinferior iliac spine and to an area on the ilium just proximal to the superior and posterosuperior rim of the acetabulum. The ligament, as a whole, spirals around to overlay the anterior aspect of the joint, attaching to the intertrochanteric line. The more lateral fork of the Y attaches to the anterior aspect of the greater trochanter, whereas the more medial fibers twist around to attach just anterior to the lesser trochanter (Fig. 16-5,*A*).

This ligament primarily checks internal rotation and extension. It allows a person to stand with the joint in extension using a minimum of muscle action; by rolling the pelvis backward, a person can "hang" on the ligaments. Note that the ligament prevents excessive movement in the direction toward the close-packed position of the hip joint. Looking at it in another way, with movement toward the close-packed position, this ligament becomes taut and twisted upon itself, causing an approxima-

(*Text continues on page 373*)

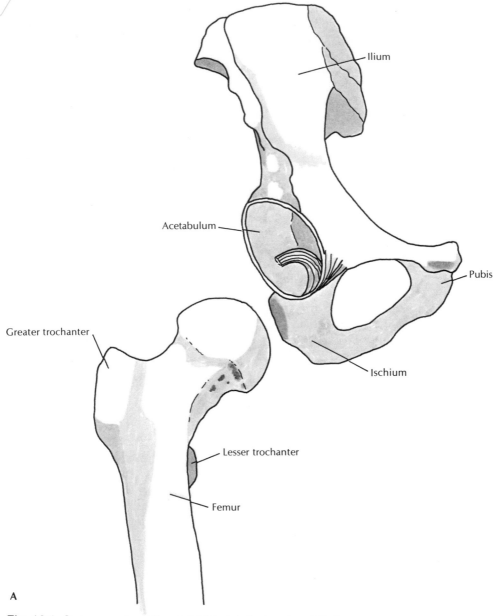

A

Fig. 16-1. Components of the right hip joint, showing (*A*) the relationship of the acetabulum to the femur, (*B*) the acetabular fossa, the proximal femur, and (*C*) the ligaments of the acetabulum

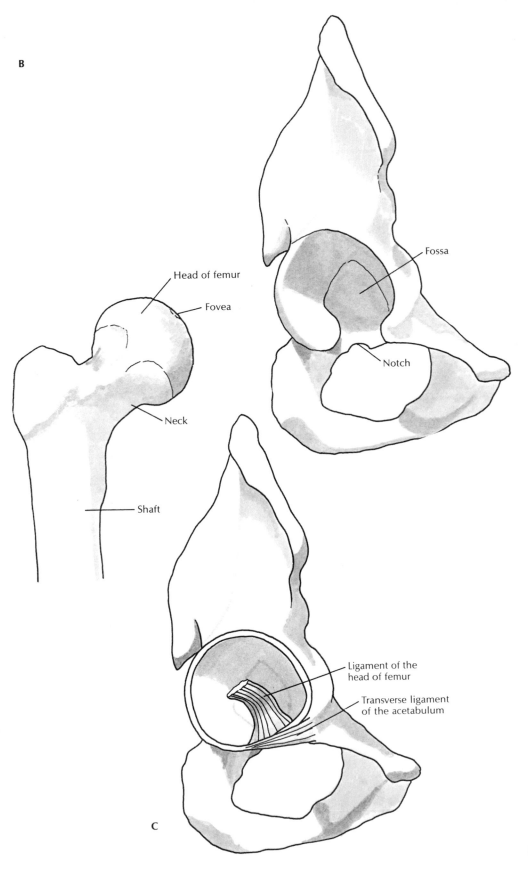

B

Head of femur

Fovea

Neck

Shaft

Fossa

Notch

Ligament of the
head of femur

Transverse ligament
of the acetabulum

C

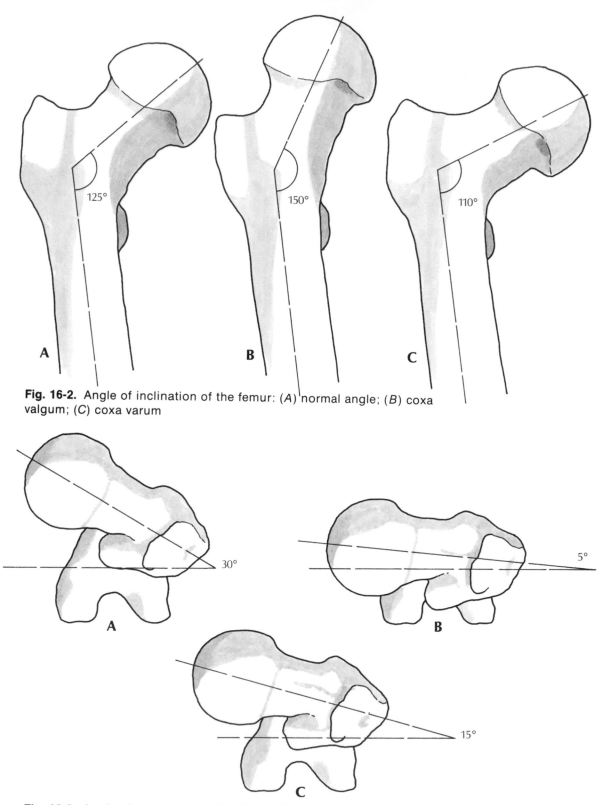

Fig. 16-2. Angle of inclination of the femur: (*A*) normal angle; (*B*) coxa valgum; (*C*) coxa varum

Fig. 16-3. Angle of torsion or declination of the femur in the transverse plane: (*A*) anteversion; (*B*) retroversion; (*C*) normal angle

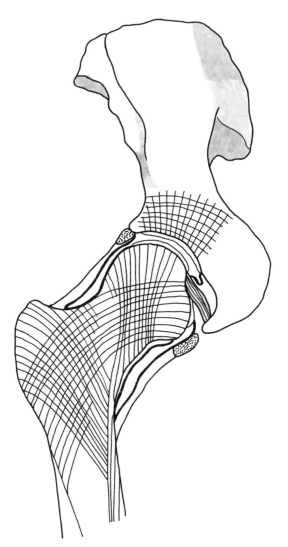

Fig. 16-4. Trabecular patterns of the upper femur

pulls tight on extension and internal rotation of the hip.

The pubofemoral ligament runs from the pubis, near the acetabulum, to the femur, just anterior to the lesser trochanter. It tightens primarily on abduction, but also helps check internal rotation of the hip (Fig. 16-5,*A*).

The ligament of the head of the femur (ligmentum teres) attaches to the roughened nonarticular area of the acetabulum inferiorly near the acetabular notch, to both sides of the notch, and to the transverse ligament that traverses the notch. It lies in the nonarticular acetabular fossa as it runs up and around the head of the femur to the fovea (Fig. 16-1,*C*).

Although it pulls tight on adduction of the hip, its mechanical function is relatively unimportant. Of more significance is its role in providing some vascularization to the head of the femur and perhaps in assisting with lubrication of the joint. The ligament of the head of the femur is lined with synovium. It is felt that this ligament may act somewhat similarly to the meniscus at the knee by spreading a layer of synovial fluid over the articular surface of the head of the femur as the head advances to contact the opposing surface of the acetabulum.

As mentioned, the *transverse ligament* crosses the acetabular notch to fill in the gap. It converts the notch into a foramen through which the acetabular artery (from the obturator artery) runs, eventually becoming the artery of the ligament of the head of the femur (Fig. 16-1,*C*).

SYNOVIUM

The synovial membrane of the hip joint lines the fibrous layer of the capsule. It also lines the acetabular labrum and, inferiorly, continues inward at the acetabular notch to line the fat pad in the floor of the acetabular fossa and to cover the ligament of the head of the femur. From the femoral attachment of the capsule at the

tion of the joint surfaces and a "locking" of the joint. Some of the lateral fibers of the iliofemoral ligament probably pull tight on adduction.

The ischiofemoral ligament attaches proximally to an area of the ischium just posterior and posteroinferior to the rim of the acetabulum. Its fibers run upward and laterally to attach to the posterosuperior aspect of the neck of the femur, where the neck meets the greater trochanter (Fig. 16-5,*B*). The ischiofemoral ligament also

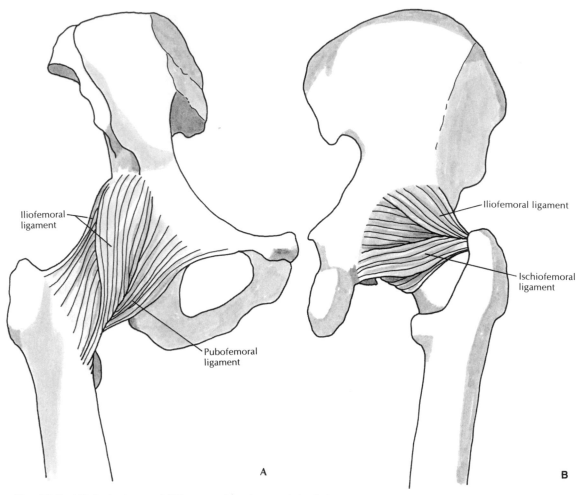

Iliofemoral
ligament

Pubofemoral
ligament

Iliofemoral ligament

Ischiofemoral
ligament

A

B

Fig. 16-5. (*A*) Anterior and (*B*) posterior views of the joint capsule of the hip joint

base neck, the synovium reflects backward proximally to line the neck of the femur.

The synovial "cavity" of the joint often communicates anteriorly with the iliopectineal bursa. It does so through a gap between the pubofemoral ligament and medial portion of the iliofemoral ligament.

BURSAE

The rather large iliopectineal bursa overlies the anterior aspect of the hip joint and the pubis, and lies beneath the iliopsoas muscle as it crosses in front of the hip joint. This bursa often communicates with the hip joint anteriorly through a space between the pubofemoral and iliofemoral ligaments. This may be a factor in the characteristic anterior pain experienced by patients with hip joint disease (Fig. 16-6).

One or more trochanteric bursae overlie the greater trochanter, reducing friction between it and the gluteus maximus, which passes over the trochanter, and the other gluteals, which attach to the trochanter. This bursa is most extensive posterolaterally to the trochanter, where

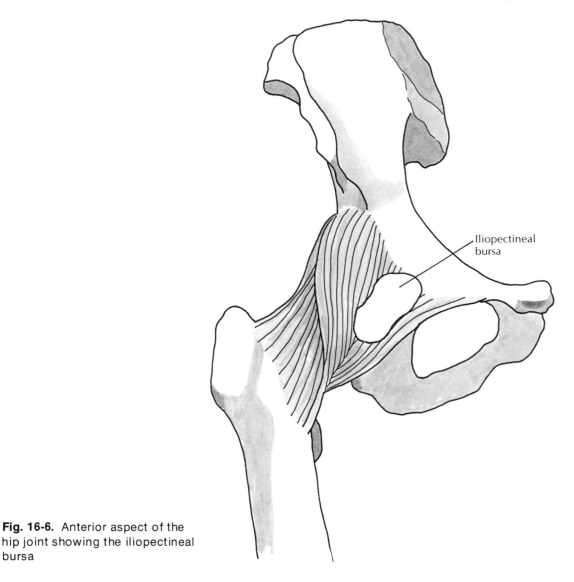

Iliopectineal
bursa

Fig. 16-6. Anterior aspect of the
hip joint showing the iliopectineal
bursa

it underlies the gluteus maximus. It is important clinically because of the prevalence of trochanteric bursitis.

BLOOD SUPPLY (Fig. 16-7)

The blood supply to the head of the femur
is of particular importance because of its
significance in common pathologic conditions at the hip, including fractures and
osteochondrosis of the femoral head
(Legg–Perthes' disease). The head of the
femur receives its vascularization from

two sources, the artery of the ligament of
the head of the femur and the arteries that
ascend along the neck of the femur. The
importance of the artery of the ligament of
the head is variable, but for the most part
it supplies only a small area adjacent to
the fovea. In as many as 20% of individuals it fails to anastomose with the other
arteries supplying the head.

The primary blood supply to the head of
the femur, then, is derived from the arteries that ascend proximally along the
neck of the femur to pierce the head just

distal to the margin of the articular cartilage. These are branches of the medial and lateral femoral circumflex arteries. The medial circumflex artery passes around posteriorly to give off branches that ascend along the posteroinferior and posterosuperior aspects of the neck. The lateral circumflex artery crosses anteriorly to give off an anterior ascending artery at about the level of the intertrochanteric line. The ascending arteries pierce the joint capsule near its distal attachment to the femur and run proximally along the neck of the femur intracapsularly. They

Fig. 16-7. Blood supply to the head of the femur

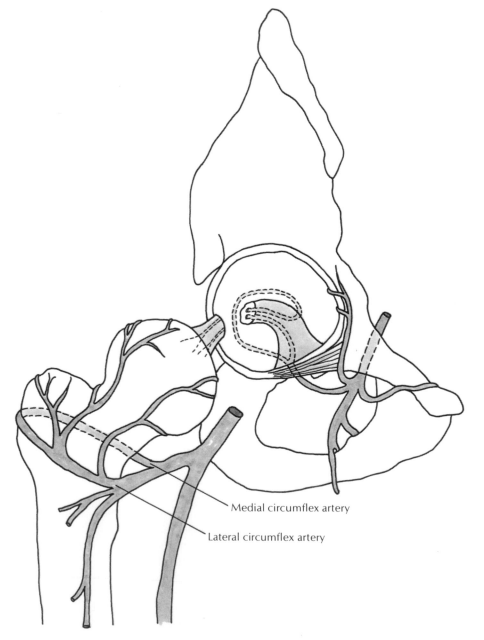

Medial circumflex artery

Lateral circumflex artery

run deep to the synovial lining of the neck. Because of their relationship to the neck, they are subject to interruption in the case of a femoral neck fracture. Also, since they are intracapsular, it is believed that increased intracapsular pressure caused by joint effusion may stop flow. This is thought to be a factor in osteochondrosis of the head of the femur and in some cases of idiopathic avascular necrosis of the head. The circumflex vessels give off extracapsular branches to the trochanteric regions of the femur. This area also receives vascularization from the superior gluteal artery and a perforating branch of the profunda.

NERVE SUPPLY

Innervation to the hip joint is supplied by branches from the obturator nerve, the superior gluteal nerve, the nerve to the quadratus femoris, and by branches from the femoral nerve, both muscular and articular. These nerves represent segments L2 through S1.

BIOMECHANICS

The hip joint, being a ball-and-socket joint, exhibits three degrees of freedom of motion. In this respect it is analogous to the glenohumeral joint. Unlike the shoulder, however, the hip is intrinsically a very stable joint. This is due, in part, to the fact that the acetabulum forms a much deeper socket than the glenoid cavity, the head of the femur comes closer to forming a full sphere than does the head of the humerus. The acetabulum, with its labrum, is able to enclose over half a sphere and to grasp passively the head of the femur to maintain joint integrity; it is difficult to pull the head from the acetabulum without removing or tearing the acetabular labrum. Coaptation of joint surfaces is also maintained, in part, by atmospheric pressure. Because of the relatively large surface

area of contact between joint surfaces, the atmospheric pressures holding the joint surfaces together may be as much as 25 kg. This is sufficient to maintain coaptation of the joint with all soft tissues about the joint removed and the limb hanging freely. It is only when the vacuum created between the joint surfaces (by the close fit) is released by, say, drilling a hole through the acetabulum, that the limb will drop free. Intrinsic stability at the joint is further enhanced by the strong ligamentous support at the hip. Since the major ligaments at the hip pull taut and are twisted upon themselves with extension, the hip joint is particularly stable in the standing position. As mentioned, the twisting of the capsule that occurs with movement toward the close-packed position effects a type of "screw home" movement at the hip in which the joint surfaces become tightly approximated. As with any joint, the close-packed position at the hip (extension–abduction–internal rotation) is the position of maximal congruence of joint surfaces.

Because the acetabulum and the neck of the femur are both directed anteriorly, their respective mechanical axes are not coincidental. There are two positions of the hip in which these axes are brought into alignment. One position is attained by flexing the hip to about 90°, abducting slightly, and rotating slightly externally. The other position is one of extension, abduction, and internal rotation. Note that the former position is the one that the hip would assume in a quadriped situation, and the latter is the close-packed position of the joint. As mentioned, in the upright position, a considerable portion of the articular cartilage of the head of the femur is exposed anteriorly. During normal use of the joint, for instance, walking, there is a relatively small contact area between acetabulum and head. This may be a factor in the prevalence of degenerative hip disease in humans; stresses of weight-bearing are born by a small surface area of cartilage, and a relatively large area of cartilage may not undergo the intermittent compression necessary for adequate nutrition (see Chapter 2, Arthrology). It should be apparent that the smaller the torsion angle at the hip (the less it is anteverted), the greater the bony stability, since the axes of the acetabulum and neck are closer to being in alignment. A smaller torsion angle also favors an increase in the effective contact area between joint surfaces, for the same reason.

Because of its intrinsic stability, the normal hip joint rarely dislocates when compared to, say, the shoulder or elbow. The shoulder, elbow, or any other joint for that matter, usually dislocates when a force is applied over the joint when it is in its close-packed position. This is not true at the hip, which will usually only dislocate when its capsule and major ligaments are lax, and its joint surfaces and bony axes are out of congruence. From this and the above discussion you might predict that the hip is most prone to dislocation when in a position of flexion (ligaments lax), adduction, and external rotation (noncongruence). Dislocation usually occurs with a force driving the femur backward on the pelvis with the hip in this position, for example, striking the knee on the dashboard of a car in a head-on collision. With such an injury, the head of the femur is driven posteriorly through the relatively weak posterior capsule.

Since the hip is freely movable in all vertical planes, it is not subject to capsuloligamentous strain from horizontal forces applied to it in most positions, even though, due to the length of the leg, these forces acting over a long lever arm are potentially quite large. However, since the hip is a weight-bearing joint, it is subject to vertical loading that must be born by its bony and cartilaginous components. In the case of a person bearing equal weight through both legs, the vertical force on each femoral head is equal to half the weight of the body minus the weight of the legs. When standing on one leg, however, the weight-bearing femoral head must support more than the weight of the body. This is because the center of gravity (at about S2) is located some distance medially to the supporting femoral head. This lever-arm through which the force is acting causes a rotary moment about the supporting femoral head with a tendency for the opposite side of the pelvis to drop. This rotary moment must be countered by the hip abductor muscles, primarily the gluteus medius, gluteus minimus, and tensor fascia lata, on the weight-bearing side. The point of application of this counterforce provided by the abductor pull is at the greater trochanter, which is considerably closer to the fulcrum (femoral head) than is the center of gravity line that represents the force produced by the body weight. Since the distance from femoral head to trochanter is about one half of the distance from femoral head to the center of gravity line, the abductors must pull with a force equal to two times the superincumbent body weight in order to prevent the pelvis from dropping to the non-weight-bearing side. The total force acting vertically at the femoral head is equal to the force produced by the pull of the abductors plus the force produced by the body weight, or up to *three times the body weight*.[10,11,22] Note that in this case "body weight" is actually the total body weight minus the weight of the supporting leg.

During stance phase of the normal gait cycle, the vertical forces acting at the femoral head are substantial. If the abductors are not strong enough to counter the forces tending to rotate or tilt the pelvis downward to the opposite side, an abnormal gait pattern results. Either the pelvis will drop noticeably to the opposite side of the weakness, usually resulting in a short swing phase on that side, or the person will lurch toward the side of weakness during stance phase on the weak side. The effect of the lurch is to shift the center of gravity toward the fulcrum (femoral head), reducing the moment arm about which the forces from the body weight may act, thereby reducing the necessary counterpull by the abductors. In fact, a marked lurch may actually shift the center of gravity lateral to the fulcrum, allowing gravity to substitute for the hip abductors, thereby preventing the pelvis from dropping to the opposite side. This lurching gait is often referred to as a "compensated gluteus medius gait." It is usually seen in patients with painful hip conditions, such as degenerative joint disease, in which there is some weakness of the abductors and in which it is desirable to reduce compressive forces acting at the joint for relief of pain. It is also seen in patients with abductor paralysis.

The "abductor lurch" may be prevented by providing an external means of preventing the pelvis from dropping toward the uninvolved side during stance phase on the involved side. This external force may be provided by use of a cane on the uninvolved side. An upward force is transmitted from the ground through the cane to counter the weight of the body tending to rotate the pelvis downward on that side. The forces acting through the cane do so about a moment arm even longer than that about which the force of gravity on the body weight acts, since the point of contact of the hand on the cane is further from the supporting femoral head than is the center of gravity line. For this reason, a relatively small force applied through the cane is required to compensate for the abductors and relieve the vertical forces acting at the involved hip. Note that the forces acting upward through the cane must be transmitted to the pelvis through contraction of the lateral trunk muscles, shoulder depressors, elbow extensors, and wrist flexors on the side of the cane.

It should be clear from the above discussion that forces of muscle contraction contribute significantly to compressive load-ing at the hip. This is not only true in a weight-bearing situation. Studies in which strain gauges have been inserted into prosthetic hips suggest that supine straight leg raising causes a compressive force to the hip that is greater than the body weight.[22] This is an important consideration in the early management of patients who have undergone an internal fixation for a hip fracture.[15]

EVALUATION

HISTORY

The hip joint is derived from segments L2 through S1. Clinically, however, pain of hip joint origin is primarily perceived as involving the L3 segment. Typically, the patient with hip joint disease complains first of pain in the midinguinal region. As the process progresses, or as the painful stimulus intensifies, pain is likely to be felt into the anterior thigh and knee. At this point pain may also be described in the greater trochanteric region and buttock as well. In some instances—and not uncommonly—pain is felt most in the knee, and the patient may actually believe the knee is at fault. Generally speaking, pain in the trochanteric region spreading into the lateral thigh is more suggestive of trochanteric bursitis. Pain in the buttock spreading into the lateral or posterior thigh is more suggestive of pain of lower spinal origin.

Because of its freedom of movement in all planes and its great stability, the hip is seldom afflicted by disorders of acute traumatic origin. The hip is a common site, however, of degenerative joint disease, and to a lesser extent, rheumatoid arthritis. Inquire as to whether the patient suffered any childhood hip disorders such as congenital dysplasia, osteochondrosis (Legg–Perthes' disease), or slipped capital epiphysis, since these may predispose to early hip degeneration. Bursitis, either trochanteric or iliopectineal, is also fairly common at the hip.

Also determine whether the patient has a history of back problems. Low back disorders may mimic hip disease and *vice versa* because of the segmental relationships. Also, hip disease often leads to back problems because of the biomechanical relationships. (Refer to Chapter 4 for a complete list of questions to be included in the history.)

PHYSICAL EXAMINATION

I. Observation

   A. *Gait*

   1. A lurch to one side during stance phase is suggestive of hip pain or abductor weakness or both on the side to which the lurch occurs.

   2. Dropping of pelvis on the opposite side of the stance leg is suggestive of abductor weakness (uncompensated) on the side of the stance leg.

   3. Development of an excessive lordosis during stance phase may suggest hip flexion contracture on the side of the stance leg.

   4. A backward lurch of the trunk during stance phase may suggest hip extensor weakness on the side of the stance leg or hip flexor weakness on the side of the swing leg.

   5. A persistent inclination of the pelvis to one side during all phases of the gait cycle, combined with a lack of heel-strike on the side of inclination, suggests an adduction contracture on the side of the inclination.

   B. *Functional activities*

   1. Loss of hip motion may result in considerable difficulty removing and donning shoes, socks, and slacks.

   2. The patient may "sacral sit" to compensate for a lack of hip flexion.

   C. *Note general posture and body build*

II. Inspection

   A. *Skin.* Usually noncontributory in common hip disorders; observe for old surgical scars.

   B. *Soft tissue*

   1. Observe for atrophy about the hip and thigh. Document thigh atrophy by girth measurements.

   2. Hip joint effusion is usually not visible due to heavy soft-tissue covering.

   C. *Bony structure and alignment.* Measure and record deviations.

   1. Use plumb bob to assess mediolateral and anteroposterior alignment in the standing position (including the spine).

   2. Assess relative heights of

      a. navicular tubercles

      b. medial malleoli

      c. fibular heads

      d. popliteal folds

      e. gluteal folds

      f. greater trochanters

      g. anterior superior iliac spines (ASISs)

      h. posterior superior iliac spines (OSISs)

      i. iliac crests

   Note: A vertical structural deviation arising from some abnormality at the hip joint or upper end of the femur is suggested if, from the floor upwards, all of the above mentioned landmarks are level up to the trochanters, but the ASISs, PSISs and iliac crests are not. Be sure to note whether the relative levels of the ASIS and PSIS on one side are the same as the levels on the opposite side. If not, the asymmetry may be due to a sacroiliac torsion rather than some abnormality at the hip joint or upper femur. If the trochanters are level and the ASIS, PSIS, and iliac crest on one side are lower by the same amount than their counterparts on the opposite side, one may suspect one of several possibilities—coxa vara on the low side, coxa valga on the high side, a shortened femoral neck on the low side or lengthened neck on the high side (rare), or cartilaginous narrowing from hip joint degeneration on the low side. The two most common of these are coxa vara and hip joint degeneration. Coxa vara is usually associated with a decreased angle of declination (torsion angle); hip joint degeneration sufficient to cause a clinically detectable vertical asymmetry will be accompanied by other symptoms and signs of degenerative joint disease (DJD) (see common lesions discussed below).

Documentation of the extent of coxa vara, hip joint narrowing, or other cause of asymmetry may be made by assessing the position of the greater trochanter relative to a line drawn from the ASIS to the ischial tuberosity (Nélaton's line). The "normal" trochanter should lie about on this line. This measurement is primarily useful in unilateral conditions in which it may be compared to the "normal" side. Documentation of total leg length discrepancy should be made by measuring from the ASIS to the medial malleolus of the same side.

III. Selective Tissue Tension Tests
  A. *Active movements.* The emphasis here should be on assessing functional activities involving use of the hip
    1. Gait

  2. Stair climbing
  3. Squatting to pick up object from floor
  4. One-legged standing (observe for dropping of pelvis to opposite side—Trendelenburg sign)
  5. Sitting, bending forward to touch floor
  B. *Passive movements*
    1. Flexion–extension
      a. These are best assessed using a Kotke hip measurement. Draw a line from PSIS to ASIS with the hip in full flexion or extension and construct a perpendicular from this line to the greater trochanter; the angle between this line and the long axis of the femur is measured in full flexion or full extension.
      b. For a general assessment, various modifications of the Thomas test may be used.
        i. Allow the knee of the extended leg to flex over the end of the table to differentiate between rectus femoris and iliopsoas or capsular tightness.
        ii. Position the patient prone over the end of the table so that both hips are flexed to 90° in the starting position. The leg to be tested for flexor tightness is extended just until the spine begins to extend. This position affords a better differentiation between how much of the movement is occurring between femur and pelvis, and how much is due to rolling of the pelvis backward.
    2. Abduction–adduction.   When

measuring, be sure to prevent lateral tilting of the pelvis.

3. Internal–external rotation
    a. Measure sitting with hips and knees flexed.
    b. Measure prone with knee flexed (this is a more "functional" measurement since the hip is extended as in walking).
    c. Limited internal rotation and *excessive* external rotation suggest retroversion (decreased angle of declination). Limited external rotation and *excessive* internal rotation suggest increased anteversion (increased angle of declination). If internal rotation is considerably limited and external rotation somewhat limited, capsular tightening is likely.

4. On all passive movements, note
    a. Range of motion (ROM). The capsular pattern of restriction is marked limitation of internal rotation and abduction, moderate limitation of flexion and extension, some limitation of external rotation and adduction.
    b. Pain
    c. Crepitus
    d. End feel

C. *Resisted movements*
    1. Resist maximal isometric contraction of muscles controlling all major hip movements, allowing no motion of the joint.
    2. Tendinitis about the hip is very rare, but resisted hip flexion may reproduce pain in the presence of iliopectineal bursitis, and resisted hip abduction, or resisted hip extension and external rotation, may re-

produce pain in trochanteric bursitis.

D. *Joint play movement tests*
    1. The same movements used for specific joint mobilization techniques are used as examination maneuvers. (see Chapter 7, Joint Mobilization Techniques).
    2. Assess
        a. Amplitude of movement: hypomobile–normal–hypermobile
        b. Irritability: pain–protective muscle spasm.

IV. **Neuromuscular Tests**
    A. If a neurologic deficit is suspected at this point in the exam, it may be appropriate to perform sensory, motor, reflex, and coordination tests (see Chapter 4).
    B. Most chronic joint conditions result in some weakness of muscles controlling the joint because of disuse and reflex inhibition. At the hip some muscle groups are so powerful that mild or even moderate weakness may not be detected by manual muscle testing. Even if detected, manual testing does not permit documentation of the extent of weakness (or strength). For this reason, it is best to test each of the major muscle groups controlling the hip—abductors, adductors, flexors, and extensors—by determining the number of repetitions that can be performed against a constant load, for example, by determining the 10 RM (repetition maximum). This allows for comparison to a "normal" side or predetermined norm, and for documentation of a baseline.

V. **Palpation**
    A. *Skin.* Palpate hip girdles and lower extremities (usually noncontributory in local lesions at or

about the hip because of heavy soft tissue covering).

1. Temperature
2. Moisture
3. Tenderness
4. Texture
5. Mobility

B. *Soft tissue*
   1. Mobility and consistency
   2. Swelling (joint effusion usually cannot be palpated at the hip)
   3. Tenderness
      a. There may be localized tenderness anteriorly if the iliopectineal bursa is inflamed or distended. It may be distended with joint effusion since it often communicates with the joint.[25]
      b. There may be localized tenderness laterally if the trochanteric bursa is inflamed.
      c. There may be areas of referred tenderness (so-called trigger points) in the related segments (L2–S1) in the presence of a lesion affecting any of the deep somatic tissues at or about the hip.

C. *Bony structures* (see under Inspection)

COMMON LESIONS

DEGENERATIVE JOINT DISEASE (DJD) (OSTEOARTHROSIS)

Degenerative joint disease at the hip often progresses to a point at which it results in significant disability. This is true at the hip more so than at any other joint. Clinically, persons with DJD of the hip frequently present to out-patient health care services because of pain and disability. Symptomatic DJD is the most common disease process affecting the hip.

The etiology of DJD of the hip varies from patient to patient. In a considerable number of people with this problem, the etiology is not entirely clear. While age is an important factor, the pathologic process of DJD is not a result of tissue changes with aging *per se*. In fact, the cartilaginous changes occuring with normal aging are seen first in the "nonarticular" areas of cartilage, whereas changes found in DJD are seen first in those areas of cartilage undergoing most frequent contact, for example, during weight bearing.[1,2,4,5,14,15,21,24] DJD is a disease of older people, because it takes a considerable length of time to cause the fatigue of tissue, such as fibrillation of articular cartilage, that is characteristic of the disease.

The asymptomic changes occurring with normal aging of articular cartilage probably result from a nutritional deficiency; the areas of cartilage not undergoing frequent intermittent compression do not undergo the absorption and squeezing out of synovial fluid necessary for adequate nutrition. This is especially true in older persons, because they tend to use their joints less frequently and through smaller ranges of movement.

The degenerative tissue changes that occur with symptomatic DJD are usually reactions to increased stress to the joint over time.[4,5,15,16,19] The tissue changes may be of a "compensatory" hypertrophic nature, such as the bony proliferation that typically occurs at the joint margins and subchondral bone or capsular fibrosis. They may also be of an atrophic nature, such as the fatigue of cartilaginous collagen fibers or the degradation of cartilage ground substance (proteoglycan). Perhaps the most disputed issue with respect to pathogenesis is whether the first tissue changes occur in the subchondral bone or in the articular cartilage. It is generally accepted, however, that regardless of which tissue changes take place first, (*1*) they take place first and foremost in the regions undergoing greatest stress with normal activities, and (2) changes in subchondral bone will, over time, result in changes in articular cartilage, and *vice versa*.[21,23] It must be emphasized at this point that normal attenuation of forces applied to a joint is dependent upon the elastic properties of subchondral bone as well as those of articular cartilage. If stresses are not normally attenuated in one of these tissues, the other will undergo increased stresses.[18,19] Thus, with subchondral bony sclerosis, the overlying articular cartilage undergoes increased stress as the subchondral bone becomes stiffer and less elastic. With fibrillation and softening of articular cartilage, increased stress is transmitted to the subchondral bone. Such abnormal stresses will inevitably lead to progression of the process (see Chapter 2, Arthrology). It is interesting to note the difference in eventual reaction to increased stress between subchondral bone and articular cartilage; subchondral bone becomes more dense (sclerotic), whereas articular cartilage breaks down. This difference reflects the differences in vascularity and regenerative capacities of the two tissues.

If we accept that in many, if not most, cases of DJD the pathogenesis is closely related to increased stress to joint tissues over time—or fatigue—we must look at conditions that may predispose the joint to increased stresses as possibly contributing to the etiology of DJD. Perhaps the most important condition at the hip to consider in this regard is congenital hip dysplasia (CHD).[2,7,15] A deficient acetabular roof and increased femoral anteversion angle are common sequellae of this condition. The resultant decrease in effective weight-bearing surface area at the joint predisposes the posterosuperolateral femoral head and superolateral acetabulum to early degenerative changes. Residual structural changes in joint components that may follow osteochondrosis or slipped femoral capital epiphysis—both of which affect younger people—may have similar effects.[16]

It is also suggested that leg length disparity may be a factor in predisposing to unilateral DJD of the hip on the side of the longer leg.[6,8] In the standing position, the pelvic obliquity produced by the leg length discrepancy would cause the long limb to assume a position of relative adduction with respect to the acetabulum. The increased adduction angulation on weight bearing results in an increased joint incongruence, causing greater stress to the lateral roof of the acetabulum. In addition, the center of gravity is shifted toward the short-leg side, increasing the moment arm about which the force of the superincumbent body weight acts at the supporting femoral head on the long-leg side (see section on biomechanics). A greater pull by the abductors on the long side then, is, required to prevent the pelvis from dropping to the short side during stance on the long side. This would increase the vertical compressive force acting at the femoral head during weight bearing on the long-leg side.

Another condition with which we must be concerned, as far as its potential to contribute to the acceleration of hip degeneration, is capsular tightness.[2,12,17] Traditionally, capsular tightness has been regarded to be more a *result* of rather than a *cause* of hip degeneration. While this is undoubtedly so, we must consider (1) the role that capsular tightening may play in accelerating the progression of the disease, and (2) what role capsular tightening may play in some cases in actually initiating the degenerative process. The hip, unlike the shoulder, is a joint that is continually brought close to its close-packed position during normal functional activities, such as walking. With every step, at push off, the hip is brought into a position of extension, internal rotation, and abduction, taking up most of the slack in the joint capsule by twisting the capsule upon itself.

This twisting of the capsule effects a compression of the joint surfaces. The compression force is normally in addition to, but acts after, the peak vertical compressive force of weight bearing. In other words, the peak compressive loading due to capsular twisting is normally not superimposed upon that of weight bearing, but rather, these forces are successively applied to the joint during the stance phase.[15,17] This is in accordance with the viscoelastic property of articular cartilage, which favors gradual loading over time as opposed to quick "shock-loading" with respect to its ability to attenuate compressive forces.[18,19,20] If, however, for whatever reason, the hip joint capsule loses extensibility, the slack will be taken up in the joint capsule sooner and the joint surfaces will become *prematurely* approximated during walking. This premature approximation causes the peak compressive loading from capsular twisting to become closer to being superimposed upon the peak compressive loading of weight bearing. It causes a greater magnitude of compressive forces to be applied to the articular cartilage over a shorter period of time, approximating a situation of shock-loading. Certain studies suggest that shock-loading, even more than loss of normal lubrication, is one of the most important factors in fatigue of articular cartilage.[20] It should also be recognized that symptoms of pain on weight bearing in the presence of hip DJD are not due to compressive forces *per se*, but result from strain to the capsuloligamentous structures as they pull prematurely tight with each step. (You will recall that articular cartilage is aneural.) Such capsular pain is enhanced by the low-grade capsular inflammation that tends to develop as the disease progresses.[2] Studies in which compressive forces have been calculated in degenerated hips before surgery and then determined after total hip arthroplasty suggest that such surgery does reduce the "flexor moment" acting at the hip from a tight capsule.[17] This may explain the often dramatic symptomatic improvement enjoyed by these patients soon after operation. In view of the above discussion, it seems that a major goal of conservative management in the earlier stages of hip DJD should be prevention and reduction of capsular tightening of the joint. Such an approach, in addition to providing symptomatic improvement, may help to slow the acceleration of the degenerative process; the effective weight-bearing surface area of cartilage is increased, and shock-loading is decreased.

We must also consider long-standing obesity as a possible contributing factor in accelerated degenerative changes at the hip. Because of the moment arm about which the force of gravity on the body weight acts at the femoral head during stance phase, *an additional 3 pounds* may act at the supporting femoral head for each added pound of body weight.

I. **History**

    A. *Onset of symptoms.* The patient is usually a middle-aged or older person who describes an insidious onset of groin or trochanteric pain. The pain is first noticed after use of the joint, such as long periods of walking, hiking, or running. The patient may relate some childhood hip problem or an old injury, but more often does not.

    B. *Site of pain.* The pain is typically felt first in the groin area. As the problem progresses, the pain is more likely to be referred further into the L2 or L3 segment, to the anterior thigh and knee. Later, other segments may become involved, with pain felt laterally and posteriorly. An occasional patient presents with a primary complaint of knee pain. This is because both the knee and the hip are largely derived embryologically from the same segment. Rarely is pain referred to below the knee in a person with only hip joint disease.

C. *Nature of pain.* The pain is noticed first at the end of the day, after considerable use of the joint; relief is obtained by rest. Later, as some low-grade inflammation develops, the patient notices some morning stiffness. At this point, pain and stiffness are noticed when getting up from sitting; the pain largely subsides after several steps (after "getting the joint loosened up"), then returns again after walking a certain distance. As the degeneration becomes more advanced, some constant aching may be noticed. The pain is increased by any amount of walking, and the patient is frequently awakened with pain at night.

With progressive capsular tightness, the patient first notices some difficulty squatting, for instance, when picking up an object from the ground. Gradually, it becomes more difficult to put on stockings and tie shoes. The ability to climb stairs may be lost in the later stages, and the patient may be able to ambulate only with the assistance of canes or crutches. Some discomfort with sitting may develop as hip flexion becomes restricted.

II. Physical Examination

A. *Observation*
  1. The patient may hesitate or have difficulty rising from sitting and initiating ambulation.
  2. An "abductor" limp will be noticed in moderate to advanced cases.
  3. The patient may have some difficulty removing shoes, socks, and slacks.
  4. Note use of aids.

B. *Inspection*
  1. Some localized (abductor or gluteal) or generalized atrophy may be noticed on the involved side. Document thigh girth, if appropriate.
  2. If significant adduction and flexion contractures are present, the patient may tend to stand with the heel raised, the hip and knee flexed, and the pelvis elevated on the involved side.
  3. If a flexion contracture and adduction contracture are present, and the patient stands with both feet flat and knees extended, the lumbar spine will be in some hyperlordosis, the pelvis will be shifted laterally toward the involved side (noticed in plumb-bob alignment), and the spine will be functionally scoliotic so as to bring the upper trunk back to the midline.
  4. Assess levels of bony landmarks for leg length equality. If unequal, attempt to determine the source of the discrepancy.
      a. Cartilagenous narrowing—Compare clinical to radiographic findings.
      b. Coxa vara/coxa valga—Malleoli, fibular heads, and trochanters are level. PSISs, ASISs, and iliac crests are lower on the varus side, higher on the valgus side. Coxa vara is often associated with retroversion; coxa valga is usually associated with increased anteversion. In coxa vara, the trochanter lies above Néla-ton's line; in coxa valga, it lies below. Compare clinical findings to radiographs.

c. Short femoral shaft—Malleoli, fibular heads, and popliteal folds are level. The greater trochanter and pelvic landmarks are lower on the short side.

d. Short tibia—The malleoli are level. The popliteal folds, fibular heads, and tibial tubercles are lower on the short side.

C. *Selective tissue tension tests*

1. Active movements

   a. Assess functional activities

      i. Squatting—Usually unable to perform in moderate to advanced cases

      ii. One-legged stance—Pelvis will drop to opposite side if abductors are significantly weak (positive Trendelenburg sign).

      iii. Stair climbing—May be restricted in advanced cases

      iv. Sit and bend forward—Usually painful or restricted

   b. Note ability to perform, pain, and crepitus.

2. Passive movements

   a. Limited in a capsular pattern of restriction

      i. May be limited by pain and spasm—acute.

      ii. May be limited by soft-tissue restriction and discomfort—chronic

   b. Note pain, crepitus, ROM, and end-feel.

3. Resisted movements—Strong and painless

4. Joint play movements

   a. Hypomobility of all joint play movements

   b. Note whether they are restricted by pain and spasm or by soft-tissue restriction.

D. *Neuromuscular tests*

1. If at this point a possible coexistent spinal lesion is suspected, motor, sensory, and reflex testing, in addition to other tests, may be warranted.

2. You may wish to assess the patient's "balance," (*e.g.,* one-legged standing with eyes closed) since this is often affected owing to alteration in afferent input from the joint capsule receptors and controlling muscles.

3. Mild to even moderate muscle weakness of the large muscle groups controlling the hip must be tested by heavy, repetitive loading. Weakness, especially of the abductors, will be found in all but minor cases.

E. *Palpation*

1. Often noncontributory

2. Possibly some warmth noted anteriorly

3. Usually some tenderness anteriorly, over trochanter, and buttock. Possibly some "trigger points" of referred tenderness elsewhere in the thigh.

F. *Other*

1. Obtain a radiographic report for comparison to clinical findings. However, early DJD can be detected clinically before radiographs show positive findings, and rather extensive changes may show on radiographs in the absence of significant symptoms.

2. Because of the loss of hip extension that is characteristic of DJD and the compensatory hyperlordosis that develops when standing, these patients are predisposed to developing back problems. A back evaluation may be warranted.

III. Management. The approach to management of patients with hip DJD will, of course, depend upon the stage of the disease as determined by the extent of the lesion and the degree of disability. For the sake of discussion we might distinguish between early and advanced cases as follows:

Early
—Pain is noticed only with fatigue.
—There is only mild limitation of internal rotation, extension, and abduction associated with pain at the extremes of these movements.
—The patient walks with little or no limp.

Advanced
—There is some constant aching; the patient is often awakened at night; there is considerable morning stiffness.
—Motion is markedly limited in a capsular pattern.
—Ambulation is performed with a marked limp or with the use of aids (canes or crutches).

The above criteria, of course, reflect the two extremes; many patients presenting with symptoms and signs fall somewhere between these. Note also that information from radiographs is not included as a criterion, since it cannot be reliably correlated to symptoms, signs, degree of disability, or prognosis.

The major difficulty facing the physical therapist with respect to management of these patients is that we rarely see the patient with *mild* DJD of the hip—and this is the patient to whom we ultimately have the most to offer. The reason for this is twofold: (*1*) considerable progression of the disease may ensue before the patient experiences sufficient pain or disability to warrant seeking medical help, and (*2*) physicians often do not refer patients with symptoms and signs of early DJD to physical therapists because therapists in the past have not met their potential in managing these patients. Too often the patient is issued a cane and advised to return if the condition worsens, at which time surgical intervention may be indicated.

A. *Management in the early stages of DJD*
1. Goals
   a. Restoration of normal joint mechanics
   b. Prevention of further progression of the disease— capsular tightness or other possible causes of increased stress to the joint.
2. Therapeutic procedures
   a. Restore normal capsular mobility with joint mobilization and active and active-assisted range of motion program. Ultrasound should be helpful in increasing capsular mobility when used during or prior to mobilization procedures.
   b. Restore normal muscle strength with progressive resistive exercise program. Emphasize especially abductor strengthening.
   c. ROM exercises to be done indefinitely, instruction in appropriate levels, and other measures to minimize compressive stress to the hip
   d. Attempt to determine if there is some underlying biomechanical or constitutional factor that may predispose the joint to abnormal stresses
      i. Obesity. For each additional pound of body weight, an additional 3

lbs. are applied to each hip joint during stance phase of normal walking. Although few physical therapists are qualified to institute a weight-loss program, you should be prepared to direct the patient to the appropriate services, upon agreement by the physician. A general conditioning program may be supervised by the therapist as an adjunct to a weight-loss program. The patient must be shown simple exercises to help maintain hip range of motion to be done indefinitely on a regular basis.

ii. Leg-length disparity. As mentioned, inequality of leg length may be a factor in development of DJD on the long-leg side. Gradual, serial elevation of the heel and sole on the uninvolved (short) side, by ¼ inch at a time, may be indicated, along with regular range of motion exercises.

iii. Congenital hip dysplasia and epiphysiolysis (slipped capital epiphysis). These conditions both result in permanent structural abnormalities that often lead to increased stress to joint surfaces at the superolateral aspect of the hip joint. Some increased congruity of joint surfaces may be achieved by elevating the heel and sole of the shoe on the uninvolved side in unilateral cases. This places the involved hip in a relative position of abduction as well as automatically shifting the center of gravity line closer to the involved hip so as to reduce the moment arm about which it acts during stance phase on the involved side.

Since these patients are more or less permanently predisposed to accelerated degenerative changes, they should be encouraged to avoid activities that may be particularly stressful to the hip. Jogging and long-distance walking should be abandoned in favor of swimming and non-weight-bearing exercises. For patients whose regular activities involve considerable walking, alternative modes of travel and perhaps use of a cane should be encouraged.

These people especially must maintain good strength and motion at their hips for maximal stabilization and maximal distribution of weight-bearing forces over joint surfaces.

B. *Management in moderate to advanced stages.* Unfortunately, the patient is often given the impression that he must simply wait until the disease progresses to a point at which surgery is indicated. Accordingly, the patient is often not referred to rehabilitative services, again because we have not demonstrated in the past that we have much to offer these patients. When they are referred to physical therapy, it is often simply for instruction in the use of a cane.

Our approach to management of these patients must be more comprehensive and more vigorous. Surgery becomes inevitable unless appropriate measures are taken in the early or moderate stages of the disease. Even so, we may simply be delaying a potentially inevitable event. But we must consider that these patients are usually middle-aged or older, and that if progression of the disease can be retarded and a satisfactory level of function maintained, the patient may very well live out his life without undergoing major surgery.

1. Goals
   a. Restoration of function to optimal level
   b. Restoration of joint mechanics to optimal level
2. Therapeutic procedures
   a. Instruct the patient in the use of the appropriate walking aid to reduce compressive loading at the hip, to relieve pain on ambulation, and to increase ambulation endurance.
   b. A raised toilet seat may be desirable.
   c. The patient may be made aware of special adaptations in shoe fasteners and devices to assist in taking on and off shoes and socks. In this regard, an occupational therapist can be of assistance.
   d. The use of other adaptive aids and devices should be instituted insofar as they may assist the patient in the ability to perform daily activities with less pain or difficulty.
   e. Primary considerations in regard to improving joint mechanics include increasing capsular extensibility and increasing the strength of the muscles controlling the hip. The basic program is outlined above under management in the early stages. In moderate or advanced stages, however, the joint is likely to be more "irritable," in that motion will tend to be limited more by pain and muscle spasm than by a pure capsular restriction. For this reason, progression of the mobilization program must often proceed more slowly. In addition, at some point in more advanced cases, motion in some planes may reach a point at which it is restricted by bony impingement because of the bony hypertrophic changes that are characteristic of the disease.

In most respects, the approach to management of these patients should closely resemble that of patients with a frozen shoulder, the primary differences being the functional considerations and the concern for reduction of compressive forces in patients with hip disease. However, there is no reason not to proceed with an intensive mobilization and strengthening program in cases of capsular hip restriction, as we do routinely with patients with capsular tightness at the shoulder. Remember that it is the tight capsule in cases of DJD at the hip that is a primary source of the patient's pain; it is a chief factor in intensifying and localizing compressive forces at the hip joint during walking.

TROCHANTERIC BURSITIS

This is one of the few other common musculoskeletal disorders affecting the hip region for which patients are often referred to physical therapy.

I. History
  A. *Onset.* The onset is usually insidious. Occasionally an acute onset is described in association with a particular activity, such as getting out of a car, during which a "snap" is felt at the lateral or posterolateral hip region. Presumably such an incident involves a snapping of a portion of the iliotibial band over the trochanter, with mechanical irritation of the intervening bursa.
  B. *Site of pain.* The pain is felt primarily over the lateral hip region. It tends to radiate distally into the L5 segment; the patient describes pain over the lateral aspect of the thigh to the knee and occasionally into the lower leg. Some patients also experience pain referred into the lumbosacral region on the side of involvement. This pain pattern closely resembles that of an L5 spinal lesion,

which is a more common disorder than trochanteric bursitis. You must differentiate by means of careful examination.
  C. *Nature of pain.* The pain is aggravated most by ascending stairs—the strongly contracting gluteus maximus causing compression of the inflamed bursa—and by rolling onto the involved side at night. Indeed, the greatest complaint is often that of being awakened at night with pain. The pain is a deep, aching, "scleratogenous" pain rather than the sharp, lancinating, dermatomal pain characteristic of L5 nerve root irritation.

II. Physical Examination
  A. *Observation.* Usually noncontributory. The lesion is not severe enough to cause a limp.
  B. *Inspection.* Usually noncontributory. If the iliotibial band is tight, the patient may stand with the pelvis shifted laterally, away from the involved side on mediolateral plumb-bob assessment, with perhaps some increased valgus of the knee on the involved side.
  C. *Selective tissue tension tests*
    1. Active movements. No functional limitations
    2. Passive movements
      a. Full passive abduction may hurt from squeezing of the bursa between the trochanter and the lateral aspect of the pelvis.
      b. A special test that often reproduces the pain is placement of the hip into full passive flexion combined with adduction and internal rotation. This compresses the inflamed bursa beneath the stretched gluteus maximus.

c. An "Ober test" may reveal iliotibial band tightness.
3. Resisted movements
   a. Resisted abduction will reproduce the pain by squeezing the bursa beneath the strongly contracting gluteals.
   b. Resisted extension and resisted external rotation may hurt if the bursa underlying the gluteus maximus is involved.
4. Joint play movements. Normal mobility and painless
D. *Neuromuscular exam.* Noncontributory
E. *Palpation.* A discrete point of tenderness will be found over the site of the lesion, usually over the posterolateral aspect of the greater trochanter. Other areas of referred tenderness are often found elsewhere in the L5 segment, usually over the lateral aspect of the thigh. No increased temperature can be detected.

III. **Management**
A. *Goals*
   1. Resolution of the chronic inflamatory process
   2. Prevention of recurrence
B. *Techniques*
   1. Temporarily avoiding continued irritation to the bursa
      a. Arranging pillows so as to avoid rolling onto the painful side
      b. Avoiding climbing stairs and long walks
      c. Ultrasound to the site of the lesion. This is a condition for which ultrasound is often dramatically effective over a course of three to six sessions. The increase in blood flow apparently assists in the resolution of the inflammatory process.

2. A tight iliotibial band may be the cause of or the result of the disorder. Full mobility of the iliotibial band should be restored as the condition resolves. Be sure that good muscle strength of the gluteals is restored, as they may weaken in long-standing cases.

ILIOPECTINEAL BURSITIS

This is somewhat more rare than trochanteric bursitis. It presents in a similar manner, but resisted hip flexion and full passive hip extension reproduce the pain. The onset is insidious. The pain is felt most in the groin, with a tendency toward radiation into the L2 or L3 segment. Since this bursa often communicates with the joint, ascertain whether involvement of the bursa is a manifestation of hip joint effusion by checking for a capsular pattern of pain or restriction.

Management of patients with iliopectineal bursitis should follow the same approach as outlined above for trochanteric bursitis.

REFERENCES

1. Barnett CH: Effects of age on articular cartilage. Res Rev 4:183, 1963
2. Cameron HU, MacNab I: Observations on osteoarthritis of the hip joint. Clin Orthop 108:31–40, 1975
3. Dee R: Mechanoreceptors of the hip joint capsule and their reflex contribution to posture. In Symposium on Osteoarthritis, pp 52–65. St Louis, CV Mosby, 1976
4. Freeman MAR: The fatigue of cartilage in the pathogenesis of osteoarthritis. Acta Orthop Scand 46:323, 1975
5. Gofton JP: Studies in osteoarthritis of the hip, I, Classification. Can Med Assoc J 104:679–683, 1971
6. Gofton JP: Studies in osteoarthritis of the hip, II, Osteoarthritis of the hip and leg length disparity. Can Med Assoc J 104:791–799, 1971

7. Gofton JP: Studies in osteoarthritis of the hip, III, Congenital subluxation and osteoarthritis of the hip. Can Med Assoc J 104:911–915

8. Gofton JP: Studies in osteoarthritis of the hip, IV, Biomechanics and clinical considerations. Can Med Assoc J 104:1007–1011

9. Hoagland FT: Osteoarthritis. Orthop Clin North Am 2(1):3–19, 1971

10. Inman VT: Functional aspects of the abductor muscles of the hip. J Bone Joint Surg 29(A):607–619, 1947

11. Lissner HR, Williams M: Biomechanics of Human Motion, pp 44–45. Philadelphia, WB Saunders, 1962

12. Lloyd–Roberts GC: The role of capsular changes in osteoarthritis of the hip joint. J Bone Joint Surg 35(B):627–642, 1953

13. Mankin HJ: Biochemical and metabolic aspects of osteoarthritis. Orthop Clin North Am 2(1):19–31, 1971

14. Mankin HJ: Biochemical changes in articular cartilage in osteoarthritis. In: Symposium on Osteoarthritis, pp 1–23. St Louis, CV Mosby, 1976

15. Morris JM: Biomechanical aspects of the hip joint. Orthop Clin North Am 2(1):33–55, 1971

16. Murray RO, Duncan C: Athletic activity in adolescence as an etiological factor in degeneration hip disease. J Bone Joint Surg 53(B):406–419, 1971

17. Paul JP: Forces transmitted at the hip and knee joint of normal and disabled persons during a range of activities. Acta Orthop Belg (Suppl) 41(1):78–88, 1975

18. Radin EL, Paul IL: Does cartilage compliance reduce skeletal impact loads? Arth Rheum 13(2):138, 1970

19. Radin EL, Paul IL: The mechanics of joints as it relates to their degeneration. In: Symposium on Osteoarthritis, pp 34–44. St Louis, CV Mosby, 1976

20. Radin EL, Paul IL: Response of joints to impact loading. Arth Rheum 14:356, 1971

21. Reiman I, Mankin HJ: Quantitative histological analysis of articular cartilage and subchondral bone from osteoarthritic and normal human hips. Acta Orthop Scand 48(1):121, 1977

22. Rydell N: Forces acting on the femoral head prosthesis: A study on strain guage supplied prostheses in living persons. Acta Orthop Scand (Suppl) 88:1–132, 1966

23. Sokoloff LS: The general pathology of osteoarthritis. In: Symposium on Osteoarthritis, pp 23–34. St Louis, CV Mosby, 1976

24. Vignon E, Arlot M, Meunier P, Vignon G: Quantitative histological changes in osteoarthritic hip cartilage. Clin Orthop 0(103):269–278, 1974

25. Warren R, Kaye JJ, Saluati EA: Arthrographic demonstration of an enlarged iliopsoas bursa complicating osteoarthritis of the hip: A case report. J Bone Joint Surg 57(A):413, 1975

17 *The Knee*

Randolph M. Kessler

REVIEW OF FUNCTIONAL ANATOMY

OSTEOLOGY

The distal end of the femur consists of two large condyles, separated posteriorly by the very deep intercondylar notch and anteriorly by the patellar groove in which the patella glides. The anterior condylar surface is referred to as the *trochlear surface of the femur*.

Looking anteriorly (Fig. 17-1), the medial condyle extends farther distally than does the lateral condyle, so that when standing with the distal surfaces of the condyles level, the femur and tibia form a valgus angle of about 10°. Both condyles have epicondyles extending from their sides. Medially, the adductor tubercle lies just superior to the medial epicondyle. The articular cartilage extends farther superiorly on the anterior surface of the lateral condyle than it does on the same aspect of the medial condyle.

Looking inferiorly (Fig. 17-2), the articular surface of the distal femur forms a U about the deep intercondylar notch. The lateral condyle extends considerably farther anteriorly than does the medial condyle, helping to prevent lateral dislocation of the patella due to a horizontal component of the direction of quadriceps pull. The medial condyle angles backward and medially. The lateral condyle lies in the sagittal plane.

Looking medially or laterally (Fig. 17-3), the condyles do not describe part of a cir-

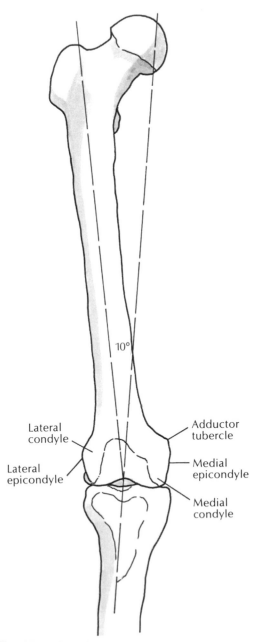

Fig. 17-1. Anterior view of the right femur

Lateral condyle

Lateral epicondyle

Adductor tubercle

Medial epicondyle

Medial condyle

10°

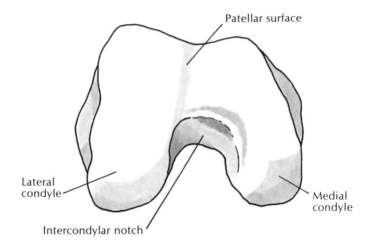

Fig. 17-2. Inferior aspect of the distal end of femur

Fig. 17-3. (*A*) Medial and (*B*) lateral aspects of distal end of the right femur

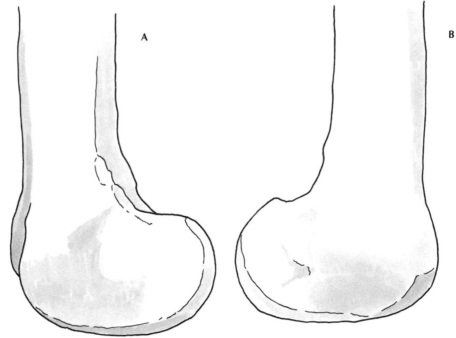

cle, but rather, their radius gradually decreases from anterior to posterior. The medial condyle is longer anteroposteriorly, with a more gradual change in radius from back to front. The small lateral condyle tends to flatten sooner, as one follows the curvature from back to front. The difference in the two condyles plays a part in the length rotation and locking

mechanism of the knee, as discussed in the section on biomechanics.

The upper end of the tibia (Fig. 17-4), consists of two large condyles with articular surfaces superiorly for articulation with the femur. Both condyles are offset posteriorly to overhang the tibial shaft. They are also angulated 5° to 10° downward anteroposteriorly. The medial tibial

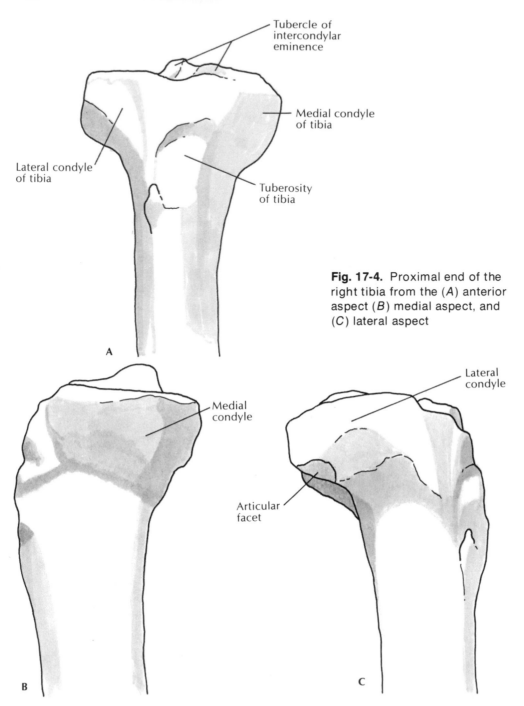

Fig. 17-4. Proximal end of the right tibia from the (A) anterior aspect (B) medial aspect, and (C) lateral aspect

condyle is larger; its superior surface is concave in all directions. The smaller lateral tibial condyle is actually convex anteroposteriorly. However, the lateral meniscus forms a concave articular surface for articulation with the convex lateral femoral condyle. Posterolaterally on the lateral tibial condyle is an articular facet for the head of the fibula, which faces somewhat downward. At the anterior-inferior junction of the tibial condyles is the tibial tuberosity, an eminence onto which the patellar tendon inserts. Superiorly, between the condyles, is the roughened intercondylar area. The medial and lateral intercondylar tubercles, or eminences, lie centrally in the intercondylar area.

The patella (Fig. 17-5) is a triangular sesamoid bone, its apex lying inferiorly, embedded in the back of the quadriceps tendon. The posterior surface of the patella is cartilage-covered for articulation in the patellar groove of the femur, between the femoral condyles. The patellar articular surface consists of a lateral facet, a medial facet, and a small odd medial facet. The patella gives extra purchase to the quadriceps tendon in producing knee extension, especially toward the limits of extension.

MENISCI

The medial meniscus is semicircular, being larger posteriorly than anteriorly. Its anterior horn inserts onto the intercondylar area of the tibia, in front of the attachment of the anterior cruciate ligament, and its posterior horn inserts in front of the attachment of the posterior cruciate ligament. Peripherally, it is attached to the joint capsule, the short capsular fibers of the medial collateral ligament, and to the outer margin of the superior aspect of the medial tibial condyle by the coronary ligament. The coronary ligament constitutes the inferior aspect of the joint capsule (Fig. 17-6).

While the medial meniscus forms part of a larger circle, the lateral meniscus forms almost all of a smaller circle. Its two horns attach quite close to each other, just in front of and just behind the intercondylar eminence. The periphery of the lateral meniscus attaches to the tibia, the capsule, and a coronary ligament, but not to the lateral collateral ligament. The lateral meniscus is more mobile than the medial meniscus, owing to its shape and less extensive peripheral attachments. A ligament usually runs from the posterior aspect of the lateral meniscus to the medial condyle of the femur. This meniscofemoral ligament runs behind the posterior cruciate, while another may run in front (Fig. 17-7). The popliteus tendon also attaches to the lateral meniscus; the attachment is said to assist in posterior movement of the meniscus during knee flexion.[24] Usually a transverse ligament connects the two menisci anteriorly.

LIGAMENTS

The medial collateral ligament is a long flat band attached above to the medial epicondyle and below to the medial aspect of the shaft of the tibia, about 4 cm below the joint line (Fig. 17-8). Its fibers run somewhat anteriorly, from top to bottom. Older descriptions often refer to *deep, shorter fibers* and *posterior oblique fibers* of the medial collateral ligaments. These are both considered part of the joint capsule (see below) in the more recent literature.[18,50] The deep capsular fibers are attached to the medial meniscus.

The medial collateral ligament becomes tight on extension of the knee, abduction of the tibia on femur, and outward rotation of the tibia on femur. Some of the anterior fibers become tight on knee flexion. The medial collateral also helps prevent anterior displacement of the tibia on the femur.

The lateral collateral ligament is a shorter, round bundle of fibers running from the lateral epicondyle to the fibular head (Fig. 17-9). It does not attach to the lateral meniscus. The popliteus tendon runs underneath the ligament between it and the meniscus. The lateral collateral is largely covered by the tendon of the biceps femoris. The lateral ligament runs slightly posteriorly from top to bottom and is tight on extension of the knee, adduction of the tibia on the femur, and outward rotation of the tibia on the femur.

The anterior cruciate ligament runs from the anterior intercondylar area of the tibia backward, upward, and laterally to

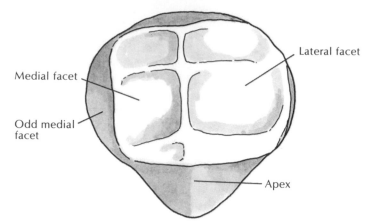

Medial facet

Odd medial
facet

Lateral facet

Apex

Fig. 17-5. Posterior aspect of the
right patella

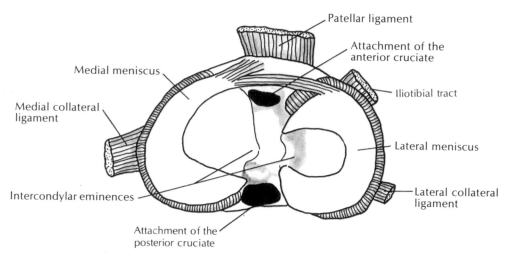

Patellar ligament

Attachment of the
anterior cruciate

Medial meniscus

Iliotibial tract

Medial collateral
ligament

Lateral meniscus

Intercondylar eminences

Lateral collateral
ligament

Attachment of the
posterior cruciate

Fig. 17-6. The superior aspect of the right tibia, showing the menisci and
tibial attachments of the cruciate ligaments

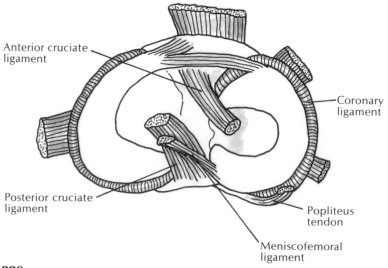

Fig. 17-7. Superior aspect
of the right tibia, showing
the ligaments

Anterior cruciate
ligament

Coronary
ligament

Posterior cruciate
ligament

Popliteus
tendon

Meniscofemoral
ligament

398

the medial aspect of the lateral femoral condyle in the intercondylar notch (Fig. 17-7). It acts primarily to check extension of the knee, forward movement of the tibia on the femur, and internal rotation of the tibia on femur. Since the anterior cruciate ligament pulls tight on internal tibial rotation and as the knee extends, some have proposed that this ligament guides the tibia into outward rotation during knee extension.[37]

The posterior cruciate ligament runs from the extreme posterior intercondylar area of the tibia forward, medially, and upward to the lateral aspect of the medial femoral condyle in the intercondylar notch (Fig. 17-7). It primarily checks backward movement of the tibia on the femur and helps check internal rotation of the tibia on the femur. It also tightens on full knee extension, although some fibers may be tight throughout the range of flexion–extension of the knee. It is aided by the popliteus muscle in checking forward sliding of the femur on tibia when squatting.

The patellofemoral ligament is a thickening of the patellar retinaculum. It passes from the adductor tubercle of the femur to the medial aspect of the patella. Its femoral attachment often becomes irritated and tender in cases of patellofemoral tracking dysfunction.

A fibrous capsule surrounds the knee joint, attaching at the margins of articular cartilage. The superior aspect of the capsule runs from the articular margin of the femur to the periphery of the menisci. The inferior fibers run a short distance from the menisci to the tibia. The inferior capsule is often called the coronary ligament.

The fibrous capsule receives extensive passive and dynamic reinforcement (Figs. 17-8 and 17-9). Passive reinforcement is provided by the above-mentioned ligaments and by what are referred to in older texts as the *deep layer* and *posterior oblique fibers* of the medial collateral ligament. These are thickenings of medial and posteromedial aspects of the joint capsule that provide added stabilization against valgus and external rotatory stresses. The posterior oblique fibers are now referred to as simply the *posteromedial capsule*. The short capsular fibers deep to the medial collateral ligament are attached to the medial meniscus. There are also some thickenings of the capsule posteriorly, referred to as the *oblique* and *arcuate popliteal ligaments*.

Dynamic capsular reinforcement is provided to all aspects of the joint capsule. Anterior reinforcement is provided by the patellar tendon, inferiorly, and quadriceps tendon, superiorly. These can be said to constitute the anterior capsule, since a fibrous capsule *per se* is absent anteriorly. Anteromedial and anterolateral reinforcement are provided by the medial and lateral patellar retinacula, which are superficial to, and may blend with, the fibrous capsule. These help stabilize the patellofemoral joint during loaded knee extension.

The distal aspect of the iliotibial band provides anterolateral reinforcement. This stabilizes against excessive internal rotation of the tibia on the femur and thus works in conjunction with the cruciates.

The pes anserinus tendons (semitendinosus, gracilis, and sartorius) and the semimembranosus tendon give medial and posteromedial reinforcement. These help prevent abnormal external rotation, abduction, and anterior displacement of the tibia on the femur. In doing so they dynamically reinforce the medial collateral ligament, the posteromedial capsule, and, to a certain extent, the anterior cruciate ligament.

Posterolateral support comes from the biceps femoris tendon. This helps check excessive internal rotation and anterior displacement of the tibia on the femur, providing reinforcement to the functions of the cruciates. It also may assist the lateral collateral ligament in preventing adduction of the tibia on the femur.

Finally, posterior reinforcement is provided by the insertions of the gastroc-

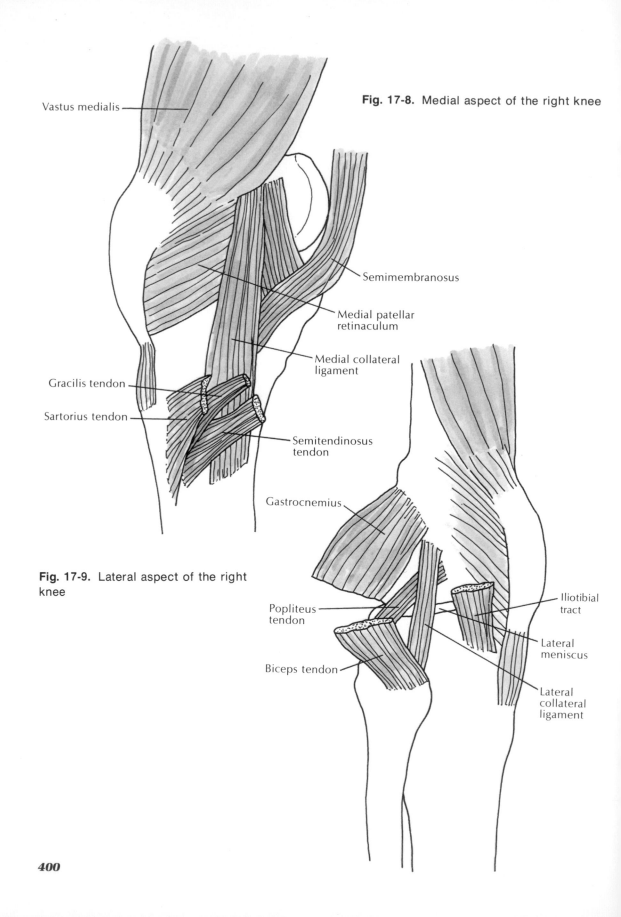

Vastus medialis

Fig. 17-8. Medial aspect of the right knee

Semimembranosus

Medial patellar retinaculum

Medial collateral ligament

Gracilis tendon

Sartorius tendon

Semitendinosus tendon

Gastrocnemius

Fig. 17-9. Lateral aspect of the right knee

Popliteus tendon

Biceps tendon

Iliotibial tract

Lateral meniscus

Lateral collateral ligament

nemius muscles and from the popliteus muscle. The popliteus helps check external rotation of the tibia on the femur and backward displacement of the tibia on the femur.

BURSAE, SYNOVIA, AND FAT PADS

The synovium of the knee joint, in addition to lining the fibrous capsule, forms several large recesses (Fig. 17-10). Anteroinferiorly, it extends inward to line the back of the infrapatellar fat pad. The medial and lateral aspects of this lining unite centrally to form the ligamentatum mucosa that extends into the joint to attach to the intercondylar notch of the femur. Anterosuperiorly, the synovium runs from the superior aspect of the patella upward beneath the quadriceps

tendon, then folds back on itself to form a pouch, and inserts on the distal femur above the condyles. This suprapatellar pouch is part of the joint cavity and provides sufficient slack in the synovium to allow full knee flexion. Posteriorly, the synovium invaginates into the intercondylar notch to pass in front of the cruciate ligaments. In this way the cruciates are intracapsular but extrasynovial.

In addition to the suprapatellar pouch, which also serves as a bursa, there are three additional major bursae anteriorly. The prepatellar bursa lies over the patella, and may become inflamed with prolonged kneeling activities (housemaid's knee). A bursa also lies between the patellar tendon and the tibia (deep infrapatellar bursa) and between the patellar tendon and skin (superficial infrapatellar bursa).

Fig. 17-10. Medial aspect of the knee, showing the synovia and bursae

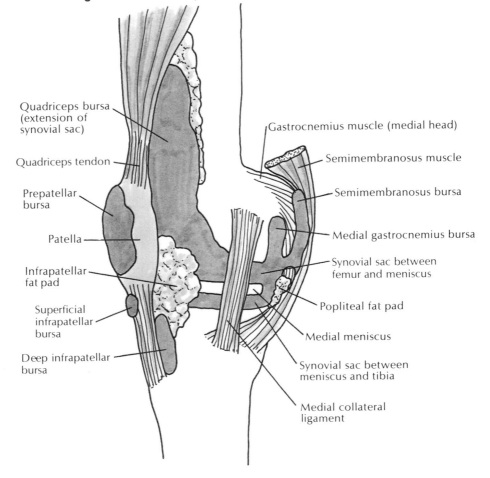

Posteriorly, a main bursa lies between the semimembranosus tendon and the medial origin of the gastrocnemius muscle. This bursa often communicates with the joint and may become swollen with articular effusion, in which case it may be referred to as *Baker's cyst*. This bursa may also extend between the gastrocnemius and the capsule, or a separate bursa may be situated here.

Bursae may also exist beneath the tendons of the pes anserinus and the iliotibial band, just proximal to their insertions. These can become irritated with high levels of activity. There may also be other bursae about the knee joint, but these are of little clinical significance.

The large infrapatellar fat pad is situated deep to the patellar tendon and in front of the femoral condyles. When the knee flexes, it fills the anterior aspect of the intercondylar notch. With the knee extended, it occupies the patellar groove and covers the trochlear surface of the femur. The back of the fat pad is lined with synovium. It is thought that as the fat pad sweeps across the condyles during knee flexion and extension, it helps to spread a lubricating layer of synovial fluid over the joint surface of the femur prior to contact with the tibia.

BIOMECHANICS OF THE FEMOROTIBIAL JOINT*

STRUCTURAL ALIGNMENT

Since the medial femoral condyle extends farther distally than does the lateral condyle, there is usually a slight valgus angulation of about 5° to 10° between the tibia and the femur. With the transcondylar axis of the femur in the frontal plane the

---

* See the section on patellofemoral joint dysfunction in this chapter for a discussion of patellofemoral biomechanics.

patella faces straight forward. In this position, the neck of the femur is directed about 20° forward as a result of the normal internal torsion of the femoral shaft with respect to the femoral neck. Also in this position, the transmalleolar axis at the ankle is rotated outward about 25° as a result of the normal external tortion of the tibial shaft, and the long axis of the foot is directed 5° to 10° outward.

MOVEMENT

The knee is normally biaxial; it flexes and extends around an axis that is horizontally oriented in the frontal plane in the standing position, and it rotates about a vertical axis. Knee flexion–extension is polycentric, the axis of movement shifting backward along a curved centroid as the knee moves from extension into flexion.

Flexion-Extension

Osteokinematics. The total range of knee flexion–extension in the healthy knee is from about 5° to 10° of hyperextension to 140° to 150° of flexion. Flexion is limited by soft-tissue approximation of the calf and posterior thigh. Extension is terminated by locking of the joint in its close-packed position as the capsules and ligaments draw tight and become twisted. As the knee approaches full extension, it also assumes a valgus angulation because the medial femoral condyle extends farther distally than the lateral condyle.

Arthrokinematics. The femorotibial joint is markedly incongruent in positions of flexion, but becomes progressively more congruent as the knee extends. In the flexed position, the small convex radius of the posterior femoral condyles contacts a relatively large radius on the tibial condyles. In fact, the lateral tibial condyle is actually a convex surface. Since the radius of curvature of the femoral condyles progressively increases anteriorly, the joint becomes more congruent as the contacting area on the femur moves anteriorly during knee extension (Fig. 17-11).

The fibrocartilaginous menisci reduce joint surface incongruency. Their mobility and deformability allow them to conform to the shape of the contacting femoral joint surfaces. The anterior segments of the menisci are somewhat mobile, whereas the posterior horns are comparatively fixed. Thus, as the knee extends and the contacting radius of the femoral condyle increases, the anterior aspects of the menisci glide forward. Conversely, as the knee flexes, the anterior segments of the menisci recede to conform to the smaller radius of curvature of the contacting femoral condyles (Fig. 17-12). By reducing joint surface incongruency, the menisci help distribute the forces of compressive loading over a greater area, thus reducing compressive stresses to the joint surfaces of the knee.

As indicated by the instant centers of motion, flexion and extension of the knee occur with a combination of rolling and sliding at the joint surfaces. The closer the instant center is to the contacting joint surfaces, the greater the amount of rolling that occurs at a particular point in the range of movement. An instant center that lies some distance from the contacting surfaces indicates considerable sliding between the surfaces. Since the normal axes of movement for flexion and extension of the knee lie within the condylar region of the femur–not on the joint surfaces or a long distance away–it follows that both sliding and rolling accompany the movement. It can be seen from the loci of normal instant centers that the axis of movement shifts farther away from the joint surface as the knee extends, indicating relatively more sliding occurring as extension takes place (Fig. 17-11).[10,11] Considering the tibia moving on the fixed femur,

Fig. 17-11. Diagram showing loci of normal instant centers and congruency during flexion and extension of the knee

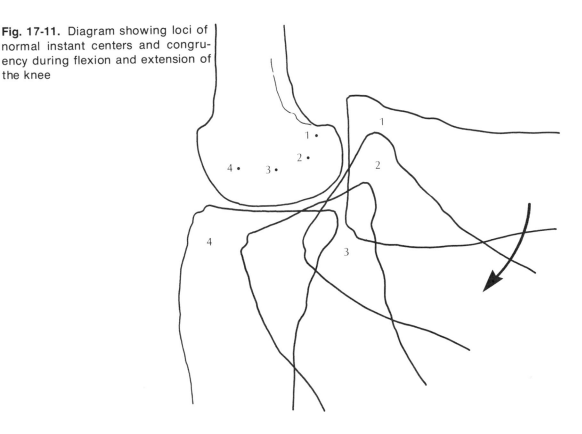

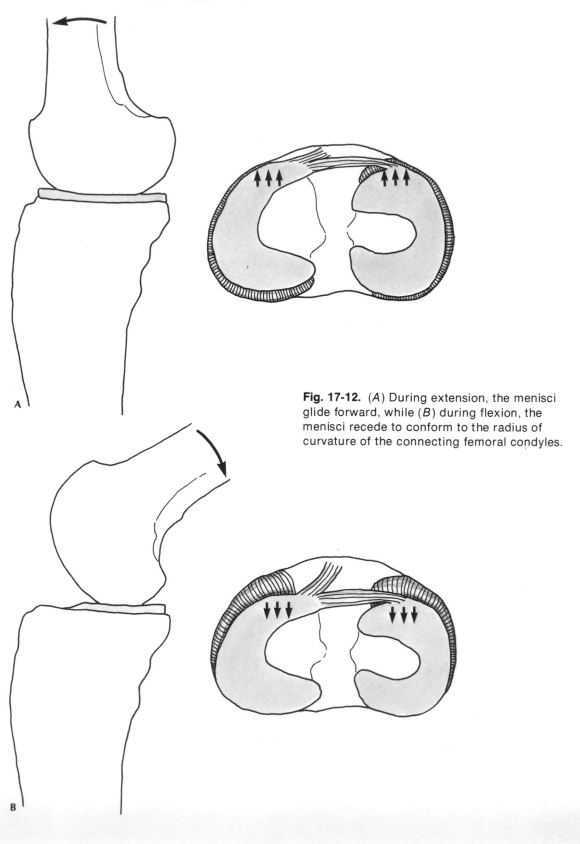

Fig. 17-12. (A) During extension, the menisci glide forward, while (B) during flexion, the menisci recede to conform to the radius of curvature of the connecting femoral condyles.

the direction of sliding and rolling of the tibial joint surface is anterior during extension and posterior during flexion.

Transverse Rotation

Because the femorotibial joint surfaces are incongruent in all positions but full extension, and because the menisci are semimobile, the knee joint can undergo some rotation in the transverse plane. This rotary movement can easily be produced actively or passivly with the knee flexed, and is important for attenuation of rotary forces acting on the knee during normal function.

There is also an automatic, or conjunct, rotation at the knee that accompanies flexion and extension of the joint. This occurs as an external rotation of the tibia relative to the femur during the final 15° to 20° of extension., and an internal tibial rotation during the initial 15° or 20° of flexion from a fully extended position. As the knee undergoes rotation, and menisci tend to move with the femur, so much of the movement occurs between the menisci and the tibia.

Several factors contribute to the occurrence of knee rotation during flexion and extension.[3,37,43,48] First, and perhaps most important, is the shape and orientation of the medial femoral condyle. Looking at the femur end on, we see that the medial condyle is curved and obliquely oriented, whereas the lateral condyle is situated in the sagittal plane (Fig. 17-2). Also of significance is the fact that the articular surface of the medial condyle is longer, in an anteroposterior direction, than that of the lateral condyle. As the tibia moves into extension the lateral side of the joint completes its movement before the medial side, because of the difference in lengths of the respective femoral articular surfaces. When this occurs, the medial side of the tibia continues to move forward along the curved medial femoral condyle, while the lateral tibial joint surface undergoes a lat-

eral spin. The net effect is an external rotary movement of the tibia on the femur. This movement reverses when the knee flexes from a fully extended position. It is believed that the cruciates also play a role in guiding rotary movement at the knee. The cruciates tighten as the knee extends and are twisted in a direction to rotate the tibia externally as they tighten.

PATHOMECHANICS

Structural Alterations

Frontal Plane. Although the knee joint normally assumes a valgus angulation, the line of application representing the weight-bearing force acting on the knee tends to bisect the joint. This is because the femoral head is offset medially from the shaft of the femur (Fig. 17-13). Excessive genu valgum causes the weight-bearing force to be shifted to the lateral side of the joint, whereas genu varum results in a medial shift of the weight-bearing force line. Such alterations in force distribution may lead to accelerated wear on one side of the joint.[9] Common factors contributing to genu valgum are iliotibial band tightness, abnormal foot pronation, and femoral anteversion. Femoral retroversion tends to result in genu varum.

Transverse Plane. In the case of increased femoral anteversion, the femoral condyles are rotated too far internally with respect to the femoral neck. Thus, with the hip joint in a neutral position, the condyles and patellae face inward, or, conversely, with the patellae and condyles facing forward, the hip joint assumes an externally rotated position. Since the tendency during gait is to maintain normal alignment of the hip joints, the individual with increased femoral anteversion tends to walk with the knee rotated inward. This inward rotation may be transmitted to the foot as a toe-in stance or as abnormal foot prona-

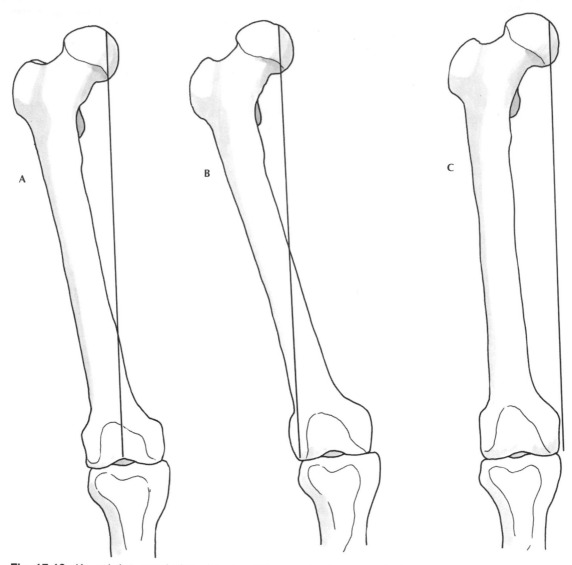

Fig. 17-13. Knee joint angulation showing (*A*) normal valgus angulation, (*B*) excessive valgus angulation, and (*C*) varus angulation

tion. At the knee, inward rotation results in a valgus angulation when the knee is semiflexed, as it is during most of the stance phase of gait. In a similar manner, abnormal retroversion of the hip causes a tendency for the patella to face outward during gait, for the knee to assume a varus position, and for the feet to either toe-out or supinate. In some individuals with torsional deviations of the femur, compensatory structural rotation of the tibia will develop. Thus, the child with femoral anteversion may also develop increased ex-

ternal tibial torsion to achieve normal foot placement. Similarly, internal tibial torsion may develop in association with femoral retroversion. Such torsional compensation at the tibia seems to enhance valgus–varus deviations.

Intrinsic Movement Abnormalities

Capsular Tightness. One of the most common causes of gross restriction of knee motion is capsular tightness. Fibrosis, and subsequent loss of extensibility of the joint capsule, frequently follows immobilization after trauma or surgery and usually accompanies the progression of chronic joint diseases, such as degenerative joint disease or rheumatoid arthritis. Capsular tightness at the knee results in a characteristic pattern of restriction in which knee extension is limited by 20° to 30°, and flexion is possible to only 80° or 100°. The functional disability resulting from capsular restriction will vary with the individual's particular activity level, but ambulation is inevitably altered, since nearly full knee extension is necessary for normal gait. The mean total range of flexion and extension required for some common activities has been studied by Laubenthal and co-workers with the following results:[25]

Activity	Mean Total Flexion–Extension Necessary
Stance phase of gait	21°
Swing phase of gait	67°
Stair climbing	83°
Sitting and rising	83°

Since capsular restriction at the knee typically allows only 50° to 80° of flexion–extension, some functional alteration is likely.

Of great significance during walking is the effect of reduced knee extension on the stresses imposed upon the articular surfaces of the joint. Normally, during stance phase of gait, peak weight-bearing forces are born with the joint just short of full knee extension, a position in which the tibiofemoral contact area is greatest, and a position in which the joint capsule has not been drawn completely tight.[9,23] Since stress equals force/unit area, the compressive stress of weight-bearing is minimized by a relatively large tibiofemoral contact area. Furthermore, the joint is not "shock loaded" by having the slack in the joint capsule suddenly taken up as the knee moves toward extension. If, however, knee extension is lacking from capsular tight-ness, the joint is unable to move to a position of maximal tibiofemoral contact, and as the knee extends, the joint capsule suddenly pulls tight; stress to the joint surfaces is increased in magnitude and the joint is shock loaded. The long term effect is likely to be accelerated wear of the joint surfaces.

Rotary Dysfunction. A more subtle yet common movement disorder affecting the knee is loss of normal rotary mechanics. The pathologic implications of rotary dysfunction at the knee have been theorized by Smillie and confirmed by Frankel and co-workers.[11,42] As mentioned, the nature and extent of rotation accompanying knee flexion and extension is governed by the shapes of the articular surfaces and is influenced by capsuloligamentous configuration. Alteration in normal rotary mechanics may reflect articular surface abnormalities or capsuloligamentous disorders. Similarly, the effect of rotary dysfunction is to produce abnormal stresses to the joint surfaces as well as capsuloligamentous structures. Smillie proposes that since normal rotary movement is small and occurs at the very limits of knee extension, full knee extension is possible in the absence of normal rotation, but at the expense of increased deformation to articular tissues. Thus, knee extension occurring without normal external tibial rotation results in abnormal stresses to the medial joint surfaces, which are oriented to move into rotation, and increased tensile stresses to the cruciates, which pull tight on extension and internal tibial rotation. Furthermore, the tibia must rotate externally as the knee approaches full extension in order to prevent the lateral side of the medial femoral condyle from contacting the medial edge of the anterior cruciate ligament.

Several types of disorders may cause altered rotary mechanics at the knee. Smillie cites meniscal displacements, such as those associated with meniscus tears, as a frequent causative factor. Since knee rotation, when combined with flexion or extension, requires meniscofemoral as well as meniscotibial movement, it is likely that alterations in structural configuration of the menisci would interfere with normal rotary mechanics. Another common cause of restricted external tibial rotation is reduced extensibility of the medial or posteromedial capsuloligamentous structures. This typically occurs following injury or surgery, in which the posteromedial capsule or medial collateral ligament may heal in an adhered or shortened state. Laxity of these same structures will also lead to abnormal rotary mechanics as external tibial rotation may be excessive or premature.[21,41] This would especially be the case if a secondary external rotation contracture developed.

In recognition of the pathomechanics and pathologic implications of rotary dysfunction at the knee, Helfet has described a simple means of clinically detecting this problem.[17] In general terms the method involves comparing femorotibial rotary alignment in a semiflexed and fully extended position. Using this test, in addition to instant center analysis, Frankel and co-workers demonstrated a positive correlation between reduced femorotibial rotation and abnormal compression of the joint surfaces during terminal knee extension.[11] In most of the patients, meniscal derangement was the underlying cause. Arthrotomy revealed abnormal wearing in localized areas of the medial articular surfaces in 22 of 30 cases. These findings confirm the nature of the kinematic abnormality associated with altered rotary mechanics and also suggest that such disorders, over a long period, may predispose to progressive degenerative joint disease.

Smillie believes that kinematic disturbance resulting from rotary dysfunction at the knee may also lead to fatigue disruption and fraying of the anterior cruciate.[42] He supports this contention with surgical case studies of isolated anterior cruciate lesions associated with chronic meniscal derangements.

The significance of rotary dysfunction at the femorotibial articulation is becoming better appreciated as our knowledge of detailed knee biomechanics improves. Because the disturbance is subtle, it is not readily recognized unless femorotibial rotary function is carefully examined. This type of assessment should become a routine component of knee examination in the rehabilitation period following capsuloligamentous injury or internal derangement.

PATHOMECHANICS OF COMMON LOADING CONDITIONS

Trauma

Knee joint injuries are commonly of traumatic origin. This stems, in part, from the fact that the knee is freely movable in only the sagittal plane (flexion–extension). Thus, forces acting to move the knee in the frontal or transverse planes are largely attenuated by internal strain to the soft tissues about the joint. Furthermore, such forces may act over the relatively long lever arms provided by the femur and the tibia, thereby increasing the potential loading of the joint structures.

Valgus–External Rotation. Because of the exposure of the lateral side of the knee to external forces, compared with that of the protected medial aspect, traumatic valgus stresses are much more common than varus stresses. Usually such forces also involve components acting in the transverse and sagittal planes, thus causing rotary and flexion–extension displacements. Since the knee is usually in some position of flexion when acted upon by a force from the lateral aspect, the direction of rotary movement is usually such that the tibia is rotated laterally with respect to the femur.

Valgus–external rotary injuries occur most frequently in contact sports—especially football—and skiing. The degree of loading of the joint is accentuated by the fixation of the foot to the ground, for example, by the cleated shoe, and by forces acting over a long lever arm, such as a ski. This does not allow rotary forces to be attenuated by movement of the foot with respect to the ground, and more of the energy is absorbed as internal strain to joint structures. Since valgus and external rotation are primarily checked by the posteromedial capsule and the capsular and superficial fibers of the medial collateral ligament, it is these structures that are most commonly damaged. The menisci, especially the medial meniscus, may be injured because of the rotary stress component. With marked separation of the medial side of the joint, the anterior cruciate ligament may be torn as well. Specifically, it has been demonstrated experimentally that, with progressive force in a valgus–external rotation direction, structures are torn in the following sequence: (1) the deep capsular fibers of the medial collateral, (2) the long superficial fibers of the medial collateral and the posteromedial capsule, and (3) the anterior cruciate ligament. A torn medial meniscus would complete the so-called terrible triad of O'Donoghue.

Hyperextension. Because the knee is used in a position close to its physiological limits of extension for most functional activities, hyperextension injuries also affect the knee quite commonly. Again, the individual involved in violent contact sports and the skier are particularly vulnerable to such injuries. Experimental studies suggest that forced hyperextension of the knee results in tearing first of the posterior capsule, followed by the anterior cruciate, then the posterior cruciate ligaments.[22]

Anterior–Posterior Displacement. Forces producing a pure translatory movement between the tibia and femur in an anteroposterior direction are somewhat less common than the above-mentioned injuries. Of these, perhaps the "dashboard injury" occurs most frequently. In such cases the victim, in a suddenly decelerating automobile, is thrust forward, striking the tibial tubercle of the bent knee on the dashboard. The tibia is forced posteriorly on the femur, stressing the posterior cruciate ligament, often to the point of rupture.

Isolated anterior cruciate tears, resulting from forces in the opposite direction, are rare. In fact, there is much controversy over the frequency of occurrence of isolated anterior cruciate lesions. When they do occur, the mechanism of injury is more likely to be a force stressing the tibia into internal rotation on the femur.[22,49]

Rotation. Forced external rotation of the tibia on the femur tends to stress the collateral ligaments and the posteromedial capsule. As mentioned above, these forces usually occur in conjunction with valgus stresses, and therefore typically affect the medial stabilizing structures.

Internal rotation of the tibia on the femur is checked by the cruciate ligaments. It is believed that forced internal rotation is the primary mechanism in isolated anterior cruciate ligament injuries.[22,49]

Forced rotation may also injure the menisci.[29] The medial meniscus, being less mobile by virtue of its attachment to the capsular fibers of the medial ligament, is much more frequently injured than the lateral meniscus. The menisci are particularly stressed when the knee is forced into rotation in an improper direction during flexion or extension of the knee. Thus, when the tibia, which is supposed to rotate internally during initial knee flexion, is forced externally as the knee goes into flexion, the menisci are caught between trying to move into flexion with the tibia and into rotation (in the wrong direction) with the femur. The result is often excessive deformation, and tearing, of a meniscus. If, as typically occurs, there is a valgus component to the rotary force, the medial meniscus is additionally stressed through its attachment to the medial ligament. Rotary stresses sufficient to produce meniscal damage do not necessarily require external forces for their production. Often the victim simply twists suddenly on the weight-bearing leg. This usually occurs during athletic endeavors, but may also take place with less vigorous activities.

Occupations or activities involving rotation of the fully flexed knee, such as wrestling or mining in cramped quarters, particularly predispose to meniscus tears. This is because when the knee is fully flexed the menisci reach their limit of posterior excursion. Rotation, which involves posterior movement of one condyle and simultaneous anterior movement of the other, may further stress one meniscus posteriorly or cause the condyle to grind over the relatively fixed meniscus.

Most traumatic medial meniscus tears affect the posterior segment of the meniscus, with the tear running in a longitudinal direction.[42] Successive injury to the same meniscus may cause the tear to extend sufficiently anteriorly to allow the lateral segment of the torn structure to flip centrally into the intercondylar region—a "bucket handle" tear (Fig. 17-14). When this occurs, it produces a mechanical block to full knee extension, and the knee is "locked." At this point, full extension can only occur at the expense of further damage to the meniscus or excessive stretching of the anterior cruciate ligament.

EVALUATION

A broad variety of common lesions affect the knee joint. Traumatic injuries may be experienced by the athlete as well as by

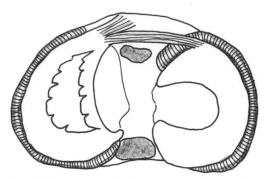

Fig. 17-14. A longitudinal tear of the medial meniscus

the more sedentary individual. Symptomatic degenerative disorders involving the knee are not uncommon in middle-aged or older individuals, and "overuse" fatigue syndromes may affect virtually any age group. The approach to evaluation of knee disorders must be sufficiently flexible to accommodate such a broad spectrum of disorders. Presented here is a relatively comprehensive assessment scheme that includes most of the evaluative procedures needed to perform a thorough clinical examination of virtually any patient presenting with a common knee disorder. Practically speaking, you will rarely ever use all of the tests and procedures outlined here in any one examination session. However, the clinician should become proficient in performing all tests, and must be cognizant of the rationale for each one in order to optomize efficiency in administering a knee examination.

HISTORY

The key to evolving a plan for an efficient yet comprehensive physical examination of the knee is the patient interview. Information elicited from the patient in the interview is necessary to gain insight into the nature and extent of the physical pathology so as to best select the appropriate objective evaluative procedures. Subjective data is also important in determining the degree of disability resulting from the presenting disorder and documenting a baseline.

Follow the format of inquiry set out in the chapter on evaluation when conducting the subjective portion of the knee exam. In addition, there are some specific questions that should be directed to patients presenting with knee problems, which are dependent upon the nature of the disorder. If the problem is of recent traumatic onset, ask

1. What was the exact mechanism of injury? Was a "pop" felt?
2. Did the knee swell? If so, how long after the injury did the swelling become noticeable and where was the swelling observed?
3. To what extent was it possible to continue activities immediately following the injury? Was it possible to walk? If the injury occurred during athletic activities was a litter or some other form of passive or assisted transport required?

If the problem is of a chronic nature, ask

1. Does the knee click, grind, grate, or pop? If so, was the onset of these symptoms associated with the onset of the present problem?
2. Has the knee ever locked, buckled, or given way? If so, under what specific circumstances? Is there some particular activity that tends to cause it?
3. Is climbing stairs, either ascending or descending, a problem?
4. Is it possible to run? What is the effect of running backward, stopping quickly, or changing directions quickly?

INTERPRETATIVE CONSIDERATIONS

Site of Pain

The knee joint receives innervation from the L3 through S2 segments and, depending on the site of pathology, pain from knee disorders may be referred into any of these segments. The majority of common knee problems affect the anteromedial or medial aspect of the joint, which is largely innervated by L3. Since the L3 segment usually does not extend much below the knee, it is rare for a patient with a common knee disorder to experience pain radiating further distally than midleg. It is more common for pain originating at the knee to be referred proximally into the anterior or anteromedial thigh. Note that the anterior aspect of the hip joint is also innervated primarily by L3 and that referred pain of hip joint origin may be very similar in site to that arising from the knee. In fact, it is not unusual, especially in the child, for a patient with a hip joint problem to complain of "knee pain."

In the patient with nontraumatic onset of pain about the knee, lesions situated elsewhere in the L3 through S2 segments must be ruled out. The two common sources of referred pain to the knee are the lumbosacral region and the hip region.

Pain felt over the posterior aspect of the knee is often due to effusion causing distension of the posterior capsule. Since the S1 and S2 segments, which innervate the posterior knee region, extend well down into the foot, posterior knee pain may be referred some distance distally.

—Pain of nontraumatic onset felt over a generalized region at the anteromedial aspect of the knee is most commonly from patellofemoral joint dysfunction. This is especially likely when the pain is aggravated most by descending stairs and prolonged sitting with bent knees.
—Localized anteromedial pain felt at the joint line, usually of sudden onset, is often related to meniscus injuries. The pain arises from the anteromedial coronary ligament. The sprain of the coronary ligament may be the sole lesion, or it may be associated with a tear of the body of the meniscus.
—Medial knee pain of traumatic onset fol-

lowing a valgus or rotary strain is usually of capsuloligamentous origin. A tear of the meniscus must also be ruled out.

Onset

Sudden Traumatic Onset. These injuries are common, especially from athletic activities involving contact or sudden changes in direction. A sudden twisting injury, in which the tibia is rotated externally on the femur without an external source of force, may tear either the capsular fibers of the medial collateral ligament (Grade I tear), the coronary ligament (peripheral attachment of the meniscus), or the body of the medial meniscus. When some external force is involved, such as in contact sports, and the knee is also forced into valgus position, the posteromedial capsule, medial collateral ligament, or anterior cruciate ligament may also be damaged.

Valgus–external rotation injuries are the most common traumatic knee disorders. In other types of injuries the mechanism should be determined, when possible, in order to estimate the nature of the stresses and which particular structure might have been traumatized.

Gradual, Nontraumatic Onset. In middle-aged and older patients, symptomatic degenerative joint disease (DJD) must be ruled out. Pain from DJD is typically noticed first near the end of the day or after long periods of walking. Later, pain and stiffness are felt upon arising in the morning, easing somewhat after getting up and about.

Possible precipitating factors, such as recent immobilization, alteration in activities, past injuries, and previous surgeries, should be considered. Patellofemoral joint dysfunction, a very common knee problem, is frequently related to quadriceps insufficiency. This may include true quadriceps weakness, as from disuse, or some increase in loaded knee-extension activities in the presence of inadequately trained quadriceps muscles. Typical activities would be hiking, bicycling, or skiing.

Effusion. Articular effusion commonly follows traumatic injury to the knee joint. This may be the result of blood filling the joint or of overproduction of synovial fluid. The time frame of the onset of effusion often provides important insight into the nature of effusion. Hemarthrosis tends to develop over a relatively short period following injury, from several minutes to a few hours; synovial effusion occurs over a longer period of time, say, 6 to 12 hours before it is noticed. Synovial effusion causes a dull, aching type of pain from the distension of the joint capsule. Hemarthrosis may be associated with more severe discomfort due to chemical stimulation of capsular nociceptors. Clinically, it is important to attempt to differentiate the nature of the effusion, since, in the case of hemarthrosis, an intra-articular fracture must be ruled out. Some relatively severe joint injuries, such as a complete rupture of the medial ligament, may not be followed by significant effusion because of leakage of fluid through the defect out from the confines of the joint capsule.

More subtle joint effusion may accompany chronic, nontraumatic knee disorders. The patient often describes posterior knee discomfort from posterior capsular distension.

Nature of Pain and Other Symptoms

Pain of traumatic origin is typically felt immediately at the time of injury. It is important to realize that, in the case of ligamentous injuries, the severity of the pain and resulting immediate disability does not necessarily reflect the severity of the injury. A minor or moderate sprain of the medial capsule or ligament is often more painful and more disabling at the time of injury than a complete rupture of the medial collateral ligament.[33] This is because, in the case of a complete rupture, there are no longer intact fibers from which pain of mechanical origin can arise. Furthermore, later development of pain from joint effusion may not be significant because of leakage of fluid through the defect. Thus, after the initial pain from the ligament's rupturing, the individual may feel relatively little pain, especially if involved in a highly motivating activity such as athletic competition.

Pain felt when sitting for long periods with the knee bent or when descending stairs is typical of patellofemoral joint problems.[4,15] These functions both involve high and prolonged patellofemoral compressive loading. Pain is felt more on descending than on ascending stairs because of greater passive tension is developed in the quadriceps mechanism during eccentric contraction than during concentric contraction. Sitting is a problem because of the prolonged nature of the resulting patellofemoral compression. Bone, being viscoelastic, undergoes "creep" or continued deformation with prolonged loading.[12] Bone is also weaker, or more likely to yield, with slowly applied loads. Thus the likelihood of trabecular breakdown is greater with loading over a long period of time than with a similar load applied quickly.

Morning pain, subsiding with initial use of the joint and then increasing again after some period of use, is typical of pain from DJD.

Buckling or giving way of the joint may suggest structural instability or functional instability. The common structural disorder causing giving way is loss of ligamentous integrity. In such circumstances the patient may cite a particular activity that is a problem; usually some activity that stresses the joint in a direction the involved ligament is supposed to check. Thus, individuals with chronic medial collateral ligament ruptures find it a problem to turn abruptly away from the involved leg because of the valgus–external rotary stress imposed on the leg.[33,41] Similarly, persons with loss of cruciate integrity may have problems descending inclines or squatting.

Functional buckling occurs as a result of reflex muscle inhibition, presumably from abnormal joint receptor activity. A common cause is internal derangement from a meniscus tear or loose body. In such cases, an abnormality in arthrokinematics resulting from the mechanical derangement may reflexly incite a sudden inhibition of the quadriceps muscles, causing the joint to give way. The patient will usually not be able to attribute the incidence of buckling to any consistent situation or activity, but will claim that the joint gives way for no apparent reason.

PHYSICAL EXAMINATION

Observation

Record any functional deficits noted throughout the patient's visit. When possible analyze and document the nature and extent of the deficit for future comparison. If the patient refers to a particular functional problem during the interview, he may be asked to attempt the particular activity or task in order to evaluate the problem more objectively. This is especially important for patients with relatively chronic problems who may not spontaneously demonstrate functional deficits during the clinic visit. Specific functions to note for patients presenting with knee disorders would include

Gait—Refer to Chapter 19, The Lumbar–Lower Extremity Scan Examination, for common gait abnormalities and possible causes. The ability to hop, run, change directions quickly, stop abruptly, and climb stairs might be specifically evaluated.
Dressing activities—The patient with restricted or painful knee motion will often have difficulty donning trousers, shorts, or stockings, and fastening shoes.

Transfer activites—Problems with standing from a sitting position are typical of gross weakness or of significant knee pain.

Inspection

Examine and record specific alterations in bony structure or alignment, soft-tissue configuration, and skin status.

I. **Inspection of Bony Structure and Alignment.** The reader should refer to the section on assessment of structural alignment in Chapter 19 for a complete discussion of this part of the examination. In many chronic knee problems, especially disorders of uncertain etiology, a complete structural assessment of the lower extremities and lumbosacral region should be carried out. In traumatic disorders of recent onset, the examination is often confined to the knee area. The following assessments are particularly relevant to examination of the knee:

A. *Standing examination*
1. Frontal alignment. The patient is viewed from behind. Use a plumbline that bisects the heels. Vertical or horizontal asymmetries in the frontal plane are detected by determining the positions of the:
—Navicular tubercles
—Medial malleoli
—Fibular heads
—Popliteal folds
— Gluteal folds
— Greater trochanters
—Posterior superior iliac spines
—Iliac crests

Document vertical disparities (leg length differences) or lateral shifts from a plumbline that bisects the heels. Note abnormal or asymmetrical valgus—varus angulations. Take care to differentiate tibial valgum or varum from genu valgum or varum; these are often confused. The knee is normally positioned in slight genu valgum since the medial condyle extends farther distally than the lateral condyle.

a. Excessive genu valgum may be documented by measuring the distance between the malleoli, with the medial femoral condyles in contact.
b. Excessive genu varum is noted by measuring the intercondylar distance at the knee with the medial malleoli.
c. Vertical disparities are documented by measuring the distance from the lowest asymmetrical landmark to the floor.
d. Horizontal deviations from the plumbline can be documented by measuring distances from the plumbline.

2. Transverse rotary alignment. The patient is viewed from the front with the feet at a normal stance width and pointed outward 5° to 10° from the sagittal plane. Assess
a. Intermalleolar line. This is normally rotated outward 25° to 30° from the frontal plane.
b. Tibial tubercles. These should be in line with the midline or lateral half of the patellae.
c. Patellae. With the feet in a normal stance position, the patellae should face straight forward.
d. Anterior superior iliac spines. A line between these

should be parallel to the frontal plane.

3. Anteroposterior alignment. The patient is viewed from the side. A plumbline facilitates assessment and measurement of deviations. In a relaxed standing position it is normal for the knee to assume a position of slight recurvatum. With the plumbline about 1 cm anterior to the lateral malleolus, the lateral femoral condyle should be slightly posterior to the plumbline. Abnormal angulation in the sagittal plane can be documented by measuring from some anatomical landmark to the plumbline.

B. *Sitting examination.* The patient sits with the legs hanging freely over the edge of the plinth. The following should be assessed:

1. Position of the patellae
   a. A laterally facing patella suggests that the medial femoral condyle is considerably longer than the lateral condyle. This is likely to be associated with a valgus angulation when the knee is straighted.
   b. The inferior pole of patella should be approximately level with the femorotibial joint line. A "high-riding" patella may be significant with respect patellofemoral joint pathology.[26]

2. Position of the tibial tubercle in knee flexion *vs.* knee extension (Helfet test)

   The tibial tubercle is pinched between the thumb and index finger to monitor its position. The position of the tubercle with respect to the patella or, better yet, the anterior ridge of the lateral femoral condyle is noted with the knee flexed, and then with the knee fully extended. The patient may be asked to repeatedly flex and fully extend the knee through 45° in order to best appreciate the extent of tibial rotation. You should note some definite external rotation of the tibia as the knee extends. The movement is subtle—but essential—and should be compared to the contralateral knee. **Note:** This is a very important test to administer, since it may allow you to detect very subtle abnormalities in knee mechanics that may predispose to chronic knee pain and, perhaps, progressive degenerative changes.

C. *Supine examination*

1. Legs straight
   a. Valgus–varus angulations may be measured with a goniometer.
   b. Leg-length disparities may be documented by measuring from the anterior superior iliac spines to the medial malleoli.

2. Knees bent at 60° angle, feet flat on the plinth
   a. Tibial lengths can be compared by noting the heights of the tibial tubercles.
   b. Leg-length disparities of more proximate origin are detected by observing the lengths of the femurs. This is done by siting, from the side, a plane across the faces of the patellae.
   c. Anteroposterior femoral tibial displacements are detected by comparing the

prominences of the tibial tubercles. This must be done before anteroposterior stability tests are carried out. In the presence of a posterior cruciate ligament rupture the tibial will sag back and the tibial tubercle will be less prominent. This will often be associated with a false positive anterior drawer test for anterior cruciate damage.

   d. An excessively prominent tibial tubercle suggests previous osteochondrosis of the tibial apophysis (Osgood-Schlatter disease). This may give rise to a high-riding patella.

II. Soft-Tissue Inspection

A. *Muscle contours*

1. Instruct the patient to maximally contract the quadriceps and calf muscle groups by fully extending the knees and plantarflexing the ankle. Carefully assess the muscle contours for obvious atrophy or asymmetries. Often significant atrophy can be observed before it is measurable by girth measurements. When asymmetries can be measured, baseline measurements should be recorded so progress can be documented.

2. Assess other muscle groups in a similar manner, including the hamstrings and the anterior and lateral compartments of the leg.

B. *Swelling.* If significant swelling exists, baseline girth measurements should be recorded when possible.

1. Generalized edema of the lower leg may accompany a variety of metabolic or vascular disorders. If occurring soon after a surgical procedure, it may indicate venous thrombosis and a physician should be notified.

   Edema persisting some time after trauma or surgery may be associated with a reflex sympathetic dystrophy.

2. Localized swelling may be articular or extraarticular:

   a. Articular effusion. This is manifest as swelling of the suprapatellar pouch and loss of definition of the peripatellar landmarks. Often the posterior capsule becomes distended, causing mild popliteal swelling. Popliteal swelling may be localized at the semimembranosus bursa, even in the case of articular effusion, since this bursa often communicates with the synovial cavity.

   b. Extraarticular. The most common site is the prepatellar bursa. This may swell after sudden or repeated trauma (Housemaid's knee). Occasionally the distal belly of a hamstring muscle will herniate through the superficial fascia when contracted. This may appear as a pronounced popliteal "swelling," but disappears when the muscle is made to relax.

III. Skin Inspection

A. *Color*

1. Localized erythema may suggest an underlying inflammatory process.

2. Ecchymosis about the knee is most commonly associated with

   a. Contusion. The injury is usually over the lateral aspect.

b. Ligamentous damage. Ecchymosis is usually noted medially.

c. Recent patellar dislocation. The ecchymosis is seen medially.

3. Cyanosis over the lower leg following trauma or surgery may be associated with a reflex sympathetic dystrophy.

4. Scars. The cause should be determined. If surgical, the reason for the surgery should be discovered.

5. Texture. In the presence of dystrophic changes the skin of the lower leg becomes smooth and glossy.

IV. **Selective Tissue Tension Tests**

A. *Active movements*

1. Weight-bearing flexion–extension. If not contraindicated by recent trauma or significant disability, the patient should be asked to perform repeated one-legged half-squats. This yields some useful information concerning the functional capacity of the part. It is also a good method by which to compare the strength of the involved knee to a normal side, when possible; manual muscle testing is usually a poor test for quadriceps strength since the examiner may not be able to manually overcome even a significantly weak muscle. Note the following:

a. The patient's ability to perform the movement. Can he fully extend the knee? How many repetitions can be performed before tiring (compare this to the opposite leg)?

b. Any tendency toward giving way

c. Patellofemoral or femorotibial crepitus. The examiner palpates at the medial and lateral patellar margins for the former, and at the femorotibial joint line for the latter. It is normal for a knee to "pop" or "snap" during this movement. A grinding similar to "sand in the joint" is more likely to indicate articular surface degenerative changes.

d. Provocation of pain. If pain is experienced, determine the point in the range of movement at which it is felt.

2. Non weight-bearing flexion–extension. If the patient is unable to perform weight-bearing flexion–extension or is unable to do it through a full range of movement, flexion and extension in a supine position are assessed. For extension ask the patient to straighten the knee; then tell him to hold it extended and attempt to raise the leg against gravity (straight leg raise). Then ask the patient to flex the knee as far as possible. The following should be noted:

a. Range of motion. If the patient is unable to fully flex or extend the knee, apply some passive overpressure to determine whether the restriction is due to pain, weakness, or true tissue restriction. The amount of passive extension should be compared to extension maintained against gravity. The degree of any "extensor lag" should be documented.

b. Crepitus during movement. If joint crepitus is present it should be determined whether it arises from the femorotibial or patellofemoral joint.

c. The presence of pain and the point in the range at which it is felt

B. *Passive movements*

1. Osteokinematic movements

    a. Flexion–extension. The knee is now passively flexed and extended, and the following noted:

        i. Range of motion. If movement is limited, determine whether the pattern of restriction is capsular or noncapsular. The capsular pattern at the knee is usually a loss of extension by 15° to 25°, with flexion possible to only 85° to 95°.

        ii. Provocation of pain

        iii. End-feel

        iv. Crepitus

    b. Knee extension with sustained internal or external rotation (McMurray's test). This test is to assess the status of the posterior segments of the medial meniscus (external rotation) or lateral meniscus (internal rotation). Nearly full range of knee flexion must be present in order to perform this test. The knee is fully flexed and the tibia fully rotated either internally or externally. Place your thumb and index finger over the medial and lateral femorotibial joint lines, maintain rotation of the tibia, and extend the knee out to 90°. The test does not pertain to extension beyond 90°. The following may indicate a positive test, though there is some question as to the reliability:[29]

        i. Provocation of a painful area of movement.

        ii. A palpable "click" elicited during the movement.

    c. Range of motion of related joints should be assessed in the presence of chronic knee problems and knee problems of uncertain etiology. Because of the biomechanical interdependency of the weight-bearing joints, a problem with one joint may lead to or be caused by a dysfunction in another.

        i. Hip range of motion, including straight leg raise

        ii. Ankle range of motion

2. Joint play movements (stress tests). The status of the capsuloligamentous structures is assessed by performing the following passive movements. Note the provocation of pain or muscle guarding and whether the movement is hypomobile or hypermobile. The latter can best be determined by comparing to a "normal" side, but experience is also very helpful. The techniques for performing these movements are illustrated in Chapter 7, Joint Mobilization Techniques.

    Note: It is very important that you take note of, and attempt to avoid eliciting, protective muscle guarding when performing the joint play tests; false negative results may mask a serious injury that warrants immediate attention.

    a. Anterior glide of the tibia on the femur (Anterior drawer test). This should be performed with the knee bent and with the knee close to full extension.[14] In the bent knee position it is necessary to determine first that the tibia is not displaced posteriorly with respect to the femur; this occurs with a posterior cruciate tear and will yield a false positive anterior glide test.

Mild to moderate hypermobility of anterior glide may exist in the presence of anterior cruciate lesion or a tear of part of the medial collateral ligament complex; gross hypermobility suggests damage to both.[14,18] If the anterior cruciate is ruptured, both condyles of the tibia can be pulled forward excessively. If only a medial ligament is damaged and the cruciate is intact, only the medial tibial condyle comes forward.[21] Differentiation is aided by performing the test with sustained internal tibial rotation and then with external rotation. If the hypermobility is extinguished by holding the tibia in internal rotation, it is likely that the cruciates are intact. If external tibial rotation abolishes the hypermobility, the medial ligaments are probably intact. Damage to both the anterior cruciate and the medial ligament is especially likely if there is significant hypermobility when the joint is tested in a position close to full extension.

b. Posterior glide of the tibia on the femur (Posterior drawer test). This is not a useful test since, if the pos-

terior cruciate ligament is ruptured, the tibia will sag back on the femur at the starting point of the test, and no hypermobility will be detected. Instead, a false positive anterior drawer sign will be elicited. Posterior cruciate laxity is thus detected on inspection of structural alignment.

c. Valgus– varus stress

   i. With the knee in full extension there should be no movement elicited, even in the presence of a ruptured collateral ligament. If there is movement, severe damage, involving at least one collateral and one cruciate, is likely.

   ii. A small amount of movement is normally present when the knee is tested in a slightly flexed position. Pain elicited on valgus stress, in the absence of hypermobility suggests injury to the capsular fibers of the medial collateral ligament or a minor injury (Grade I) to the superficial fibers of the medial collateral. Valgus hypermobility suggests a medial collateral ligament injury (Grade II or Grade III). Marked valgus hypermobility indicates accompanying cruciate damage. Varus hypermobility or pain is rare because the lateral collateral is seldom injured.

d. Internal and external rotation of the tibia on the femur

      i. These can be performed with the patient supine and the knee in various positions of flexion. Hypermobile external rotation suggests damage to one of the collaterals, usually the medial collateral ligament. Pain on external rotation may be elicited in the presence of a coronary ligament sprain, or a medial capsuloligamentous injury; findings on valgus stress are used to differentiate. Hypermobile or painful internal rotation is usually associated with cruciate injuries.

     ii. When tested in a prone position with the knee bent to 90°, joint distraction or compression can be maintained to help differentiate between ligamentous injuries and injuries to the menisci or coronary ligaments (Apley's test). Pain elicited during external rotation with distraction suggests a collateral ligament injury. Pain on internal rotation with distraction may indicate a cruciate injury. Pain on rotation with compression, not elicited when the joint is distracted, suggests a problem with a meniscus or a meniscal attachment (coronary ligament).

  e. Patellar mobility
    i. Medial–lateral
    ii. Superior–inferior

  f. Anteroposterior glide of the proximal tibiofibular joint.

C. *Resisted movements.* Lesions involving the muscles or tendons crossing the knee joint are not uncommon and are best detected by assessing the effect of maximal isometric contraction of the structure to be tested. Tendinitis most commonly affects the insertion of the iliotibial band, one of the pes anserinus tendons, or the insertion of the biceps femoris. The quadriceps are often contused in athletic activities, especially football.

Provide manual resistance to the isometric contraction and determine whether the contraction is strong or weak and whether it is painless or painful. The most important movements to resist are the following:

Knee flexion—for the biceps femoris and pes anserinus tendons

Knee extension—for the iliotibial tendon and quadriceps muscles

External rotation of the tibia on the femur—for the iliotibial tendon

Internal rotation of the tibia on the femur—for the pes anserinus tendons

If lesions involving other muscles or tendons are suspected, the appropriate resisted movements should be tested. In cases of relatively chronic tendinitis brought on by repetitive minor trauma, such as by long distance running, pain may not be elicited on resisted movement testing unless the patient has recently engaged in the provoking activity. To avoid false negative findings, you may wish to have the patient perform the relevant activity just prior to testing. Also, testing repeated contractions of the suspected structure may increase the likelihood of eliciting discomfort in chronic cases.

V. **Neuromuscular Testing.** Resisted movements, as described above, are used primarily to detect painful lesions of muscles or tendons, and give only general information pertaining to muscle strength. If it is desirable to detect or quantify subtle losses in muscle strength—as may arise from disuse or segmental neurologic deficits—or strength increases resulting from training, repeated loading of the muscle to near-fatigue levels must be carried out. This is especially true for large-muscle groups such as the quadriceps and calf muscles. Various exercise equipment may be used for this purpose. A particularly convenient, though expensive, method is use of an isokinetic apparatus which gives a torque-curve readout. A simpler but very useful method for the quadriceps and calf groups is to ask the patient to perform repeated half-squats and toe-raises, respectively, in a standing position.

Manual tests for smaller groups, used especially to detect myotomal weaknesses associated with nerve root lesions, are described in Chapter 19, Lumbar—Lower Extremity Scan Examination.

VI. **Palpation.** Clinically, palpation is best carried out in conjunction with inspection and is organized similarly.

A. *Bony structures and soft-tissue attachments.* Note any abnormalities in size, position, or integrity of bony structures; determine the existence of tenderness, especially at tendon and ligament attachments, with the realization that deep tenderness is often referred. With the patient sitting at the edge of the plinth, legs hanging freely, palpate the following:

1. Patella
   a. Note its size, shape, and position. A small, high-riding patella may be a predisposing factor in patellofemoral joint problems.
   b. Palpate the superior and inferior poles where the quadriceps and patellar tendons attach for tenderness.
   c. Passively hold the knee extended, push the patella medially, and palpate the medial articular facets on the back side of the patella for tenderness.

2. Femoral condyles
   a. Note the prominence of the anterior aspect of the lateral condyle.
   b. Palpate the adduction tubercle, a major site of attachment for the medial retinaculum, as well as the site of insertion for the adductor magnus.

3. Proximal tibia
   a. Palpate the area of insertion of the pes anserinus and medial collateral ligament.
   b. Palpate the tibial tubercle, onto which the patellar tendon inserts.
   c. Palpate the lateral tibial tubercle, where the iliotibial band inserts.

4. Fibular head. The lateral collateral ligament inserts at its apex.

B. *Soft-tissue palpation*
   1. Muscles. Palpate the various muscle groups about the knee for
      a. Mobility. This is especially important after surgery or prolonged immobilization, which may lead to the development of adhesions between muscle planes or between muscles and other tissues.

b. Continuity. Occasionally severe trauma may cause palpable ruptures of muscles or tendons.

c. Consistency. Prolonged disuse and reflex sympathetic dystrophy predispose to "stringy," fibrotic muscles. Contusions of the quadriceps often resolve with heterotopic bone formation, which may be palpable.

2. Ligaments

a. Anteromedial coronary ligament (anteromedial border of the medial meniscus). This is palpated at the anteromedial joint line. It becomes more prominent here when the tibia is passively rotated internally with respect to the femur. This is a site of point tenderness following medial meniscus tears or isolated coronary ligament sprains.

b. Medial collateral ligament. The palpating finger follows the medial joint line from its anterior aspect a short distance posteriorly until it is felt to be obliterated by the anterior margin of the medial collateral ligament. The posterior margin of the ligament can be similarly palpated where it crosses the joint line. The examiner should estimate the course of the ligament and palpate along its extent. It cannot be distinguished as a discrete structure because of its flat configuration. Localized tenderness will usually correspond well with the site of medial collateral ligament injuries.

c. Lateral collateral ligament. This is best palpated with the patient's ankle crossed over the opposite knee. It is felt as a well-defined, round structure crossing the lateral joint line between the femur and fibular head. This is one of the few sites at which a ligamentous rupture is palpable; however, at the lateral collateral ligament this is a rare occurrence.

3. Tendons

a. Patellar tendon. This is easily palpated from the inferior pole of the patella to its insertion on the tibial tubercle.

b. Iliotibial band. From its insertion on the lateral tibial tubercle, the blunt, posterior edge of the iliotibial band can be felt well up into the lateral thigh region.

c. Biceps femoris. This is a very prominent tendon, easily felt at the posterolateral corner of the knee, inserting into the fibular head.

d. Medial retinaculum. The retinaculum is flat and cannot be distinguished as a distinct structure. It is palpated in a generalized area between the adductor tubercle and the medial border of the patella. It is often tender in cases of patellofemoral joint dysfunction.

e. Pes anserinus tendons. The pes anserinus tendons join to give a flat tendinous insertion on the anteromedial aspect of the proximal tibia 5 to 7 cm below the joint line.

i. The semitendinosus tendon is easily felt as a prominent, cordlike structure at the posteromedial corner of the knee.

ii. The gracilis tendon is more difficult to distinguish, but can be felt as a "piano wire" between the semitendinosus tendon, posteriorly, and the sartorius tendon, anteriorly.

iii. The sartorius tendon is a large, blunt structure crossing the posteromedial aspect of the knee, anterior to the semitendinosus and gracilis tendons.

f. Gastrocnemius heads. These are palpated deep in the popliteal fossa.

4. Palpation for effusion. When a large volume of fluid accumulates within the confines of the synovial cavity, fluid is easily seen and palpated at the medial and lateral patellar margins, and distension of the posterior aspect of the joint is noted. Smaller quantities of fluid may be detected by

a. Milking the fluid distally out of the suprapatellar pouch with one hand while palpating along the medial and lateral patellar margins with the other. Fluid will be felt to drain beneath the palpating fingers, and the patella may be felt to float up off the femoral condyles. Compare to the opposite knee.

b. After having milked the fluid distally, as described above, tap the patella posteriorly with the free hand.

If fluid has caused the patella to "float," a "click" will be felt as it is pushed down onto the femoral condyles. Palpate for distension of the semimembranosus bursa, which often communicates with the joint.

C. *Skin palpation.* The skin about the knee area and the distal aspect of the leg should be palpated lightly with the back of the hand. The examiner should note:

1. Temperature. Localized areas of increased temperature may signify underlying inflammation. In reflex sympathetic dystrophy or other vascular problems, the leg may feel abnormally cool.

2. Tenderness. Burning dysesthesias may be associated with neural disorders, such as nerve root impingements, or they may arise as referred tenderness from deep somatic pathologies.

3. Moisture. Hyperhidrosis is common with reflex xympathetic dystrophy. Abnormalities in skin moisture may also be associated with other vascular or metabolic disorders.

4. Mobility. Skin mobility is often impaired by adhesion following surgery or prolonged immobilization, and especially with development of a reflex sympathetic dystrophy.

SUMMARY OF EVALUATION PROCEDURES

The knee evaluation presented here is lengthy when considered in the context of a busy clinical practice. The experienced examiner rarely administers all of the tests discussed but chooses the appropriate examination procedures based upon the patient interview and the general nature of the problem. To improve efficiency when administering a knee examination, the clinician must organize the tests according to patient positioning; the standing tests are done first, then the sitting tests, the supine tests, and finally the prone tests. The conceptual scheme of organizing the exam presented here must be translated into a more practical scheme based upon patient positioning. Therefore, for each position, the relevant observations, inspection procedures, selective tissue tension tests, neuromuscular tests, and palpation procedures must be carried out before asking the patient to change positions. The following outline summarizes the knee evaluation according to patient positioning. It can be used as a checklist when administering the exam and as the basis for devising a knee evaluation form tailored to a particular clinical setting.

I. Standing
  A. Observation
    1. Gait
    2. Dressing
    3. Special functions—running, stair climbing, abrupt stop, abrupt turn, hopping, squatting, etc.
  B. Inspection
    1. Standing structure and alignment
    2. Soft-tissue contours
    3. Swelling
    4. Skin
  C. Selective tissue tension tests—active weight-bearing flexion–extension
  D. Neuromuscular tests
    1. Repeated half-squats (L3) (same as weight-bearing flexion–extension)
    2. Repeated toe-raises
II. Sitting on edge of plinth
  A. Inspection
    1. Patellar alignment and positioning
    2. Femorotibial rotary alignment in flexion *vs.* extension (Helfet test)
    3. Muscle contours with maximal isometric contraction
    4. Skin
  B. Resisted movements
    1. Extension
    2. Flexion
    3. Internal tibial rotation
    4. External tibial rotation
  C. Neuromuscular tests—resisted hip flexion (L2,L3)
  D. Palpation
    1. Bony structures and soft-tissue attachments
    2. Tendons
    3. Ligaments
III. Supine
  A. Inspection
    1. Tibial lengths (knees bent)
    2. Anteroposterior tibial alignment (knees bent)
    3. Femoral lengths (knees bent)
    4. Leg length measurement (anterior superior iliac spine to medial malleolus)
    5. Valgus–varus angulation
    6. Swelling or atrophy (take girth measurements)
    7. Skin
  B. Selected tissue tension tests
    1. Non-weight-bearing flexion–extension—measured with goniometer
    2. McMurray's test (extension with sustained rotation)
    3. Joint play movements
      a. Anteroposterior glide
      b. Valgus–varus tilt
      c. Internal–external rotation
      d. Patellar mobility
      e. Superior tibiofibular joint
    4. Ankle range of motion
    5. Passive hip flexion–extension, abduction–adduction, and straight leg raise
  C. Neuromuscular tests
  D. Palpation
    1. Muscles

2. Effusion
3. Skin
IV. Prone
   A. Inspection
     1. Soft tissues
     2. Skin
   B. Selected tissue tension tests
     1. Apley test (tibial rotation with distraction or compression)
     2. Passive hip internal–external rotation
     3. Resisted knee flexion
   C. Palpation
     1. Muscles
     2. Skin

COMMON LESIONS AND THEIR MANAGEMENT

LIGAMENTOUS INJURIES

History

The patient will invariably recall the traumatic event; you should attempt to determine the exact mechanism of injury.

Onset.   One of the most common mechanisms occurs when a football player is tackled from the side with the foot planted and the knee slightly flexed. The victim is usually struck while trying to turn or "cut" away. The forces on the knee include a valgus stress, external rotation of the tibia on the femur, and usually an anterior movement of the tibia on the femur. With sufficient force, the medial capsule is torn first, followed by the medial collateral ligament, then by the anterior cruciate ligament.[21] The medial meniscus is invariably torn as well, completing the "terrible triad of O'Donoghue."

A minor medial ligament sprain is a common lesion that usually results from an external rotation strain of the tibia on the femur. An external force may or may not be involved.

A force against the anterior thigh, tending to drive the femur backward on the tibia, while the knee is close to full extension, tends to stress the anterior cruciate ligament. This is especially true if the tibia is in a position—or forced into a position—of internal rotation with respect to the femur. In fact, forced internal rotation of the tibia on the femur in itself may tear the anterior cruciate ligament. Internal rotary strains are thought by some to be the primary cause of isolated anterior cruciate ligament lesions.[22,49] A force driving the tibia backward on the femur will stress the posterior cruciate ligament. This seems to be true regardless of whether or not the knee is flexed, since the posterior cruciate remains relatively taut in most positions of the knee. An example of such an injury is the not uncommon "dashboard injury"; a car suddenly stops and a passenger (not wearing a seatbelt) continues forward, striking the tibial tubercle of his bent knee against the dashboard, thus driving the tibia backward on the femur.

In the case of a force driving the knee into hyperextension, the posterior capsule tends to give way first, then the posterior cruciate ligament, and finally the anterior cruciate ligament.[22]

It is not uncommon in cases of severe ligamentous injuries for the patient to attempt to continue activities (*e.g.*, return to the field in a football game) immediately following the injury. This is especially true in the case of a complete rupture of the medial collateral ligament, since no fibers remain intact from which pain can arise. The pain often subsides after a few minutes if the patient is in a highly motivating situation. No effusion ensues since the capsule is usually torn, allowing the fluid to leak out of the joint cavity. In partial ligamentous injuries, the individual is less likely to continue activity because of persisting pain following the injury.

In severe injuries the patient may describe painful effusion occurring within a few minutes after injury; this is highly suggestive of hemarthrosis, and an intra-articular fracture must be ruled out by the physician.

Slower development of effusion over, say, several hours suggests synovial effusion due to capsular irritation. This is common with mild and moderate ligamentous injuries.

Site of pain. The patient usually will point to a localized area that corresponds well to the site of the tear as being the primary site of pain. The exception is an isolated tear of the anterior cruciate, which is relatively rare and may result in more generalized discomfort.

In the case of effusion, especially hemarthrosis, the entire knee area is likely to be painful; the patient is less able to localize the site of injury. Also, in severe injuries involving several structures, localization is less likely because of generalized pain.

The knee is largely innervated by the L3 segment, although it also receives contributions from L4 to S2. Referred pain into these segments is a possibility, although this does not seem to occur as frequently with acute ligamentous lesions as it does with chronic, degenerative problems.

Nature of pain and disability. In the absence of significant effusion, the pain is described as a continuous, deep, fairly localized pain, which is increased by any movement tending to further stress the ligament (partial tear). When considerable effusion exists, a more intense, aching, throbbing pain is described that is aggravated by weight-bearing and virtually any movement. Hemarthrosis is, as a rule, more painful than synovial effusion.

If a moderately severe tear or complete rupture is left to heal, the pain will largely subside. The patient may walk quite comfortably but states that he is unable to perform some particular activity such as running, jumping, cutting, walking downstairs, or squatting without having the knee give way. If carefully assessed, the particular disabilities will correspond to activities that tend to move the knee into directions that the stretched or ruptured ligament is meant to check. Some examples include

1. Inability to turn quickly—Medial or lateral collateral ligament
2. Inability to run forward well—Anterior cruciate ligament
3. Inability to go downstairs easily, squat, or run backward—Posterior cruciate ligament or posterior capsule

A medial collateral ligament rupture will usually result in considerable disability, whereas isolated cruciate tears may cause little or no disability if quadriceps muscle function is good.[42]

Physical Examination

In the acute stage, once joint effusion, considerable pain, and significant muscle guarding have developed, it may prove very difficult to carry out some of the evaluation procedures. In any case, the knee must be examined, sparing the patient as much discomfort as possible and ensuring that no harm is imposed by the tests. The value of immediate, on-the-spot examination prior to the onset of effusion cannot be overemphasized.

I. **Acute Lesion with Effusion**
   A. *Observation.* The patient may hobble into the office, perhaps using crutches. The knee is held slightly flexed with only toe-touched weight-bearing, if any. Removal of the shoe, sock and trousers is carried out with difficulty.
   B. *Inspection.* Joint effusion is obvious, especially in the suprapatellar region. The patient stands with the leg held semi-flexed, often unable to place the heel on the floor.
      1. The Helfet test cannot be administered because the knee cannot be fully extended.

2. Girth measurements at the suprapatellar region are increased from effusion.

3. Some redness of the skin over the knee may be noticed. The skin may be somewhat shiny from being stretched.

C. *Selective tissue tension tests*

1. Active movement
   a. Weight-bearing flexion–extension is impossible.
   b. In supine, active movement is limited in a capsular pattern because of joint effusion, with pain especially at the extremes of both motions. Passive overpressure is met with a muscle-spasm end-feel

2. Passive movements
   a. Flexion–extension is limited in a capsular pattern (about 15° loss of extension and 60° to 90° loss of flexion) with no crepitus and a muscle spasm end feel.
   b. McMurray's test must usually be deferred because of insufficient knee flexion.

3. Resisted movements
   a. These should be strong and painless, barring concurrent tendon injury.
   b. Quantitative determination of muscle strengths must be deferred because of the acute condition.

4. Passive joint play movements. (Be aware of possible false negative results from muscle guarding.)
   a. Anterior glide. This may be painful if the anterior cruciate or posteromedial capsule is sprained. The posterolateral capsule is rarely involved, except in severe injuries. Gross hypermobility suggests a tear of the anterior cruciate and medial stabilizing structures. Mild to moderate instability may indicate an isolated anterior cruciate tear or a medial capsuloligamentous tear (anterior cruciate if internal tibial rotation is also hypermobile, medial capsule if external rotation is hypermobile).
   b. Posterior glide. Pain or hypermobility suggests a posterior cruciate lesion.
   c. Valgus–varus tilt. Gross hypermobility on valgus stress suggests a rupture of the medial capsule and the medial collateral ligament. Mild instability suggests that only the deeper medial capsular fibers are torn. Pain in the absence of instability suggests a mild to moderate sprain. Varus stress will reproduce pain from a lateral collateral ligament injury.
   d. Internal–external tibial rotation
      i. Pain or instability on internal rotation suggests a cruciate lesion (anterior or posterior) or a posterolateral capsular lesion. Compare to other tests in order to differentiate.
      ii. Pain or instability on external rotation associated with pain or instability on valgus stress suggests a medial capsular lesion, medial collateral ligament lesion, or both. Pain on external tibial rotation without associated pain

on valgus stress may result from a coronary ligament sprain. A lateral collateral ligament lesion may also lead to pain on external rotation, but this lesion is rare.

iii. Apley's test should produce more rotary pain with distribution than with compression in the presence of a ligament injury.

e. Patellar mobility cannot be validly assessed if significant effusion is present.

f. Superior-tibiofibular joint. Joint play movement here may be painful in the case of a lateral collateral ligament sprain.

D. *Palpation*

1. There is likely to be localized tenderness at the site of the tear. There may be referred tenderness in nearby areas as well.

2. Effusion is easily confirmed by the tap test or by emptying the suprapatellar pouch while palpating at the lateral patellar margins. Posterior capsular distension may also be noted. Hemarthrosis may accompany (*1*) a cruciate tear, (*2*) a meniscus tear extending to the peripheral attachment, (*3*) a severe capsular tear, or (*4*) an intra-articular fracture.

3. The joint is warm and slightly moist.

II. **Acute Lesions Without Effusion.** Although most ligament injuries at the knee are followed by the development of some effusion, there are cases in which it does not. The absence of significant effusion should not be taken to imply that the injury is mild. On the contrary, complete medial capsular ruptures, usually occurring with tearing of all or part of the medial collateral ligament, may not be followed by much joint effusion, since the fluid escapes the confines of the joint capsule through the defect.

The primary difference between a patient presenting with effusion and one presenting without are that in the absence of effusion

1. The patient will enter with less of a gait disturbance. The knee will not be maintained in as much flexion, and he may be able to walk without aids.

2. The available range of motion will be greater.

3. Effusion is not noted on inspection and palpation of the joint.

Generally, the patient who does not develop much joint swelling has less pain and disability. The clinician must carefully assess joint play movements to determine whether the absence of effusion reflects a minor lesion or a very severe injury. Information acquired during the patient interview will also be instructive.

If it is determined that significant instability is present on one or more joint play movements, a physician experienced in dealing with such injuries must be notified immediately, since immediate surgery may be indicated.

III. **Chronic Ligament Ruptures.** Unfortunately, patients occasionally present with chronic ligament ruptures. The primary complaint is functional instability or giving way of the knee with particular activities. Objectively, the patient may walk in without a limp or obvious disability. The only significant findings may be

1. Difficulty performing some specific function such as running,

turning sharply, squatting, descending stairs, or running backward.

2. Quadriceps muscle atrophy, especially if the joint was swollen or immobilized.[8]
3. Hypermobility on one or more joint play movements.
4. A positive Helfet test.

Laxity of one of the medial stabilizing structures—the medial capsule or medial collateral ligament—is most likely to result in some disability. These are often combined with anterior cruciate ruptures. The result is instability of anterior glide and external rotation of the tibia on the femur. Functionally, the individual is unable to turn away from the involved side without the leg giving way, a real problem for a young, active individual. The medial meniscus may be torn at the time of injury or some time later from abnormal joint mechanics. The meniscus tear will compound the instability and the tendency for the knee to buckle.

Management

The approach to management of ligamentous injuries must be dependent upon several factors, including the patient's age and desired activity level, and the nature of the pathology. Relative to the pathology, you must know the severity of the injury and whether the lesion is acute or chronic. Traditionally the severity of ligamentous lesions are graded as follows:

Grade I: Mild sprain, with no gross loss of integrity of the ligament fibers. On examination there is no joint play hypermobility.

Grade II: Moderate tear, with partial loss of integrity of the ligament, manifested as mild joint play instability

Grade III: Severe tear, or complete rupture of the ligament, resulting in moderate to marked joint play hypermobility

This classification is useful for general communication purposes, but it cannot be used as an absolute guide to clinical management; it does not adequately represent the broad continuum of ligamentous injuries, nor does it take into account other individual factors such as the patient's age, activity level, motivational status, or the stage of the lesion.

The stage of the lesion—how acute or chronic it is—is also somewhat of an arbitrary designation. For the sake of this discussion, we will base this classification on specific clinical criteria that hopefully reflect the nature of the existing inflammatory process.

Acute lesion
—The patient is unable to bear weight without pain and a significant limp.
—There is significant loss of knee motion with a painful, muscle spasm end feel.
—There is obvious swelling or effusion.

Chronic lesion
—The patient can walk with minimal pain and without a significant limp.
—Knee motion is relatively free, or, if restricted, it is limited by stiffness (nonpainful end-feel).
—There is little or no swelling.

Subacute lesion
—Some combination of acute or chronic criteria

 I. **Mild Sprains (Grade I)**
   A. *Acute stage*
     1. Control of inflammation and effusion. Most ligament injuries at the knee affect tissues that are fairly superficially situated and can therefore be affected directly by superficial thermal modalities. The patient should be instructed to apply ice

packs frequently over the site of the injury to minimize the hyperemic phase of the inflammatory process and the associated localized swelling and enzymatic activity.

The use of a compressive bandage about the knee may also help minimize local tissue swelling as well as joint effusion. The patient should be carefully instructed in wrapping techniques to avoid tourniquet effects. Frequent elevation of the part should also be encouraged to prevent and reduce fluid stasis, which may increase or prolong swelling.

The knee must be protected from additional stress in order to optimize the healing reponse. The patient should use crutches with minimal weight-bearing until he can bear weight without pain, and until knee extension through a full range is possible.

2. Maintenance of optimal function as healing ensues. Unnecessary loss of strength and range of motion must be minimized without imposing inappropriate stresses on the healing tissue. The patient should be instructed in gentle active range of motion of the knee through the pain-free range, to be carried out several times throughout the day. Isometric strengthening exercises for the quadriceps and hamstring groups should also be instituted and gradually progressed as healing takes place.

B. *Subacute to chronic stage*

1. Assist in resolution of inflammation and promote healing response. Once the hyperemic phase of inflammation has subsided, some intermittent increase in blood flow to the part may speed the healing phase. Since the medial ligaments at the knee are fairly superficial, increased blood flow may be affected with superficial heating agents such as hot packs, warm whirlpools, or infrared radiation. Deeper heating may be accomplished with various forms of diathermy. Ultrasound is most effective in heating tissues adjacent to bone.

The use of friction massage directly to the site of the lesion, and applied transversely to the direction of the ligament fibers, may help prevent adherence of the healing ligament to adjacent tissues. This may also help align newly produced collagen along the normal lines of stress, that is, in line with the longitudinal axis of the ligament. Take care not to friction at the proximal attachment of the medial collateral ligament. Occasionally periosteal disruption here results in the development of a bony outcropping (Pelligrini–Stieda syndrome). Although this is undoubtedly an inevitable result of the original injury, the use of massage may be held suspect should some medicolegal question develop.

2. Restoration of normal function. Range of motion activities should be gradually progressed, avoiding provocation of pain at the site of injury. In most minor sprains, range of motion returns easily as effusion abates.

Strengthening exercises should also be gradually progressed. Once full painless knee extension is possible, isotonic exercises should be initiated. The most important exercise for most individuals is resistance over the final 20° of extension to regain strength of the vastus medialis muscle. Resisted straight leg raising may also be effective in this regard. Athletes, or other individuals placing unusual demands upon the functional capacity of the knee, must undergo a more rigorous retraining program. For these individuals, especially, exercises should approximate the type of loading normally imposed on the joint. Most athletic activities, as well as routine activities of daily living, involve relatively high rate loading conditions. Isokinetic exercise equipment, with variable speed adjustments, provide a convenient means of providing high speed resistant to various muscle groups, while at the same time monitoring the percent of maximal torque output. Such exercises not only result in strengthening but also optimize the training effect of the exercise program.

As normal osteokinematic range of motion and strength are regained, the therapist must also ascertain that normal arthrokinematics are also restored. Most importantly, one must determine, using the Helfet test, that normal femorotibial rotary function returns. Occasionally one finds that the patient regains knee extension without concurrent return of external tibial rotation, presumably because of residual tightness or adherence of part of the medial joint capsule. This may be a source of persistent chronic knee pain or eventual degenerative changes following otherwise benign traumatic knee disorders. If such rotatory restrictions are detected, mobilization procedures should be instituted to correct them (see external tibial rotation in Chapter 7, Joint Mobilization Techniques).

Resumption of normal activity levels should be carefully supervised by the clinician in charge of the rehabilitation program. As pain subsides and as motion returns, the patient should be instructed to gradually increase weight bearing on the leg. Crutches should not be discarded, however, until full knee extension is possible, both passively and actively, against gravity. Running, jumping, and athletic activities must not be allowed until strength is near normal, range of motion is full, and normal femorotibial rotation has returned. Such activities must be very gradually progressed from straight-ahead jogging to straight-ahead running, then running with gentle turns, and finally running with abrupt stops and turns. It must be emphasized here that clinical signs of healing, such as restoration of strength and range of motion with no pain on stress testing, in no way signify return of normal strength to the injured ligament.[30] Restoration of ligamentous strength requires a maturation process of collagen aggregation and realignment that may take from several months to a year following injury.[2,32] Any advantages of returning to activities involving intermittent high loading of the knee must be weighed against the risk of the still weakened structure giving way prematurely, possibly resulting in a more serious injury than that originally suffered. In making judgments of appropriate activity levels, the desires of the coach and the highly motivated young athlete must often take second priority to knowledge of the rate and mechanisms of tissue healing.

II. Moderate Sprains (Grade II)

A. *Acute stage.* If it is determined that slight hypermobility exists on one or more joint play movements, considerably more protection of the part is warranted to optimize residual stability of the knee. It is most important to make sure that gross instability (a Grade III injury) is not being masked by protective muscle guarding. Inability to test joint play without eliciting significant muscle guarding may warrant retesting the knee under anesthesia.

Management of an acute Grade II injury should follow the same approach as that discussed for more mild sprains, the primary difference being that the knee must be better protected. The means by which this is accomplished will vary according to (*1*) the reliability of the patient and (2) the degree of ongoing supervision during the healing phase. For the patient who will not be followed on a daily or twice daily basis in, say, a sports medicine clinic, or for the patient in otherwise unreliable situations, relatively rigid immobilization of the knee may be indicated. This may be in the form of a "knee cage," which is typically an adjustable canvas splint with rigid metal stays, or a plaster splint. Plaster splints may be complete cylinder splints, bivalved cylinder splints, or a posterior semi-cylinder splint held in place with an elastic wrap. The advantage of the knee cage and the posterior splint is that a compressive bandage may be worn under the splint to control effusion; the wrap can be reapplied for adjustment when necessary.

Weight bearing must be restricted to the weight of the lower leg only, by using crutches and a three-point crutch gait. The gait pattern should approximate normal walking as much as possible. Gradual resumption of weight-bearing should not be initiated until 2 or 3 wk following injury, when the acute inflammatory process has subsided and some fibrous healing of the defect has taken place. The use of crutches should continue until knee extension can be performed against gravity through a full range of movement, and until at least 3 to 4 wk following injury.

When a removable splint is used, gentle range of motion may be initiated under carefully supervised conditions once symptoms and signs of acute inflammation have subsided, usually several days following injury. The knee must not be moved into the painful ranges. Pain-free, isometric quadriceps contractions should be started as soon as possible after injury to minimize quadriceps muscle wasting—a significant contributing factor in prolonged debilitation.

B. *Chronic stage.* In cases of Grade II ligament sprains, protection from forces that would stress the injured ligament should continue for 3 to 6 wk. This allows sufficient time for a fibrous scar to develop and will minimize the degree of residual laxity. At this point, rehabilitation should follow the guidelines discussed under Grade I injuries with the following additional considerations: (*1*) after more prolonged immobilization, capsular fibrosis may lead to some persistent loss of knee motion; (*2*) the degree of muscle weakness is usually greater; (*3*) there is more likelihood of some residual femorotibial rotary dysfunction; and (*4*) activities must be resumed much more gradually.

1. The stiff knee. Persistent loss of knee motion will usually be in a capsular pattern. Restoration of capsular extensibility will be facilitated by the use of ultrasound as a heating agent, followed by specific joint mobilization procedures. The use of joint distraction mobilizations at the limits of knee extension and inferior patellar glide at the limits of knee flexion are often particularly effective mobilization techniques (see Chapter 7, Joint mobilization techniques). When knee extension is regained, but knee flexion remains limited to 90° to 100°, extracapsular restric-

tions should be considered. The most common extracapsular restricting factor is loss of patellar mobility, especially loss of inferior glide. This occurs most frequently after surgeries that involve, in some way, the extensor mechanism, but may also follow prolonged immobilization after traumatic knee injuries. The problem is often surprisingly resistant to active stretching; as the patient attempts to flex his knee, abnormal femoropatellar mechanics causes a protective reflex contraction of the quadriceps, and the patient ends up fighting against his own muscles. Passive inferior glide of the patella, performed at the limit of knee flexion, is very effective in such cases.

Occasionally a sprained medial collateral ligament heals adhered to the medial femoral condyle, keeping it from sweeping across the condyle as the knee flexes. This typically results in a persistent loss of knee flexion to 90°. This problem is sometimes difficult to overcome. The use of friction massage to the site of adherence followed by stretching may gradually free the adhered tissue. Manipulative rupturing of the adherence should be avoided since there is no control against imposing trauma to the ligament proper.

2. Femorotibial rotary dysfunction. This is often a problem after prolonged immobilization of the knee for any reason. In the case of moderate ligament sprains two types of rotary dysfunction may be de-

tected. The first is restriction of external tibial rotation during knee extension, as discussed above under Grade I injuries. This is relatively easily managed, when due to capsular lightness or adherence, by external rotary mobilization procedures. The second and more serious type of rotary dysfunction is hypermobility of external tibial rotation resulting from some residual laxity of the medial or posteromedial capsule. This may present as increased external rotation of the tibia with the knee flexed, and little external rotary movement noted as the knee extends since it is already "pre-rotated." An actual external rotary contracture may thus develop in which the tibia remains excessively rotated externally in all positions of flexion–extension. Though little can be done conservatively for the hypermobility, the contracture should be corrected by internal rotary mobilization.

C. *Return to normal activities.* Again, it should be emphasized that, following ligamentous injury, a clinically healed ligament is not necessarily a strong ligament.[6,32] Experiments to date suggests that many months, and probably a year, of using the part are necessary to stimulate collagen maturation to a point of normal ligamentous strength.[2,32] The individual who enters high-stress activities prematurely is susceptible to two possible modes of ligamentous failure: (*1*) sudden rupture (Grade III) resulting from a single high-loading event or (*2*) gradual fatigue yielding of the ligament from

the cumulative effect of loads that the ligament is not yet able to withstand. The end point of both is often an unstable knee that may permanently restrict many recreational activities. Such long-term disadvantages must be weighed against what are often relatively short-term advantages of the young athlete returning to competition the same season of the injury. Unfortunately, for the college-level or professional athlete, the consequences of not returning to action as soon as possible are often unacceptable when considered in the context of future career opportunities.

Ideally, the rehabilitation program should involve a supervised, gradual progression of activity levels as discussed for Grade I injuries. High-loading activities, such as those involving violent contact or unexpected and uncontrolled changes in direction of movement, should be deferred for 6 to 12 mo following Grade II injuries.

III. **Severe Injuries (Grade III)**

A. *Acute stage.* When the presence of moderate to marked instability on one or more joint play movement tests is detected on examination of the knee, an orthopaedic surgeon should be consulted immediately. Surgical apposition of the torn ligamentous ends will optimize residual stability.[6] At the knee this is critical. Early surgery, performed prior to atrophy and adherence of the torn ends to adjacent tissues, is preferred over late reconstructive procedures.[7,34,39,40]

There is some dispute among authorities over whether surgical repair for isolated anterior cruciate ligament ruptures in the absence of a fracture or meniscus tear is warranted. First, it is pointed out by many that isolated anterior cruciate lesions are extremely rare.[21,22] Smillie proposes that if only the anterior cruciate is involved little functional impairment ensues if adequate quadriceps function is restored.[42] Perhaps the greatest problem faced in repairing a torn anterior cruciate, or in related reconstructive procedures, is the precarious blood supply to the ligament. Strict, prolonged immobilization is necessary to assure healing following surgery. However, the debilitating effects of such prolonged immobilization often negate advantages the surgery may offer. Newer surgical reconstruction and augmentation procedures may offer a solution to this dilemma.

B. *Chronic stage*

When complete ruptures are not detected and appropriately managed in the early stages, chronic instability will result. Whether this leads to functional instability will depend on the ligament involved and the individual's activity level. When the medial collateral ligament is ruptured the anterior cruciate is often injured concurrently; even if not, the cruciate will usually undergo eventual fatigue yielding because of the resulting abnormal joint mechanics. The instability resulting from involvement of these two ligaments usually causes an unacceptable degree of disability; the individual can do little more than walk in a straight line on level ground. Changes in direction and negotiating uneven terrain result in unexpected giving way of the

involved leg. The individual with an isolated cruciate rupture may have very little disability, depending upon quadricep function and the person's activity level.

Conservative attempts at managing chronic ligament ruptures should be primarily directed towards optimizing compensatory muscle functioning. The quadriceps must be lengthened to above-normal levels. For anteromedial rotatory instability, resulting from combined medial collateral and anterior cruciate ruptures, the pes anserinus and medial hamstring groups should also be developed.

MENISCUS LESIONS

Meniscus lesions affecting the knee are common injuries, especially in athletes. When a tear of the body of the meniscus is diagnosed, treatment is usually surgical since the relatively avascular menisci have limited capacity for repair. Tears confined to the body of a meniscus cannot heal. Tears of the body of a meniscus extending to the periphery may heal by the infiltration of granulation tissue into the defect from the peripheral vascularized region of the meniscus. However, such healing is usually incomplete or, if it is complete, the meniscus will usually have increased in size and may no longer function normally. A torn meniscus left untreated may well lead to early degenerative changes because of the resulting alteration in knee mechanics.

Tears or sprains localized to the periphery, such as coronary ligament sprains, do heal, and surgery for these lesions is usually not required unless the meniscus has been rendered grossly unstable.

Once it has been determined through examination that a meniscus lesion exists, it is important that the injury be classified as a tear confined to the periphery or a tear involving the body of the meniscus. Often arthroscopy or arthrography will assist the physician in making this distinction. Most tears involving the body of the medial meniscus are accompanied by an anteromedial coronary ligament sprain, but the converse is not necessarily true. If only a coronary ligament tear is present, the physical therapist will assume a primary role in management whereas physical therapy is usually indicated post-surgically only for a tear of the body of a meniscus.

History

Onset. The menisci move with the tibia on flexion–extension and with the femur on rotation. If, during flexion, external tibial rotation is forced instead of the internal rotation that should normally occur, abnormal stresses are applied to the menisci with the possibility of a tear occurring. The same, of course, applies to the case of forced internal tibial rotation during knee extension. Similarly, flexion or extension taking place in the absence of the normal rotary movement that should accompany it may result in a meniscus tear. The medial meniscus, being less mobile, is more susceptible to injury. Since tibial rotation is not possible in the fully extended knee, the history is one of twisting on a semi-flexed knee. Again, athletes, especially those wearing cleated shoes and involved in contact sports, are particularly prone to suffering meniscus injuries, occasionally in conjunction with ligament tears.

Meniscus tears may also occur with hyperflexion of the knee, especially during weight bearing. In this position, the femoral condyles have rolled back to articulate with the posterior aspects of the tibial articular surfaces. The menisci, then, must recede backward during flex-

ion, but can only recede to a certain point before capsuloligamentous attachments restrict further movement of the menisci. If further flexion is forced once the menisci have reached their limit of backward movement, the menisci are susceptible to being ground between the femoral and tibial joint surfaces. This is especially true if rotation is forced in hyperflexion, since a rotary movement entails further backward movement of one condyle. Certain occupations, such as mining, in which one must move about in a squatting position, may predispose to development of meniscal tears from this mechanism. In athletics, the wrestler is classically prone to this type of injury.

Site of pain. The victim will usually feel "something give" in the joint, often with an accompanying deep, sickening type of pain. If not masked by other injuries or extensive effusion, the patient will often be able to point to the spot on the joint line corresponding to the site of the tear where the coronary ligament has been sprained.

Nature of pain and disability. The onset is usually sudden with an immediate deep pain associated with giving way of the joint. If hemarthrosis occurs, the typical severe, generalized pain arising within minutes of the injury is reported. If a longitudinal tear of the medial meniscus extends anteriorly past the midpoint of the meniscus, the lateral portion may slip over the dome of the medial femoral condyle. This grossly interferes with normal knee mechanics, with a resultant immediate locking of the joint so that the last 20° to 30° of extension are lost. An injury involving such immediate locking is usually preceded by one or more previous minor incidences of giving way followed by effusion. Finally, the developing longitudinal tear extends anteriorly far enough to cause such locking.

The person sustaining a meniscus tear is very hesitant to resume activity immediately following the injury, unlike the person suffering a ligamentous sprain. Synovial effusion, causing a generalized pressure sensation, may arise within hours following injury. Effusion nearly always accompanies a medial meniscus tear. It does not always accompany a lateral tear.

In the case of an untreated meniscus tear the acute stage may completely subside with restoration of motion. The person may resume normal activities with little or no pain. The complaint, however, is one of intermittent buckling of the joint for no apparent reason, even during simple walking. Occasional or persistent "clicking" of the joint may be reported. Chronic or intermittent effusion may also occur, probably from altered joint mechanics resulting in undue stress to the joint capsule.

Physical Examination

I. **Acute Stage**
  A. *Observation*
    1. The patient may hobble in on crutches with the knee held slightly flexed and touching down only the toe.
    2. Obvious effusion may be present.
    3. The patient may have difficulty removing the shoe, sock, and trousers.
  B. *Inspection*
    1. Effusion may be noted, especially in the suprapatellar region.
    2. The patient stands with the knee held semi-flexed.
    3. The Helfet test *may not* be performed because of incomplete extension.
    4. The suprapatellar girth measurement may be increased from effusion.
    5. The skin may appear slightly red and shiny.
  C. *Selective tissue tension tests*
    1. Active movements
      a. Weight-bearing flexion–extension is impossible.
      b. Flexion–extension in supine reveals
        i. A capsular pattern if effusion is present
        ii. Considerable loss of extension if the knee is locked, causing a distorted capsular pattern if effusion is present, a noncapsular pattern if little or no effusion is present
      c. Passive overpressure reveals a muscle-guarding end-feel at the extremes of flexion and extension.
      d. If the knee is locked, a springy-rebound end-feel will be noted moving into extension.
    2. Passive movements
      a. These are essentially the same as indicated above for active movement, with perhaps slightly greater range of movement.
      b. McMurray's test may not be performed if considerable effusion restricts flexion, since it is only applicable from full flexion to 90°. If flexion is possible, a painful click may be elicited on combined external rotation and extension if a tear exists in the posterior portion of the medial meniscus, or on combined internal rotation and extension if a posterior lateral meniscus lesion exists.
    3. Resisted movements. These should be strong and painless unless a tendon or muscle has also been injured. Quantative strength measurements cannot be made because of the acute condition.

4. Passive joint play movements
    a. Rotation opposite the side of the lesion may be painful, especially during Apley's test with compression applied. Distraction with rotation should relieve the pain.
    b. Otherwise, these should be relatively normal unless a ligamentous injury also exists.
D. *Palpation*
    1. Tenderness will be present at the joint line where a sprain of the peripheral attachment has occurred. This usually corresponds quite well with the side and site of the tear.
    2. Effusion, as mentioned, nearly always accompanies a medial meniscus tear, but not always a lateral tear. The tap test and emptying of the suprapatellar pouch will confirm the presence of minor effusion.
    3. The joint is warm, and the skin somewhat moist.

II. Chronic Tear
A. *History*. The patient describes intermittent giving way of the joint, often followed by some effusion, especially if the medial meniscus is at fault. There may be a history of locking with manipulative reduction by the patient, a friend, or physician, followed by immediate relief of pain and restoration of extension. The younger, active person is usually suffering a longudinal tear, beginning posteriorly and gradually extending anteriorly. The older person may have a "degenerative" horizontal tear, with sliding occurring between the upper and lower portions. Clicking is noted by the patient when the femoral condyle passes over a centrally protruding piece of a meniscus.

B. *Objective signs* may include
    1. Quadriceps atrophy, especially involving the vastus medialis
    2. Full range of motion, but perhaps some difficulty or apprehension when performing weight-bearing flexion–extension
    3. Possibly a positive Helfet test owing to altered joint mechanics
    4. Possibly a positive McMurray test if the posterior segment of meniscus is torn.
    5. Pain on forced extension if the anterior segment of meniscus is torn
    6. A positive Apley test when the joint is compressed, but not when it is distracted
    7. Tenderness to palpation at the joint line, usually corresponding to the site of the lesion
    8. Perhaps some mild chronic effusion
    9. Quantitative quadriceps weakness compared to the other leg.

III. Coronary Ligament Sprain
A. *History*. The patient usually describes a twisting injury followed by some minor swelling and pain over the anteromedial knee region. Rarely is the victim significantly disabled immediately following the injury, and he usually does not seek medical attention in the acute stage.

The acute symptoms usually subside within a few days. If the meniscus maintains good mobility during healing, the individual will have no further problems. However, often the coronary ligament becomes adhered to the anteromedial margin of the medial tibial condyle as it heals, resulting in reduced mobility of this part of the meniscus. In such cases, the individual develops a more chronic problem characterized by intermittent twinging of the pain when the adhered tissue is stressed, usually with activities involving external rotation of the tibia on the femur. It is the persistent nature of the problem that eventually prompts the individual to seek medical assistance even though the disorder is otherwise minor

B. *Objective findings*

  1. The consistent findings on physical examination are

   a. Point tenderness over the anteromedial joint line

   b. Pain on external rotation of the tibia on the femur, but no pain on valgus stress

  2. Occasionally forced extension hurts, as well. Rarely is effusion present by the time the person is seen clinically. There may be some minimal quadriceps atrophy if the problem has been long-standing.

Management of Meniscus Injuries

Acute tear of the body of a meniscus. If this is suspected on examination, the referring physician should be consulted and notified of the positive findings. The patient is probably a surgical candidate. If surgery is not planned, treatment in the acute stage is essentially the same as that discussed in this chapter for an acute, minor ligamentous sprain. Weight bearing must not be allowed on a locked knee and should be restricted on a knee that cannot fully extend because of effusion. Extension must not be forced in the locked knee, since, if the displaced piece of meniscus does not slip back, extension may occur only at the expense of the anterior cruciate ligament or articular cartilage.

Chronic tear of the body of a meniscus. Again, the physician should be notified if this is suspected. If surgery is not contemplated, the goal is restoration of optimal joint mechanics: mobilization, strengthening, and instruction in appropriate activity levels are necessary. A particular motion, especially extension, must not be encouraged if the restriction is due to an intra-articular block, as from a displaced piece of meniscus.

Coronary ligament tear. We usually see individuals with coronary ligament tears in the chronic stage only, since the acute pain and disability are usually not severe. The persistent intermittent knee pain is the result of adherence of the anteromedial coronary ligament to the underlying tibia; the adhesion is broken with some sudden movement, then adherence recurs during healing.

The objective of treatment is to gradually restore mobility to this part of the meniscus. This is accomplished through the use of ultrasound and transverse friction massage applied directly to the site of the lesion. Five to ten minutes of massage, over three to four treatment sessions are usually sufficient. Attention should be paid to quadriceps weakness if present. The patient may be instructed in self-administered friction massage, to be applied before activity.

PATELLAR TRACKING DYSFUNCTION (CHONDROMALACIA PATELLAE)

Disorders of the patellofemoral joint constitute a large percentage of chronic knee problems of nontraumatic origin. Unfortunately, nonacute patellofemoral joint dysfunctions tend to be referred to as "chondromalacia patellae," which literally means *softening of the articular cartilage of the patella*. Since articular cartilage is not a pain sensitive structure, the term "chondromalacia" does not adequately describe the clinically significant features of the pathology nor does it take into account etiologic considerations. In fact, surgical studies suggest that surface chondromalacia *per se* is a relatively normal characteristic of most adult patellae and probably has little relationship in cause or effect to symptomatic knee problems.[1,16,28,35,38,44]

Biomechanical Considerations

The patella is a triangular sesamoid bone receiving attachment medially from above by the quadriceps tendon, laterally from the patellar retinacula, and inferiorly from the patellar tendon. The patella glides inferiorly with respect to the femoral condyles when the knee flexes, and superiorly when the knee extends.

Because the medial femoral condyle extends further distally than the lateral condyle does, most knee joints assume a slight valgus angulation in the standing position (Figs. 17-1, 17-13, and 17-15). The direction of pull of the quadriceps musculature tends to be in line with the femur, whereas the pull of the patellar tendon is in line with the long axis of the tibia. The angle formed between the line of pull of the quadriceps muscle and the patellar tendon is often called the *Q angle*.

The vector that represents the pull on the patellar tendon during loaded knee extension can be resolved into a longitudinal component and a lateral component (Fig. 17-15). The longitudinal component is in line with the direction of pull of the quadriceps and in line with the long axis of the femur. The lateral vectorial component causes a tendency for the patella to be pulled laterally with respect to the long axis of the femur during loaded knee extension.

As the patella glides inferiorly and superiorly during knee flexion and extension, it should do so in line with the long axis of the femur. It is important then that excessive lateral patellar movement does not occur. Prevention of excessive lateral patellar movement during loaded knee extension is dependent upon structural and

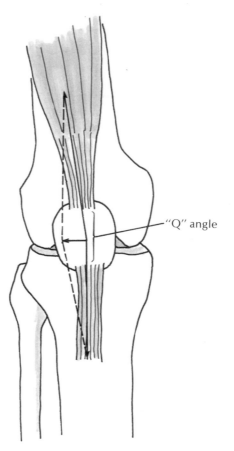

Fig. 17-15. Pull of the patellar tendon during loaded knee extension, showing the "Q" angle, and longitudinal and lateral vectoral components

dynamic mechanisms of patellar stabilization. Structural factors include

1. *Lateral femoral condyle* which, because it is prominent anteriorly, provides some abutment against lateral patellar movement (Fig. 17-2).
2. *Deep patellar groove of the femur*, in which the patella glides when the knee is in positions of flexion.
3. *Angle between the pull of the quadriceps and the pull of the patellar tendon.* When the knee is in positions of flexion, there is an angle between the pull of the quadriceps and the pull of the patellar tendon, projected onto the sagittal

plane (Fig. 17-16). The result of these pulls, represented vectorially, is a patellofemoral compressive force that holds the patella tightly against the patellar groove of the femur, disallowing extraneous movement.

It should be noted that the structural stabilizing mechanisms mentioned here are primarily operational in positions of some knee flexion. As the knee approaches full extension, the patella begins moving superiorly out of the deep part of the patellar groove of the femur. In this position the sagitally projected angulation between the quadriceps muscle and patellar tendon decreases, thus reducing the patellofemoral compressive force that holds the patella firmly in the groove. As the knee moves into extension, especially when loaded, dynamic patellar stabilizing factors play an essential role.

The most important dynamic factor necessary to assure normal patellofemoral joint function is contraction of the vastus medialis muscle. The distal fibers of the vastus medialis originate from the medial aspect of the distal femur and run almost horizontally to insert on the medial aspect of the patella. They attach to the patella by way of the medial retinaculum. The horizontal orientation of these fibers of the vastus medialis allows them to prevent excessive lateral movement of the patella during loaded knee extension (Fig. 17-17).

Etiology

Chronic patellar tracking dysfunction is a condition in which the patella tends to be pulled too far laterally each time the knee is extended under load. We can now consider possible causative factors, both structural and dynamic. Structural factors might include the following:

1. An increase in the valgus angulation between the quadriceps muscle and the patellar tendon, often referred to as an

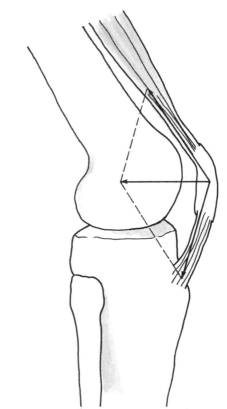

Fig. 17-16. Patellofemoral compression forces in the sagittal plane with the knee in a flexed position

increased *Q angle* (Fig. 17-15). Common causes are (*1*) increased femoral anteversion, (*2*) increased external tibial torsion, and (*3*) increased foot pronation.

2. A lateral femoral condyle that is not sufficiently prominent anteriorly. This results in a loss of the abutment effect normally provided by the lateral condyle (Fig. 17-18).

3. A small, high-riding patella, often called *patella alta*. The more superiorly the patella moves on the femur during knee extension, the less time it spends in the deep portion of the patellar groove where it is better stabilized.

Dynamically, the most important cause of reduced lateral patellar stabilization is vastus medialis insufficiency. This com-

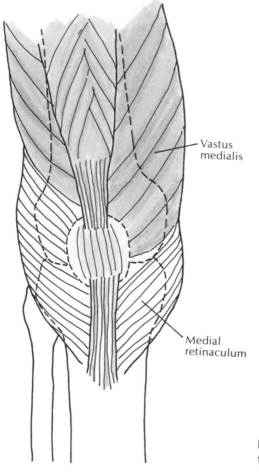

Vastus medialis

Medial retinaculum

monly occurs from disuse atrophy associated with immobilization or following injury to the knee. It may also occur when an individual increases activities involving loaded knee extension, and the vastus medialis is not adequately conditioned to meet the added loads imposed on the extensor mechanism.

Pathology

In order to best understand the clinical manifestations of patellar tracking dysfunction, we must first discuss the pathologic implications of excessive lateral patellar movement. As the patella moves against the femoral condyles, the contact area on the back of the patella varies with the position of the knee. During normal knee function, both the medial and lateral facets of the patellar articular surface receive compressive stresses from contact with the femur. The small odd medial facet, however, only makes contact at extremes of knee flexion, a position that the knee seldom assumes during normal

Fig. 17-17. Orientation of the fibers of the vastus medialis

Fig. 17-18. Femoral condyles, showing (A) normal prominence of the lateral condyle and (B) insufficient prominence of the lateral condyle anteriorly

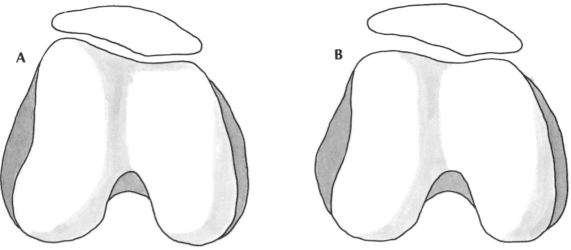

A

B

daily activities (Fig. 17-19).[16] Thus, during normal use of the knee, the odd medial facet is nonarticulating and does not receive much compressive stress. Because of this, the subchondral bone is less dense, softer, and weaker at the odd medial facet, compared with that of the rest of the patella (Fig. 17-20).[36,45-47]

If the patella is pulled too far laterally during loaded knee extension, movement of the patella will follow the contour of the patellar groove of the femur. This causes the patella to undergo some rotation in the transverse plane, bringing the odd medial facet into a contacting position (Fig. 17-21). Under such conditions the relatively weak subchondral bone of the odd medial facet may not be able to withstand the loads imposed upon it. This results in an increase rate of trabecular microfracturing, which may incite a low-grade, painful inflammatory response. Trabecular breakdown may be further enhanced by shear stresses between the soft odd medial facet and the stiffer medial facet during compressive deformation.[47] For a particular load, the odd medial facet would deform more than the medial facet, resulting in shearing when the two are compressed simultaneously. This would cause the pathologic process to progress into the medial facet of the patella.

Excessive lateral patellar movement during repeated knee extension may also cause abnormal tensile stresses to the medial retinaculum of the knee. This could also be a source of low-grade inflammation and pain associated with patellar tracking dysfunction.

Clinical Manifestations

The patient presenting with patellar tracking dysfunction usually demonstrates characteristic symptoms and signs consistent with the etiologic and pathologic factors mentioned. The consistent subjective complaints of a patient presenting with patellar tracking dysfunction include

1. A gradual onset of pain. The patient often describes some recent increase in activities involving loaded knee extension, or he may report some knee injury or disuse preceding the onset of the problem.
2. Pain is felt primarily in a generalized area over the medial aspect of the knee and in the peripatellar regions.
3. The pain is aggravated by activities involving increased patellofemoral compressive stresses. These typically include walking down stairs and sitting with the knee bent for long periods of time. Slowly applied loads, such as those involved with sitting with the knees bent, are likely to cause more discomfort than high strain rate loading such as running or walking. This is because bone is stronger under fast strain rates for loads of equal magnitude.

The objective findings on physical examination of patients with patellar tracking dysfunction might include

1. Some structural predisposing factor, such as an increased Q angle or a high-riding patella. Common causes of an increased Q angle include iliotibial band tightness, femoral anteversion, external tibial torsion, and increased foot pronation.
2. Femoropatellar crepitus during weight-bearing knee movements if the tissue breakdown has spread to surface layers of articular cartilage
3. Discomfort when the patella is passively moved laterally, if the medial retinaculum is irritated
4. Tightness of the lateral retinaculum noted when the patella is moved medially
5. Visible vastus medialis atrophy when the patient is asked to strongly contract the quadriceps muscles
6. Tenderness to deep palpation of the backside of the medial patella and to palpation of the adductor tubercle, where the medial retinaculum attaches

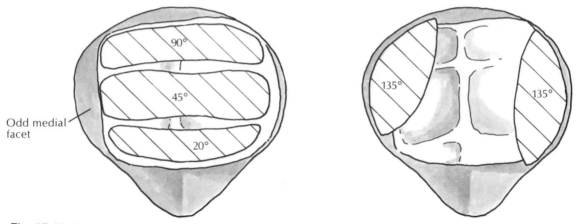

Odd medial facet

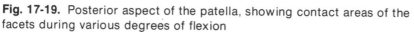

Fig. 17-19. Posterior aspect of the patella, showing contact areas of the facets during various degrees of flexion

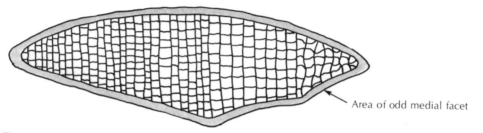

Area of odd medial facet

Fig. 17-20. Diagram of subchondral bone density of the patella. Density is reduced in the area of the odd medial facet.

Fig. 17-21. Diagram depicting (*A*) normal loading and (*B*) abnormal pull of the patella laterally during loaded knee extension. The medial facet is brought into a contacting position.

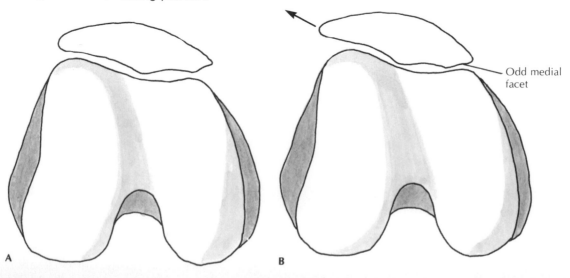

Odd medial facet

Management

Treatment of patellar tracking dysfunction must take into consideration etiologic and pathologic factors. The most important early measure is the reduction of activities involving high or prolonged patellofemoral compressive loads. This is necessary in order to prevent continued tissue trauma. The patient must understand the deleterious affects of such activities as climbing stairs or bent-knee sitting, since these activities do not necessarily cause immediate pain.

Particular attention should be paid to strengthening the vastus medialis. This may be necessary to correct vastus medialis insufficiency or as an attempt to compensate for structural causes of patellar tracking dysfunction. In order to strengthen the vastus medialis, resistance must be applied to the terminal 5° or 10° of knee extension. Since bone is stronger under fast loading conditions, the exercises should be performed with a rapid loading cycle. This will minimize the possibility that the exercise program will inflict additional trauma. Exercise equipment that allows variable speed and isokinetic resistance lends itself well to this type of loading.

Assess the extensibility of the lateral retinaculum by noting the excursion of medial patellar movement with the knee close to full extension. If the lateral retinaculum appears tight, it should be stretched using the same technique as used to test its mobility. The effectiveness of stretching procedures may be enhanced by prior or simultaneous heating with ultrasound.

If the condition is associated with abnormal foot pronation and does not respond to the treatment measures mentioned, you should consider stabilization of the foot to control pronation. This may be accomplished with various orthotic devices, such as a contoured arch support, or shoe modifications, such as a medial heel wedge or lateral sole wedge.

If a tight iliotibial band is found to contribute to functional valgus deviation at the knee, institute procedures to stretch the iliotibial band. These are best done passively with the patient lying on his side. The examiner sits behind the patient's pelvis to stabilize it against rolling backward. He positions the leg to be stretched with the hip in extension and neutral rotation, and flexes the knee to about 90°. Supporting under the patient's knee and preventing hip rotation or knee extension, the examiner stretches the iliotibial band by adducting the extended hip toward the plinth.

There are few patients with patellar tracking dysfunction who do not respond satisfactorily to a well-designed and appropriately instituted conservative treatment program. Common causes of failure include (1) inadequate restriction of activities in the early stages of treatment or (2) inadequate or inappropriate quadriceps strengthening. Typical faults include

1. Resisting through too great an arc of movement. Only the terminal 5° to 10° of extension should be resisted; resistance to knee extension applied at greater ranges of flexion causes excessive patellofemoral compression stress and may perpetuate the problem.

2. Exercises may be performed too slowly. Subchondral bone is weakest—and therefore is more likely to breakdown—under slowly applied loads. Since there is some patellofemoral compression with terminal extension exercises, the loading cycles should be performed quickly to prevent additional trauma to the subchondral bone of the patella.

3. Insufficient resistance to terminal extension exercises. Few patients understand isometric exercises well enough to effectively strengthen muscles through their use. Some external load is necessary for more accurate monitoring of work performed and improve-

ment. It is necessary to work the muscle close to fatigue in order to effect strengthening. "Quad sets" alone are usually inadequate.

4. Lack of attention to underlying contributory biomechanical abnormalities. The most common contributory abnormalities are a tight iliotibial band and abnormal foot pronation.

The rare patient who does not respond satisfactorily to a well-instituted conservative program may be a surgical candidate.[5,16,20] Surgery may involve loosening of a tight lateral retinaculum or reduction of the Q angle by moving the attachment of the patellar tendon medially. Occasionally the medial structures of the extensor mechanism are tightened as well. If the surface layers of the patellar articular cartilage are grossly disturbed, the surgeon may shave the back side of the patella. If shaved to vascularized subchondral bone, a more congruous layer of fibrocartilage will develop as part of a healing response.

REFERENCES

1. Abernathy PJ, Townsend PR, Rose RM, Radin EL: Is chondromalacia patellae a separate clinical entity? J Bone Joint Surg 60(B):205–210, 1978
2. Adams A: Effect of exercise upon ligament strength. Res Q 37:163–167, 1966
3. Barnett CH: Locking at the knee joint. J Anat 87:91–95, 1953
4. Bentley G: Chondromalacia patellae. J Bone Joint Surg 52(A):221–232, 1970
5. Bentley G: The surgical treatment of chondromalacia patellae. J Bone Joint Surg 60(B):74–81, 1978
6. Clayton ML, Metes JS, Abdulla M: Experimental investigations of ligamentous healing. Clin Orthop 61:146–153, 1968
7. D'Arcy J: Pes anserinus transposition for chronic anteromedial rotational instability of the knee. J Bone Joint Surg 60(B):66–70, 1978
8. de Andrade JR, Grant C, Dixon A: Joint distension and reflex muscle inhibition in the knee. J Bone Joint Surg 47(A):313–321, 1967
9. Engin AE, Korde MS: Mechanics of normal and abnormal knee joint. J Biomechanics 7:325–334, 1974
10. Frankel VH: Biomechanics of the knee. In Ingiversem et al (eds): The Knee Joint. New York, Elsevier-Dutton, 1971
11. Frankel VH, Burstein AH, Brooks DB: Biomechanics of internal derangement of the knee. J Bone Joint Surg 53(A):945–962, 1971
12. Frankel VH, Burstein AH: Orthopaedic Biomechanics. Philadelphia, Lea & Febiger, 1971.
13. Frankel VH, Hang Y: Recent advances in the biomechanics of sports injuries. Acta Orthop Scand 46:484–497, 1975
14. Furman W, Marshall JL, Girgis FG: The anterior cruciate ligament: A functional analysis based on postmortem studies. J Bone Joint Surg 58(A):179–185, 1976
15. Goodfellow J, Hungerford DS, Woods C: Patellofemoral joint mechanics and pathology. 2. Chrondromalacia patellae. J Bone Joint Surg 58(B):291–299, 1976
16. Goodfellow J, Hungerford DS, Zindel M: Pattelofemoral joint mechanics and pathology. Functional anatomy of the patellofemoral joint. J Bone Joint Surg 58(B):287–290, 1976
17. Helfet A: Disorders of the Knee. Philadelphia, JB Lippincott, 1974
18. Hughston JC, Andrews JR, Cross MJ, Moschi A: Classification of knee ligament instabilities. Part I. The medial compartment and cruciate ligaments. J Bone Joint Surg 58(A):159–172, 1976
19. Hughston JC, Andrews JR, Cross MG, Moschi A: Classification of ligament instabilities. Part II. The lateral compartment. J Bone Surg 58(A):173–179, 1976
20. Insall J, Falvo KA, Wise DW: Chondromalacia patellae, a prospective study. J Bone Joint Surg 58(A):1–8, 1976
21. Kennedy JC, Fowler PJ: Medial and anterior instability of the knee. J Bone Joint Surg 53(A):1257–1270, 1971
22. Kennedy JC, Weinberg HW, Wilson AS: The anatomy and function of the anterior cruciate ligament, as determined by clinical and morphological studies. J Bone Joint Surg 56(A):223–234, 1974
23. Kettelkamp DB: Clinical implications of

knee biomechanics. Arch Surg 107:406–410, 1973

24. Last RJ: The popliteus muscle and the lateral meniscus. J Bone Joint Surg 32(B):93–99, 1950

25. Laubenthal KN, Smidt GL, Kettelkamp DB: A quantitative analysis of knee motion for activities of daily living. Phys Ther 52:34–42, 1972

26. Marks KE, Bentley G: Patella alta and chondromalacia. J Bone Joint Surg 60(B):71–73, 1978

27. MacConaill MA: The function of intraarticular fibrocartilage, with special references to the knee and inferior radioulnar joints. J Anat 66:210–227, 1932

28. Meachim G, Emery IH: Quantitative aspects of patellofemoral cartilage fibrillation in Liverpool necropsies. Ann Rheum Dis 33:39–47, 1974

29. Nicholas JA: Injuries to the menisci of the knee. Orthop Clin North Am 4(3):647–664, 1973

30. Noyes FR: Functional properties of knee ligaments and alterations induced by immobilization. A correlative biomechanical and histological study in primates. Clin Orthop 123:210–242, 1977

31. Noyes FR, DeLucas JL, Torvik PJ: Biomechanics of anterior cruciate ligament failure: An analysis of strain-rate sensitivity and mechanisms of failure in primates. J Bone Joint Surg 56(A): 236–253, 1974

32. Noyes FR, Torvik PJ, Hyde WB, Delucas JL: Biomechanics of ligament failure. II. An analysis of immobilization, exercise, and reconditioning effects in primates. J Bone Joint Surg 56(A):1406–1418, 1974

33. O'Donoghue DH: Treatment of acute ligamentous injuries of the knee. Orthop Clin North Am 4(3):617–645, 1973

34. Oretorp N, Gillquist J, Tiljedahl S: Long term results of surgery for non-acute anteromedial rotary instability of the knee. Acta Orthop Scand 50:329–336, 1979

35. Outerbridge RE: The etiology of chondromalacia patellae. J Bone Joint Surg 43(B):752–757, 1961

36. Raux P, Townsend PR, Miegel R, Rose RM, Radin EL: Trabecullar architecture of the human patella. J Biomech 8:1–7, 1975

37. Shaw JA, Eng M, Murray DG: The longitudinal axis of the knee and the role of the cruciate ligaments in controlling transverse rotation. J Bone Joint Surg 56(A):1603–1609, 1974

38. Shoji H: Chondromalacia patellae: Histological and biochemical aspects. NY State J Med 74:507–510, 1974

39. Slocum DB, Tarson RL, James SL: Late reconstruction procedures used to stabilize the knee. Orthop Clin North Am 4(3):679–689, 1973

40. Slocum DB, Tarson RL: Pes anserinus transplantation. J Bone Joint Surg 50(A):226–242, 1968

41. Slocum DB, Tarson RL: Rotatory instability syndrome of the knee. Its pathogenesis and a clinical test to demonstrate its presence. J Bone Joint Surg 50(A):211–225, 1968

42. Smillie IS: Injuries of the Knee Joint. New York, Churchill Livingstone, 1978

43. Steindler A: Kinesiology of the Human Body. Springfield Charles C Thomas, 1955

44. Storigord J: Chondromalacia of the patella: Physical signs in relation to operative findings. Acta Orthop Scand 46:685–694, 1975

45. Townsend PR, Miegel RE, Rose RM, Raux P, Radin EL: Structure and function of the human patella: The role of cancellous bone. J Biomed Mater Res 7:605–611, 1976

46. Townsend PR, Raux P, Rose RM, Miegel RE, Radin EL: The distribution and anisotrophy of the stiffness of cancellous bone in the human patella. J Biomech 8:33–367, 1975

47. Townsend PR, Rose RM, Radin EL, Raux P: The biomechanics of the human patella and its implications for chondromalacia. J Biomech 10:403–407, 1977

48. Turner W (ed): Anatomical Memoirs of John Goodsir. Edinburgh, Adam & Black, 1968

49. Wang YJB, Rubim RM, Marshall JL: A mechanism of isolated anterior cruciate ligament rupture. Case report. J Bone Joint Surg 57(A):411–413, 1975

50. Warren LF, Marshall JL: The supporting structures and layers on the medial side of the knee. An anatomical analysis. J Bone Joint Surg 61(A):56–62, 1979

18 *The Ankle and Hindfoot*

Randolph M. Kessler

FUNCTIONAL ANATOMY OF THE JOINTS

OSTEOLOGY

The *tibia* flares at its distal end. As a result, the cross section of the bone changes from triangular, in the region of the shaft, to quadrangular in the area of the distal metaphyseal portion of the bone. Medially is a distal projection of the tibia, the medial malleolus; laterally is the fibular notch, which is concave anteroposteriorly for articulation with the distal end of the fibula. Along the medial side of the posterior surface is a groove for the passage of the tibialis posterior tendon. The term *posterior malleolus* is often used to refer to the distal overhang of the posterior aspect of the tibia (Fig. 18-1).

The lateral surface of the medial malleolus and the inferior surface of the tibia have a continuous cartilaginous covering for articulation with the talus. The articular surface of the inferior end of the tibia is concave anterposteriorly. Mediolaterally, it is somewhat convex, having a crest centrally that corresponds to the central groove in the trochlear surface of the talus. This, then, is essentially a sellar joint surface. It is slightly wider anteriorly than posteriorly. The articular surface of the medial malleolus is comma-shaped, the "tail" of the comma being situated posteriorly (Fig. 18-1).

The fibula, which is quite narrow in the region of its shaft, becomes bulbous at its distal end (Fig. 18-2). This distal portion of the bone, the lateral malleolus, is triangular in cross section. When viewed from a lateral aspect, the fibula is somewhat pointed distally. The lateral malleolus extends farther distally and is situated more posteriorly than the medial malleolus. The medial aspects of the lateral malleolus is covered by a triangular cartilaginous surface for articulation with the lateral side of the talus. Above this surface, the fibula contacts the tibia in the fibular notch of the tibia. The apex of this triangular surface points inferiorly. There is a fairly deep depression in the posteroinferior region of the lateral malleolus called the *malleolar fossa* that can be easily palpated. The posterior talofibular ligament attaches in this fossa. There is a groove along the posterior aspect of the lateral malleolus through which the peroneus brevis tendon passes.

The talus constitutes the link between the leg and the tarsus (Fig. 18-3). It consists of a body, anterior to which is the head. The body and head of the talus are connected by a short neck.

The superior surface of the body is covered with articular cartilage for articulation with the inferior surface of the tibia. This articular surface is continuous with the articular surfaces of the medial and lateral aspects of the talus. The superior surface is somewhat wider anteriorly than posteriorly. It is convex anteroposteriorly and slightly concave mediolaterally, corresponding to the sellar surface of the inferior end of the tibia mentioned above. In this sense, the superior talar articular sur-

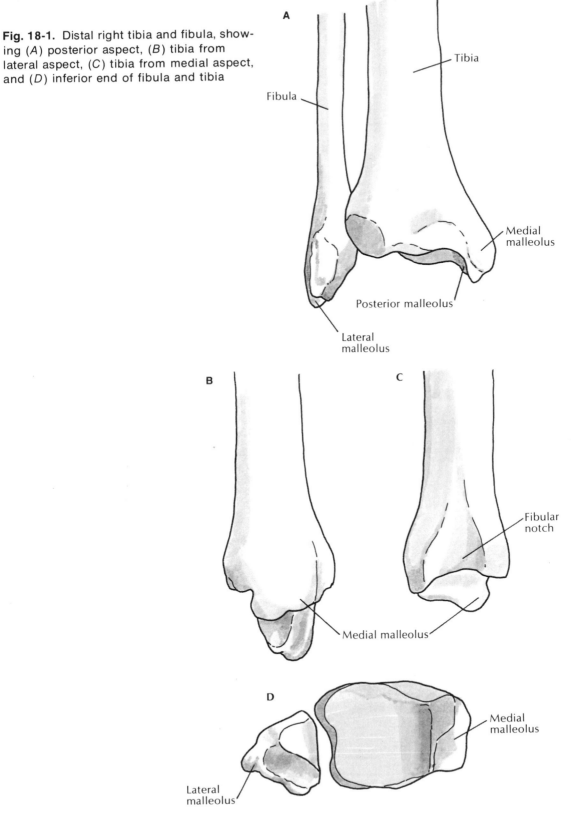

Fig. 18-1. Distal right tibia and fibula, showing (A) posterior aspect, (B) tibia from lateral aspect, (C) tibia from medial aspect, and (D) inferior end of fibula and tibia

A

Fibula

Tibia

Medial malleolus

Posterior malleolus

Lateral malleolus

B

C

Fibular notch

Medial malleolus

D

Medial malleolus

Lateral malleolus

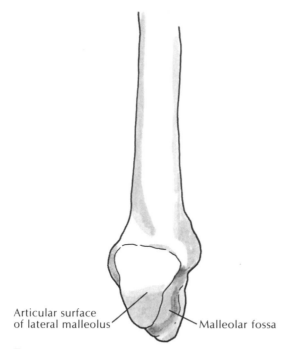

Fig. 18-2. Medial aspect of distal right fibula

Articular surface of lateral malleolus

Malleolar fossa

face is trochlear, or pulleylike and is often referred to as the *trochlea*.

The lateral aspect of the body of the talus is largely covered by articular cartilage for articulation with the distal end of the fibula (Fig. 18-4). This articular surface is triangular, the apex situated inferiorly. Just below this apex is a lateral bony projection to which the lateral talocalcaneal ligament attaches.

The articular surface of the medial aspect of the talus is considerably smaller than that of the lateral side, and it faces slightly upwards (Fig. 18-5). It contacts the articular surface of the medial malleolus on the tibia. It is comma-shaped, the tail of the comma being situated posteriorly. The roughened area below the medial articular surface serves as an attachment for the deltoid ligament. The medial and lateral talar articular surfaces tend to converge posteriorly, lending to the wedge shape of the trochlea. It should be emphasized, however, that the lateral

articular surface of the talus is perpendicular to the axis of movement at the ankle joint, whereas the medial surface is not. This has important biomechanical implications, which are discussed in the following section.

If you view the profiles of the lateral and medial sides of the trochlea, you see that the lateral profile is a section of a circle, whereas the medial profile may be viewed as sections of several circles of different radii; the medial profile is of smaller radius anteriorly than posteriorly.[19] More precisely stated, the contour medially is of gradually increasing radius anterioposteriorly, forming a carteloid profile. The importance of this is described in the section on biomechanics.

Posteriorly, the body of the talus is largely covered by a continuation of the trochlear articular surface as it slopes backward (Fig. 18-6). At the inferior extent of the posterior aspect is the nonarticular posterior process. The posterior process consists of a lateral and a smaller medial tubercle, with an intervening groove through which passes the tendon of the flexor hallucis longus. The posterior talofibular ligament attaches to the lateral tubercle. The medial talocalcaneal ligament and a posterior portion of the deltoid ligament attach to the medial tubercle.

The neck and head of the talus are positioned anteriorly to the body. They are directed slightly medially and downward with respect to the body. The head is covered with articular cartilage anteriorly, for articulation with the navicular, and inferiorly, for articulation with the spring ligament (plantar calcaneonavicular ligament).

The inferior surface of the talus has three cartilage-covered facets for articulation with the calcaneus (Fig. 18-7). The posterior facet, which is the largest of these, is concave inferiorly. The medial and anterior articular facets are continuous with each other and with the inferior articular surface of the head. Both the me-

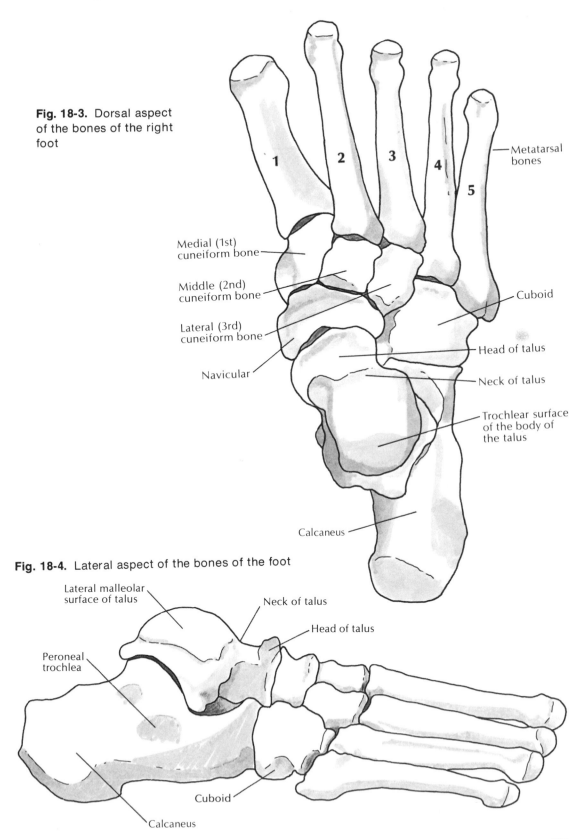

Fig. 18-3. Dorsal aspect of the bones of the right foot

Metatarsal bones

1 2 3 4 5

Medial (1st) cuneiform bone

Middle (2nd) cuneiform bone

Lateral (3rd) cuneiform bone

Navicular

Cuboid

Head of talus

Neck of talus

Trochlear surface of the body of the talus

Calcaneus

Fig. 18-4. Lateral aspect of the bones of the foot

Lateral malleolar surface of talus

Neck of talus

Head of talus

Peroneal trochlea

Cuboid

Calcaneus

451

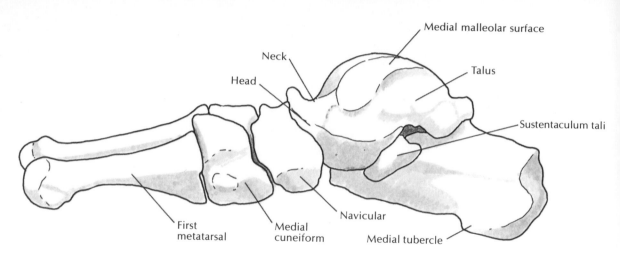

Fig. 18-5. Medial aspect of the bones of the foot

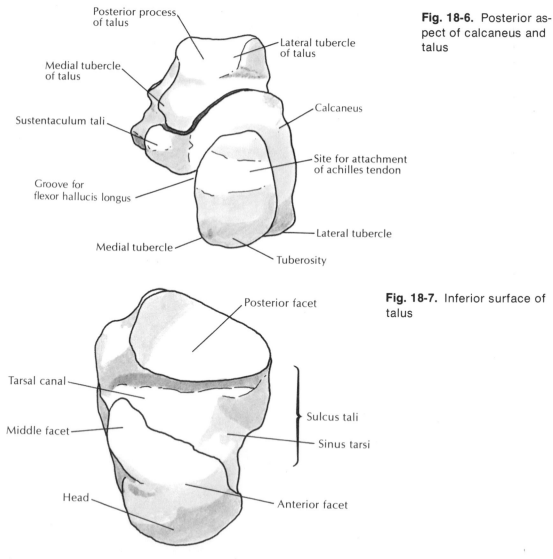

Fig. 18-6. Posterior aspect of calcaneus and talus

Fig. 18-7. Inferior surface of talus

dial and the anterior facets are convex inferiorly and articulate with the superior aspect of the sustentacula tali of the calcaneus. A deep groove, the sulcus tali, separates the posterior and medial facets on the inferior aspect of the talus. This groove runs obliquely from posteromedial to anterolateral. Where it is the deepest—posteromedially—it forms the *tarsal canal*; where it widens and opens out laterally, it is referred to as the *sinus tarsi*. The interosseus talocalcaneal ligament and the cervical ligament occupy the sinus tarsi.

The calcaneus is situated beneath the talus in the standing position and provides a major contact point with the ground. It is the largest of the tarsal bones. The calcaneus articulates with the talus superiorly, and with the cuboid anteriorly. Posteriorly it projects backward, providing considerable leverage for the plantar flexors of the ankle. The superior aspect of the calcaneus bears the posterior, medial, and anterior facets for articulation with the corresponding facets of the talus (Fig. 18-8). The posterior facet is convex, whereas the medial and anterior facets are concave. The medial and anterior facets are situated on the superior aspect of the sustentaculum tali, which is a bony projection of the calcaneus that overhangs medially. As with the corresponding facets on the talus, the medial and anterior facets of the calcaneus are usually continuous with each other. The medial and anterior facets are separated from the posterior facet by the *sulcus calcanei*, which forms the bottom of the sinus tarsi and tarsal canal, thereby corresponding to the sulcus tali of the talus.

The posterior aspect of the large posterior projection of the calcaneus contains a smooth superior surface, which slopes upward and forward, and a rough inferior surface, which slopes downward and forward. The upper surface is the site of attachment for the Achilles tendon (Fig. 18-6). The lower surface blends inferiorly with the tuber calcanei, which is the point of contact of the calcaneus with the ground in the standing position.

The tuber calcanei on the inferior aspect of the calcaneus consists of a medial tubercle and a lateral tubercle, of which the medial is the larger. Anterior to the

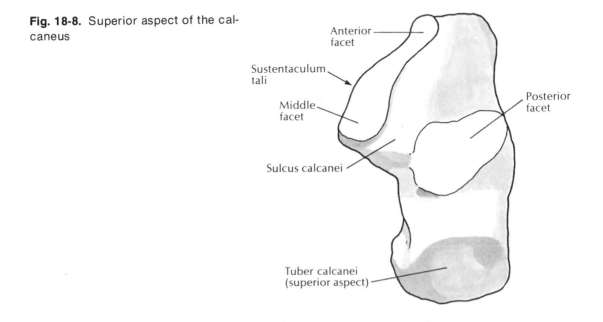

Fig. 18-8. Superior aspect of the calcaneus

Anterior facet

Sustentaculum tali

Middle facet

Sulcus calcanei

Posterior facet

Tuber calcanei (superior aspect)

tuber calcanei is a roughened surface for the attachment of the long and short plantar ligaments (Fig. 18-9). At the anterior extent of the inferior surface of the calcaneus is the anterior tubercle, which also serves as a point of attachment for the long plantar ligament. On the inferior aspect of the medially projecting sustentaculum tali is a groove through which runs the flexor hallucis longus tendon.

The lateral aspect of the calcaneus is nearly flat. There is a small prominence, the peroneal trochlea, that is located just distal to the lateral malleolus (Fig. 18-4). The peroneus brevis tendon travels downward and forward, just superior to this trochlea, while the peroneus longus tendon passes inferior to it. The calcaneofibular ligament attaches just posterior and slightly superior to the peroneal

Fig. 18-9. Plantar surface of the foot

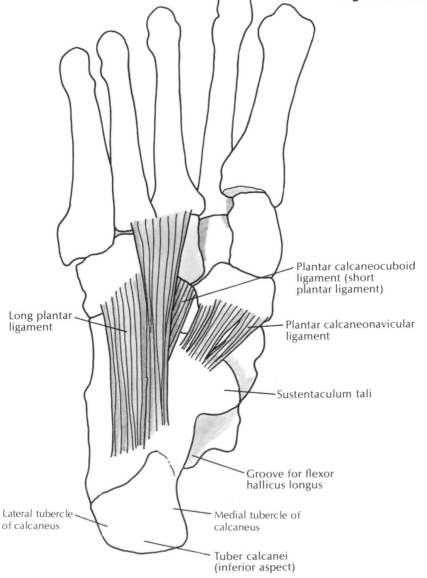

Long plantar ligament

Plantar calcaneocuboid ligament (short plantar ligament)

Plantar calcaneonavicular ligament

Sustentaculum tali

Groove for flexor hallicus longus

Lateral tubercle of calcaneus

Medial tubercle of calcaneus

Tuber calcanei (inferior aspect)

trochlea, at which point there may be a rounded prominence.

From the anterosuperior extent of the medial aspect of the calcaneus, the sustentaculum tali projects in a medial direction (Fig. 18-8). The sustentaculum tali may be palpated just below the medial malleolus.

On the narrowed anterior aspect of the calcaneus is the cartilage-covered articular surface that contacts the cuboid bone. This is a sellar joint surface, being concave superinferiorly and convex mediolaterally (Fig. 18-3).

The remainder of the tarsus includes the navicular and cuboid bones, which contact the talus and calcaneus, respectively, and the three cuneiforms, which articulate with the first three metatarsals (Fig. 18-3). The cuboid extends distally to contact the remaining two metatarsals. (These bones will not be considered in detail here, but will be referred to in the biomechanics section of this chapter.)

LIGAMENTS AND CAPSULES

The Inferior Tibiofibular Joint

This is a syndesmosis, and lacks articular cartilage and synovium. The distal fibula is situated in the fibular notch of the lateral aspect of the distal tibia and bound to it by several ligaments (Figs. 18-10 and 18-11). The anterior and posterior tibiofibular ligaments pass in front of and behind the syndesmosis. They are both directed downward and medially to check separation of the two bones. The inferior transverse ligament is a thickened band of fibers that is closely related to the posterior tibiofibular ligament. It passes from the posterior margin of the inferior tibial articular surface downward and laterally to the malleolar fossa of the fibula. This ligament is lined inferiorly with articular cartilage where it contacts the posterolateral talar articular surface during extreme plantar flexion. The interosseus

Fig. 18-10. Lateral view of the ligaments of the right talocrural and proximal tarsal joints

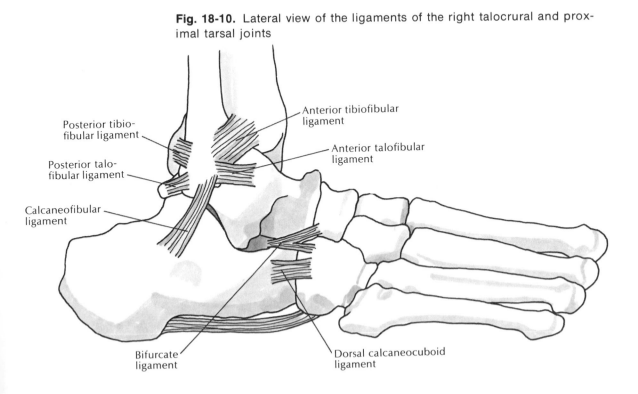

Posterior tibio-fibular ligament

Posterior talo-fibular ligament

Calcaneofibular ligament

Anterior tibiofibular ligament

Anterior talofibular ligament

Bifurcate ligament

Dorsal calcaneocuboid ligament

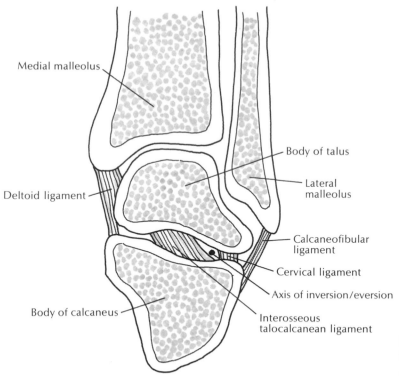

Fig. 18-11. Coronal section through the talocrural and subtalar joints

ligament is a continuation of the interosseus membrane of the tibia and fibula. It extends between the adjacent surfaces of the bones at the syndesmosis. The tibia and fibula are separated at the syndesmosis by a fat pad.

The ligaments of the inferior tibiofibular articulation are oriented to prevent widening of the mortise. They are also important in preventing posterior displacement of the fibula at the syndesmosis, which tends to occur when the leg is forcibly internally rotated on the tarsus. It should be realized that complete sectioning of the inferior tibiofibular ligaments alone allows only a minimal increase in the intermalleolar space.[1] This is because the two bones are indirectly held together by their mutual connections to the talus, by way of the medial and lateral ligaments of the ankle. Significant diastasis, then, is usually accompanied by rupture of one or more of the talocrural ligaments, usually the deltoid ligament.

The Ankle Joint (Ankle Mortise or Talocrural Joint)

This joint is formed by the superior portion of the body of the talus fitting within the mortise, or cavity, formed by the combined distal ends of the tibia and fibula. The medial, superior and lateral articular surfaces of the talus are continuous, as are those of the medial malleolus, distal end of the tibia, and lateral malleolus.

The fibrous capsule attaches at the margins of the articular surfaces of the talus below and to the tibia and fibula above, except anteriorly, where a portion of the dorsal aspect of the neck of the talus is enclosed within the joint cavity. The capsule extends somewhat superiorly between the distal ends of the tibia and fibula, to just below the syndesmosis. The fibrous capsule is lined by a synovial membrane throughout its entirety. The capsule is well supported by ligaments, especially medially and laterally.

The medial ligaments are collectively referred to as the *deltoid ligament* (Fig. 18-12). The anterior portion of the deltoid ligament consists of the tibionavicular ligament, superficially, and the deeper anterior tibiotalar fibers. The tibionavicular ligament blends with the plantar calcaneonavicular (spring) ligament inferiorly. The middle fibers of the deltoid ligament constitute the tibiocalcaneal ligament, with some tibiotalar fibers deep to it. The posterior tibiotalar ligament forms the posterior portion of the deltoid ligament. The deltoid ligament as a whole attaches proximally to the medial aspect of the medial malleolus and fans out to achieve the distal attachments described above. In this way, it is somewhat triangular in form, with the apex at its proximal attachment.

The lateral ligaments, unlike those of the medial side, are separate bands of fibers diverging from their proximal attachment at the distal end of the fibula (Fig. 18-10). The anterior talofibular ligament—the most frequently injured ligament about the ankle—passes medially, forward and downward, from the anterior aspect of the fibula to the lateral aspect of the neck of the talus. The calcaneofibular ligament runs from the tip of the lateral malleolus downward and backward to a small prominence on the upper lateral surface of the calcaneus. It is longer and narrower than the anterior and posterior talofibular ligaments. The posterior talofibular ligament passes from the malleolar fossa medially, and slightly downward and backward to the lateral tubercle of the posterior aspect of the talus.

It should be noted that the proximal attachments of both the medial and lateral ligaments of the ankle are near the axis of movement for dorsiflexion and plantarflexion. For this reason, these ligaments are not pulled tight to any significant extent during normal movement at the talocrural joint.[18] Also, the calcaneofibular ligament, which crosses both the talocrural and the talocalcaneal joints, runs parallel to, and inserts close to, the axis of movement at the subtalar joint. It, then,

Fig. 18-12. Medial view of the ligaments of the talocrural and proximal tarsal joints

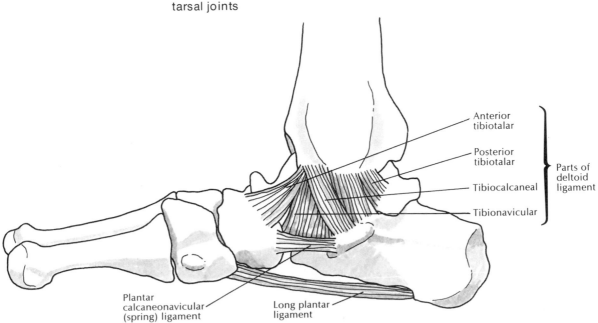

Anterior tibiotalar

Posterior tibiotalar

Tibiocalcaneal

Tibionavicular

Parts of deltoid ligament

Plantar calcaneonavicular (spring) ligament

Long plantar ligament

plays little or no role in restricting inversion at the subtalar joint. This is true in all positions of dorsiflexion and plantar flexion, since it maintains a parallel orientation to the subtalar axis throughout the range.

The ligaments about the talocrural joint primarily function to restrict tilting and rotation of the talus within the mortise, and to restrict forward or backward displacement of the leg on the tarsus. The main exception to this is the tibiocalcaneal portion of the deltoid ligament, which is so oriented as to help check eversion at the subtalar joint as well as an "eversion tilt" of the talus in the mortise.

In the neutral position, the anterior talofibular ligament can check posterior movement of the leg on the tarsus and external rotation of the leg on the tarsus because it is directed forward and medially. With the foot in plantar flexion, the anterior talofibular ligament becomes more vertically oriented and is in a position to check inversion of the talus in the mortise. This ligament is the most commonly injured of the ligaments of the ankle, the mechanism of injury usually being a combined plantar flexion–inversion strain.

The calcaneofibular ligament is directed downward and backward when the foot is in the neutral position. When the foot is dorsiflexed, the ligament becomes more vertically oriented and is in a better position to check inversion of the tarsus with respect to the leg.

The posterior talofibular ligament is oriented so as to check internal rotation of the leg on the tarsus and forward displacement of the leg on the tarsus.

The deltoid ligament, considered as a whole, contributes to restriction of eversion, internal rotation, and external rotation, as well as forward and backward displacement of the tarsus. However, sectioning of the deltoid ligament alone apparently results primarily in instability into eversion of the tarsus on the tibia, the other motions being checked by other ligaments, as described above.

The Subtalar Joint

Functionally, the subtalar joint includes the articulation between the posterior facet of the talus and the opposing articular surface of the calcaneus, as well as the articulation between the anterior and medial facets of the two bones. These articulations move in conjunction with one another. Anatomically, the anterior and medial articulations are actually part of the talocalcaneonavicular joint; they are enclosed within a joint capsule separate from that of the posterior talocalcaneal articulation.

The joint capsules of the posterior portion of the talocalcaneal joint and the talocalcaneonavicular portion of the subtalar joint are separated by the ligament of the tarsal canal. This ligament runs from the underside of the talus, at the sulcus tali, downward and laterally to the dorsum of the calcaneus, at the sulcus calcanei. Since it is situated medially to the axis of motion of inversion–eversion at the subtalar joint, it checks eversion.[33] This ligament is often referred to as the *interosseous talocalcaneal ligament* (Fig. 18-11).

More laterally, in the sinus tarsi, is the cervical talocalcaneal ligament. It passes from the inferolateral aspect of the talar neck downward and laterally to the dorsum of the calcaneus. It occupies the anterior part of the sinus tarsi. Since the cervical ligament lies lateral to the subtalar joint axis, it restricts inversion of the calcaneus on the talus.[33]

Also, within the lateral aspect of the sinus tarsi, bands from the inferior aspect of the extensor retinaculum pass downward, as well as medially, to the calcaneus. These bands are considered part of the talocalcaneal ligament complex. They help check inversion at the subtalar joint.

Talocalcaneonavicular Joint

This joint includes the articulation between the anterior and medial facets of the talus and calcaneus (described above as part of the subtalar joint), the articulations between the inferior aspect of the head of the talus and the subjacent spring ligament, and the articulation between the anterior aspect of the head of the talus and the posterior articular surface of the navicular. The combined talonavicular and talo-spring ligament portion of this joint is essentially a compound ball-and-socket joint; the head of the talus is the ball, while the superior surface of the spring ligament and the posterior surface of the navicular form the socket. It should be noted that the superior surface of the spring ligament is lined with articular cartilage. The talonavicular portion of this joint constitutes the medial half of the transverse tarsal joint.

The talocalcaneonavicular joint is enclosed by a joint capsule, the posterior aspects of which traverses the tarsal canal, forming the anterior wall of the canal. The capsule is reinforced by the spring ligament inferiorly, the calcaneonavicular portion of the bifurcate ligament laterally, and the tibionavicular portion of the deltoid ligament medially (Figs. 18-10 and 18-12).

The spring ligament passes from the anterior and medial margins of the sustentaculum tali forward to the inferior and inferomedial aspect of the navicular. As mentioned, its superior surface articulates with the underside of the head of the talus. This ligament maintains apposition of the medial aspects of forefoot and hindfoot and in so doing helps to maintain the normal arched configuration of the foot. Laxity of the ligament allows a medial separation between calcaneus and forefoot, with the forefoot assuming an abducted position with respect to the hindfoot. At the same time, the foot is allowed to "untwist," which effectively lowers the normal arch of the foot, and the talar head is allowed to move medially and inferiorly. Further discussion of the twisted configuration and arching of the foot is included in the section on biomechanics.

The Calcaneocuboid Joint

The lateral portion of the transverse tarsal joint is the calcaneocuboid joint. The calcaneocuboid joint is a sellar joint in that the calcaneal joint surface is concave superoinferiorly and convex mediolaterally (Figs. 18-3 and 18-4); the adjoining cuboid surface is reciprocally shaped. This joint is enclosed in a joint capsule distinct from that of the talocalcaneonavicular joint and constitutes the medial half of the transverse tarsal joint. The joint capsule is reinforced inferiorly by the strong plantar calcaneocuboid (short plantar) ligament and the long plantar ligament. The short plantar ligament runs from the anterior tubercle of the plantar aspect of the calcaneus to the underside of the cuboid. The long plantar ligament runs from the posterior tubercles of the calcaneus forward to the bases of the fifth, fourth, third, and sometimes second metatarsals (Fig. 18-9). Both of these ligaments support the normal arched configuration of the foot by helping to maintain a twisted relationship between the hindfoot and forefoot.

Dorsally, the joint capsule is reinforced by the calcaneocuboid band of the bifurcate ligament.

SURFACE ANATOMY

Bony Palpation

Medial Aspect. The medial malleolus is easily palpated and observed as a large prominence medially. About 2 cm distal to the medial malleolus, the sustentaculum tali can be felt, especially if the foot is held everted. The tibiocalcaneal portion of the deltoid ligament passes from the malleolus to the sustentaculum tali.

Moving the palpating finger about 5 cm directly anterior to the sustentaculum, you can locate the *navicular tubercle* as a prominence on the medial aspect of the arch of the foot. The tibionavicular portion of the deltoid ligament attaches just above the tubercle. Just superior, and perhaps slightly posterior, to the navicular tubercle, the medial aspect of the *talar head* can be palpated as a less prominent bony landmark. These two landmarks are important in assessing the structure of the foot with regard to the degree of twisting of the forefoot in relation to the hindfoot (the degree of "arching" of the foot).

Dorsal Aspect. At the level of the malleoli, the anterior aspects of the distal ends of the tibia and fibula can be felt. The junction of the two bones, at the syndesmosis, can usually be distinguished, although it is considerably obscured by the distal tibiofibular ligament which overlies it. With the foot relaxed in some degree of plantar flexion, the dorsal aspect of the talar neck can be felt just distal to the end of the tibia. With the foot held inverted and plantarly flexed, the anterolateral aspect of the articular surface of the talus can be easily felt just distal and somewhat lateral to the syndesmosis. Between the dorsal aspect of the talar neck and the most prominent aspect of the dorsum of the foot further distally, which is the first cuneiform, is the navicular bone, the dorsal aspect of which can be palpated.

Lateral Aspect. The lateral malleolus lies subcutaneously and so is easily palpated. The fairly flat lateral aspect of the calcaneus also has little soft-tissue covering and can be felt throughout its extent. About 3 cm distal to the tip of the malleolus, a small prominence can be felt on the calcaneus. This is the peroneal tubercle. The peroneus brevis tendon passes superior to the tubercle, whereas the peroneus longus passes inferiorly. Occasionally a small prominence can be palpated just posterior to the peroneal tubercle; this is the point of insertion of the calcaneofibular ligament.

Just distal, and slightly anterior, to the malleolus, a rather marked depression can be felt if the foot is relaxed. This is the lateral opening of the sinus tarsi. Traversing the lateral aspect of the sinus tarsi are the inferior bands of the extensor retinaculum and the cervical talocalcaneal ligament.

Moving the palpating finger around dorsally and slightly superiorly from the sinus tarsi, you can feel the lateral aspect of the neck of the talus where the often-injured anterior talofibular ligament attaches.

Posterior Aspect. At the posterior aspect of the heel is a prominent crest running horizontally between the upper and lower posterior calcaneal surfaces. The Achilles tendon gains attachment to the upper surface; the lower surface, covered by a fat pad, slopes forward to the medial and lateral tubercles on the inferior aspect of the calcaneus.

Palpation of the posterior aspect of the talus is obscured by the Achilles tendon, which overlies it prior to inserting on the calcaneus.

Inferior Aspect. Palpation of the inferior aspect of the calcaneus is made difficult by the thick skin and fat pad that cover it. The weight-bearing medial tubercle can be vaguely distinguished posteriorly in most people. Traction osteophytes (heel spurs) occasionally develop just anterior to the calcaneal tubercles where the long plantar ligament attaches.

Tendons and Vessels

Medial Aspect. The tendons of the tibialis posterior, flexor digitorum longus, and flexor hallucis longus muscles cross behind the medial malleolus. The tibialis posterior is the most anterior of these and is best visualized or papated when plantar flexion and inversion are performed against some resistance. Posterior to the tibialis posterior tendon is the flexor digitorum longus tendon, which is less prominent. Palpation of the flexor digitorum is facilitated by providing some resistance to toe flexion. The flexor hallucis longus tendon is deeper and runs farther posteriorly; it is not usually palpa-

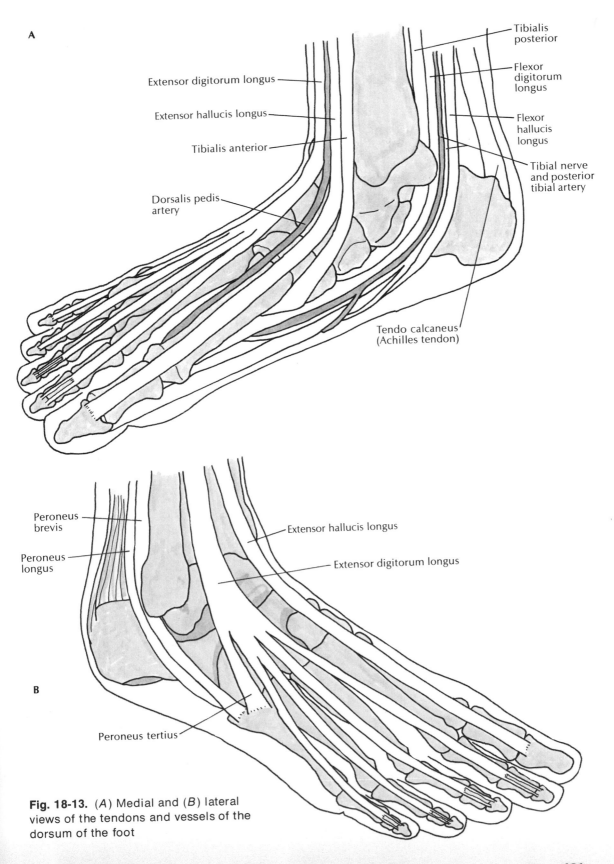

A

Extensor digitorum longus

Extensor hallucis longus

Tibialis anterior

Dorsalis pedis
artery

Tibialis
posterior

Flexor
digitorum
longus

Flexor
hallucis
longus

Tibial nerve
and posterior
tibial artery

Tendo calcaneus
(Achilles tendon)

Peroneus
brevis

Peroneus
longus

Extensor hallucis longus

Extensor digitorum longus

B

Peroneus tertius

Fig. 18-13. (*A*) Medial and (*B*) lateral
views of the tendons and vessels of the
dorsum of the foot

461

ble. Between the flexor digitorum and flexor hallucis longus tendons runs the posterior tibial artery. Its pulse is palpable behind the malleolus. The tibial nerve, which usually cannot be palpated, runs deep and posterior to the artery.

Just anterior to the medial malleolus is the long saphenous nerve; it can usually be visualized and palpated.

Dorsal Aspect. Running along the medial side of the dorsum of the ankle is the tendon of the tibialis anterior, which is the most prominent tendon crossing the dorsal aspect of the foot. It is made especially prominent by resisting inversion and dorsiflexion of the foot. It attaches to the medial aspect of the base of the first metatarsal.

Just lateral to the tibialis anterior tendon, the extensor hallucis longus tendon can easily be seen and palpated as the subject extends the big toe.

Running lateral to the extensor hallucis longus tendon, passing distally from where it emerges at the ankle, is the dorsalis pedis artery. Its pulse can best be palpated over the dorsum of the foot, at about the level of the navicular and first cuneiform bones.

Further laterally, the common tendon of the extensor digitorum longus is seen and felt when the subject extends the toes. Its four branches can be distinguished where they develop, just distal to the ankle.

If the subject everts and dorsiflexes the foot, the tendon of the peroneus tertius is usually observable just proximal to its insertion at the dorsum of the base of the fifth metatarsal.

Lateral Aspect. The peroneus longus and peroneus brevis tendons cross behind the lateral malleolus, the brevis running more anteriorly. The brevis passes superior to the peroneal tubercle on the lateral aspect of the calcaneus; the longus passes inferior to the tubercle. Some resistance should be applied to plantar flexion and eversion of the foot when palpating these tendons.

Posterior Aspect. The Achilles tendon is quite prominent and is easily seen and felt proximal to its insertion on the calcaneus. Deep to the tendon, between the tendon and the upper surface of the posterior calcaneus, is the retrocalcaneal bursa. There is also a calcaneal bursa between the Achilles tendon and the skin. These bursae cannot be distinguished on palpation.

BIOMECHANICS

The structural relationships and movements that occur at the ankle and hindfoot are complex. From a clinical standpoint, however, it is important that the clinician have at least a basic understanding of the biomechanics of this region. The joints of the foot and ankle constitute the first movable pivots in the weight bearing extremity once the foot becomes fixed to the ground. Considered together, these joints must permit mobility in all planes in order to allow for minimal displacement of a person's center of gravity with respect to the base of support when walking over flat or uneven surfaces. In this sense, maintenance of balance and economy of energy consumption are, in part, dependent upon proper functioning of the ankle–foot complex. Adequate mobility and proper structural alignment of these joints are also necessary for normal attenuation of forces transmitted from the ground to the weight-bearing extremity. Deviations in alignment and changes in mobility are likely to cause abnormal stresses to the joints of the foot and ankle, as well as to the other weight-bearing joints. It follows that detection of biomechanical alterations in the ankle–foot region is often necessary for adequate interpretation of painful conditions affecting the foot and ankle, as well as conditions affecting the knee, hip, or lower spine, in some cases.

STRUCTURAL ALIGNMENT

In the normal standing position, the patella faces straight forward, the knee joint axis lies in the frontal plane and the tibial tubercle is in line with the midline—or lateral half—of the patella. In this position, a line passing between the tips of the malleoli should make an angle of about 20° to 25° with the frontal plane.[3,17,19] This represents the normal amount of tibial torsion; the distal end of the tibia is rotated outward with respect to the proximal end. The lateral malleolus is positioned inferiorly with respect to the medial malleolus such that the intermalleolar line makes an angle of about 10° with the transverse plane.[19] The joint axis of the ankle mortise joint corresponds approximately to the intermalleolar line. With the patellae facing straight forward, the feet should each be pointed outward about 5° to 10°.

If, when the feet are in normal standing alignment, the patellae face inward, increased femoral anteversion, increased external tibial torsion, or both, may be present. Clinically, the fault can be differentiated by assessing rotational range of motion of the hips and estimating the degree of tibial torsion by noting the rotational alignment of the malleoli with respect to the patellae and tibial tubercles. In the presence of increased hip anteversion, the total range of hip motion will be normal but skewed such that internal rotation is excessive and external rotation is restricted proportionally. Similar considerations hold for a situation in which the patellae face outward when the feet are normally aligned; femoral retroversion, internal tibial torsion, or both, are likely to exist.

With respect to the frontal plane, normal knee alignment may vary from slight genu valgum to some degree of genu varum. Since in most individuals the medial femoral condyle extends further distally than the lateral condyle, slight genu valgum tends to be more prevalent. At the hindfoot, the calcaneus should be positioned in vertical alignment with the tibia. A valgus or varus heel can usually be observed as a bowing of the Achilles tendon. A valgus positioning of the calcaneus on the talus is associated with pronation at the subtalar joint, whereas a varus hindfoot involves supination.

When considering the structure of the foot as a whole, it is helpful to compare it to a twisted plate (Fig. 18-14); the calcaneus, at one end, is positioned vertically when contacting the ground, whereas the metatarsal heads are positioned horizontally when making contact with a flat surface.[26] Thus, in the normal standing position on a flat, level surface, the metatarsal heads are twisted 90° with respect to the calcaneus.

To demonstrate this, you can construct a model by taking a light rectangular piece of cardboard and twisting it so that one end lies flat on a table and the opposite end is perpendicular to the table top. Note the "arching" of the cardboard. This is analogous to the arching of the human foot. It should be realized that the term *arch* here applies to the configuration of the structure, which is dependent upon the fact that it is twisted upon itself. It does not refer to *an arch* in the true architectural sense, in which the arched configuration is dependent upon the shapes of the component "building blocks." In the foot, both situations exist. On the medial side, there is little architectural arching and, therefore, little inherent stability of the medial arch. The medial arch is dependent almost entirely upon the twisted configuration of the foot, which is maintained statically by the short and long plantar ligaments, and dynamically by the anterior and posterior tibialis muscles. In contrast, the lateral side of the foot represents a true architectural arch (Fig. 18-15).[26] Here the cuboid, being wedged between the calcaneus and metatarsals, serves as the

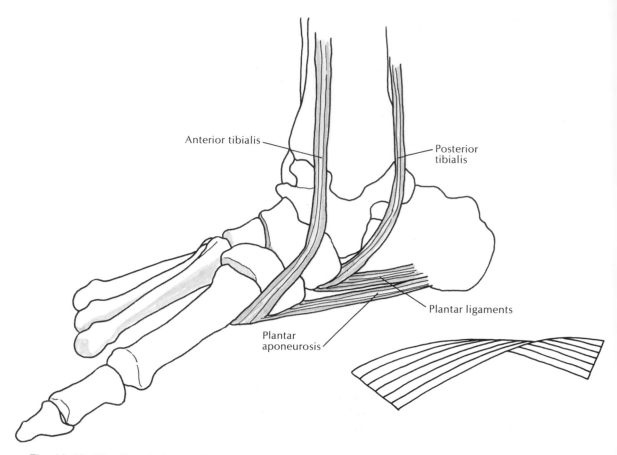

Fig. 18-14. The "twisted plate," which generates the medial arch

structural keystone. Only a small component of the lateral arch is a result of the twisted configuration of the foot.

Referring back to the cardboard model, notice that when the cardboard is allowed to untwist—by inclining the vertical end in one direction and keeping the other end flat on the table—the arch flattens. Inclining the vertical end in the opposite direction increases the twist and increases the arch. In the foot, inclination of the vertical component of the structure, the calcaneus, will result in similar untwisting or twisting; this results in a respective decrease or increase in the arching of the foot, if the metatarsal heads remain in contact with the ground (Fig. 18-16). The person who stands with the heel in a valgus position will have a relatively "flat" or untwisted foot, whereas a person whose heel is in a varus position when standing will appear to have a "high" arch because of increased twisting between hindfoot and forefoot. The former situation is often referred to as a *pronated foot* or *flatfoot*, while the latter is called a *supinated foot* or *pes cavus*. In the situation of the heel remaining in a vertical position but the metatarsal heads inclined on, say, an uneven surface, the effect will also be to twist or untwist the foot and therefore, to raise or to lower the arch. For example, if the inclination is such that the first metatarsal head is on a higher level than the fifth, the forefoot supinates on the hindfoot, untwisting the foot and lowering the arch. Note that supination of the forefoot with the hindfoot fixed is the same as pronation of the hindfoot with the forefoot fixed; they both involve untwisting of the tarsal skeleton from motion at the subtalar, transverse tarsal, and tarsal–metatarsal joints.

Reference is often made to a *transverse* *arch* of the foot, distinguishing it from the *longitudinal arch*. The cardboard model should help to make it clear that some transverse arching results from the twisted configuration of the foot. This is

Fig. 18-15. (*A*) The lateral arch of the foot is a true arch. The calcaneus forms the ascending flank, the cuboid is the true keystone, and the fourth and fifth metatarsals are the descending flank. (*B*) The medial arch of the foot is not a true arch.

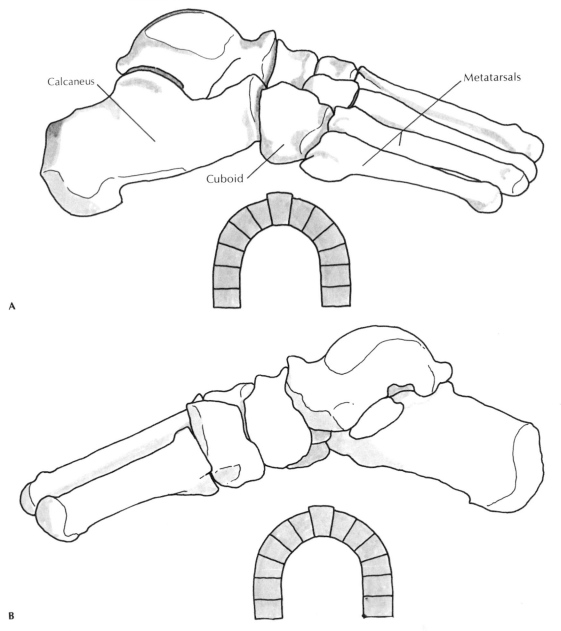

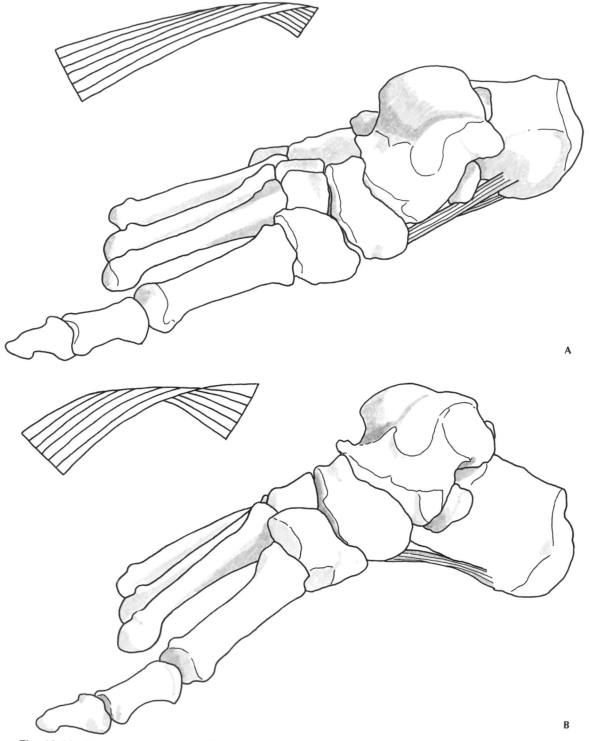

Fig. 18-16. The medial arch. (*A*) When it is allowed to "untwist," the arch flattens; (*B*) when the medial arch is "twisted," the arch increases.

simply a transverse component of the arch discussed above. This transverse component will increase and decrease along with twisting and untwisting of the foot. There is also a structural component to the transverse arching of the foot, resulting from the contours and relationships of the tarsals and metatarsals. It must be realized, however, that at the level of the metatarsal heads in the standing individual, no transverse arch exists, since each of the heads makes contact with the floor.

ARTHROKINEMATICS OF THE ANKLE–FOOT COMPLEX

The Ankle Mortise Joint

The superior articular surface of the talus is wider anteriorly than posteriorly, the difference in widths being as much as 6 mm.[3,19] The articular surfaces of the tibial and fibular malleoli maintain a close fit against the medial and lateral articular surfaces of the talus in all positions of plantar flexion and dorsiflexion. As the foot moves from full plantar flexion into full dorsiflexion the talus rolls backard in the mortise. It would seem, then, that with ankle dorsiflexion the malleoli must separate in order to accomodate the greater anterior width of the talus. This separation could occur as a result of a lateral shift of the fibula, a lateral bending of the fibula, or both. However, it is found that the amount of separation that occurs between the malleoli during ankle dorsiflexion varies from .0 to only 2 mm, which is much less than would be expected considering the amount of wedging of the superior articular surface of the talus. There appears to be a significant discrepancy between the difference in anterior and posterior widths of the trochlea of the talus and the amount of separation which occurs between the tibial and fibular malleoli with ankle dorsiflexion.

In understanding this apparent paradox, we must look more closely at the structure of the trochlea and the type of movement the talus undergoes during ankle dorsiflexion. If we examine both sides of the trochlea we see that the lateral articular surface, which articulates with the fibular malleolus, is longer in its anteroposterior dimension than the medial articular surface. The reason for this is that the lateral malleolus moves over a greater excursion, with respect to the talus, during plantar flexion–dorsiflexion, than does the medial malleolus. This is partly because the axis of motion is farther from the superior trochlear articular surface laterally than medially. The corollary to this (and this is true of essentially all joints with sellar surfaces) is that the relatively track-bound movement that the talus undergoes on plantar flexion–dorsiflexion at the ankle is not a pure swing, but rather an impure swing; it involves an element of spin, or rotation, that results in a helical movement. Another way of conceptualizing this movement is to consider the talus as a section of a cone whose apex is situated medially rotating within the mortise about its own long axis, rather than a truly cylindrical body undergoing a simple rolling movement within the mortise (Fig. 18-17). As a result of this, the intermalleolar lines projected onto the superior trochlear articular surface at various positions of plantar flexion and dorsiflexion are not parallel lines. Therefore, the degree of wedging of the trochlea does not reflect the relative intermalleolar distances in dorsiflexion and plantar flexion of the ankle. The true intermalleolar distances are represented by the length of these nonparallel lines projected onto the superior trochlear surface. The projected line with the foot in plantar flexion is only slightly shorter, if at all, than that for dorsiflexion, and the necessary separation of the malleoli during dorsiflexion is minimal.[19]

Up to this point, we have been speaking of the ankle mortise joint axis as a fixed axis of motion. This has been done for the sake of simplicity and convenience using

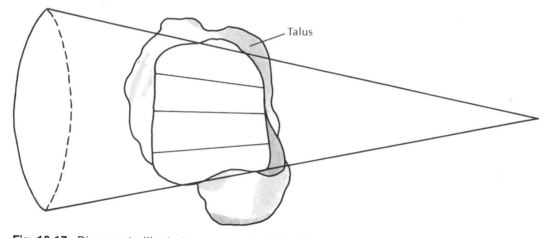

Talus

Fig. 18-17. Diagram to illustrate movement of the talus as a section of a cone, whose apex is situated medially, rotating within the mortise about its own long axis

the approximate center of movement as the joint axis. But, as mentioned in Chapter 2, Arthrology, no joint moves about a stationary joint axis. As indicated by instant center analysis of ankle joint motion, this is true of the ankle mortise joint as well.[31] The surface velocities determined from the instant centers of movement show that when moving from full plantar flexion to full dorsiflexion, there is initially a momentary distraction of the tibiotalar joint surfaces, followed by a movement of combined rolling and sliding throughout most of the range, and terminating with an approximation of joint surfaces at the position of extreme dorsiflexion. These findings are consistent with the fact that the close-packed position of the ankle mortise joint is dorsiflexion; the tightening of the joint capsule that occurs with movement of any joint into its close-packed position produces an approximation of the joint surfaces.

The Subtalar Joint

As discussed previously, this is a compound joint with two distinct articula-tions. From the outset, movement at this joint is somewhat difficult to conceptualize because the posterior articulation between the talus and calcaneus is concave superiorly on convex inferiorly, while the anteromedial articulation is convex on concave. Understanding talocalcaneal movement is perhaps facilitated by considering it analogous to movement at the proximal and distal radioulnar joints. The radioulnar joints, like the talocalcaneal joints, move in conjunction with one another and have only one degree of freedom of motion. The posterior calcaneal facet moving against the opposing concave talar surface can be compared with the radial head moving within the radial notch of the ulna. As this movement occurs, the anteromedial facet of the talus must move in relation to the concave anteromedial surface of the calcaneus, just as the head of the ulna must move within the ulnar notch of the radius at the distal joint of the forearm. In at least some individuals, this type of movement at the subtalar joint is accompanied by a slight forward displacement of the talus during pronation and a backward displacement on supination, thus making the total movement a helical, or screwlike, motion.[27]

The Transverse Tarsal Joints: Talonavicular and Calcaneocuboid Joints

Although perhaps some movement occurs between the cuboid and navicular bones, we will consider movement of these two bones acting as a unit with respect to the calcaneus and the talus. The configuration of the talonavicular articulation is essentially that of a ball-and-socket joint. Because of this configuration, it potentially has three degrees of freedom of movement, allowing it to move in all planes. However, because the navicular is closely bound to the cuboid bone laterally, its freedom of movement is largely governed by the movement allowed at the calcaneocuboid joint.[9] The calcaneocuboid joint, having a sellar configuration, has two degrees of freedom, each of which occurs about a distinct axis of motion. The axis of motion with which we shall be most concerned is the axis of pronation and supination. This axis is similar in location and orientation to the subtalar joint axis, the major difference being that it is not inclined as much vertically. It passes through the talar head, backward, downward, and laterally. Such an orientation allows a movement of inversion–adduction–plantarflexion (supination) and eversion–abduction–dorsiflexion (pronation) of the forefoot. In the standing position, movement and positioning at the transverse tarsal joint occurs in conjunction with subtalar joint movement; when the subtalar joint pronates, the transverse tarsal joint supinates, and *vice versa*. Pronation of the forefoot close packs and locks the transverse tarsal joint complex, whereas supination results in loose packing and a greater degree of freedom of movement.[26]

OSTEOKINEMATICS OF THE ANKLE–FOOT COMPLEX

Terminology

At this point, some terms related to movement and positioning of various components of the ankle and foot must be clarified. Throughout this chapter the following definitions will hold:

Inversion–Eversion—Movement about a horizontal axis lying in the sagittal plane. Functionally, pure inversion or eversion rarely occurs at any of the joints of ankle or foot. More often they occur as a component of supination or pronation.

Abduction–Adduction—Movement of the forefoot about a vertical axis or the movement of the free foot that results from internal or external rotation of the hindfoot with respect to the leg.

Internal–External Rotation—Movement between the leg and hindfoot occurring about a vertical axis. Pure rotations do not occur functionally, but rather occur as components of pronation and supination.

Plantarflexion–Dorsiflexion—Movement about a horizontal axis lying in the frontal plane. Functionally, these usually occur in conjunction with other movements.

Pronation–Supination—Functional movements occurring around the obliquely situated subtalar or transverse tarsal joint axis. At both of these joints, pronation involves abduction, eversion, and some dorsiflexion; supination involves adduction, inversion, and plantar flexion of the distal segment on the proximal segment. This is because these joint axes are inclined backward, downward, and laterally. It must be appreciated that when the metatarsals are fixed to the ground, pronation of the hindfoot (su ᵃʳ joint) involves supination of t front (transverse tarsal joint)

Pronated Foot–Supinated Foot—Traditionally, a pronated foot (in the standing position) is one in which the arched configuration of the foot is reduced; the hindfoot is pronated while the forefoot is supinated. In a supinated foot (standing) the arch is high, the hindfoot is supinated and the forefoot is pronated.

Valgus–Varus—Terms used for alignment of parts. *Valgus* denotes inclination away from the midline of a segment with respect to its proximal neighbor, whereas *varus* is inclination toward the midline. At the hindfoot and forefoot, valgus refers to alignment in a pronated position and varus to alignment in a supinated position.

Orientation of Joint Axes and the Effect on Movement

In the normal standing position, the axis of movement for the knee joint is horizontal and in a frontal plane. With flexion and extension of the free-swinging tibia, movement will occur in a sagittal plane. The ankle mortise joint axis is directed backward mediolaterally about 25° from the frontal plane, and downward from medial to lateral about 10° to 15° from horizontal. Movement of the free foot about this axis results in combined plantar flexion, adduction, and inversion or combined dorsiflexion, abduction, and eversion. Note that the above statements relate the movements at the respective joints to the orientations of the joint axes when the foot and leg are swinging freely In this position, movements at one joint may occur independently of the other.

We must be more concerned, however, with what happens when the foot becomes fixed to the ground and movement occurs simultaneously at the joints of the lower extremities. This is the situation during weight-bearing activities, or normal functional activities, involving the leg. The obvious question in this regard would be:

How is it possible to move both the tibia and femur in the sagittal plane, such as when performing a knee bend with the knee pointed forward, when movement is occurring at the ankle and knee about two nonparallel axes? The heavy-weight lifter largely avoids the problem by pointing the knees outward, thereby using external rotation and abduction at the hip. This brings the knee and ankle axes closer to parallel alignment. The fact remains, however, that it is possible to perform a deep knee bend with the knee directed forward, and through a considerable range. Since the knee joint axis lies horizontally in the frontal plane, we would not expect a problem here, since it is ideally oriented to allow rotation of the bones in the sagittal plane. It would seem, then, that by performing such a knee bend, an internal rotatory moment must be applied to the ankle, since the ankle joint axis is externally rotated with respect to the frontal plane. Surely our ankle mortise joints cannot be expected to withstand such stresses during daily activities. This apparent problem can be resolved by considering the orientation of the joint axis and associated movements at the subtalar joint.

The axis of motion for the subtalar joint is directed backward, downward, and laterally.[6,19,27] The degree of inclination and mediolateral deviation of the axis varies greatly among individuals. The average deviation from the midline of the foot is 23°, whereas the average deviation from the horizontal is 42°. Because the axis of motion for the subtalar joint deviates from the sagittal plane and from the horizontal plane, movement at this joint involves combined eversion, dorsiflexion, and abduction, or combined inversion, plantar flexion, and adduction. Note that pure abduction and adduction of the foot are movements that would occur about a vertical axis and that inversion and eversion occur about a purely horizontal axis. Since the subtalar axis is positioned about midway between horizontal and vertical, it follows that movement about this axis would include elements of adduction–abduction as well as eversion–inversion.

Now we can once again consider a situation of simultaneous knee and ankle flexion in the sagittal plane with the foot fixed, (*e.g.,* a deep knee bend). It was indicated that with such a movement, an internal rotatory moment of the tibia on the talus would be applied to the ankle. Because the subtalar axis allows an element of movement about a vertical axis (rotation in the horizontal plane), this internal rotatory moment can be transmitted to the subtalar joint. Internal rotation of the tibia on the foot is, of course, equivalent to external rotation of the foot on the leg, which we refer to as abduction of the foot. Subtalar movement is essentially uniaxial, so that any movement occurring at the joint may occur only in conjunction with its component movements, that is, abduction can only occur in conjunction with eversion and dorsiflexion, the three together constituting pronation at the subtalar. Thus we can say that with the foot fixed, simultaneous dorsiflexion of the ankle and flexion of the knee, keeping the leg in the sagittal plane, requires pronation at the subtalar joint. As a corollary to this, we say that with such a movement, if pronation at the subtalar joint is restricted, an abnormal internal tibial rotatory stress will occur at the ankle mortise joint, or an internal femoral rotatory stress will be placed upon the knee, or both.[6] The need for subtalar movement can be reduced by moving the leg out of the sagittal plane—by pointing the knee outward—bringing the knee and ankle axes into closer alignment.

Similar considerations apply to the situation of an individual rotating his leg over a fixed foot. Any rotation imparted to the tibia is transmitted to the subtalar joint (Fig. 18-18). For example, if you rotate the leg externally over a foot that is fixed to the ground, the subtalar joint undergoes a movement of supination. This is analogous to movement about a mitered hinge; movement of one component about a vertical axis is transmitted to the second component as movement about a horizontal axis. Supination causes the calcaneus to assume a varus position, which, since the metatarsals remain flat on the ground, increases the twist in the foot and raises the arch.[17] The opposite occurs with internal tibial rotation; pronation of the hindfoot causes a relative supination of the forefoot; the foot untwists and the arch flattens. You can easily observe this on yourself when attempting to rotate the leg with the foot fixed to the ground. With respect to the structural alignment, then, an individual with excessive internal tibial torsion will tend to have a pronated hindfoot (calcaneus in valgus position) and a forefoot that is supinated with respect to the hindfoot. The resultant untwisting of the foot causes a flatfoot upon standing. The person with excessive external tibial torsion will tend to have a varus heel and a high arch.

The degree of twisting and untwisting of the foot also varies with stance width.[26] When standing with the feet far apart, the heel tends to deviate into a valgus position with respect to the floor, and the metatarsal heads remain flat; the metatarsals assume a position of supination with respect to the heel, thereby untwisting the foot. The opposite occurs when standing with the legs crossed.

It should be noted that when standing with the hindfoot in pronation and the forefoot in supination, the medial metatarsals assume a position closer to dorsiflexion.[17] Since the joint axis of the first metatarsal is obliquely oriented—from anterolateral to posteromedial—dorsiflexion of the first metatarsal involves a component of abduction away from the midline of the foot. Therefore, in a pronated foot, the first metat is usually positioned in varus. On t hand, a person with "metatarsu

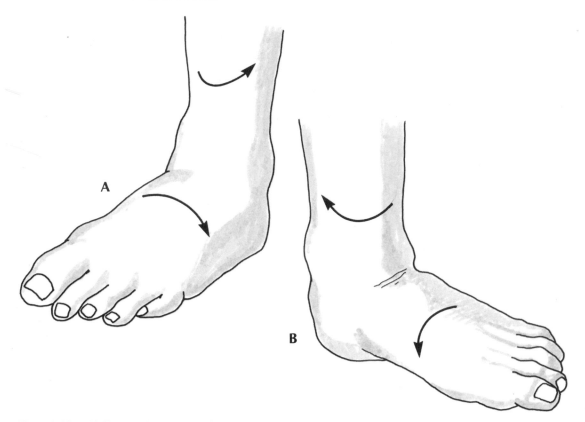

Fig. 18-18. (*A*) External rotation of the tibia over the fixed foot imparts a movement of supination to the foot, increasing the arch; (*B*) internal tibial rotation flattens, or pronates, the fixed foot.

varus," a condition in which the first metatarsal deviates into varus position, the foot will tend to assume a pronated position. This is because in order for the first metatarsal to be in a varus angle, it must also be in some dorsiflexion. This causes supination of the forefoot, which necessitates pronation of the hindfoot, in order for the individual to stand with the metatarsal head and calcaneus in contact with the ground.

The Ankle and Foot During Gait

As clinicians we must be concerned with the function of the joints of the ankle and foot during normal daily activities. The prime consideration here, of course, is walking. Again, because these are weight-bearing joints and because the foot becomes fixed to the ground during the stance phase, we must be aware of the biomechanical interrelationships between these joints and the other joints of the lower extremity.

During the gait cycle, the leg progresses through space in a sagittal plane. In order to minimize energy expenditure, the center of gravity must undergo minimal vertical displacement. Minimization of vertical displacement of the center of gravity is largely accomplished by angular movement of the lower extremity components in the sagittal plane, that is, flexion–extension at the hip, knee, and ankle complex. The hip has no trouble accommodating such movement since it is multiaxial, allowing some movement in all vertical planes. The knee, although essentially uniaxial, allows flexion and extension in the sagittal plane because its axis of movement is perpendicular to this plane and horizontally oriented. The ankle mortise joint, however, cannot allow a pure sagittal movement between the leg and foot because its axis of motion is not perpendicular to the sagittal plane; it is rotated outward about 25°. During the normal gait cycle, however, movement between the foot and leg in the sagittal plane does occur. This is only possible through participation of another joint, the subtalar joint. Movement of the tibia in a parasagittal plane over a fixed foot requires simultaneous movement at the subtalar and ankle mortise joints. This is consistent with the fact that no muscles attach to the talus. Those muscles that affect movement at the ankle mortise joint also cross the subtalar joint, moving it as well.

In considering the various movements occurring at each of the segments of the lower extremity during gait, it is convenient to speak of three intervals of stance phase; these are (*1*) the interval from heel-strike to foot-flat, (*2*) midstance (foot-flat), and (*3*) the interval from the beginning of heel-rise to toe-off.

During the first interval, each of the segments of the lower extremity rotates internally with respect to its more proximal neighboring segment; the pelvis rotates internally in space, the femur rotates internally on the pelvis, and the tibia rotates internally on the femur (Fig. 18-19,*A*).[22,23,32] It follows that the entire lower limb rotates during this phase and that distal segments rotate more, in space, than the more proximally situated segments. At the point of heel-strike, the foot becomes partially fixed to the ground, so that only minimal internal torsion between the heel and the ground takes place. Much of this internal rotation is absorbed at the subtalar joint as pronation (Fig. 18-19,*B*).[35,36] Internal rotation of the leg with respect to the foot, occurring at the

subtalar joint, makes the axis of the ankle mortise joint more perpendicular to the plane of progression. This allows the ankle mortise joint to provide for movement in the sagittal plane, which, of course, is the plantar flexion occurring at the ankle during this interval (Fig. 18-19,*C*). Note that the foot tends to deviate slightly medially in this stage of stance phase. This is because the obliquity of the ankle axis, in the coronal plane, imposes a component of adduction of the foot during plantar flexion.

At heel-strike, a moment arm equal to the distance between the point of heel contact and the ankle joint develops. The reactive force of the ground acting on the foot at heel-strike across this moment arm will tend to swing the tibia forward in the sagittal plane. This results in some flexion at the knee, which is consistent with the fact that the tibia is rotating internally with respect to the femur. Knee flexion, from an extended position, involves a component of internal tibial rotation.

Note that at heel-strike, the hindfoot moves into pronation while the tibialis anterior muscle contracts to bring the forefoot into supination. This causes the foot to untwist, the transverse tarsal joint to unlock, and the joints to assume a loose-packed position. The foot at this point is in a position favorable for free mobility and is, therefore, at its greatest potential to adapt to variations in the contour of the ground.[9,36]

Once the foot becomes flat on the ground, movement at the ankle mortise joint changes abruptly from plantar flexion to dorsiflexion.[28,30] Through the early period of foot-flat, during which most of dorsiflexion occurs, the segments of the lower extremity continue to rotate internally. This rotation is transmitted to the joints of the ankle, since the foot is now fixed to the ground. Some internal rotation of the tibia automatically occurs at the ankle mortise joint during dorsi with the foot fixed, since the joint

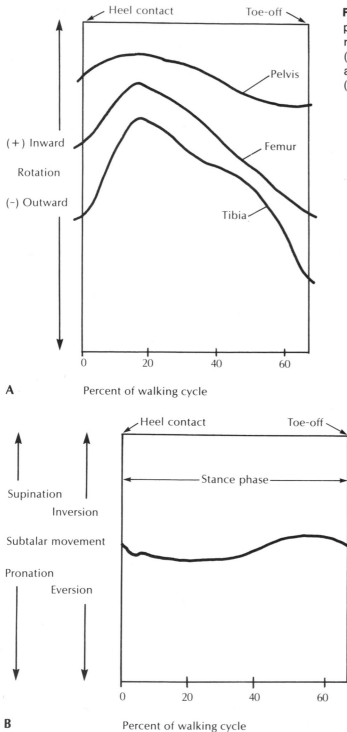

Fig. 18-19. The compositive curves show (A) transverse rotations of the pelvis, femur, and tibia (stance phase), (B) subtalar rotation; and (C) ankle mortise rotation (sagittal plane).

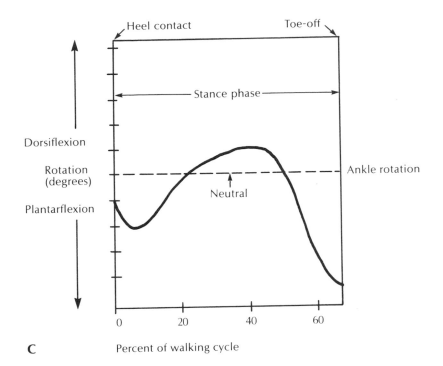

C   Percent of walking cycle

inclined about 15° from horizontal, downwards and laterally. However, most of the internal rotation takes place at the subtalar joint as a component of pronation.[6,36]

Throughout most of the period during which the foot is flat on the ground, the segments of the lower extremity rotate externally; the more distal segments rotate externally to a greater degree than their proximal neighbors.[24] Again, because the foot is fixed to the ground, the tibia rotates externally with respect to the foot. This occurs as supination at the subtalar joint. The change during foot-flat, from internal rotation to external rotation, takes place after most of ankle dorsiflexion is complete.

Because the forefoot is fixed to the ground, the inversion occurring at the subtalar joint imposes pronation at the transverse tarsal joint, causing a close-packing or locking of the tarsus. Consistent with this, the peroneus longus muscle contracts, maintaining a pronated twist of the metatarsals and bringing the foot as a whole toward its twisted configuration. The foot at this point is being converted into an intrinsically stable lever capable of providing for the thrust of pushing off.

During the final interval of stance phase, from heel-rise to toe-off, the segments of the lower limb continue to rotate externally. This external rotation of the tibia is again transmitted to the subtalar joint as supination of the hindfoot. With contraction of the calf muscle, the ankle begins plantar flexion, creating a thrust for push-off. This again creates a moment arm acting on the knee, this time moving the tibia into extension with respect to the femur. Note that this is consistent with the external rotation of the tibia occurring during this phase, since knee extension involves a component of external tibial rotation.

The extension of the metatarsophalangeal joints, occurring with heel-rise, causes a tightening of the plantar aponeurosis through a windlass effect, since the distal attachment of the aponeurosis crosses the plantar aspect of the joints (Fig. 18-20).[18] This tightening of the aponeurosis further raises the arch and adds to the rigidity of the tarsal skeleton.

It should be emphasized that during this final phase of stance, the joint movements that occur automatically convert the foot into a stable lever system and require little, if any, muscle contraction in order to accomplish this.

In summary, then, the transverse rota-

tions of the segments of the lower extremity that occur during stance phase of the gait cycle are transmitted to the ankle joints. This is because during the stance phase the foot is relatively fixed to the ground so that rotation between the foot and the ground is minimal. The ankle mortise axis is inclined slightly vertically (about 15° from the horizontal axis) while the subtalar joint axis is situated about

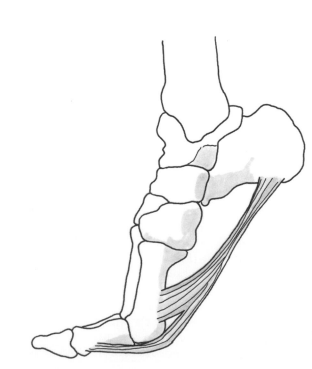

Fig. 18-20. (A) The foot is flat; (B) toe standing causes the aponeurosis to tighten. Tightening the plantar aponeurosis raises the arch and adds to rigidity of tarsal skeleton.

A

B

midway between horizontal and vertical. Both joints are able to "absorb" rotatory movements transmitted to the ankle because of the vertical inclination of the joint axes. With the foot fixed to the ground, the tibia rotates slightly internally at the ankle mortise during dorsiflexion and externally during plantar flexion. Internal rotation of the talus with respect to the calcaneus occurs as pronation, while external rotation results in supination at the subtalar joint. Also, once the foot becomes flat on the ground, the metatarsal heads become fixed and the twisting and untwisting of the foot becomes dependent upon the position of the hindfoot. At heel-strike, the tibia rotates internally, pronating the hindfoot, while the tibialis anterior contracts to supinate the forefoot; this results in an untwisted foot. During midstance, as the tibia rotates externally and the subtalar joint gradually supinates, the foot becomes twisted. This twisting is further increased by tightening of the plantar aponeurosis. The twisted configuration results in maximal joint stability with minimal participation of the intrinsic foot muscles. It is the twisted foot, then, that is best suited for weight bearing and propulsion. During midstance there is little activity of the intrinsic muscles in the normal foot because the twisted configuration confers a passive, or intrinsic, stability upon the foot. However, in the flatfooted person, considerably more muscle action is required since the foot is relatively untwisted.[26] The flatfooted person must rely more on extrinsic stabilization by the muscles. An untwisted configuration is desirable in situations in which the foot must be mobile, such as in adapting to surface contours of the ground. Consistent with this is the fact that at heel-strike, the foot assumes an untwisted state in preparation for conformation to the contacting surface.

A relatively common condition that illustrates the biomechanical interdependency of the weight-bearing joints is femoral anteversion. An individual with femoral anteversion must stand with the leg internally rotated in order to position the hip joint in normal (neutral) alignment. Conversely, if the leg is positioned in normal alignment with the patella facing straight forward, the hip joint assumes a position of relative external rotation. External rotation at the hip decreases the congruity of the joint surfaces. During stance phase, as the femur externally rotates on the pelvis, the hip of the person with femoral anteversion will tend to go into too much external rotation. As the slack is taken up in the part of the joint capsule that pulls tight on external rotation, the joint receptors sense the excessive movement. To avoid excessive joint incongruity and to prevent abnormal stress to the joint capsule, the person with femoral anteversion must *internally* rotate during stance phase. This internal rotation is transmitted primarily to the subtalar joint, which is best oriented to accommodate transverse rotations. Internal rotation at the subtalar joint causes pronation of the hindfoot; the foot untwists and the arch flattens. Thus, femoral anteversion predisposes to pronation of the foot. Also, because of the internal rotatory movement transmitted through the knee, femoral anteversion may also be a causative factor in certain knee disorders. For example, internal rotation imposed upon a semiflexed knee causes the knee to assume an increased valgus position. This may predispose to patellar tracking dysfunction (see Chapter 17, The Knee). Since there is a tendency for the individual with femoral anteversion to walk with increased hip joint incongruity, the force of weight bearing is transmitted to a smaller area of contact at the articular surface of the hip. The result may be accelerated wear of the hip joint surfaces, perhaps leading to degenerative hip disease.

Femoral anteversion provides a good example of how a structural abnormality in one region may lead to localized biomechanical disturbances as well as altered mechanics at joints some distance away. This, again, is especially true of the lower extremity, and should emphasize that when evaluating many patients with foot disorders it may be appropriate, if not necessary, to examine the structure and function of the knee, hip, and lower back. Conversely, foot or ankle dysfunction may precipitate disturbances in more proximal joints.

EXAMINATION

The L4, L5, S1, and S2 segments contribute to the ankle and foot. Symptoms arising in the more proximal regions of these segments may refer to the ankle and foot, the most common of which might be parethesias arising from lumbar nerve root irritation. Actual pain of more proximal origin is rarely felt in the foot. Rather, foot and ankle pain usually arises from local pathology. Pain arising from tissues of the foot or ankle may be referred a short distance proximally, but almost never to the knee or above.

The common lesions affecting the ankle are of acute, traumatic onset, whereas those affecting the foot are more likely to be chronic disorders resulting from stress overload. Because of the biomechanical interdependency of the weight-bearing joints, we must often direct attention to the structure and function of more proximally situated joints when evaluating patients with chronic or subtle foot disorders. Similarly, examination of the foot may well be in order in cases of disorders affecting more proximal regions.

HISTORY

A patient interview designed to elicit specific information related to the patient's pain, functional status, and other associated symptoms, as set out in the chapter on evaluation of musculoskeletal disorders, should be carried out. The following are general concepts that apply to information that may be elicited when interviewing patients with common foot or ankle disorders.

—If the disorder was of an acute, traumatic onset, attempt to determine the exact mechanism of injury. Plantar flexion-inversion strains are more likely to result in capsuloligamentous injury, whereas forces moving the foot into dorsiflexion and external rotation (abduction) are more likely to produce a fracture.

—If the disorder is of a more chronic nature and of insidious onset, attempt to determine whether a change in activity level or footwear may be associated with the onset of the problem. Also inquire about the effect of changing footwear. For example, you might determine the effect of variations in heel height, including whether the problem is affected, for better or for worse, by going barefoot.

—Chronic stress overload (fatigue) disorders may be classified as (1) those due to high levels of activity in which the frequency or high rate of tissue stress is such that the body is unable to keep up with the increased rate of tissue microtrauma (the rate of tissue breakdown exceeds the rate of repair and the tissue gradually fatigues); (2) those that occur with normal activity levels and are due to some structural or biomechanical abnormality that subjects the affected tissue to mildly increased stresses over a long period of time. Such stresses may produce pain on an intermittent basis and, over a long period of time, may induce tissue hypertrophy. Since these are mild stresses acting over a long period, the body is able to respond by laying down an excessive amount of tissue in an attempt to strengthen itself against these abnormal stresses.

Tissue hypertrophy such as corns and callouses may, in itself, lead to pain by allowing localized areas of stress concentration.

Patients incurring tissue damage from high stresses acting over a relatively short time period are typically individuals who have increased their activity level significantly. Often, but not always, the patient will blame a particular activity for contributing to the onset of the problem. Keep in mind that in such instances the patient may or may not be correct; the particular disorder may have been developing over some period of time, perhaps as a result of a biomechanical abnormality, and may simply be aggravated by a particular activity. By evaluating the mechanical effects of activities that reproduce the pain, you often find important clues as to the nature of a particular disorder.

Shoes tend to provide support for the twisted or arched configuration of the foot to varying degrees. A high heel causes the toes to dorsiflex when standing with the feet in contact with the ground. This raises the arch by tightening the plantar aponeurosis that crosses the plantar surface of the metatarsophalangeal joints (Fig. 18-20). Heels also reduce the passive tension on the Achilles tendon and gastrocnemius– soleus group and, by effectively reducing the toe lever-arm of the foot, reduce the active tension developed in the gastrocnemius– soleus muscle– tendon complex. Most shoes also provide some contoured base of support for the "arch" of the foot. This maximizes the contacting surface area of the foot and, therefore, distributes the stresses of weight bearing over most of the sole of the foot. Proper contouring of a shoe also minimizes the amount of tension that needs to be developed in the plantar aponeurosis, long and short plantar ligaments, tarsal joint capsules, and intrinsic muscles to maintain a normal twisted configuration to the foot. When you go

barefoot, the effects of the heel and contoured support are lost. This usually creates no problem in a person with good bony alignment and ligamentous support. However, in a person with a tendency toward pronation (untwisting of the foot) the added tension to the plantar ligaments may lead to pain. Or, if the ligaments are already lax, increased intrinsic muscle activity will be necessary. If such prolonged muscular activity is necessary, pain may also arise from muscular fatigue. These individuals are often more comfortable wearing shoes than going barefoot. Even individuals with normal foot structure may experience some foot pain with lower heel heights if they are accustomed to wearing a shoe with a heel. Lowering the heel reduces the support provided by the plantar aponeurosis, putting more tension on the plantar ligaments and joint capsules and calling for increased activity of the intrinsic muscles of the foot. This is why flat-soled shoes, especially, must have well-contoured "arch supports."

Shoes also provide an interface for shear and compressive stresses. Foot pain arising from localized pressure concentration, from shear stresses between the skin and an exterior surface, or from shearing between skin and subcutaneous tissue may be alleviated by going barefoot. This is primarily true in cases in which such stresses occur over all but the soles of the feet. Pain from pressure concentration over the sole of the foot, as frequently occurs over the head of the second metatarsal, may be reduced by wearing shoes, since the contouring of the shoe may serve to distribute the pressures of weight bearing over a broader area.

Complaints of cramping of the foot may accompany muscular fatigue usually associated with some biomechanical disturbance. Cramping may also accompany intermittent claudication from arterial insufficiency. Claudication should always be suspect when the patient relates a history of pain or cramping of the feet, and usually of the lower leg, after walking some distance, but the pain is relieved with rest. Cramping may accompany disc protrusions, presumably from altered conduction of fibers subserving motor control or muscle reflexes. This cramping is noticed more often at night.

PHYSICAL EXAMINATION

I. Observation

    A. *General appearance and body build.* Weight bearing stresses will be increased in the presence of obesity.

    B. *Activities of daily living — Dressing, grooming, gait, and transfer activities (see gait analysis discussion under Lumbar – lower extremity scan exam).* With localized foot or ankle disorders, usually only the gait is affected. Observe the patient walking with and without shoes. An antalgic gait associated with foot or ankle lesions is typically one in which heel-strike or push-off, or both, are lacking. This results in a shortened stride on the affected side, which is accentuated at faster paces. Chronic disorders may produce no obvious gait disturbances. However, look carefully for more subtle gait deviations, indicating a possible biomechanical abnormality of one or more of the weight-bearing joints that may be related to a foot problem. It is of primary importance to observe for abnormal rotatory movements of the weight-bearing segments; to assess rotations of the hindfoot into pronation and supination, look at

        1. The patellae to judge rotary movements of the femur

        2. The position of the malleoli with respect to each other or the tibia

        3. The position of the calcanei

        4. The degree of toeing-in or toeing-out

II. Inspection

    A. *Skin and nails*

        1. If areas of redness or actual skin breakdown are noted, suggesting excessive shear or compression forces, document the size of the involved area to serve as a baseline measurement. This can easily be done by tracing the perimeter of the involved area on a piece of acetate (such as old radiographic film).

        2. Excessive dryness or moisture may suggest abnormal vascularity or abnormal sympathetic activity to the part, or both.

        3. Note the site and size of hypertrophic skin changes, such as corns and callouses. These suggest mildly increased shear or compression forces acting over a longer period of time than those that might produce localized inflammation or actual breakdown. Keep in mind that a painful callous is one in which the underlying tissue is in the process of breaking down.

        4. Diffuse ecchymosis may be associated with common ankle sprains as well as more serious trauma.

        5. Inspect the toe nails for splitting, overgrowth, inappropriate trimming, and inflammation of the nail beds.

    B. *Soft tissue*

        1. Swelling (see under palpation)

        2. Wasting of isolated or generalized muscle groups

        3. General contours

    C. *Bony structure and alignment*

        1. Note toe deformities such as claw toes, hammer toes, and varus – valgus deviations.

            a. Claw toes are usually associated with a pes cavus deformity and may accompany certain neurologic disorders. The metatarsophalangeal joints are positioned in extension and the interphalangeal joints in flexion. Contracture of the long toe-extensors causes extension of the toes, which increases the passive tension on the long toe-flexors. The intrinsic muscles are overbalanced, both actively and passively, by these muscle groups.

b. Hammer toes are a result of capsular contracture of the proximal or distal interphalangeal joints. The involved joint or joints are fixed in some degree of flexion.

c. A valgus deformity of the first metatarsolphalangeal joint is a common disorder. It may be associated with a varus deviation of the first metatarsal, a pronated foot, or both. The toe may be rotated, with the toe nail pointed inward.

2. Assess the length of the metatarsals. A line across the metatarsal heads should form a smooth parabola, with the second metatarsal being the longest. A shortened first metatarsal may lead to increased weight bearing by the second and sometimes the third metatarsal, resulting in tissue hypertrophy, pain, or both.

3. Navicular tubercle. An imaginary straight line passes from the medial malleolus to where the head of the first metatarsal meets the ground. The navicular tubercle should be within one third of the perpendicular distance between this line and the ground.

4. The calcanei should be positioned vertically with little or no inward or outward bowing of the Achilles tendon.

5. The general configuration of the foot should be assessed in standing and sitting positions.

a. When standing, an untwisted foot is one in which the hindfoot is in pronation and the forefoot in supination. The calcaneus will be in valgus position and the navicular tubercle will be sunken and often prominent. The talar head also becomes prominent medially, and the forefoot often assumes an abducted position with respect to the hindfoot. There is often an associated valgus deformity of the first metatarsal-phalangeal joint.

With excessive twisting of the foot—pes cavus—the calcaneus assumes a varus position, and the medial arch is well formed, with the navicular tubercle positioned well superiorly. There is often a tendency toward clawing of the toes in a cavus foot.

b. When sitting, the foot should relax into a position of plantar flexion, inversion, and adduction. A "supple" or "mobile" flatfoot will take on a more normal configuration in sitting with the force of weight bearing relieved. A "fixed" or "structural" flatfoot will maintain its planus (untwisted) state.

6. Perform a complete structural exam of the remainder of the lower extremities, the pelvis, and the lower back, as discussed in the next chapter. Any structural deviations or asymmetries should be noted, and the possible effects on the biomechanics of the foot considered.

7. Inspect the shoes, inside and out, for wear patterns that may offer clues as to the presence of persistent biomechanical disturbances and localized areas of pressure. Also inspect for other possible sources of pain arising from the shoe, such as nails protruding through the insole, and prominent seams.

   a. On the outer sole, the wear pattern should be displaced somewhat laterally at the heel. Over the front sole, the wear pattern should be spread fairly evenly across the area corresponding to the level of the first, second, and third metatarsophalangeal joints, with less wear laterally. There should be an even wear pattern across the rest of the medial side of the sole. Areas of localized excessive wear should be noted as well as abnormal wear patterns.

   b. The upper of the shoe should show a gently curved transverse crease line at the level of the metatarsophalangeal joints. Excessive curling of the vamp of the shoe and the front part of the sole may occur in a shoe that is too long, too narrow, or both. A crease line that runs obliquely, from forward and medial to backward and lateral, may arise from a stiff first metatarsophalangeal joint.

   Localized prominences of the upper commonly occur medially in the presence of hallux valgus or dorsally with hammer toes or claw toes. Such prominences should be noted.

   Inspect for excessive overhanging of the upper with respect to the sole. This is likely to be observed medially in shoes of patients with pronation of the hindfoot.

   Viewed from behind, the cup formed by the counter of the shoe should rise vertically and symmetrically from the sole. Inclination of the counter medially, with bulging of the lateral lip of the counter will be seen in shoes of patients with pronated feet.

   Areas of excessive scuffing of the upper should be noted. Scuffing of the toe of the shoe may occur with weak dorsiflexors or restriction of motion toward dorsiflexion.

   c. When inspecting the inside of the shoe, feel along the inner surface of the seams for prominent areas that may give rise to pressure concentration. Also feel along the entire surface of the inner sole for prominent areas that might be caused by protruding nails.

   The wear pattern on the inside of the shoe should also be examined. There should be evidence of an even distribution of pressure over the medial and lateral sides of the heel counter, over the inner sole at the heel, and over the inner sole at the metatarsal heads.

III. Selective Tissue Tension Tests

A. *Active movements (functional movements)*

1. Barefoot walking
   a. Normal gait
   b. On toes. If unable, determine whether it is because of pain, weakness, or restriction of motion. The heel should invert and the arch should rise.
   c. On heels. If unable, determine whether it is because of pain, weakness, or restriction of motion.
2. Standing with feet fixed
   a. Externally rotate the leg with respect to the foot. This should cause some varus deviation of the heels and raising of the arches. Compare one foot to the other.
   b. Internally rotate the legs on the feet. This should result in some valgus deviation of the heels and flattening of the arches. Compare one foot to the other.
3. Standing, keeping knees extended
   a. Evert the feet by standing on medial borders of feet.
   b. Invert the feet by standing on lateral borders of feet.
4. Sitting, with legs hanging freely. Compare range of motion of one foot to the other. Assess pain, range of motion, and crepitus.
   a. Dorsiflexion
   b. Plantar flexion
   c. Inversion
   d. Eversion
   e. Toe movements

B. *Passive range of motion*

1. Sit with legs hanging freely. Compare range of motion of one foot to the other. Note the presence of pain or crepitus. Note abnormalities or asymmetries in range of motion. Note the presence of pathologic end-feels.
   a. Hindfoot
      i. Dorsiflexion
      ii. Plantar flexion
      iii. Inversion
      iv. Eversion
   b. Forefoot
      i. Dorsiflexion
      ii. Plantar flexion
      iii. Pronation (eversion)
      iv. Supination (inversion)
      v. Abduction
      vi. Adduction
   c. Toes
      i. Flexion–extension
      ii. Abduction–adduction
2. Supine
   a. Hip flexion–extension
   b. Knee flexion–extension
3. Prone. Hip internal–external rotation

C. *Resisted movements (maximal isometric contractions)*

1. With the patient sitting with legs hanging freely, assess presence of pain or weakness.
   a. Tibialis anterior (dorsiflexion–inversion)
   b. Tibialis posterior (plantar flexion–inversion)
   c. Peroneus tertius (dorsiflexion–eversion)
   d. Peroneus longus and brevis (plantar flexion–eversion)
   e. Toe extensors
   f. Toe flexors

D. *Joint play movements.* Assess for

hypermobility or hypomobility and presence or absence of pain. (See Chapter 7, Joint Mobilization Techniques.)

1. Distal tibiofibular joint—anterior–posterior glide
2. Ankle mortise joint
   a. Distraction of talus
   b. Anterior and posterior glide of talus. (Anterior glide is an important test for integrity of the anterior talofibular ligament.)
3. Subtalar joint
   a. Distraction of calcaneus
   b. Dorsal rock of calcaneus, plantar rock of calcaneus
   c. Inversion–eversion tilts of calcaneus
4. Transverse tarsal joint—dorsal–plantar glides
5. Naviculocuneiform joint—dorsal–plantar glides
6. Cuneiform–metatarsal joints
   a. Dorsal–plantar glides
   b. Pronation–supination twists
7. Cuboid–fifth metatarsal joint—dorsal–plantar glides
8. Intermetatarsal articulations—dorsal–plantar glides
9. Metatarsophalangeal and interphalangeal joints
   a. Dorsal–plantar glides
   b. Internal–external rotations
   c. Medial–lateral tilts
   d. Distraction

IV. **Neuromuscular Tests.** There are few localized neurologic problems that affect the foot. If a disorder affecting a relevant nerve root (L4, L5, S1, or S2) is suspected, or if a problem affecting a peripheral nerve supplying the foot is suspected, the necessary sensory, motor, and reflex testing should be performed. The segmental and peripheral nerve innervations, as well as the related reflexes, are listed in Chapter 4, Assessment of Musculoskeletal Disorders.

V. **Palpation**
A. *Skin*
   1. Moisture or dryness. Abnormal moisture, usually associated with pain and joint restriction, may accompany a reflex sympathetic dystrophy. Vascular disorders may also cause changes in the moisture or texture of the skin.
   2. Texture
   3. Mobility. Skin mobility may be restricted after prolonged immobilization, especially following a surgical procedure.
   4. Temperature. Inflammatory lesions will often result in increased skin temperature over the site of the lesion. Fairly precise documentation of the degree of inflammation may be made by using a thermister probe. This often offers a convenient guide as to the effect of treatment procedures on the state of the lesion as well as a guide to the state of the inflammatory process in general. For example, a baseline reading can be documented and measurements taken before and after each treatment session (these must be taken over precisely the same point and at the same time of day). You can expect a slight elevation of, say, 1°C after any treatment that imposes some mechanical stress, such as mobilization, massage, or exercise. However, it is important that the elevation does not persist over more than a few hours. If so, the treatment program may be too vigorous. If some decline in temperature is noted, it may be

a sign that resolution is taking place. Thermister readings, as with most tests, are significant when compared to a normal side.

B. *Soft tissue*

 1. Swelling
    a. Localized extra-articular swelling may accompany ankle sprains, usually involving the lateral aspect of the ankle below the lateral malleolus.
    b. Localized articular effusion of the ankle mortise joint manifests as a loss of definition over the malleolar regions. Subtle joint effusion can be detected by applying firm pressure with the thumb and index fingers over the regions below the medial and lateral malleoli simultaneously. This will force the fluid into the anterior capsular region and cause a fullness over the dorsum of the ankle.
    c. Generalized edema of the foot may follow major trauma, or it may accompany systemic, more generalized vascular or metabolic disorders.
 2. Mobility
 3. Consistency
 4. Pulses
    a. The pulse of the dorsalis pedis artery may be palpated just lateral to the tendon of the extensor hallucis longus over the dorsum of the foot.
    b. The pulse of the posterior tibial artery is palpated behind the tendons of the flexor digitorum longus and flexor hallucis longus post-

erosuperior to the medial malleolus.

 5. Other specific tendons, ligaments, and muscles should be palpated, as indicated by findings to this point in the exam. A guide to palpation of these structures is included in the section on surface anatomy in this chapter.

C. *Bony structures and tendon and ligament attachments*

 1. Palpate joint margins to assess structural alignment and to note any hypertrophic changes.
 2. Palpate tendon and ligament attachments as indicated in the section on surface anatomy.

COMMON LESIONS AND THEIR MANAGEMENT

The common disorders affecting the foot are in the majority of cases the result of some biomechanical disturbance. As indicated in the preceding section, such biomechanical disorders may be of local origin, or the primary problem may involve one of the other weight-bearing segments. For this reason, evaluation of chronic, subtle foot disorders requires that structural and functional assessments of the other weight-bearing joints be made. Similarly, evaluation of patients with problems in these other regions may necessitate examination of the foot. In understanding the rationale of the evaluative and treatment procedures related to foot disorders, it is essential that the practioner have a basic knowledge of the biomechanics of the foot and how they relate to the mechanics of the other weight-bearing joints.

Because the numerous joints of the foot contribute to make it a very mobile structure as a whole, it has the ability to attenuate the energy of forces applied to it.

For this reason, traumatic lesions affecting the foot are relatively rare. On the other hand, the common lesions affecting the ankle are usually of traumatic origin.[4] While the individual joints making up the ankle are relatively trackbound or uniaxial, the ankle complex allows some movement in the sagittal, frontal, and transverse planes. However, transverse rotations are of limited range because they do not occur about a true vertical axis. Also, eversion is normally quite restricted because the fibular malleolus extends distally to create an abutment that limits this movement. Forces that move the ankle past its physiologic limits of motion will tend to cause damage, usually to the osseus or ligamentous components of the ankle complex, or to both. Excessive forces to the ankle producing such damage are often the result of forces from the ground acting over the lever arm provided by the foot, or by forces of the center of gravity of the body acting over the lever arm of the lower extremity with the foot fixed. Because of these lever arms over which forces acting on the ankle may be applied, and because certain ankle motions are normally limited, the ankle is often the site of acute traumatic injuries such as sprains and fractures.

Except in situations in which there is malalignment of bony constituents, such as following healing of a fracture, or in situations in which there is marked restriction of movement of one of the ankle joints, such as following arthrodesis of the subtalar joints, degenerative joint disease affecting the ankle is rare. Rheumatoid arthritis often affects the foot, but less often the ankle.

Both the foot and ankle may be the site of fatigue disorders. Such disorders result from abnormally high stresses occurring over relatively short periods of time, or mildly abnormal stresses occurring over a long period of time. The former situation usually occurs in athletes or others who have undergone an abrupt increase in activity level. In such cases, the degree of microtrauma affecting certain tissues exceeds the rate at which the body is able to repair itself; the result is a fatigue yielding of the involved tissue. Examples are stress fractures, blisters, and many of the tendinitis conditions affecting this region. Lower stresses occurring over longer periods of time tend to result in tissue hypertrophy that may contribute to certain painful disorders. Typical examples are heel spurs and various callous formations.

ANKLE SPRAIN

The most common lesion affecting the ankle is a sprain or tear of one of the ligaments.[4,13] The anterior talofibular ligament is the most commonly sprained ligament at the ankle and is probably the most commonly sprained ligament in the body. The next most frequently sprained ligaments at the ankle are the calcaneocuboid and the calcaneofibular ligaments. Portions of the deltoid ligament may also be sprained, but more often a forceful eversion stress will result in an avulsion of the tibial malleolus rather than damage to the ligament.[5,7]

I. **History**
   A. *Onset of pain.* The patient will invariably recall the traumatic incident. The common mechanism of injury for an anterior talofibular ligament sprain is a plantar flexion–inversion stress.[15,16,21,29] Typical examples include a jumper coming down upon the lateral border of the plantarly flexed foot, a person wearing high-heeled shoes or walking on uneven ground who catches a toe on the lateral side of the foot, or a person stepping off a curb or step who rolls over the lateral side of the plantarly flexed foot. If the forefoot is forced into supination or adduction, the calcaneocuboid

ligament may be injured instead or as well. The calcaneofibular ligament restricts inversion with the foot in a more neutral or dorsiflexed position. It may be injured along with the talofibular ligament if, at the time of injury, the person retains good contact of the foot with the ground, but continues to force the foot into inversion.

When torn, the deltoid ligament is usually injured because the foot is forced into external rotation and eversion with respect to the leg. As mentioned, it is more common for a portion of the tibial malleolus to avulse with the deltoid ligament attachment. The anterior tibiofibular ligament may be torn with a similar mechanism, since as the talus rotates within the mortise, it tends to wedge the tibia and fibula apart, producing a diastasis.[1,5,7] In order for the talus to rotate enough to produce a diastasis and to tear the anterior tibiofibular ligament, the deltoid ligament is torn or the tibial malleolus is avulsed as well.[1]

B. *Site of pain.* This usually corresponds well with the approximate location of the injury. Some pain may be referred distally into the foot or proximally into the lower leg.

C. *Nature of pain or disability.* Similar to ligamentous lesions at the knee, the degree of pain and disability immediately following an injury to an ankle ligament does not necessarily correlate well with the severity of the lesion.[20] A person sustaining a mild or moderate sprain may describe more pain and be more reluctant to continue a particular activity than one who completely ruptures a ligament.

This is because in the event of a rupture, there is complete loss of continuity of the structure and there are no longer intact fibers to be stressed and from which pain can be elicited.

Repeated episodes of anterior talofibular ligament sprains are not uncommon. Usually the initial injury results in somewhat more pain and disability than with subsequent occurrences. These individuals typically describe intermittent giving way of the ankle, often during athletic activities, followed by pain and effusion lasting for a few days.[11,34]

II. Physical Examination

A. *Observation.* A patient seen soon after injury may hobble into the office walking with a characteristic "foot flat," short-stance gait; both heel-strike and push-off are lacking. If the pain is more severe, the patient may present walking with the aid of crutches or hopping in on one leg.

B. *Inspection.* Localized swelling over the region of the involved ligament is usually present within several hours following the injury. Since the anterior talofibular ligament and the deep fibers of the deltoid ligament blend with the ankle mortise joint capsule, there may be some associated articular effusion. Within a day or so following most ankle sprains, there is diffuse ecchymosis in the region of the injury, which may extravasate distally into the foot.

C. *Selective tissue tension tests*

1. Active movements. In the acute stage there is likely to be considerable difficulty in heel and toe walking and other weight-bearing activities involving ankle movements. The examiner must exercise judgment in requesting these movements to avoid undue discomfort or stress to the part.

2. Passive movements/joint play movements (key objective tests)

a. If the ankle mortise joint capsule has been stressed with subsequent articular effusion, the ankle movements will be limited in a capsular pattern; plantar flexion will be slightly more restricted than dorsiflexion.

b. In the case of a mild or moderate ligamentous sprain, pain will be reproduced with movements which stress the involved ligament. There will usually be an associated muscle-spasm end-feel. Painless hypermobility will be noted in the presence of chronic ruptures. Acute ruptures will also demonstrate hypermobility; however, a false negative finding may be elicited because of protective muscle spasm. Take care to assure maximal relaxation of the part when performing passive movements. The common ligaments injured and the passive movements used to test their integrity are

i. Anterior talofibular. (a) Combined plantar flexion – inversion – adduction of the hindfoot and (b) anterior glide of the talus on the tibia[4,25]

ii. Calcaneocuboid ligament. Combined supination – adduction of the forefoot

iii. Calcaneofibular ligament. Inversion of the hindfoot in a neutral position of plantar flexion – dorsiflexion

iv. Deltoid ligament. (a) Anterior fibers – combined plantar flexion – eversion – abduction of the hindfoot and (b) middle fibers – eversion of the hindfoot

3. Resisted movements. These should be strong and painless. Occasionally the peroneal tendons are strained in conjunction with an inversion ligamentous strain. In this case, isometric resistance to eversion will be strong and painful.

D. *Neuromuscular tests.* Noncontributory

E. *Palpation*

1. Tenderness will usually correspond to the site of the lesion in acute injuries. There is also likely to be diffuse tenderness in the presence of marked swelling from extravasation of blood into the tissues.

2. Joint effusion from synovitis or extra-articular swelling will be palpable in the acute stages.

3. Skin temperature will be elevated over the region of the involved structure in the acute stages.

III. Management

A. *Acute sprains—immediate measures.* At this early stage, there is little that needs to be done to, or for, the patient that he cannot do on his own. Ice, elevation, compression, mobility exercises, and strengthening can be carried out easily at home by most patients. This does, however, require very clear and precise instruction by the therapist. Do not spare words or time in assuring that the patient understands exactly what he should or should not be doing with the ankle. A follow-up visit after 2 or 3 days should be scheduled so that a reassessment can be made and the program appropriately progressed. At this point, there should be evidence of reduction of the acute inflammatory process; pain, temperature, and swelling should be decreased. It is important, in the subacute stage, to carefully reassess joint play movements, since at this stage you can determine more easily whether there has been some loss of integrity of the involved structure. Often in the acute stage, muscle spasm precludes accurate determination of the extent of the damage.

1. Reduced stress to the ligament to allow healing without undue lengthening.
   a. Ankle strapping will help reduce movement in response to mild (non-weight-bearing) stresses. Swelling should have stabilized by the time of application. A felt or foam rubber "horseshoe" should be used to fill in the submalleolar depressions so as to obtain even compressions of the area with application of tape or an elastic bandage.
   b. Crutches should be used to relieve stress and pain during ambulation. A three-point, partial weight-bearing crutch gait should be instituted; non-weight bearing is usually not necessary and should be avoided because of its non-functional nature.
2. Reduction of the acute inflammatory process to reduce pain and to prevent undue tis-

sue damage from localized pressure and proteolytic cellular responses
   a. Ice—To decrease bloodflow and reduce capillary hydrostatic pressure, thereby reducing extravasation of blood fluids
   b. Compression—Increased external pressure to the area will minimize capillary leakage by effectively reducing the volume of the tissue spaces. This can be maintained by appropriate application of an elastic bandage with a horseshoe pad below the malleolus.
   c. Elevation—Reduces capillary hydrostatic pressure to minimize fluid loss and assists the venous and lymphatic return.
3. Prevention of residual disability
   a. Insitute motion of the part in planes that do not stress the healing ligament to minimize residual loss of movement and optimize circulation in the area.
   b. *Isometric exercises* to the muscles in the area should be started as early as pain allows to maintain strength of the muscles of the lower leg and foot.

B. *Acute sprains—subsequent measures*
   1. Mild sprains. In the case of a simple sprain, in which there is no hypermobility on the associated passive movement tests, gradual return to normal activities should be allowed as the inflammatory process resolves. Weight bearing should be increased and the crutches discarded, usually by the fifth

day. Range of motion, strength, and joint play should be restored to normal. Most patients may regain normal motion and strength with careful instruction in home exercises. Before discharging the patient from care, the therapist must ascertain that normal joint play has returned. If it has not, the restricted movements must be restored with passive joint mobilization techniques. Friction massage, initiated in the subacute stage, may promote healing of the ligament in a mobile state and prevent adherence to adjacent tissue.

As the swelling subsides in the subacute stage, strapping should be substituted for the elastic bandage to provide support and to increase proprioceptive feedback as the patient resumes functional use of the part. Use of strapping should continue until good strength, range of motion, and joint play are restored. The athlete should continue to strap the ankle when participating in vigorous activities. Studies suggest that ankle strapping does play a role in preventing ankle sprains.[14] This is probably not due to actual mechanical support provided by the tape, since movement of the bones within the skin (to which the tape is adhered) is probably still sufficient to allow a ligament to be stretched. However, the added proprioceptive input provided by the tape may enhance protective reflexes (such as contraction of the peroneal muscles) in response to forces tending to stress the ankle ligaments.

Return to vigorous activity must be gradual. Clinical evidence of healing does not indicate that a ligament has regained normal strength. In fact, maturation of the new collagen layed down during healing may take weeks or months. The necessary stimulus for maturation and restoration of normal ligamentous strength is stress to the ligament produced by functional use of the part. This induces formation of the appropriate collagen cross-links and realignment of the new collagen fibers along the normal lines of stress. However, the ligament must not be overstressed before normal strength is regained, since it is susceptible at this point to reinjury. The athlete should begin by jogging, then running, in straight lines. When normal muscle strength and joint motion have been regained, figure-of-eight patterns that impose some lateral stress to the part may be initiated. Gradually, the patient should progress to sharp cutting drills. When these can be performed well and without pain, competitive activity may be resumed.

Also during the later stages of rehabilitation, balance drills should be instituted to facilitate the restoration of normal protective reflexes.[10,12] Progression may proceed from challenging one-legged standing to one-legged standing on a rocking board to one-legged standing on a board supported on half a sphere (free to tilt in all planes).

2. Moderate sprains and complete ruptures. The related literature reflects some con-

troversy regarding the management of ruptured ligaments at the ankle. Most authorities would agree that injuries involving extensive damage, with rupture of both the anterior talofibular and calcaneofibular ligaments, should be repaired surgically to restore passive stability to the ankle.[2,34] Good results are favored by early surgery, since the torn ends will tend to atrophy and retract with time, making apposition and suturing technically difficult or impossible. Similar considerations apply to rupture of the deltoid ligament.

There is more divergence of opinion, however, with respect to management of isolated ruptures, in which some hypermobility of anterior glide of the talus in the mortise is demonstrable. While some favor early surgical intervention to suture the torn ends and minimize residual structural instability, others favor early return to function following some period of restricted activity and immobilization. There is evidence from studies by Freeman that suturing of the ligament does result in a more stable joint, but in the end, the functional status of those undergoing surgery is really no better than those treated "conservatively."[10,11,12] In fact, those treated nonoperatively returned to normal function significantly sooner than those undergoing surgery, if they were not immobilized in plaster for a prolonged period of time. Of those treated conservatively, there was very little difference in residual mechan-

ical stability between those who were immobilized in plaster for 6 wk and those treated with strapping and early mobilization. The incidence of residual pain and swelling several months following injury was highest in the surgical group. The only way to guarantee increased mechanical stability following rupture of the anterior talofibular ligament is to reappose the torn ends with sutures. However, it seems that the residual disability resulting from prolonged immobilization in those treated with surgery outweighs whatever advantage this form of management may have in producing a more stable ankle. Further studies by Freeman suggest that there is no correlation between mechanical instability, as determined by stress radiographs, and the incidence of residual disability resulting from chronic swelling and pain.

Conservative (nonsurgical) management of patients in whom there is evidence of actual loss of integrity of the ligament should follow the same approach as management for less serious injuries; the primary difference should be that those ankles with more extensive damage will need to be protected, by crutches and strapping, somewhat longer, perhaps as long as 2 weeks. However, early motion and strengthening at painfree intensities should be initiated as resolution of the acute inflammatory process ensues. Also, in cases of more extensive damage, return to normal and, especially, to vigorous activity levels should be more gradual.

Again, it must be emphasized that although new collagen is layed down within the first week or two following injury, it takes months for this new tissue to mature to normal strength. During the period of maturation, the ligament is weaker than normal and, therefore, more susceptible to reinjury.

C. *Chronic, recurrent ankle sprains.* Following initial injury, especially to the anterior talofibular ligament, a certain number of patients will go on to suffer recurrent giving way of the ankle, with subsequent pain and swelling. There are three possible causes of this to be considered and to which assessment should be directed

1. Healing of the ligament with adherence to adjacent tissues. In this situation, the healed ligament does not allow the joint play necessary for normal functioning of the part.[7] With repetitive stress to the tightened structure, pain and swelling will result from a fatigue phenomenon. With forceful stress to the structure, the adhesion will rupture, producing another sprain. This type of problem will present as a painful, minor restriction on passive plantar flexion–inversion of the hindfoot, and on anterior glide of the talus. Treatment consists of deep, transverse friction massage to the ligament and specific joint mobilization in the directions of restriction. Normal mobility to the ligament is thereby gradually restored.

2. Loss of protective reflex muscle stabilization. Normally, stress to some aspect of a joint capsule or to a joint ligament results in firing of specific receptors in the structure, through a reflex arc, to produce contraction of the muscles overlying the stressed structure. This "booster" mechanism of dynamic joint stabilization protects joint ligaments from injury under conditions of heavy loading. Thus, when the anterior talofibular ligament is stressed, the peroneus tertius is called to reduce the load to the ligament. Damage to a ligament with subsequent immobilization may result in interference of this protective mechanism. Freeman has shown good results in management of such cases by instituting a program of balance training (as described above). You must also make sure that good muscle strength has been restored.

3. Gross mechanical instability of the joint. If both the anterior talofibular ligament and the calcaneofibular ligament are ruptured, or if there has been extensive capsular disruption with an anterior talofibular ligament rupture, the resultant mechanical instability of the joint may not allow certain functional weight-bearing activities to be performed without giving way. Such cases will present with obvious hypermobility on joint play movement tests. If an aggressive muscle strengthening and balance training program is not sufficient to compensate for the instability, surgical reconstruction may be contemplated.

Thus, you should direct assessment of

the chronically unstable ankle toward determining if there is some residual increase or decrease in joint play, if good muscle strength has been regained, and whether the person is able to balance well during one-legged standing under various unstable conditions (*e.g.*, on a tilt board). It is important to realize that giving way of the joint is not necessarily the result of structural instability, and that some degree of structural instability can be compensated for by muscle strengthening or balance training.

PROBLEMS RELATED TO FOOT PRONATION

Pronation of the hindfoot with respect to the forefoot is a relatively common disorder that may or may not give rise to foot pain. Also, because of the biomechanical interplay between the foot and other weight-bearing segments, the pronated foot may result in dysfunction in other regions of the lower extremity, especially the knee. Similarly, a pronated foot may be caused by some local structural abnormality of the tarsal skeleton, or it may be caused by some structural deviation in segments either distal or proximal to the hindfoot.

Pain resulting from a pronated foot is usually of the fatigue type from prolonged increased stress on the affected tissues. In some patients, pain may arise with normal activity levels, while others may get along well until they engage in some activity, such as jogging, involving increased stress levels or frequency. Pain of local origin usually has its source in one of the plantar structures responsible for maintaining the twisted configuration of the foot—the plantar aponeurosis, the short plantar ligament, or the long plantar ligament. Pain may also arise from fatigue of the intrinsic muscles of the foot, in which activity may be increased in an attempt to prevent undue stress to the plantar aponeurosis and ligaments. In association with increased tensile stress to the plantar

aponeurosis, a calcaneal periostitis may develop from the added pull to the proximal attachment of the aponeurosis on the plantar surface of the calcaneus. Excessive pulling on the periosteum in this region occasionally results in a bony outcropping (heel spur) that in itself may give rise to localized pressure to the overlying soft tissue. You should consider periostitis and eventually osteophyte formation as resulting from increased stress to the plantar aponeurosis. It must be emphasized that spurring can develop in the absence of pain, and that a cartilaginous spur may be present that is not visible in radiographs. Another source of local pain occurring in association with a pronated foot is pressure from the shoes against the talar head or the navicular, which become prominent medially when the foot untwists.

A pronated foot may be the cause of, or be associated with, pain in the forefoot, leg, or the knee. Pain from pressure over the first one or two metatarsal heads may result from increased weight bearing over the medial side of the forefoot. This occurs if the talar head and navicular drop downward and inward, shifting the center of gravity line medially. Since hallux valgus often accompanies pronation of the hindfoot, either as a cause or as a result, pressure over a prominent first metatarsophalangeal joint may also occur with increased pronation of the foot. Leg pain may result from increased tension on the anterior or posterior tibialis muscles, which are dynamic supporters of the arch of the foot. Chronic periostitis at the proximal attachment of these muscles may result, and is often referred to as *shin splints*. The knee tends to assume a valgus position when the foot pronates. Such an angulation tends to increase the lateral pull on the patella during loaded quadriceps contraction. This may predispose to pain from patellar tracking dysfunction at the knee (see Chapter 17, The Knee).

As mentioned, pronation of the hindfoot

may occur from some local structural disorder or from structural deviations elsewhere. The common local causes are capsuloligamentous laxity and bony abnormalities. Capsuloligamentous laxity may be a hereditary condition or it may accompany some specific disease state, such as rheumatoid arthritis. The common *bony* anomaly resulting in flatfoot is tarsal coalition, in which the talus and calcaneus are fixed to one another in a pronated orientation through fibrous or osseous union. The common malalignment problems affecting other regions that predispose to abnormal pronation of the hindfoot are femoral anteversion, internal tibial torsion, a shortened Achilles tendon, and adduction of the first metatarsal. The excessive internal rotation imposed by anteversion of the femur or internal tibial torsion during stance phase is at least partially absorbed by the subtalar joint, bringing the hindfoot into pronation. In the presence of a short Achilles tendon, the midtarsal joint attempts to compensate for lack of dorsiflexion at the ankle; in order to do so, the foot must untwist to unlock the midtarsal joints. Because of the oblique orientation of the first cuneiform–first metatarsal joint, adduction of the first metatarsal also involves a component of dorsiflexion. This effectively supinates the forefoot, which necessitates a compensatory pronation of the hindfoot in order to get the foot flat on the ground. Each of these possible causes must be considered when examining the patient with a pronated foot.

Finally, we must remember that abnormal foot pronation during gait is not always associated with a "pronated foot" seen on structural examination with the patient standing. The typical example is an individual with increased tibial varum. The foot usually appears normal or even supinated during relaxed standing. However, when running or walking there is a tendency to heel-strike on the lateral border of the heel, and the foot must undergo increased hindfoot pronation in order for the heel to become flat on the ground. So, even though the foot appears not to be pronated, it will be subject to increased pronatory stresses. Similar considerations apply to the individual with femoral anteversion or external tibial torsion, in which cases the cause of pronation is not localized to the foot itself.

I. **History**
   A. *Onset of pain* is usually insidious, since the tissue pathologies associated with biomechanical abnormalities such as a pronated foot are typically fatigue phenomena. Often the onset can be related to some increased activity level, such as long-distance running. Another common predisposing factor is a period of disuse, such as immobilization of the foot in a cast. In such cases, the muscles of the foot weaken, and when activity is resumed, they no longer contribute their share to stabilizing the arch of the foot. This results in increased stress to the capsuloligamentous structures. Occasionally, a change in footwear, for example, to lower heel height, can be related to the onset. Lowering the heel height increases the tension on the Achilles tendon, which may in turn result in increased pronation of the hindfoot in the same way as described for a shortened Achilles tendon. A lowered heel also results in reduced dorsiflexion of the toes during the stance, decreasing the windlass effect on the plantar aponeurosis and reducing the twisted configuration of the foot.
   B. *Site of pain.* Foot pain associated with abnormal pronation usually is felt over the plantar aspect of the foot. Pain from calcaneal periostitis and heel spurs is fairly

well localized over the bottom of the heel, often more medially; it may be referred anteriorly into the sole of the foot. Pain from fatigue stress to the plantar ligament or aponeurosis is felt over the sole of the foot, usually more medially. Keep in mind that the bony and soft-tissue pathologies referred to above may occur concurrently.

Forefoot pain arising secondary to a pronated foot condition may be felt in the region of the medial metatarsal heads, if due to abnormal weight distribution, or it may be felt over the medial aspect of the first metatarsophalangeal joint, if caused by pressure over the joint resulting from a hallux valgus deformity.

Knee pain related to a pronated foot is typically from patellofemoral joint problems (see section on patellar tracking dysfunction in Chapter 17).

C. *Nature of pain.* Pain is from increased stress to the plantar ligaments, fascia, capsules, or calcaneal periosteum under conditions in which increased untwisting of the foot takes place. This typically occurs in a person whose foot undergoes an abnormal degree of pronation during stance phase, or whose foot remains in a pronated position during prolonged standing. The muscles controlling the twist, or arch, of the foot will protect these structures for a certain period of time. However, once the muscles fatigue, more stress is transmitted to the ligaments and fascia, which are responsible for the passive stabilization of the arched configuration of the foot. In some cases, this may occur with normal activity levels, such as after walking some distance or after standing for a long period of time. In others, increased activity, such as long-distance running, provides the added stress to bring on the pain. Once a low-grade inflammation develops, the pain is brought on with less stress and may be relatively continuous during weight bearing. In these more severe cases, pain is typically pronounced upon initial weight bearing, subsiding somewhat as the muscles contract more to protect the painful structures, then increasing again as the muscles fatigue.

II. **Physical Examination**

A. *Observation and inspection of structural alignment.* Evidence of excessive pronation of the foot and associated biomechanical abnormalities may be noted when the patient walks or stands.
1. Flattening of the medial arch. The region of the navicular and the talar head may appear to be prominent medially and depressed inferiorly.
2. Adduction of the first metatarsal, perhaps with a valgus deformity of the first metatarsophalangeal joint
3. Valgus position of the heel maintained throughout stance phase
4. Internal tibial torsion. The feet may be pointed inward while the patellae face straight forward.
5. Femoral anteversion. The patellae face inward when the feet are in normal alignment. This must be differentiated from external tibial torsion, which may present similarly. External tibial torsion is evidenced by an increased external rotation of the intermalleo-

lar line with respect to the frontal plane (in excess of about 25°). Femoral anteversion is suggested when the total range of motion at the hip is about normal, but the range of internal rotation is increased and the range of external rotation is proportionally decreased.

6. Genu valgum. This often exists in conjunction with femoral anteversion.

B. *Inspection*

1. Structural alignment (see above)

2. Skin. Inspect for signs of pressure over the navicular tubercle, first metatarsophalangeal joint, and the medial metatarsal head. Look at the patient's foot as well as at the shoe.

3. Soft tissue. Inspect for muscle atrophy that may relate to loss of dynamic support of the arch of the foot.

C. *Selective tissue tension tests*

1. Active movements. If inspection of structural alignment reveals a pronated position of the hindfoot, observe the effect of raising up on the toes and externally rotating the leg over the fixed foot. Both of these movements should decrease the pronation, and cause an increased twisting and arching of the foot. If not, a rigid flatfoot, caused by some fixed structural abnormality such as tarsal coalition, probably exists.

2. Passive movements. Unless a rigid flatfoot exists (a relatively rare condition) a pronated foot is usually a hypermobile foot. Hypermobility, especially of the midtarsal joints, may be noted.

a. If a tight heel cord or restricted ankle mortise joint capsule is a contributing cause, dorsiflexion of the hindfoot will be restricted. One must lock the foot by supinating the calcaneus and pronating the forefoot when testing ankle dorsiflexion to avoid misinterpreting movement of the forefoot as being movement at the ankle. There should be about 10° to 20° of dorsiflexion. If dorsiflexion and plantar flexion are both restricted, the joint capsule is probably at fault. If dorsiflexion is restricted with the knee straight, but not with the knee bent, the gastrocnemius is tight. If dorsiflexion is restricted regardless of the position of the knee, the soleus is probably at fault.

b. If anteversion of the hip is a contributing factor, hip range of motion will be relatively normal but skewed toward internal rotation with restriction of external rotation.

c. Joint play movements of the tarsal joints are likely to be hypermobile.

d. Pain from low-grade inflammation of the plantar fascia or ligaments, or from calcaneal periostitis, may be reproduced by passively everting the heel, supinating the foot, and dorsiflexing the toes.

3. Resisted movements. Usually noncontributory

D. *Neuromuscular tests*. Determine whether weakness, either neurogenic or atrophic, of any of the muscles controlling movement and stability of the foot exists.

E. *Palpation.* Localized tender areas may exist that relate to areas of low-grade inflammation occurring in response to abnormal tissue stresses. As usual, the finding of localized tenderness to palpation, in itself, must not be taken to be diagnostic of any specific disorder because of the common phenomenon of referred tenderness associated with lesions of deep somatic tissue.

Typical areas of tenderness associated with abnormal foot pronation might include the calcaneal attachment of the plantar fascia and long plantar ligament, especially at the medial tubercle; the plantar fascia, usually over the medial aspect of the sole of the foot; the navicular tubercle; the short plantar ligament, between the sustentaculum tali and the navicular tubercle; the medial one or two metatarsal heads; and the medial aspect of the first metatarsophalangeal joint.

Areas of skin or subcutaneous tissue hypertrophy may be distinguished on palpations as localized indurated regions. Such callouses, associated with pronation, might be found over the medial one or two metatarsal heads or over the medial aspect of the first metatarsalphalangeal joint.

III. **Management.** Symptoms arising in association with abnormal foot pronation are the result of increased stress to some pain sensitive tissue. Proper management, then, must involve selective reduction of abnormal stresses. The approach used must be in accordance with findings on evaluation, including information relating to the patient's activity level. In de-

veloping a program of management, it must be kept in mind that the tissue pathology resulting in the painful condition may be due to normal stresses occurring at too great a frequency, or abnormally high stresses occurring at normal frequencies or some combination thereof. Either situation may result in tissue fatigue in which the rate of tissue breakdown exceeds the rate at which the tissue is able to repair itself. However, the approach to management will differ, depending upon which condition prevails. Generally speaking, management of conditions associated with pronation of the foot involves measures to reduce either the frequency or magnitude of stresses, or both.

In the case of the pronated foot, forces are typically increased by structural malalignments that cause changes in the direction in which forces occur and changes in the degree of movement of skeletal parts during functional activities. The most common postural malalignment causing abnormal foot pronation is probably increased femoral anteversion, which is usually accompanied by increased genu valgum (knock knees). As mentioned earlier, the other common structural deviations predisposing to increased pronation of the foot are adduction of the first metatarsal and increased internal tibial torsion. Each of these conditions results in untwisting of the tarsal skeleton during ambulation, such that a greater tensile stress is imposed upon the plantar ligaments, fascia, and joint capsules. Under such conditions, the foot loses the normal passive stability normally produced by becoming twisted during stance phase. To compensate, the intrinsic muscles of the foot must contract more to prepare the foot for push-off. Pain may arise from increased stress to the plantar capsuloligamentous structures, from fatigue of the abnormally contracting muscles, or from both.

The individual with longstanding pronation from a congenital structural malalignment or from a malalignment acquired early in life, is likely to have a permanent hypermobility of the joints of the foot. The ligaments and joint capsules will have been elongated from the chronic increased stresses applied to them throughout development. By the time they are adults, these people are not likely to have pain arising from the already lengthened ligaments and fascia during normal activity levels. They are, however, likely to have feet that tire easily from increased activity of the intrinsics and other muscles supporting the arch during gait. They are also more predisposed to developing problems elsewhere, such as metatarsalgia, hallux valgus, and patellofemoral joint dysfunction.

Persons with more subtle structural deviations resulting in an increased tendency toward pronation are likely to have problems only with increased activity levels, such as long distance running, that increase the magnitude and frequency of pronatory stresses. The mobility of the joints of the foot in these people allowed by the capsules and ligaments is likely to be fairly normal. It is especially important in patients experiencing pain suggestive of increased pronation, but who have relatively normal structural alignment, to consider nonstructural causes. The most common of these would include a tight heel cord and inappropriate footwear. It is these patients, having subtle structural deviations or nonstructural causes of increased pronation, who are likely to experience pain and develop pathologies associated with increased strain to specific tissues. The most common tissues involved are the supporting plantar structures of the foot, including the periosteum of the plantar aspect of the calcaneus, and the Achilles tendon.

A. *Techniques*

1. Instruction in appropriate activity levels. As with any common musculoskeletal disorder, appropriate instruction in exactly what the patient should and should not do, and to what degree, is an essential component of the treatment program too often overlooked. With respect to problems related to increased foot pronation, this is especially important in the person experiencing problems primarily with increased activity levels. Treatment of the long-distance runner experiencing pain from plantar fasciitis, Achilles tendinitis, or other pronation-related disorders, simply involves advising the patient to not run so much. But this is not adequate management of the problem since, as with any disorder, we must be concerned primarily with restoring optimal function. From the patient's standpoint, optimal function may be running long distances! The role of the therapist should be first to decide whether the patient's functional expectations are realistic. The individual with considerably increased femoral anteversion, knock knees, and hypermobile flatfeet probably should not be engaging in activities, such as long distance running, that involve high frequency, weight-bearing

stresses. Posture, however, should not prevent him from engaging in other vigorous conditioning exercise such as swimming and bicycling.

If there are no gross structural malalignments predisposing to pronation-type problems, the therapist must then determine what can be done to reduce the stresses to the involved tissues, to allow them to heal and to prevent further pathology and pain. As far as healing is concerned, the most important step to be taken is to reduce the stresses that caused the problem. The most reliable method of doing this is to reduce the activity level. The long-distance runner experiencing chronic, persistent pain, must be advised to markedly reduce, or stop, running for a period of 1 to 2 wk to allow the tissue to heal. Complete immobilization, however, is seldom, if ever, indicated for fatigue disorders such as these. During this period of relative rest the therapist should determine what can be done to reduce stresses when the activity is resumed. Other procedures to help restore the involved tissue to its normal state may also be instituted.

2. Muscle strengthening and conditioning. Strengthening and endurance exercises for the intrinsic muscles of the foot, as well as for the extrinsic muscles, such as the anterior and posterior tibialis that help maintain a twisted configuration of the foot, are important in the management of virtually all foot problems resulting from abnormal pronation. Im-proving the function of these muscles will allow the individual with the hypermobile flatfoot to stand or walk for longer periods of time before muscle fatigue sets in. It will also help relieve strain on the plantar fascia and ligaments, in those suffering from strain of these structures, by increasing the dynamic support of the arch, thereby allowing the muscles to take a greater portion of the load.

3. Strapping. Strong muscles are of little use unless they contract with sufficient force and at the appropriate time to perform the desired function. Abnormal foot pronation can be controlled to varying degree by contraction of the muscles that affect an increased twisted configuration of the foot. Most important among these are the anterior and posterior tibialis muscles and the peroneus longus. Theoretically, muscle function can be enhanced by providing additional input along the afferent limb of the reflex arcs that normally invoke muscle contraction during functional activities. One method of doing so is to strap the part in a manner that will cause increased tension to the straps, and therefore the skin, when movement occurs in the undesired direction. The added afferent input from the tension and pressure produced by the straps serves to enhance activity of muscles that normally check the undesired movement. This is apparently the means by which ankle strapping helps to "stabilize" the ankle against inversion

sprains.[13] Although empirically there seems to be evidence for the efficacy of such procedures, electromyogram studies have yet to be performed to substantiate the proposed mechanism.

A strapping technique described by Stanley Newell of Seattle, and others, is designed to restrict abnormal foot pronation. It may be used to protect the passive stabilizing structures of the foot, such as the plantar fascia and associated structures, during the rehabilitation phase following injuries to them. It may also be used to assess what effect more permanent stabilizing measures, such as orthotic devices or shoe modification, may have.

Technique—The foot and large toe are wrapped with foam underwrap. Using a roll of 1½ in wide athletic tape, a ¾ in wide circumferential anchor strap is applied to the base of the large toe and a 1½ in wide anchor applied around the forefoot about ¼ in proximal to the base of the fifth metatarsal. From this point in the procedure, the arched configuration of the foot must be maintained by holding the first metatarsal in plantar flexion and adduction, or by dorsiflexing the large toe. With the arch maintained, two to four straps are applied from the medial side of the large toe anchor, along the medial side of the foot, around the back of the calcaneus, and along the lateral border of the foot to the lateral aspect of the forefoot anchor. The straps are then secured with circumferential straps applied in the same manner as the anchors. Occasionally, excessive pressure is applied to the digital branch of the lateral plantar nerve, proximal to the base of the fifth metatarsal, in which case the position of the forefoot anchor must be adjusted. The patient may be instructed in the procedure or asked to return for daily reapplication of the wrap.

4. Ultrasound and friction massage. These may be important treatment measures in cases of plantar fasciitis, Achilles tendinitis, and tibialis periostitis. The resultant increased blood flow may assist in the healing process. Transverse frictions will promote the development of a mobile structure and help prevent adhesions as healing ensues.

5. Achilles tendon stretching. This is especially important when evaluation reveals a tight heel cord as a possible contributing cause of the patient's problem, and in cases of Achilles tendinitis. One must take care to assure that the stretching force is applied to the hindfoot since using the forefoot as a lever to stretch the heel cord will result in dorsiflexion of the transverse tarsal joint in addition to dorsiflexion at the ankle mortise joint. This may result in hypermobility of the transverse tarsal joint, which may add further to a tendency toward pronation of the foot.

In the more acute stages of Achilles tendinitis, you must not be overly vigorous in restoring mobility to the heel cord since the condition could be aggravated. However, since most cases of Achilles tendinitis are fatigue disorders, an acute stage never exists. Some gentle stretching may be initiated carefully from the outset since the slow, short-termed stress produced by such stretching procedures in no way approximates the high frequency, high strain-rate stresses which produce this type of disorder. In fact, early stretching, performed judiciously, will help prevent the fibers from healing in a shortened state.

6. Shoe inserts and modifications. When abnormal foot pronation is due to some structural malalignment, whether marked or subtle, only surgery can remedy the true cause of the disorder. However, nonsurgical management is effective in the majority of cases. In order to optimize function, while at the same time preventing stresses sufficient to cause painful pathology, the excessive untwisting of the foot must be reduced. This can be accomplished by altering the orientation of the segments of the foot as they contact the ground during stance phase or by producing direct support to the arched configuration of the foot, or both.

   If the joint capsules and ligaments of the foot are not elongated, as in the hypermobile flatfoot accompanying gross malalignment, the twist in the foot during stance phase can be increased by increasing the pronatory orientation of the forefoot or by increasing the supinatory orientation of the hindfoot. This can be done by providing a lateral wedge for the forefoot or a medial wedge for the heel. A trial, temporary insert can be made by cutting such a wedge from a piece of 1/8 in to 3/16 in felt to fit inside the shoe. However, if it is to be used on a permanent basis, the wedge should be incorporated into the sole or heel of the shoe by one experienced in shoe modifications, or incorporated into an orthosis.

   If the tarsal joints of the foot are lax, then the twisted configuration cannot be restored by indirect means such as wedging, since these rely upon taking up the slack in the joint capsules to effect a twisting of the tarsal skeleton. In the case of a hypermobile, pronated foot, some direct support must be provided to prevent the head of the talus and navicular from dropping downward and medially in a pronatory fashion. For the severely pronated foot, such an arch support may be used in conjunction with wedging of the sole or heel. Such wedging may be built into the orthosis or into the shoe. Regardless of the type of shoe modification or insert used, in order to be effective the calcaneus must be stabilized by a firm shoe counter or a calcaneal cup built into an orthosis. If the calcaneus is not held firmly, it will tend to compensate for attempts to increase the twist of the foot by rolling further over into a valgus position (pronation). Thus, many orthoses now in use have a heel cup incorporated into the orthosis itself, obviating the need for an extra-firm shoe counter. Such an orthosis can be used, for example, in athletic shoes, which often do not have very stiff counters.

When chondromalcia at the knee occurs as a result of abnormal pronation of the foot, the use of arch supports or shoe modification may be a necessary component of the treatment program.

The progression of a hallux valgus deformity may also be retarded by use of orthoses or shoe modifications, if the adduction of the first metatarsal is a result of abnormal foot pronation.

In cases of metatarsalgia, if reducing the degree of pronation with appropriate orthotic devices or shoe modification does not adequately relieve the pressure over the metatarsal heads, a metatarsal insert may be used. This simply reduces the stress to the metatarsal heads by increasing the weight-bearing surface area behind the heads. Metatarsal pads are available "ready-made" with an adhesive backing, or a metatarsal support may be incorporated into an arch supporting orthosis. To place the pad properly in the shoe, tape it to the patient's foot in place just behind the metatarsal heads with the widest dimension of the pad forward. Outline the bottom of the pad with lipstick or some substance that will leave a mark on the insole of the shoe when the patient steps down. The patient then puts on the shoes and walks about to make sure it is reasonably comfortable, realizing, of course, that it will at first feel somewhat peculiar. The shoes are then removed and the pad adhered to the insole of the shoe in the appropriate place as indicated by the marks left on the insole by the lipstick.

Because orthotic fabrication and shoe modifications are technical skills that require considerable time and training, it is usually not practical for the therapist to incorporate these skills into his practice. Since foot problems and related disorders are common and because alteration of footwear is often an important component of management of these problems, it is important that the therapist develop a close working relationship with an orthotist, podiatrist, or other professional possessing these skills.

REFERENCES

1. Alldredge RH: Diatases of the distal tibiofibular joint and associated lesions. JAMA 115:2136, 1940
2. Anderson KJ, LeCocq JF: Operative treatment of injuries to the fibular collateral ligament of the ankle. J Bone Joint Surg 36(A):825, 1954
3. Barnett CH, Napier JR: The axis of rotation at the ankle joint in man: Its influence upon the form of the mobility of the fibula. J Anat 86:1, 1952
4. Cedell CA: Ankle lesions. Acta Orthop Scand 46:425–445, 1976
5. Cedell CA: Supination—Outward rotation injuries of the ankle. Acta Orthop Scand (Suppl) 110:1–148, 1967
6. Close JR, Inman VT, Poor PM, Todd FN: The function of the subtalar joint. Clin Orthop 50:159–179, 1967

7. De Souza Dias DL, Foerster TP: Traumatic lesions of the ankle joint: The supination external rotation mechanism. Clin Orthop 100:219– 224, 1974

8. Dwyer FC: Causes significance and treatment of stiffness in the subdeltoid joint. Med Proc R Soc 69(2):97– 102, 1976

9. Elftman H: The transverse tarsal joint and its control. Clin Orthop 16:41– 46, 1960

10. Freeman M: The etiology and prevention of instability of the foot. J Bone Joint Surg 47(B):678– 685, 1965

11. Freeman M: Instability of the foot after injuries to the lateral ligament of the ankle. J Bone Joint Surg 47(B):669– 677, 1965

12. Freeman M: Treatment of ruptures of the lateral ligament of the ankle. J Bone Joint Surg 47(B):661– 668, 1965

13. Fulp MJ: Ankle joint injuries. J Am Podiatry Assoc 65(9):8, 1975

14. Garrick JG, Requa RK: Role of external support in the prevention of ankle sprains. Med Sci Sports 5:300, 1973

15. Gerbert J: Ligament injuries of the ankle joint. J Am Podiatry Assoc 65(8):802– 815, 1975

16. Gross AE, MacIntosh DL: Injuries to the lateral ligaments of the ankle: A clinical study. Can J Surg 16:115, 1973

17. Hicks JH: The mechanics of the foot. I. The joints. J Anat 87:345, 1953

18. Hicks JH: The mechanics of the foot. II. The plantar aponeurosis and the arch. J Anat 88:25, 1954

19. Inman VT: The Joints of the Ankle. Baltimore, Williams & Wilkins, 1976

20. Jackson, DW: Ankle sprains in young athletes: Relation of severity and disability. Clin Orthop 101:102, 1974

21. Kleiger B: Mechanisms of ankle injury. Orthop Clin North Am 5:153– 176, 1974

22. Lamoreux L: Kinematic measurements in the study of human walking. Bull Pros Res 10– 15:3– 84, 1971

23. Leonard MH: Injuries of the lateral ligaments of the ankle: A clinical and experimental study. J Bone Joint Surg 31(A):373, 1949

24. Level AS, Inman VT, Blosser JA: Transverse rotation of the segments of the lower extremity in locomotion. J Bone Joint Surg 30(A):859– 872, 1948

25. Lindstrand A: New aspects in the diagnosis of lateral ankle sprains. Orthop Clin North Am 7(1):247– 249, 1976

26. MacConnaill MA, Basmajian JV: Muscles and Movements: A Basis for Human Kinesiology, pp 74– 84. Baltimore, Williams & Wilkens, 1969

27. Manter JT: Movements of the subtalar and transverse tarsal joints. Anat Rec 80:397, 1941

28. Murray MP, Draught AP, Kory RC: Walking patterns in normal men. J Bone Joint Surg 46(A):335– 360, 1964

29. Nicholas JA: Ankle injuries in athletes. Orthop Clin North Am 5:153– 176, 1974

30. Peiyer E, Wright DW, Mason L: Human locomotion. Bull Pros Res 10– 12:48-105, 1969

31. Sammarco GJ, Burstein AH Frankel VH: Biomechanics of the ankle: A kinematic study. Orthop Clin North Am 4:75– 95, 1973

32. Saunders JB, Dec M, Inman VT, Eberhart HD: The major determinants in normal and pathological gait. J Bone Joint Surg 35(A):543– 558, 1953

33. Smith JW: The ligamentous structures in the canalis and sinus tarsi. J Anat 92:616, 1958

34. Staples OS: Ruptures of the fibular collateral ligaments of the ankle: Result study. Immediate surgical treatment. J Bone Joint Surg 47(A):101– 107, 1975

35. Subotnick SI: Biomechanics of the subtalar and midtarsal joints. J Am Podiatry Assoc 65(8):756– 764, 1975

36. Wright DG, Desai SM, Henderson WH: Action of the subtalar and ankle complex during stance phase of walking. J Bone Joint Surg 46(A):361, 1964

19 The Lumbar–Lower Extremity Scan Examination

Randolph M. Kessler

A common problem in the clinical examination of patients presenting with chronic, insidious musculoskeletal problems of the low back and lower extremities is not knowing to which area to direct physical examination procedures after completing the history portion of the exam. The reason for this is twofold: (1) chronic musculoskeletal disorders affecting the low back and the various regions of the lower limbs often present with similar pain patterns, and (2) biomechanical disorders affecting the back and various lower extremity regions often coexist. The former is a result of the common phenomenon of referred pain that is characteristic of most common musculoskeletal disorders; localized pain arising from deep somatic tissues is usually perceived in an area not corresponding well to the exact site of pathology. Thus, patients with "low-back pain" usually feel discomfort primarily in the upper buttock or sacroiliac regions, patients with trochanteric bursitis often have significant pain in the posterior hip and lateral thigh areas, and those with patellar chondromalacia frequently feel pain over the medial aspect of the distal thigh and upper leg. Also, as the severity of the pathology increases, there is greater likelihood that pain may be perceived throughout a distribution corresponding to any or all of the relevant sclerotome. So, if a relatively acute disorder affects a tissue innervated primarily by the L5 segment, the patient may feel pain in any or all of those regions also innervated by L5.

A typical example would be the individual with moderate to advanced degenerative hip disease who invariably experiences pain in the groin, spreading into the anterior thigh and to the knee—the L3 sclerotome. This occurs because the anterior aspect of the hip joint capsule, from which the pain primarily arises, is innervated largely by the L3 segment. Similarly, the person with involvement of the L3 segment of the spine from, for example, facet joint or disc pathology, may feel pain that spreads in the same distribution as that described above for hip joint disease. It may not be obvious from subjective information alone whether the hip, the low back, or both are involved. Likewise, it is often difficult to determine on the basis of subjective information alone whether a patient has trochanteric bursitis, an L5 spinal disorder, or both; the trochanteric region is innervated primarily by L5, and pain arising in conjunction with trochanteric bursitis is often felt down the lateral aspect of the thigh and dorsum of the leg (the L5 scleratome), as may be the case with pain originated at the L5 spinal level.

Another classic example of localization of pain to distant regions of a relevant sclerotome occurs in the child with a hip joint disorder, such as a slipped capital femoral epiphysis, who feels pain primarily in the knee; both the hip and the knee joints are innervated largely by L3. Because delocalization and reference of pain are common phenomena, the subjective account of pain distribution does not provide a reliable indication of the true site of pathology. Additional objective information is often required.

The prevalence of coexistent disorders or abnormalities of the low back and lower extremity regions is largely a result of the biomechanical interdependency of the weight-bearing joints in the closed kinetic chain. Normal attenuation of the energy introduced to the weight-bearing joints by the vertical displacement of the center of gravity requires that the overall displacement of the center of gravity be minimized, which in turn requires normal movement of the weight-bearing joints during stance phase of gait. Loss of critical movement at any of weight-bearing joints will cause increased energy input to the entire weight-bearing skeleton from the force of the body weight acting over a greater distance, the result being added vertical compressive loading during stance phase. Similarly, energy input to the weight-bearing joints in a horizontal plane is normally attenuated by joint movements. With the foot fixed to the ground, in order for the body to be normally moved through space in the presence of reduced critical movement at any joint, compensation is required at some other joint. Such an alteration in function is likely to result in added stresses to the compensating joint. Thus, the patient with loss of hip extension tends to walk with greater extension of the lower lumbar joints and the person with loss of ankle dorsiflexion undergoes greater-than-normal extension movements at the knee. Since the close-packed positions of the spine and knee are extension, these abnormalities are likely to cause increased subchondral compressive stresses and increased capsular tensile stresses to the knee and spinal joints.

Less obvious are the results of abnormalities in transverse rotation of the weight-bearing joints during stance phase of gait. From heel-strike to foot-flat the pelvis, thigh, and leg normally undergo internal rotatory movements, the distal segments more so than their supradjacent neighbors. The segments of the leg similarly undergo external rotation during foot-flat to toe-off. Since the foot is relatively fixed to the ground, however, it does not rotate. This means that the ankle–foot complex must absorb the rotatory movements imposed from above—internal rotation is absorbed by pronation of the foot, and external rotation is transmitted to the foot as a supinatory movement. The reader should observe the result of rotating the leg over the foot that is fixed to the ground; internal rotation causes the calcaneous to shift into valgus position, and the medial arch to lower (pronation of the hindfoot), whereas external rotation brings the heel into varus position and raises the arch (supination of the hindfoot). It should also be noted that internal rotation of the thigh with the knee slightly bent causes an increased valgus angulation at the knee. This is of practical significance because the knee remains slightly bent during all phases of the gait cycle.

Again, because attenuation of the forces of the body weight moving over the fixed foot requires a normal contribution of movement from all weight-bearing joints, abnormalities of function at any one joint may affect the function of one or more of the others in the chain. A common example occurs in the person with increased femoral anteversion, who tends to walk with excessive internal rotation during stance phase of gait. This results in abnormal valgus angulation at the knee and increased foot pronation. The former may predispose to patellar tracking problems, while the latter may lead to a variety of problems, including plantar fasciitis, heel spurs, hallux valgus, metatarsalgia, and fatigue of the intrinsic foot musculature (see Chapter 18, The Ankle and Hindfoot).

On the other hand, a primary problem of abnormal foot pronation may lead to excessive internal rotatory and valgus stresses to the knee and increased internal rotation of the hip during gait. It should be clear that the best approach to management of pathologies resulting from such biomechanical derangements would be one which takes into consideration primary etiologic factors. This often requires that evaluating procedures be directed to areas other than simply the primary region of involvement.

The above considerations should help emphasize the need to evaluate all of the weight-bearing joint regions in many, if not most, chronic musculoskeletal disorders affecting the low back or lower limb. A further factor to consider in this regard is the common phenomenon of summation of otherwise subliminal afferent input from coexistent minor disorders involving tissues innervated by the same or adjacent spinal segments. A common example is the person who stresses the joint capsules of the low back excessively throughout the day and who also has some low-grade inflammation of the trochanteric bursa. Noxious input from both areas may summate at the dorsal horn of the spinal cord, and other central neural connections, to cause more low-back pain as well as more lateral thigh pain than would be present if either disorder existed by itself. In this particular example the clinician must differentiate between the possibility of one lesion referring pain into another part of the relevant segment and two distinct pathologies within the same segment. This cannot be determined without evaluating both the low back and the hip regions. Pain arising from the summation of input from different sites of the same segment will, of course, be more likely to occur in the patient with multisegmental restrictions of motion of the lower spine, since with daily activities, the soft tissues (joint capsules and ligaments) of the spine will be stressed more, causing an increase in afferent input to the relevant spinal levels.

In such cases, the threshold to pain arising from minor disorders affecting tissue in the lower limbs innervated by the corresponding spinal segments is probably reduced. Any back pain is likely to be enhanced by such segmentally related pathologies. Most persons, by their middle-age or later, develop some lower-lumbar facet-joint capsular restriction secondary to disc narrowing or other causes. Thus, middle-aged or older individuals with chronic low-back or lower-limb pathologies should always be examined for coexistent segmental disorders that may be contributing to the amount of pain the person experiences.

In summary, the low back–lower extremity scan exam may be used to

1. Determine the area of involvement in cases in which relatively vague subjective information fails to suggest the site of pathology. This is not an uncommon occurrence and is related to the fact that pain of deep somatic origin may be referred into any of or all of the relevant sclerotome.
2. Examine for the presence of some distant biomechanical derangement that may be related, in cause or effect, to the patient's primary physical pathology that causes his pain.
3. Rule out the possibility of some segmentally related disorder that may, by the mechanism of summation of segmentally related afferent input, contribute to the patient's pain perception.

The scan exam is oriented, then, toward detecting gross or subtle biomechanical abnormalities and toward determining the presence of common lumbar or lower-extremity musculoskeletal disorders. Essential to the detection of significant biomechanical derangements are careful assessment of function (gait analysis), evaluation of bony structure and alignment, and examination of joint mobility. These examination procedures are combined with the key objective tests for the common chronic disorders affecting the lower back and lower extremities, to constitute the lumbar–lower extremity scan exam. A discussion of the common pathologies and their primary clinical manifestations will facilitate understanding and interpretation of the examination procedures involved in the scan exam.

COMMON LESIONS OF THE LOW BACK AND LOWER EXTREMITIES AND THEIR PRIMARY CLINICAL MANIFESTATIONS

THE LUMBOSACRAL REGION

I. **Acute (Severe) Posterolateral Disk Prolapse (Outer annulus or posterior longitudinal ligament still intact)**
   A. *Subjective complaints*
      1. Sudden onset of unilateral lumbosacral pain, often with gradual buildup of pain intensity. Occasionally the patient denies a sudden onset and notes first experiencing pain upon rising in the morning. There may be some aching into the leg.
      2. Worse with sitting and upon rising from a long period of recumbency; somewhat relieved with recumbency
   B. *Key objective signs*
      1. Functional lumbar deformity, with a loss of lordosis and usually a lumbar scoliosis with the convexity to the involved side
      2. Marked, painful restriction of spinal movement, especially forward and backward bending
      3. Positive dural mobility tests. Usually positive leg raising tests bilaterally.

II. **Acute Facet-Joint Derangement**
   A. *Subjective complaints*
      1. Sudden onset of lumbosacral pain and deformity; little or no leg discomfort
      2. Pain is aggravated by being up

and about, relieved by sitting or recumbency
   B. *Key objective findings*
      1. Marked lumbar deformity. Loss of lordosis and lumbar scoliosis with convexity to side of involvement
      2. Lumbar extension and side bending to the side of involvement are painfully restricted. Forward bending and contralateral side bending are slightly restricted.
      3. Negative dural signs

III. **Localized Unilateral Facet-Joint Capsular Tightness**
   A. *Subjective complaints*
      1. Often a history of past episodes of acute low-back dysfunction
      2. Aching in the lumbosacral region, aggravated by long periods of standing, walking, or activities involving prolonged or repetitive lumbar extension. Also worse with increased muscular tension, such as during periods of emotional stress, and worse in the evening than in the morning.
   B. *Key objective findings*
      1. Possible subtle predisposing biomechanical factor such as a leg-length disparity
      2. Possible minor restriction of side bending to the involved side, and deviation of spine toward the involved side on forward bending and away from the involved side on extension
      3. Discomfort on quadrant tests when localized to the involved segment

IV. **Multisegmental Bilateral Capsular Restriction of Lumbar Facet Joints— Degenerative Joint Disease (DJD)**
   A. *Subjective complaints*
      1. The patient is middle-aged or older.

2. Often a long history of intermittent back problems
3. Aching across the lower back and hip girdles is made worse with long periods of standing or walking. The back is stiff in the morning, somewhat better at midday, and aching again by evening. Possibly some intermittent aching into one or both legs.
B. *Key objective findings*
1. Some loss of the normal lumbar lordosis
2. Restriction of spinal motion in a generalized capsular pattern of limitation. Marked restriction of spinal extension, moderate restriction of side bending bilaterally, mild to moderate restriction of rotations and forward bending.

V. **Lower Lumbar Disk Extrusion with Nerve Root Impingement**
A. *Subjective complaints*
1. Sudden or gradual onset of lumbosacral pain and unilateral leg pain. The patient may describe an onset suggestive of an acute posterolateral prolapse (see above) with progressive loss of back pain and increase in leg pain.
2. The leg pain may be relatively sharp and is usually felt down the posterolateral thigh and into the anterior lateral or posterior aspect of the lower leg. The leg pain may be aggravated by sitting or by being up and about, and is relatively relieved by rest.
B. *Key objective findings*
1. Mild to moderate loss of lumbar movement, usually toward extension and in movements toward the side of involvement; occasionally occurs away from the involved side.

2. Mild segmental neurologic deficit
3. Positive dural mobility signs

VI. **Acute Sacroiliac Dysfunction**
A. *Subjective complaints*
1. Sudden onset of unilateral sacroiliac pain, often associated with some twisting motion
2. Occasional spread of pain to the posterior thigh
3. Pain is usually aggravated by activities involving combined hip and spine extension, such as standing erect (posterior torsional displacement). Less often it is aggravated by combined hip and spine flexion, such as sitting (anterior torsional displacement).
B. *Key objective findings*
1. Posterior torsional displacement (most common)
   a. Tendency to stand with the hip, knee, and low back slightly flexed on the involved side. If so, the knee landmarks and the greater trochanter will be lower on the involved side than on the uninvolved side. The posterior superior iliac spine (PSIS) and iliac crest will also be lower on the involved side, more so than the knee landmarks and trochanter. The anterior superior iliac spine will not be as low on the involved side as the knee and trochanteric landmarks. The pelvis will be shifted away from the involved side.

   If the patient stands with the legs straight, all of the landmarks up to, and including, the trochanters will be level. The PSIS and iliac crest will be lower on the involved side than on the uninvolved side, but the anterior superior iliac spine (ASIS) will be higher. The pelvis will appear to be rotated forward on the involved side.

b. The anterior torsion strain test will be quite painful; the posterior torsion test will be less painful.

c. Contralateral straight leg raising may cause some pain, which is relieved when the involved leg is raised.

2. Anterior torsional displacement (rare)

a. Tendency to stand with the hip and knee in more extension on the involved side than on the uninvolved side. The pelvis may be shifted toward and inclined away from the involved side. If the patient stands in this manner, the knee landmarks and trochanter will be lower on the uninvolved side. The PSIS and iliac crest will also be lower on the uninvolved side, more so than the knee landmarks and trochanter. The ASIS will not be as low on the uninvolved side as the other landmarks.

If the patient can stand erect, the trochanters and landmarks below will be level. The PSIS and iliac crest will be higher on the involved side; the ASIS will be lower on the involved side.

b. Posterior torsion strain will be quite painful, anterior torsion strain will be less painful.

c. Ipsilateral straight leg raise test may cause some pain, which is relieved when the opposite leg is raised.

VII. Chronic Sacroiliac Hypermobility

A. *Subjective complaints*

1. History suggestive of intermittent acute sacroiliac dysfunction with gradual progression to more chronic sacroiliac and posterior thigh pain. Development may be associated with past pregnancy.

2. Pain is aggravated by prolonged or repetitive activities involving

a. Combined hip and spine extension or hip extension with contralateral hip flexion

b. Combined hip and spine flexion or hip flexion with contralateral hip extension

B. *Key objective findings*

1. Possible signs of sacroiliac asymmetry on assessment of structural alignment (see above under acute sacroiliac dysfunction).

2. Pain or crepitus on one or more sacroiliac stress tests.

THE HIP

I. Degenerative Joint Disease

A. *Subjective complaints*

1. Gradual, progressive onset of hip pain and dysfunction

2. The pain is felt first and most in the groin region. With progression, pain may spread to the anterior thigh, posterior hip, and lateral hip regions.

3. Pain is first noticed after long periods of weight-bearing activities. Later, pain and stiffness are noted upon rising in the morning, easing somewhat by midday, then increased again by evening.

B. *Key objective findings*
1. Tendency to stand with hip and knee flexed and lumbar spine hyperextended. The pelvis is shifted toward the involved side.
2. Gait abnormality characterized by tendency to incline the trunk toward the involved side during stance phase
3. Painful limitation of hip motions in a capsular pattern of restriction; marked limitation of internal rotation and abduction, moderate restriction of flexion and extension, mild to moderate restriction of adduction and external rotation

II. Trochanteric Bursitis
A. *Subjective complaints*
1. Insidious onset of lateral hip pain, often spreading into the lateral thigh, aggravated most by climbing stairs or, occasionally, by sitting with the involved leg crossed over the uninvolved leg.
2. Occasionally an acute onset is described, associated with a "snap" felt in the hip region (the iliotibial band snapping over the greater trochanter.)

B. *Key objective findings*
1. Pain on resisted hip abduction
2. Pain on approximation of the knee on the involved side to the opposite axilla
3. Possible pain on stretch of the iliotibial band
4. Possible pain on full passive hip abduction

III. Iliopectineal Bursitis
A. *Subjective complaint.* Gradual, usually nontraumatic, onset of anterior hip pain, made worse by activities involving extreme or repetitive hip extension.

B. *Key objective findings*
1. Pain on resisted hip flexion

2. Pain on full passive hip extension
3. Possible pain on full hip flexion

THE KNEE

I. Acute Medial Ligamentous Injury
A. *Subjective complaints*
1. Sudden onset of knee pain, usually associated with some athletic activity. There may or may not have been some external force acting on the knee at the time of injury in the case of a partial tear.
2. Gradual buildup of swelling over several hours in the case of a partial tear; little swelling in the case of a complete rupture
3. The patient often attempts to continue the activity in which he was engaged in the case of a complete rupture, but much less so in the case of a partial tear.

B. *Key objective findings*
1. Antalgic, toe-touch gait in the acute phase of a partial tear; less severe gait disturbance or no gait disturbance for a complete rupture
2. Effusion with limitation of motion in a capsular pattern in the case of a partial tear; little swelling and relatively free range of motion if a complete rupture
3. Pain and spasm on valgus and external rotary stress if a partial tear; painless hypermobility in the case of a complete rupture

II. Acute Meniscus Tear
A. *Subjective complaint.* Essentially the same as for a partial ligamentous tear. The individual is very hesitant to continue to engage in the activity.

B. *Key objective findings*
1. The same as for a partial ligament tear except no pain on stress tests
2. Point tenderness over the anteromedial joint line
3. Disproportionate loss of extension (locked knee) if a mechanical block to movement is created by a displaced piece of the meniscus

III. Lateral Patellar Tracking Dysfunction (Chondromalacia patellae)
A. *Subjective complaints*
1. Gradual onset of medial knee pain aggravated especially by descending stairs and sitting for long periods of time
2. The onset may be associated with an increase in some activity involving repeated loaded knee extension

B. *Key objective findings*
1. There may be some predisposing structural factor such as anteversion of the hip, genu valgum, a small patella, a high-riding patella, or a diminution in the prominence of the anterior aspect of the lateral femoral condyle.
2. There may be some atrophy of the vastus medialis.
3. Lateral glide of the patella may cause some medial discomfort.
4. Palpation of the medial aspect of the back side of patella may cause discomfort.
5. Femoropatellar crepitus may be noted on weight-bearing knee flexion–extension.

IV. Chronic Coronary Ligament Sprain (Adhesion)
A. *Subjective complaint.* Sudden medial knee pain associated with some weight-bearing twisting movement, followed by persistent aching or twinging of pain over the medial knee region.

There is usually no significant disability.
B. *Key objective findings*
1. Point tenderness over the anteromedial joint line
2. Pain on passive external rotation of the tibia on the femur. No pain on valgus stress

V. Tendinitis — Biceps, Iliotibial, or Pes Anserinus
A. *Subjective complaint.* Gradual onset of pain, almost always associated with long-distance running or some other athletic activity. The pain is lateral for biceps or iliotibial tendinitis and medial for pes anserinus tendinitis. There is little that reproduces the pain except the activity that caused the problem.
B. *Key objective findings*
1. Pain on resisted knee flexion and external tibial rotation in the case of biceps tendinitis
2. Pain on resisted knee extension and external tibial rotation in the case of iliotibial tendinitis
3. Pain on resisted knee flexion and internal rotation for pes anserinus tendinitis
4. Pain on straight leg raising for biceps tendinitis
5. Point tenderness over the site of the lesion, usually at the tenoperiosteal junction
6. Pain on iliotibial band extensibility test for iliotibial tendinitis

THE ANKLE AND FOOT

I. Acute Ankle Sprain
A. *Subjective complaints*
1. Sudden onset of lateral ankle pain, associated with a plantar flexion–inversion strain, usually during some athletic activity. Continued participation in

the activity, at the time of injury, is usually not possible.

2. Gradual development of lateral ankle swelling over the subsequent several hours with continued difficulty in weight bearing

B. *Key objective signs*

1. Obvious limp associated with traumatic arthritis of the ankle mortise joint (Table 19-1)
2. Swelling and often marked ecchymosis over the lateral aspect of the ankle
3. Pain is reproduced on
   a. Plantar flexion–inversion stress
   b. Anterior glide of the talus in the mortise

II. Chronic Recurrent Ankle Sprains

A. *Subjective complaint.* History of acute ankle sprain (see above) followed by one or more episodes of the ankle's giving way during activities involving jumping or quick lateral movements. Pain, swelling, and dysfunction associated with subsequent episodes are usually not as severe as that occurring with the original injury.

B. *Key objective findings.* These are variable, depending upon the causative factors. Consider the following possible causes and the related clinical manifestations.

1. True structural instability (rare). Hypermobility of anterior glide of the talus in the mortise
2. Residual ligamentous adhesion. Hypomobility or pain on anterior glide of the talus in the mortise
3. Alteration in proprioceptive neuromuscular protective response. Poor balance reactions on one-legged standing

III. Achilles Tendinitis and Bursitis

A. *Subjective complaint.* Usually a gradual onset of posterior ankle pain that may be associated with some increase in activity level. The pain is made worse when wearing lower-heeled shoes, and is improved with higher heels.

B. *Key objective findings*

1. Pain on strong resisted or repetitive resisted ankle plantar flexion
2. Pain on extreme hindfoot dorsiflexion
3. Tenderness to palpation over the distal Achilles region

IV. Medial Metatarsalgia

A. *Subjective complaint.* Pain over the first two metatarsal heads after long periods of weight bearing. The onset is usually insidious, occasionally associated with a change in foot wear

B. *Key objective findings*

1. Pressure metatarsalgia
   a. Often associated with a pronated or pronating foot
   b. The first metatarsal may be abnormally short.
   c. The medial metatarsal heads may be tender to deep palpation.
2. Tension metatarsalgia (from increased tension on the distal insertion of the plantar fascia)
   a. Usually associated with a pronating foot
   b. The pain may be reproduced by everting the hindfoot while supinating the forefoot and dorsiflexing the toes

THE SCAN EXAM TESTS

GAIT ANALYSIS

The reader should refer to Tables 19-1 and 19-2 for an overview of the primary gait abnormalities associated with various common lumbar or lower extremity pathologies or structural deviations. These tables emphasize the biomechanical interplay among the weight-bearing regions. A careful assessment of gait is an essential component of the evaluation of chronic low back and lower extremity disorders, since it is, of course, the most important functional requirement of these regions and also because many biomechanical abnormalities will not be evident on other parts of the examination.

When evaluating chronic disorders, most of which are the result of stress overloads, it is important to realize which functional abnormalities are present and to appreciate that these are not always manifest as obvious static deviations or deformities. For example, a person's foot may undergo excessive pronation while walking, but the foot may not necessarily appear "pronated" on assessment of bony structure and alignment during standing. Experience in gait analysis is invaluable in understanding the pathomechanics and, in some instances, the etiologies of many common chronic disorders. For this reason it also leads to greater sophistication in devising and implementing treatment strategies, since many chronic disorders are temporarily relieved by "symptomatic" treatment but will inevitably recur unless the underlying causes are dealt with.

Tables 19-1 and 19-2 are organized to serve as a guide to the clinical assessment of gait abnormalities associated with the common disorders affecting the low back and lower extremities. After having documented the salient features of some abnormal gait pattern, the clinician may consult the tables to estimate what the underlying physical dysfunction may be and to see what the common causes are. This information should then be correlated with findings from the remainder of the physical examination.

ASSESSMENT OF STRUCTURAL ALIGNMENT

Static alterations in skeletal alignment are significant if they are relatively pronounced or if they are acquired. In either case, they affect a considerable reduction in the stresses that may be imposed upon related tissues without pain or degenerative changes. Congenital skeletal deviations, as long as they fall within relatively normal limits, are usually insignificant under normal activity levels, since the related tissues automatically adapt to the various stresses they must withstand as the musculoskeletal system develops. However, such "normal" deviations may make the patient more susceptible to certain stress-overload pathologies under conditions of increased activity, such as recreational or competitive athletics. To avoid omitting crucial assessments, the examination of structural alignment may be organized into the following three components: (*1*) frontal alignment, (*2*) sagittal alignment, and (*3*) transverse (rotary) alignment. The primary assessments of each are carried out with the patient in a relaxed standing position, the low back and lower extremities well exposed (shorts are best), the feet at a normal base width and pointed slightly (about 5° to 10°) outward. The patient is instructed to look straight ahead and to keep the arms to his side.

I. Frontal Alignment. The patient is viewed from behind.

    A. *Horizontal asymmetry* is best detected by use of a plumb bob. The plumb bob is hung so that it barely clears the ground, and the patient positioned as close as possible to the plumb line, without touching it, and with the plumb bob bisecting his heels.

    1. It should be noted, first, whether the plumb line bisects the legs, pelvis, and lower spine. If there is a lateral shift of the pelvis with respect to the plumb line, consider the following possibilities:

    a. A shorter leg on the side of the shift; this will be

(*Text continues on page 518*)

Table 19-1. Effects of Common Pathologies on Gait—Sagittal Plane (Patient Viewed From the Side)

Gait Disturbances	NATURE OF DISTURBANCE: COMMON CAUSES				
	Painful or Restricted Ankle Plantar Flexion	Painful or Restricted Ankle Dorsiflexion	Painful or Restricted Knee Extension	Painful or Restricted Hip Extension	Painful or Restricted Low-Back Extension
Common causes	1. Capsular restriction, e.g., postimmobilization 2. Traumatic arthritis, e.g., post-ankle-sprain	1. Capsular restriction, e.g., postimmobilization 2. Heel-cord tightness, e.g., postimmobilization 3. Traumatic arthritis, e.g., post-ankle-sprain	1. Capsular restriction, e.g., DJD or post-immobilization 2. Traumatic arthritis, e.g., post-sprain 3. Locked knee, e.g., bucket-handle meniscus tear	1. Capsular restriction, e.g., DJD 2. Iliopectineal bursitis	1. Multisegmental capsular restriction, e.g., DJD 2. Posterior disk prolapse 3. Acute facet-joint dysfunction
PATTERN OF GAIT DISTURBANCE					
Loss of heel-strike a. Toe-touch gait b. Flatfooted gait	X		X (if painful or locked) X (if stiff)		
Loss of plantar flexion following heel-strike with accelerated stance phase	X		X (if stiff)		
Loss of dorsiflexion during foot-flat stage of stance → premature heel-rise, exaggerated hip and knee flexion during early swing phase		X	X (if stiff)		

Loss of push-off and heel-rise		X	X
Shortened stance phase on involved side		X	X (stance shortened bilaterally)
Tendency toward increased knee extension during stance	X (if stiff)		
Trunk lurch forward during stance		X	X (if painful)
Knee held in increased flexion during stance	X (early and late stance)	X	X
Loss of hip extension during stance	X	X	X
Loss of low-back extension during stance; trunk held in forward position			X (if painful)
Tendency toward increased low-back extension during stance			X (if stiff)

Table 19-2. Effects of Common Pathologies on Gait—Frontal Plane and Transverse Planes (Patient Viewed From the Front or Back)

Gait Disturbances	NATURE OF DISTURBANCE: COMMON CAUSES				
	Pronation Deformity or Functional Pronation Deviation of Hindfoot	Painful or Restricted Ankle or Knee Flexion or Extension	Valgus Deformity or Functional Valgus Deviation of Knee	Varus Deformity or Functional Varus Deviation of Knee	External Tibial Torsion
	1. Congenital hypermobility of foot (flexible deformity) 2. Tarsal coalition (fixed deformity) 3. Increased femoral anteversion (functional) 4. Genu valgum (functional) 5. Loss of hindfoot dorsiflexion, e.g., tight heel cord	See Table 19-1	1. DJD of lateral knee (deformity) 2. Increased femoral anteversion (functional → structural) 3. Increased foot pronation (functional) 4. Tight iliotibial band (functional)	1. DJD of medial knee (deformity) 2. Increased femoral retroversion (functional)	1. Congenital (structural) 2. Acquired compensation for femoral anteversion
PATTERN OF GAIT DISTURBANCE					
Toeing inward					
Lowered navicular (flatfoot)	X				
Valgus deviation of heel	X		X		
Toeing outward		X			X (uncompensated)
Patella facing outward during swing phase				X (if 2° retroversion)	
Patella facing inward during swing phase					
Patella facing inward during stance	X		X (if 2° anteversion)		X (if compensated)
Patella facing outward during stance					
Pelvis rotates excessively externally (contralateral side forward) during stance					
Pelvis shifted ipsilaterally					
Pelvis shifted contralaterally					
Trunk inclined ipsilaterally during stance					
Trunk inclined contralaterally during stance					

	Internal Tibial Torsion	Increased Femoral Anteversion or Functional Internal Rotary Deviation of Femur	Increased Femoral Retroversion or Functional External Rotary Deviation of Femur	Painful or Restricted Hip Abduction and Internal Rotation	Restricted Hip Adduction	Painful or Restricted Lumbar Lateral Deviation
NATURE OF DISTURBANCE: COMMON CAUSES	1. Congenital (structural) 2. Acquired compensation for femoral retroversion	1. Congenital (structural) 2. Increased foot pronation (functional) 3. External tibial torsion (compensatory)	1. Congenital (structural) 2. Internal tibial torsion (compensatory)	Capsular restriction, e.g., hip DJD	Tight iliotibial band	1. Posterolateral disk protrusion 2. Acute facet joint dysfunction (unilateral)

	Internal Tibial Torsion	Increased Femoral Anteversion or Functional Internal Rotary Deviation of Femur	Increased Femoral Retroversion or Functional External Rotary Deviation of Femur	Painful or Restricted Hip Abduction and Internal Rotation	Restricted Hip Adduction	Painful or Restricted Lumbar Lateral Deviation
PATTERN OF GAIT DISTURBANCE	X (uncompensated)	X (uncompensated)				
		X (if compensated for by external torsion)				
		X (if compensated for by external torsion)				
			X (uncompensated)	X		
			X			
		X				
		X				
	X (if compensated)		X			
		X				
				X		
					X	
				X		X (rare)
						X

checked for later on assessment of vertical symmetry.

b. Tight hip abductors (almost always the iliotibial band) on the side opposite the shift. This is often associated with a valgus deviation of the knee on the tight side. Iliotibial band extensibility should be checked later.

c. Loss of hip abduction on the side of the shift. The most common cause is a capsular restriction secondary to degenerative hip disease. Hip range of motion should be assessed later to determine if a capsular pattern of restriction exists.

2. Note obvious valgus/varus deviations or asymmetries.

a. Bilateral genu valgum (knock knees) is often associated with femoral anteversion, foot pronation, or both.

b. Unilateral genu valgum is often associated with iliotibial band tightness, lateral compartment DJD of the knee, unilateral femoral anteversion, or unilateral foot pronation.

c. Bilateral genu varum (bowed legs) is often associated with femoral retroversion.

d. Unilateral genu varum is often associated with medial degenerative knee disease or unilateral femoral retroversion.

e. Tibial varum or valgum should be differentiated from genu varum or valgum.

f. Calcaneal valgum is usually associated with foot pronation, genu valgum, femoral anteversion, or some combination thereof. It is evidenced by inward bowing of the Achilles tendon.

g. Calcaneal varum may be present with foot supination, femoral retroversion, genu varum, or some combination, and is seen as outward bowing of the Achilles tendon.

3. Note obvious asymmetries in muscle bulk. The calves or hamstrings on one side may be atrophied in the presence of a chronic S1 or S2 radiculopathy.

4. Note lateral spinal curvatures. A lumbar scoliosis may be associated with

a. A lateral pelvic inclination. The lumbar convexity will be toward the side on which the pelvis is lower.

b. A lateral pelvic shift. The convexity will be on the side toward which the pelvis is shifted.

c. Acute spinal derangements (disc prolapse or facet-joint dysfunction). The lumbar convexity is usually toward the side of the problem, except in some prolapses in which protruding disc material is medial to the sensitive structure (*e.g.,* nerve root).

d. Asymmetrical lumbar degenerative changes, with asymmetrical disc narrowing and facet-joint tightness. The convexity is usually away from the side of the degeneration.

e. A structural thoracolumbar scoliosis. Ask the patient to bend forward to observe for a fixed rotary component, typical of structural curves.

The lumbar convexity is usually to the left, with a left rotary component; the thoracic convexity is to the right, with a right rotary component. These curves, unless severe, are generally asymptomatic.

B. The presence of segmental vertical asymmetries (leg-length disparities) is best determined by comparing the heights of the key bony landmarks listed below. This is usually done by palpating similar prominences or contours with the same finger of both hands, then assessing the relative heights of the palpating fingers. For each of the landmarks, it is not so important that the examiner feel some precise point as it is that he feel the same prominence or contour with both palpating fingers.

1. Medial malleoli. The most common cause of one being lower than the other is a foot that is more pronated on the lower side. Check transverse alignment later and correlate this with the position of the calcaneus, since with foot pronation the calcaneus will tend to be in a valgus position.

2. Fibular heads and popliteal folds. If the malleoli are level and these not level, disparity in tibial length should be suspected. Inquire about a previous fracture or other possible causative factors.

3. Greater trochanters. If the ankle and knee landmarks are level, but the trochanters are not level, the shaft of one femur is probably shortened, barring severe degenerative changes of the knee. Again, inquire about previous fractures.

4. Posterior superior iliac spines. If the ankle and knee land-marks as well as the trochanters are level, but the PSISs are not, consider the possibility of (*1*) tortional asymmetry in the sacroiliac joints, (*2*) valgus–varus asymmetry in the proximal femur, (*3*) and advanced degenerative changes of one hip joint, as the most common causes.

a. The most common torsional displacement at the sacroiliac joint is a backward torsion of the ilium on the sacrum, in which case the PSIS on the involved side will be lower than the opposite PSIS, but the ASIS on the involved side will be higher. One should, then, check the relative heights of the ASISs.

b. In the case of femoral valgus or varus asymmetry, both the PSIS and the ASIS will be higher on the side that is in relative valgus position. You might also use Néla-ton's line to confirm the existence of valgus/varus asymmetry. Assess the position of the greater trochanter with respect to a line formed from the ASIS to the ischial tuberosity; with a valgus femur the trochanter will fall more inferiorly with respect to Nélaton's line compared to a varus femur. It should be realized that valgus angulation of the femur is usually associated with increased anteversion and a relatively mobile hip joint, whereas a varus femur is usually associated with retroversion and a more stable hip joint.

c. Advanced degenerative changes of a hip joint, sufficient to cause noticeable lowering of the pelvis on the involved side, will invariably be associated with a capsular restriction of motion at the hip. Internal rotation and abduction are markedly restricted, flexion and extension are moderately restricted, and adduction and external rotation are somewhat limited.

5. Iliac crests. If these are not level, look for the cause of asymmetry at some lower segment (see above). **Note:** Asymmetry in height of landmarks at any level should result in a corresponding asymmetry of all landmarks situated more superiorly. If not, combined segmental asymmetries must be suspected (one asymmetry compensating for, or adding to, another.)

II. **Sagittal Alignment.** The patient is viewed from the side. Note obvious abnormalities or asymmetries in flexion–extension positioning of the lower extremity joints and spine. It should be realized that a fairly broad range of "normal" variation exists in sagittal alignment. For some people, it is normal to stand with the ankles, hips, and knees slightly flexed and the spinal curves somewhat flattened. For others it might be normal to stand with the lower extremity joints well extended and with more accentuation of the spinal curves. Any "deviation" must be considered in light of other findings. Asymmetries can be considered to be more reliably significant.

A. *Abnormal extension (e.g., hyperextension) of the knee* and other weight-bearing segments is most often the result of restricted ankle dorsiflexion, as from a tight heel cord or capsular ankle restriction. A less common and more serious cause of severe "back knee" is neuropathic arthropathy such as may occur with tertiary syphilis.

B. *Abnormal flexion of the knee* and other segments occurs with a greater variety of disorders, including

1. Restricted ankle plantar flexion (rare), the most common cause of which is capsular restriction following immobilization.

2. Restricted extension of the knee from
   a. Capsular restriction, occurring acutely with traumatic arthritis (effusion) or chronically following immobilization or surgery.
   b. An internal derangement, such as a bucket-handle meniscus tear, causing a mechanical block to knee extension

3. Restricted hip extension, most commonly resulting from degenerative hip disease and the associated capsular pattern of restriction.

4. Restricted low-back extension caused by
   a. An acute spinal derangement, such as a posterior disc prolapse or acute facet-joint dysfunction.
   b. Multisegmental capsular restriction associated with degenerative spinal changes.

III. **Transverse Rotary Alignment.** The patient is viewed from the front. The stance width should be normal and the feet slightly (5° to 10°) pointed outward. Obvious foot deformities, such as hallux valgus, should be noted. Hallux valgus is often associated with abnormal foot pronation which, in turn, often occurs in conjunction with transverse rotary abnormalities of more proximal segments. Assessment of segmental rotary alignment is performed, working upward from the feet, by examining the positioning and symmetry of the following landmarks:

A. *Navicular tubercles.* Assess the positions of the navicular tubercles compared to a line from the medial malleolus to the point where the first metatarsal contacts the ground. The tubercle should fall just on, or below, this line. The individual with a static (*i.e.*, resting) pronation deviation of the foot will have a navicular tubercle that falls well below the line. This is a true flatfoot and will invariably be associated with a valgus heel. Abnormality in bony alignment must be confirmed since many individuals have considerable bulk of the medial soft tissues of the foot, which gives the foot a flattened appearance. When a true flatfoot is detected, determine whether it is structural (fixed) or functional (mobile). To do so, ask the patient to raise up on the balls of the feet or to attempt to externally rotate the legs over the stationary foot; in both cases, the arch will be seen to rise significantly if the pronated position of the foot is functional. The common cause of a structurally pronated foot is tarsal coalition. The common causes of a mobile flat foot are congenital ligamentous laxity and femoral anteversion. It must be appreciated that a person who does not have static pronation deviation of the foot, as evidenced on examination of structural alignment, may still have a problem from abnormal foot pronation during gait. On the other hand, it should be realized that an individual with a static pronation deviation of the foot does not necessarily have a pronation problem, especially if the deviation has existed since childhood. The tissues of the foot will have adapted to the increased pronatory stresses during development.

B. *Intermalleolar line.* A line passing through the tips of the medial and lateral malleoli should make an angle, opening laterally, of about 25° with the frontal plane when the knee axis is situated in the frontal plane (*i.e.*, when the patellae are facing straight forward). **Note:** 25° corresponds to the lateral malleolus being about 4 cm posterior to the medial malleolus when the intermalleolar distance is 10 cm, or about 3.5 cm posterior for a 9 cm intermalleolar width, or about 3 cm posterior for an 8 cm width.

1. If the angle is excessive, you must suspect increased external tibial torsion or increased femoral anteversion. It is not unusual for these to coexist, the two having a mutual compensatory effect to cancel abnormal toeing inward (from femoral anteversion) or toeing outward (from external tibial torsion). Compensation would occur during development. The presence of femoral anteversion is best determined clinically by assessing hip rotational range of motion in the prone position. An anteverted hip is a very mobile hip that appears to have an increase in internal rotation at the expense of a loss of external rotation.

2. Similarly, if the angle the intermalleolor line makes with the frontal plane is diminished

when the patellae face straight forward, there may be an increase in femoral retroversion or abnormal internal tibial torsion. A retroverted hip is a less mobile hip that will appear to have a loss of internal rotation, with external rotation perhaps somewhat increased.

C. *Patellae.* With the feet pointed slightly outward the patellae should face straight forward.
1. If the patellae face inward, suspect increased femoral anteversion, increased external tibial torsion, or both (see above).
2. If the patellae face outward when the feet are in a normal position, the cause may be femoral retroversion, internal tibial torsion, or both (see above).

D. *Anterior superior iliac spines.* These should be positioned in a frontal plane. If the pelvis is rotated (one ASIS more anterior than the other) the common causes to be considered are
1. A fixed (structural) spinal scoliosis, the rotary component of which is transmitted to the pelvis through the sacrum by way of the lumbar spine.
2. Torsional asymmetry of the sacroiliac joints. The pelvis will appear to be rotated forward on the side on which the ilium is in more anterior torsion with respect to the sacrum.

REGIONAL TESTS

I. Lumbosacral Tests
A. *Active movements.* With the patient standing, the examiner demonstrates the movement to be performed as verbal instructions are given.
1. Forward bending. Ask the patient to bend the head forward, then the middle back, and finally the low back.
   a. If the patient has a relatively acute back problem and this movement is extremely difficult to perform —the patient tending to support his body weight by placing his hands on his thighs or a nearby plinth— a posterior disk prolapse should be suspected.
   b. If the patient has a relatively acute back problem but is able to bend forward reasonably well, with only mild discomfort and restriction, an acute facet-joint dysfunction or less severe disk prolapse might be considered. It is not unusual to see variations in lateral deviations of the spine as the patient bends forward in either instance. For example, the spine may start out deviated in the upright position and the deviation may disappear during forward bending. Or, the spine may be erect on standing and deviate as forward bending proceeds, and the deviation may or may not resolve by the end point of the movement. Such patterns may occur with movement abnormalities resulting from either disk or facet-joint derangements.
   c. If the patient does not have an acute problem, the examiner should observe the spine during forward bend-

ing from the back, then from the side.

When viewing from behind, look for lateral deviation of the spine during movement. A deviated arc of movement is more likely to be due to an alteration of intervertebral disk mechanics, whereas a deviation that exists up to the end point of movement is more likely the result of a unilateral or asymmetrical capsular restriction or a fixed scoliosis. If a fixed scoliosis exists, a rotary component will be present; the side of the convexity will appear higher than the side of the concavity in the forward-bent position.

When viewing from the side, assess the continuity of movement at the various spinal segments. The overall spinal curve should be relatively smooth; flattened areas may reflect segmental hypomobility whereas angular areas may be associated with segmental hypermobility.

With full forward bending of the lumbar spine, the normal lumbar lordosis should be straightened, but usually not reversed. Inadequate straightening of the lordosis may occur with localized or generalized capsular restriction. Reversal of the lumbar lordosis may suggest hypermobility.

2. Side bending. Ask the patient to side bend the head, shoulders, middle back, and then lower back first to one side, and then to the opposite side. Symmetry of movement may be judged by comparing the distance from the fingertip to the fibular head on either side, and by observing the degree of spinal curvature occurring with movements in either direction. Symmetry of movement, however, is only significant with respect to the starting position; if the resting position of the spine involves a right side-bending curve, then "normal" movement would be a greater degree of side bending to the right than to the left. As with forward bending, you should also assess the continuity of segmental movement. In cases of chronic disorders, some passive overpressure should be applied at the extremes of side bending to see if pain or other symptoms are reproduced. Reproduction of pain on passive overpressure is most likely to occur when a capsular restriction exists on the side to which the movement is performed.

a. In acute spinal derangements, such as a posterolateral disk protrusion or unilateral facet-joint derangement, lumbar side bending may be absent to one side (usually toward the involved side), especially if a functional spinal deviation exists in the erect position.

b. With multisegmental capsular restriction, side bending will be moderately restricted in both directions.

c. With localized unilateral capsular restrictions, side

bending will be only slightly limited toward the involved side.

3. Rotations. Stand behind the patient and place one hand over the ASIS and the other over the PSIS to stabilize the pelvis. Ask the patient to turn toward the side on which the examiner contacts the PSIS. Symmetry of movement is assessed by observing the lateral curvature of the lower spine that occurs during rotating; the spine will be seen to bend opposite the direction of rotation. The same considerations apply to assessment of rotation as discussed under side bending.

4. Extension. From behind the patient, place a hand over both of the patient's ASISs to stabilize and ask the patient to bend the head, shoulders, middle back, and then lower back backward. The lumbar lordosis should be seen to increase from the resting position as the patient extends. Note deviations toward one side.

    a. In the case of an acute spinal derangement lumbar extension will be negligible, most of the observable backward bending occurring at higher levels.

    b. With multisegmental capsular restriction lumbar extension will also be markedly limited due to premature close packing of the facet joints.

    c. The spine may be seen to deviate away from the side of a localized unilateral capsular restriction.

B. *Passive movements*

    1. Quadrant test. This is a provo-

cation test for a localized capsular restriction that may not cause an obvious restriction of motion or pain on active movement tests. Stand to the patient's side and place one arm across the patient's chest to grasp the opposite shoulder and the other hand over the lower back, with the thumb over the region of the mammillary process of about L2 on the side closest to the examiner. Use the upper arm to bring the patient's trunk around into side bending, rotation, and extension, while applying counterpressure forward and inward with the other thumb. This maneuver localizes a close-packing movement to the facet joint immediately superior to the examiner's thumb and, therefore, localizes a stress to the capsule of that joint. The remaining joints caudal to the first segment tested are examined in the same manner, in an attempt to reproduce the patient's symptoms. The opposite side of the spine may then be tested. This test is less likely to reproduce nerve root symptoms, by reducing the size of the intervertebral foramen, as it may in the cervical spine, since the lumbar intervertebral foramina are quite large in diameter compared to the exiting nerve roots.

2. Sacroiliac provocation/mobility tests. These may reproduce pain from a sacroiliac disorder, and a snap might be elicited if the joint is abnormally mobile. (Little or no movement should occur at this joint.)

a. Backward torsion strain. The patient lies on his side with the side to be tested on top. Flex the upper knee toward the patient's abdomen, then hold it flexed with your upper thigh or pelvis in order to free the hands. One hand is placed over the patient's ASIS, the forearm directed diagonally in the posterocaudal direction with respect to the patient. The opposite hand is placed over the patient's ischial tuberosity, the forearm directed in an anterocephalad direction. Produce a force-couple movement to rotate the ilium backward on the sacrum while simultaneously moving the patient's hip and knee into more flexion with your pelvis or anterior thigh.

b. Forward torsion strain. The patient lies prone. Stand at the side to be tested. The more cephalad hand is placed over the sacrum, with the fingers pointing toward the patient's head. With the opposite hand grasp around medially to the anterior aspect of the patient's knee. Push downward on the inferior aspect of the sacrum while simultaneously lifting the patient's leg into extension to move the ilium, by way of the hip joint capsule, into a forward strain on the sacrum.

3. Dural mobility tests. These tests may reproduce symptoms (usually pain) in the case of a disk prolapse, in which a bulging disk may approximate the anterolateral aspect of the dural sac of the caudal equina, or in the case of a disk extrusion, in which the protruded disk material may be adjacent to some part of the dural investment of a nerve root. The dura can be moved in a cephalad direction by flexing the neck or in a caudal direction by applying tension to the femoral or sciatic nerves. The femoral nerve and its contributing nerve roots are stretched by prone knee flexion, the sciatic nerve and its roots by straight leg raising. Additional tension is applied to the sciatic nerve by dorsiflexion of the ankle.

Dural mobility tests for the sciatic nerve roots may be done sitting or supine. It is often best to perform them in both positions and to correlate the results. Sitting increases the likelihood of obtaining a positive test in the case of a minor prolapse, since it is a position of relatively high intradiscal pressure. However, measurements to be used by which to judge improvement are best taken in the supine position by measuring the distance, from the lateral malleolus to the plinth, at which pain is produced on straight leg raising.

A true positive dural mobility test will reproduce back pain, hip girdle pain, leg pain, or some combination thereof, and pain should be felt somewhere between 30° and 60° of straight leg raising. At angles less than 30° there is very little movement of the nerve roots, and by 60° the dura will have already moved sufficiently to have caused reproduction of pain. Also, above 60° you cannot rule out the possibility that reproduction of pain is due to movement of the spinal column as the pelvis tilts backward. The examiner must be prepared to differentiate between pulling on tight hamstrings and reproduction of leg pain from dural impingement. Possible mechanical effects from movement of the spine or sacroiliac joint can be ruled out by seeing if ankle dorsiflexion further accentuates the pain produced; if so, it is likely to be a true positive dural sign.

The sitting tests are done with the patient sitting at the edge of the plinth. First move one knee toward extension, noting any guarding of the movement and inquiring as to reproduction of symptoms. If pain is produced, the leg is held just up to the painful point and the effect of ankle dorsiflexion and neck flexion assessed. The opposite leg is similarly tested.

The supine tests are carried out in a similar manner by moving first one leg and then the other into flexion with the knee straight. Again, the effects of ankle dorsiflexion and neck flexion are assessed.

The pattern of positive results yields some clues as to the relationship between the protrusion and the pain-sensitive structure (*e.g.*, dura or dural covering of a nerve root).

a. In the case of prolapsed or extruded material that is anterior to the pain-sensitive tissue, ipsilateral leg raising, contralateral leg raising, and neck flexion may all hurt.

b. If the protruded material is medial to the nerve root as it exits from the dural sac (rare), leg raising may hurt bilaterally, but neck flexion may be painless.

c. If the protrusion is lateral to the exiting nerve root, ipsilateral leg raising may reproduce symptoms, neck flexion may or may not be painful, and contralateral leg raising will be painless.

C. *Neuromuscular tests.* These are tests for segmental interference of neural conduction, the most common cause of which is a disk extrusion in the lumbar spine. Other causes of neurologic deficit in the legs are rare but are usually more serious. Any multisegmental deficit should be viewed with some suspicion, since nerve root impingement from a disk protrusion rarely involves more than one root, the occasional exception being an L5–S1 protrusion which may affect the L5 and S1 roots.

1. Sensory (dermatomal) tests. Subtle sensory deficits are best detected by assessing vibratory perception with a tuning fork. This is because pressure tends to affect the large myelinated fibers that mediate vibratory and proprioceptive sensation first. Gross sensory testing may be carried out using a wisp of cotton or a pin.

The key sensory areas to test are in the distal part of the limb, since these are the areas where there is relatively little overlap of segmental innervation. These include

L4—Medial aspect of the big toe
L5—Web space between the first and second toes

S1—Below the lateral malleolus

S2—Distal Achilles tendon region

These areas should be tested first; then test the various aspects of the leg and thigh. If a significant deficit is detected proximal to the foot, you must be sure that more serious pathologies have been ruled out, since it is rare for involvement of one root to cause an obvious deficit in the thigh or leg because of overlapping dermatomes.

When performing sensory tests, test a small area on one limb. Ask the patient if he feels the expected sensation (vibration, touch, or pinprick); Then test the corresponding area on the opposite limb and ask the patient again if he feels it. Ask the patient if the intensity of stimulus felt is about the same on both sides. Proceed in this fashion for all of the areas to be tested. Sensory tests are most easily carried out with the patient supine.

2. Motor (myotomal) tests. Because most limb muscles receive innervation from more than one segment, only subtle motor dysfunction will be noted in the case of segmental deficits resulting from disc protrusions. Significant motor loss should suggest a more serious pathology. Key muscles should be tested for each segment. Large muscle groups, such as the quadriceps and calf muscles, must be tested by repetitive resistance against a load, since even in the presence of loss of segmental input to such muscles, sufficient tension may still be produced to prevent the examiner from detecting weakness by overcoming the contraction. Key muscle groups may be tested for each of the segments contributing to the limb.

L2—Hip flexors, tested in the sitting position

L3—Knee extension, tested by repetitive one-legged half-squats in the standing position

L4—Ankle dorsiflexion, tested in the supine position

L5—Ankle dorsiflexion–eversion and large-toe extension, tested in the supine position

S1,S2—Ankle plantar flexion, tested by repeated toe-raising in the standing position

S1,S2—Knee flexion, tested in the prone position

For each muscle group, absolute strength is judged as normal or weak and compared to the contralateral side.

3. Deep-tendon reflexes (DTRs). Segmented neurologic deficits may result in diminution of deep-tendon reflexes on the involved side. When examining DTRs, primarily observe for asymmetry of responses from one side to another. Difficulty eliciting reflexes on both sides is no indication of pathology so long as there is no asymmetry in response.
   a. Knee jerk reflex—L3, L4
   b. Ankle jerk reflex—S1, S2
   c. Note that L5 does not contribute to these reflexes.

II. **Hip Tests**
   A. *Active and passive movements*
      1. Flexion–extension. The patient lies supine with both

knees bent and is instructed to pull one leg up toward the opposite axilla. Apply overpressure at the end point of movement and instruct the patient to extend the opposite hip. The test is repeated, reversing the direction of movement for each leg. Note pain or restriction of movement.

    a. If the hip joint capsule is tight, flexion is limited to about 90° to 120° and extension limited by 20° to 45°.

    b. Pain at the extremes of flexion and extension, with relatively full movement, may be present in cases of iliopectineal bursitis.

    c. Pain only at the extremes of flexion toward the opposite axilla may occur with sacroiliac dysfunction or with trochanteric bursitis.

    d. Pain only at the extremes of extension, with the opposite hip flexed, may be present in cases of sacroiliac dysfunction.

    e. Relatively acute back problems may be irritated by flexion or extension, since some lower spinal movement will occur near the end point of either movement.

2. Abduction–adduction. The patient lies supine and is instructed to abduct and adduct the leg as far as possible. Apply some passive overpressure at the end points of movement.

    a. Capsular restriction will result in rather marked limitation of abduction and mild limitation of adduction.

    b. Full motion, with pain at the extremes of adduction, abduction, or both may be present in cases of trochanteric bursitis.

3. Internal–external rotation. The patient lies prone with knees bent. Simultaneously rotate both of the patient's hips externally, then internally.

    a. In cases of capsular restriction, internal rotation will be markedly restricted and external rotation less restricted.

    b. An anteverted hip will be quite mobile, with more internal rotation than normal and perhaps a slight loss of external rotation.

    c. A retroverted hip is less mobile with less-than-normal internal rotation and perhaps a slight increase in external rotation.

4. Iliotibial band stretch. The patient lies on his side with the side to be tested on top. The examiner is at the patient's backside and sits on the plinth with his back against the patient's pelvis to stabilize it. Grasp the patient's leg, bend the knee to 90°, and extend the hip as far as possible. While preventing the knee from bending and the hip from rotating, attempt to approximate the patient's knee to the plinth, keeping the hip extended. The examiner must support beneath the patient's knee to keep from imposing an uncomfortable valgus stress across the knee.

    a. If the iliotibial band is tight, you will have considerable difficulty touching the patient's knee to the plinth.

    b. The movement will reproduce pain associated with trochanteric bursitis or tendinitis at the tibial insertion of the iliotibial band (runner's knee).

B. *Resisted movements*

1. Resisted hip flexion is tested isometrically during sitting for the presence of iliopectineal bursitis. (This is done also as a test for the integrity of the L2 myotome.)
2. Resisted hip abduction is tested with the patient supine for presence of trochanteric bursitis.

III. Knee Tests

A. *Structural alignment*

1. Femorotibial. Assess the position of the tibial tubercles with respect to the patellae in the sitting, bent-knee position. The tubercle usually lines up with the midline or lateral half of the patella. Of most importance here is symmetry.
   a. A tubercle that is positioned too far medially may be suggestive of posteromedial capsular tightness, as may occur with healing of a sprain or rupture of one of the cruciate ligaments.
   b. A tubercle that is situated too far laterally may suggest laxity (*e.g.*, rupture) of the posteromedial capsule or medial collateral ligament.
2. Femoropatellar. Assess the position and size of the patellae with the patient sitting and the knees bent over the edge of the plinth. The patellae should face straight forward and the inferior poles of the patellae should be about level with the femorotibial joint line. A small, high-riding, outward-

facing patella may predispose to a lateral patellar tracking disorder.

B. *Active–passive movements*

1. Flexion–extension. These can be assessed at the same time as hip flexion and extension and, in a weight-bearing situation, while testing the L3 myotome.
   a. If a capsular restriction exists, flexion will be limited to 90° to 100° and extension will be lacking by 20° to 30°.
   b. Loss of knee extension, in the presence of full flexion, is most often due to an internal derangement such as a bucket-handle meniscus tear.
   c. During weight-bearing movements, the examiner should palpate at the femoropatellar joint and at the femorotibial joint for crepitus that may indicate degenerative changes. Snapping and popping during movement is common, but a continuous grinding, suggestive of sand in the joint, is more significant.
2. Passive internal–external rotation. With the patient supine, and using a handhold at the foot, rotate the tibia internally and externally on the femur, with the knee close to full extension.
   a. Hypermobility of external rotation suggests a medial ligament or posteromedial capsule rupture.
   b. Hypermobility of internal rotation may be associated with a cruciate rupture.
   c. Pain on external rotation may be present in the case of a coronary ligament

sprain or medial collateral ligament sprain. A valgus stress can be used to differentiate, since this will stress the medial collateral but not the coronary ligament.

3. Dynamic tibial rotary function. With the patient sitting, first assess the positions of the tibial tubercles (see above), then passively extend each knee repetitively, over the final 25° of extension. Rotation of the tibia during extension is assessed by observing the tibial tubercle during the movement; normally, the tubercle should be seen to rotate laterally through an angle of 10° to 15° during the final phase of extension. The involved side must be compared to the opposite knee. Loss of dynamic tibial rotation may be due to

a. The tibia being already rotated at the starting position. This is determined on assessment of structure (see above).

b. Tightness or adhesion of the medial capsuloligamentous structures, such as may occur with healing of a sprain during immobilization.

c. An internal derangement such as a meniscus displacement or a cartilaginous loose body.

4. Patellar glide. Move the patella passively, medially, and laterally, as far as possible. At the extremes of medial movement you may palpate the underside of the medial patella with firm sustained pressure. In the case of chronic patellar tracking disorders, lateral glide may be painful if the medial re-

tinaculum is irritable, and the underside of the medial aspect of the patella may be tender.

C. *Resisted movements*

1. Internal–external rotation. The patient is prone with the knee bent. Grasp the tibia around the malleoli and instruct the patient to resist your attempt to rotate the leg in either direction.

a. Resisted internal rotation will reproduce pain from pes anserinus tendinitis.

b. Resisted external rotation may reproduce pain from iliotibial band tendinitis or biceps tendinitis. Resisted knee flexion will hurt for the latter but not the former.

2. Knee flexion (also a test for the S1–S2 myotomes). Flexion of the tibia is isometrically resisted in the prone position. This may reproduce pain from pes anserinus tendinitis or biceps tendinitis.

IV. **Ankle and Foot Tests**

A. *Active–passive movements*

1. Flexion–extension. The patient lies supine and is instructed to dorsiflex and plantar flex both feet simultaneously for comparison. Passive over-pressure is applied at the extremes of plantar flexion, across the forefoot, in an inversion direction. Passive over-pressure is applied to hindfoot dorsiflexion by dorsiflexion of the calcaneus.

a. Loss of both plantar flexion and dorsiflexion is usually the result of a capsular restriction of ankle mortise movement.

b. Isolated loss of dorsiflexion is usually due to heel-cord tightness.

c. Pain from Achilles tendinitis may be reproduced at the extremes of dorsiflexion with passive overpressure.

d. Pain from an anterior talofibular ligament sprain or adhesion may be reproduced on plantar flexion–inversion with passive overpressure.

2. Anterior glide of the talus in the mortise. The patient is supine. Place one hand over the dorsum of the distal tibia and cup the other hand around the back of the calcaneous. The talus, by way of the calcaneous, is pulled forward in the mortise and the movement is compared to the opposite side.

   a. Hypermobility will be present in the case of a chronic anterior talofibular ligament rupture.

   b. Pain will be reproduced from a talofibular ligament sprain or adhesion.

3. Hindfoot inversion–eversion. The range of calcaneal inversion and eversion is assessed and the two feet are compared. Capsular restriction will result in a greater loss of inversion than eversion.

4. Forefoot twisting and untwisting. The calcaneous is held inverted and the forefoot maximally pronated (twisted). The calcaneous is then everted and the forefoot supinated (untwisted). With the foot held untwisted, the toes are moved into sustained dorsiflexion.

   a. Twisting of the foot will be limited in capsular restriction of the tarsal skeleton (rare except following immobilization).

   b. Untwisting of the foot may reproduce pain from a calcaneocuboid ligament sprain, which often occurs in conjunction with an anterior talofibular sprain.

   c. Untwisting of the foot with sustained toe dorsiflexion may reproduce pain from plantar fasciitis or calcaneal periostitis, since this stretches the plantar fascia.

CLINICAL IMPLEMENTATION OF THE LUMBAR–LOWER EXTREMITY SCAN EXAM

Gait analysis and a comprehensive assessment of structural alignment should be included in the assessment of virtually all chronic disorders of the low back and lower extremities. It is rare, however, to include all of the regional tests discussed during any one examination; tests are chosen as indicated by subjective information and findings on gait analysis and inspection of structural alignment. The clinician must be prepared to judge which tests might be relevant in a particular case—a judgment that is facilitated by experience.

In order for the scan exam to be of practical use in a busy clinical setting, the clinician must be able to perform the examination within a reasonable period of time, say, 15 minutes or less. This requires knowledge of which tests are to be performed, understanding of the rationale for each test, skill in appropriately carrying out each test, and ability to interpret the results.

Clinically, the tests of the scan exam must be carried out according to the patient's position in order to minimize time requirements and to prevent omission of crucial tests. The following is a summary of the tests included in a complete lumbar–lower extremity scan exam, according to the position of the patient. This format should be followed in the clinical implementation of the scan exam.

I. **Standing**
   A. *Gait analysis*
      1. Sagittal
      2. Frontal
      3. Transverse
   B. *Inspection of structural alignment and soft tissue*
      1. Frontal—from behind
      2. Sagittal—from the side
      3. Transverse (rotatory)—from the front
   C. *Functional tests*
      1. Active lumbar movements
         a. Forward bending
         b. Side bending
         c. Rotation
         d. Backward bending
      2. Lumbar quadrant tests
      3. Standing unilateral half squats
         a. Assess strength for quadriceps function and L3 myotome.
         b. Palpate the femoropatellar and femorotibial joints for crepitus.
      4. Standing unilateral toe raises. Assess strength for gastroc-soleus function and S1–S2 myotomes.

II. **Sitting**
   A. *Alignment*
      1. Position of patellae
      2. Rotary position of tibia
   B. *Functional tests*
      1. Dural mobility
         a. Knee extension and ankle dorsiflexion
         b. Neck flexion
      2. Reflexes
         a. Knee jerks
         b. Ankle jerks
      3. Resisted hip flexion

      a. Assess strength for L2 myotome.
      b. Assess irritability for iliopectineal bursitis.
   4. Tibial rotary mechanics

III. **Supine**
   A. *Functional tests*
      1. Dural mobility
         a. Straight leg raising and ankle dorsiflexion
         b. Neck flexion
      2. Hip and knee flexion and extension range of motion
      3. Hip abduction–adduction range of motion
      4. Resisted hip abduction
      5. Knee internal–external rotation movements
      6. Patellar glide, medially and laterally
      7. Ankle dorsiflexion–plantar flexion range of motion
      8. Resisted ankle dorsiflexion—L4 myotome
      9. Resisted dorsiflexion–eversion—L5, S1 myotomes
      10. Resisted large toe extension—L5 myotome
      11. Hindfoot inversion–eversion and forefoot twisting and untwisting. Dorsiflex toes when untwisted.
   B. *Sensory testing of foot and leg*

IV. **Sidelying.** Functional tests
   A. Sacroiliac posterior torsion
   B. Iliotibial band extensibility

V. **Prone.** Functional tests
   A. Sacroiliac anterior torsion
   B. Hip internal–external rotation range of motion
   C. Resisted knee rotations
   D. Resisted knee flexion
      1. Assess strength—S1, S2 myotomes
      2. Assess irritability—biceps or pes anserinus tendonitis

Appendix
Component Motions, Close-Packed Positions, and Capsular Patterns

In the close-packed position, the joint capsule and major ligaments are twisted, causing the joint surfaces to become firmly approximated. This is a direct result either of the conjunct rotation that necessarily accompanies a diadochal movement into this position or of the spin that accompanies an impure swing into the position. From this it follows that movement into or out of a close-packed position is never accomplished by a pure chordate swing alone. **Note:** Habitual movements of daily activities usually involve motions that move a joint closer to or farther from a close-packed position. A typical example would be the motions occurring at the hip when walking.

Consider the relationship between the close-packed position at a particular joint and the capsular pattern of restriction, as described by Cyriax, at the same joint: The more intimate the anatomic and functional relationship between the joint capsule and major supporting ligaments, the more likely the close-packed position will be the most restricted position of the joint in a capsular pattern of restriction. Thus, in the hip and shoulder joints, in which the major ligaments blend with the joint capsule, movements into the close-packed position are the first to be lost with a capsular pattern of restriction. In the knee, however, in which the ligaments are easily

distinguished from the capsule, flexion may be the most limited in a capsular restriction, whereas extension constitutes the close-packed position.

THE TEMPOROMANDIBULAR JOINT

Note: Both temporomandibular joints are involved in every jaw movement, forming a bicondylar arrangement.

Component Motions

Opening of the mouth

1. The head of the mandible first rotates around a horizontal axis (rolls dorsally) in relation to the disk (lower compartment).
2. This movement is then combined with gliding of the head anteriorly (and somewhat downward) in contact with the lower surface of the disk.
3. At the same time, the disk glides anteriorly (and somewhat downward) toward the articular eminence of the glenoid fossa (upper compartment). The forward gliding of the disk ceases when the fibroelastic tissue attaching to the temporal bone posteriorly has been stretched to its limits.
4. Thereafter there is some further hinging and gliding anteriorly of the head of

533

the mandible until it articulates with the most anterior part of the disk and the mouth is fully opened.

Closing of the mouth. The movements are reversed.

Protrusion. The disks glide anteriorly in the upper compartment (simultaneously on both sides). Both condyles glide anteriorly and slightly downward but do not rotate.

Retraction. The movements are reversed.

Lateral movements. Anterior gliding occurs in one joint while rotation around a cranial–caudal axis occurs in the other joint. One condyle glides downward, forward, and inward while the other condyle in the fossa rotates and glides ipsilaterally.

Note: When the jaw is moved from side to side (as in chewing) a movement involving a shuttling of the condylar-disk assembly occurs in the concave parts of the fossa.

Rest Position

The mouth is slightly open. The teeth of the mandible and maxillae are not in contact but slightly apart.

Close-Packed Position

In this centric relation or apex of the force position, the condyles and disk assembly are in a seated apex relationship to the mandibular fossa. The heads of the condyles are at their most retruded position. The precise location of this position depends on the structure of the fossa and the condyle. Since this position is a dynamic one, it also depends on the pull made by the closing muscles.

Potential Close-Packed Position

This is full or maximal opening. **Note:** The potential close-packed position is one in which the joint is also very congruent and stable but is less commonly assumed.

Capsular Pattern of Restriction

In bilateral restriction, lateral movements are most restricted; opening of the mouth and protrusion are both limited; closing of the mouth is most free. **Note:** In unilateral capsular restrictions, contralateral excursions are most restricted. In mouth opening, the mandible will deviate toward the restricted side.

UPPER EXTREMITY

THE SHOULDER (GLENOHUMERAL JOINT)

Component Motions

Flexion (elevation in the sagittal plane)

1. At full elevation of the humerus, whether accomplished through coronal abduction or sagittal flexion, the humerus always ends up back in the plane of the scapula, *as if* it had been elevated through a pure swing; that is, at an angle midway between the sagittal and coronal planes. Since sagittal flexion is an impure swing, the humerus tends to undergo a lateral conjunct rotation on its path to full elevation. If this were allowed to occur, however, the humerus would end up such that the medial condyle pointed backward, rather than forward, with the capsule of the glenohumeral joint completely twisted. This essentially would involve a premature close-packing that would prevent full elevation. To avoid this, the humerus must rotate medially on its long axis during the complete arc of sagittal flexion. The rotation occurs because the anterior aspect of the joint capsule pulls tight on flexion, while the posterior capsule remains relatively lax.
2. Downward (inferior) glide of the head of the humerus on the glenoid.

Abduction

1. Lateral rotation of the humerus on its long axis to counter the medial conjunct rotation that tends to occur during this impure swing (see *Flexion*). In this case, the posterior capsule pulls tight during abduction, effecting a lateral rotation of the humerus.
2. Inferior glide of the humeral head on the glenoid.

External rotation. Anterior glide of the head of the humerus.

Internal rotation. Posterior glide of the head of the humerus.

Horizontal adduction. Posterior glide of the humeral head.

Horizontal abduction. Anterior glide of the humeral head.

Close-Packed Position

Combined horizontal abduction, and external rotation.

Capsular Pattern of Restriction

External rotation is most limited; abduction, quite limited; internal rotation and flexion, somewhat limited (relatively free).

ACROMIOCLAVICULAR JOINT

Component Motions

1. Allows widening and narrowing of the angle (looking from above) between the clavicle and the scapula. Narrowing occurs during protraction; widening occurs during retraction (about 10° total, according to Kapandji). Occurs about a vertical axis.
2. Allows rotation of the scapula *upward,* such that the inferior angle of the scapula moves away from the midline; or *downward,* such that it moves to-

ward the midline. Occurs about a horizontal axis lying in the sagittal plane. Actually, very little A-C joint motion is involved in this rotation of the scapula. While about 30° occurs with elevation of the clavicle at the sternoclavicular joint, much of the remaining 30° occurs because of axial rotation of the clavicle; since the clavicle is S-shaped anteriorposteriorly, an axial rotation converts the S to a supero-inferior attitude, the distal end pointing more or less upward. This occurs as a result of tightening of the coracoclavicular ligaments as the scapula begins to rotate upward (the coracoid rotating downward).
3. Allows rotation of the scapula such that the inferior angle swings anteriorly and posteriorly. As the scapula moves upward and forward on the thorax, the inferior angle swings posteriorly. This occurs about an axis lying horizontally in the frontal plane and probably is accompanied by considerable length rotation at the sternoclavicular joint as well.

Close-Packed Position

A combination of upward rotation of the scapula relative to the clavicle, and narrowing of the angle between scapula and clavicle as seen from above. This occurs during elevation of the arm and during horizontal adduction.

Capsular Pattern

Primarily pain into the close-packed position, such as when horizontally adducting the arm.

STERNOCLAVICULAR JOINT

Component Motions

1. Allows length rotation of the clavicle, as discussed under Acromioclavicular Joint above: about 50° total. This oc-

curs during elevation of the arm, and somewhat during protraction and retraction.

2. Allows upward and downward swing of the clavicle such as during shoulder shrugging or elevation of the arm. This occurs about an axis passing through the costoclavicular ligament, so that with elevation the clavicular articular surface slides inferiorly on the sternum; and with depression, superiorly: about 30° total.

3. Allows forward and backward swing of the clavicle, such as with protraction and retraction. This occurs about an axis lying somewhat medial to the joint, so that the clavicular articular surface slides foward on protraction: about 45° to 60° total motion.

Note: To emphasize the interplay of all joints involved with shoulder movements, the components of shoulder abduction in the frontal plane, one of the more complex shoulder movements, are reviewed here.

With the arm at the side in the resting position, the glenoid faces almost equally anteriorly and laterally. The humerus rests in the "plane of the scapula," or in alignment with the glenoid, such that the medial humeral condyle points about 45° inward and backward.

During the first 30° or so of abduction what happens to the scapula is variable, but during this time it becomes "set" or fixed against the thoracic wall in preparation for movement. From 30° to full elevation, for every 15° of movement about 10° occurs at the glenohumeral joint and 5° at the scapulo-thoracic joint. The scapula must rotate upward as well as forward around the chest wall. The early part of this movement occurs as a result of elevation at the sternoclavicular joint, as well as movement at the acromioclavicular joint, such that its angle narrows (looking from above) and the scapula rotates slightly upward on the clavicle. This close-packs the A-C joint but also draws

the coracoclavicular ligaments tight, because of the downward movement of the coracoid relative to the clavicle. Thus, between, say, 90° and 120°, motion stops at the A-C joint. Further elevation from scapular rotation is possible only because the coracoclavicular ligaments pull the clavicle into long-axis rotation.

The S-shape of the clavicle becomes oriented supero-inferiorly such that the distal end of the clavicle points somewhat upward, allowing the A-C joint to maintain apposition as the scapula continues to rotate upward. This clavicular rotation occurs, of course, at the S-C joint.

Since the convex humeral head is moving in relation to the concave glenoid cavity to allow upward swing of the humerus, it must glide inferiorly in the glenoid. The humerus must move out of the plane of the scapula in order to be elevated in the frontal plane; it must undergo an impure swing. As with any impure swing, a conjunct rotation occurs, in this case a medial rotation. However, the posterior and inferior capsular fibers cannot allow this amount of rotation, so in order for the humerus to come back into the plane of the scapular on full elevation, it must rotate laterally on its long axis. This lateral rotation is necessary for clearance of the greater tuberosity under the acromial arch.

The clinically important considerations are that elevation is impossible without appropriate S-C and A-C movements, especially rotation of the clavicle on its long axis, without inferior glide of the humeral head, and without lateral rotation of the humerus on its long axis.

Furthermore, one must consider the motions occurring in the thoracic and lower cervical spines on shoulder movement. For example, bilateral elevation of the arms requires considerable thoracic extension; the person with a significant thoracic kyphosis will not be able to perform this movement throughout the full range. On unilateral elevation the upper thoracic spine must side-bend toward, the lower thoracic away from, the side of motion.

THE ELBOW

Component Motions

Extension

Superior glide of ulna on trochlea
Pronation of ulna relative to humerus
Abduction of ulna relative to humerus
Distal movement of radius on ulna
Pronation (inward rotation) of radius relative to humerus

Flexion

Inferior glide of ulna on trochlea
Supination of ulna relative to humerus
Adduction of ulna relative to humerus
Proximal movement of radius on ulna
Supination (outward rotation) of radius on humerus

Close-Packed Position

Extension.

Capsular Pattern

More limitation of flexion than extension.

FOREARM

Prosupination

Pronation—supination.

Proximal radioulnar joint and radiohumeral joint. This movement is essentially one of pure spin of the head of the radius on the capitellum and therefore one of roll and slide of the radius in the radial notch of the ulna and annular ligament.

Distal radioulnar joint. Here the radius is said to rotate around the head of the ulna, being largely a sliding movement. However, functionally the ulna also tends to move, backward and laterally during pronation and forward and medially during supination. We must therefore consider as component movements during pronation:

Palmar glide of the radius on ulna
Inward rotation of radius on ulna (looking palmarly)
Dorsal glide of ulna on radius
Outward rotation of ulna on radius (looking palmarly)
Abduction of ulna on humerus

The reverse would naturally occur on supination.

Capsular Pattern

Involvement of the distal radioulnar joint produces little limitation of movement, but there is pain at the extremes of pronation and supination.

THE WRIST

Radiocarpal Joint

Palmar flexion

Dorsal movement of proximal carpals (scaphoid and lunate) on radius and disk
Distraction of radiocarpal joint

Dorsiflexion

Palmar movement of proximal carpals on radius (the scaphoid also spins—supinates—on the radius at full wrist dorsiflexion)
Approximation of scaphoid and lunate to radius and disk

Radial deviation

Approximation of scaphoid to radius
Ulnar slide of the proximal carpals on the radius (this movement is quite limited and is somewhat increased by the tendency for the scaphoid to extend [slide palmarly and supinate] on the radius)

Ulnar Deviation

Distraction of scaphoid from radius
Radial slide of proximal carpals on radius

Ulnomeniscotriquetral Joint

This joint is primarily involved with pronation and supination of the forearm. During pronation and supination, the disk moves with the radius and carpals and must therefore sweep around the distal end of the ulna. During flexion and extension, the disk stays with the radius and ulna and movement occurs between the disk and the carpals. In this situation the disk acts as an ulnar extension of the distal radial joint surface to become, functionally, part of the radiocarpal joint.

During wrist radial deviation there is considerable distraction of the triquetrum and pisiform from the ulna, with approximation on ulnar deviation.

Midcarpal Joint

Palmarflexion

Dorsal slide of hamate and capitate on triquetrum and lunate
Palmar slide of trapezoid on scaphoid

Dorsiflexion. From full flexion to neutral, the reverse of the above takes place. At neutral the hamate, capitate, and trapezoid become close-packed on the scaphoid, and these four bones tend to move together in a palmar slide and supinatory spin on the radius, lunate, and triquetrum. **Note:** The scaphoid acts as a proximal carpal from neutral into palmarflexion and as a "distal carpal" from neutral into full dorsiflexion. Also note the supination and radial deviation that tends to occur on extreme dorsiflexion of the wrist.

Radial Deviation. There is some ulnar slide of the hamate and capitate on the trique-

trum and lunate, with considerable distraction of the base of the hamate from the lunate.

The trapezoid slides radially on the scaphoid.

Ulnar Deviation. This is the reverse of radial deviation. **Note:** The entire carpus might be divided into four functional units: (1) Hamate, capitate, trapezoid always acting as distal carpals; (2) scaphoid, acting as proximal carpal into flexion and distal carpal into extension; (3) triquetrum and lunate, always acting as proximal carpals; and (4) trapezium, acting primarily in its articulation with the first metacarpal of the thumb, playing little part in movements at the wrist.

Close-Packed Position

Of the wrist as a whole, extension (dorsiflexion) with radial deviation.

Capsular Pattern

Equal limitation of palmarflexion and dorsiflexion.

THE HAND

"Intermetacarpal Joints"

While these are not true synovial joints, movement does take place between the heads of the metacarpals on grasp and release.

Grasp. The metacarpals form an "arch" through the following movements:

Palmar movement of 2nd relative to 3rd, 4th relative to 3rd, and 5th relative to 4th metacarpal head.
Supination of 4th and 5th metacarpals, perhaps slight pronation of the 2nd.

Release. The arch is flattened through the reverse of the above movements.

Component Motions of the Metacarpophalangeal Joints

Flexion

Palmar glide of the base of the phalanx on the head of the metacarpal

Supination of the phalanx on the metacarpal, especially with grasp or pinch

Ulnar deviation of the phalanx on metacarpal, especially with grasp or pinch

Approximation of the phalanx and the metacarpal

Extension. Reverse of flexion.

Radial deviation

Radial slide of the base of the phalanx on the head of the metacarpal

Ulnar deviation, ulnar slide of the base of the phalanx

Component Motions of the Interphalangeal Joints

Flexion

Palmar glide of the base of the more distal phalanx on the head of the more proximal phalanx

Distraction of the distal phalanx on proximal phalanx

Supination of the distal phalanx on the more proximal phalanx (more at DIP than PIP)

Radial deviation of the distal phalanx on the more proximal phalanx

Extension. The reverse of flexion.

Component Motions of the Trapezio Metacarpal Joint

This is a sellar joint with the trapezium concave in the plane of the palm and convex perpendicularly.

Extension (radial deviation)

Ulnar slide of the base of the 1st metacarpal on the trapezium

A slight amount of lateral rotation (supination) occurs

Flexion. The opposite of extension.

Abduction (away from the plane of the palm). Palmar slide of the base of the first metacarpal.

Adduction. Dorsal slide of the base of the metacarpal.

Opposition. This is a combined movement with considerable conjunct rotation as a consequence of the impure swing and is easily visible by the rather marked medial rotation which occurs, allowing the thumb pad to oppose the pads of the fingers. It is typical for relatively more conjunct rotation to take place at a sellar joint such as this or the interphalangeal joints or humeroulnar joint than at ovoid joints.

Close-Packed Positions

Trapezio metacarpal joint: *opposition*
Metacarpophalangeal joint: *flexion*
Interphalangeal joints: *extension*

Capsular Patterns

Trapezio metacarpal joint: abduction and extension limited, flexion free
Metacarpophalangeal joint: more restricted in flexion than extension
Interphalangeal joints: more restricted in extension, some restriction of flexion

THE LOWER EXTREMITY

HIP

Component Motions

Flexion. Posterior and inferior glide of femoral head in acetabulum.

Abduction. Inferior glide of femoral head in acetabulum.

External Rotation. Anterior glide of femoral head.

Internal Rotation. Posterior glide of femoral head.

Close-Packed Position

Internal rotation with *extension* and *abduction.*

Capsular Pattern

Internal rotation and abduction are most restricted; flexion and extension are restricted; external rotation is relatively free.

KNEE

Component Motions

Flexion

Medial rotation of tibia on femur during first 15° to 20° of flexion from full extension
Posterior glide of tibia on femur
Inferior movement of patella
Inferior movement of fibula

Extension. The reverse of flexion.

Analysis of knee motion. The knee primarily moves about a single axis that lies horizontally in the frontal plane. If the tibia moves on a stationary femur, roll and slide occur in the same direction, but in the case of the femur moving on a fixed tibia, roll and slide occur in opposite directions. Toward the last 10° to 20° of extension, almost a pure roll takes place, the rolling phase being somewhat longer on the lateral side. Moving into flexion, the rolling motion between the joint surfaces gradually becomes more and more a sliding motion. Thus, the articular contact point on the femur gradually moves backward (while moving into flexion); the articular contact point on the tibia moves backward during the first phase of flexion, then gradually narrows down to a point (in the case of the femur moving in the tibia).

A length rotation also occurs between the femur and tibia during flexion and extension at this joint. This rotation is a necessary part of the normal joint kinematics and may be lost in certain pathologic conditions, such as a torn meniscus or adhered capsule. Considering the case of the femur moving on the tibia during the last, say, 30° of extension, the femur must rotate inward in order for close-packing and full extension to occur. There are many explanations for this phenomenon. Most include the fact that because the lateral femoral condyle is smaller, it reaches its close-packed congruent position in extension before the medial condyle does. In order for the medial condyle to continue movement, it must slide backward around an axis passing somewhere through the lateral femoral condyle. The resultant rotation of the *lateral* condyle forces the anterior segment of the lateral meniscus forward over the convex lateral tibia condyle such that the lateral femoral condyle is no longer congruent and may continue into somewhat more extension. Of course, this all happens simultaneously and continues until the knee becomes locked in its close-packed position of full extension (about 5° of hyperextension). In this position, the cruciates are pulled tight and twisted so as to prevent internal rotation of the tibia on the femur. The collaterals also become twisted relative to each other (the medial ligament passing downward and forward, the lateral ligament passing downward and backward) so as to prevent outward rotation of the tibia on the femur. Both sets of ligaments prevent further extension with help from the soft tissues posteriorly.

Close-Packed Position

Extension with lateral rotation.

Capsular Pattern

Flexion is most restricted; extension is somewhat restricted.

ANKLE (MORTISE)

Component Motions

Dorsiflexion. (1) Backward glide of talus on tibia; (2) spreading of distal tibiofibular joint.

Plantarflexion. The reverse of dorsiflexion.

Close-Packed Position

Dorsiflexion.

Capsular Pattern

Dorsiflexion and plantarflexion are both limited; plantarflexion slightly more so, unless the heel cord is tight.

SUBTALAR JOINT

Component Motions

This joint is essentially bicondylar. Of interest is the fact that the posterior facet of the talus on the calcaneus is a concave on convex surface, while the combined anterior and medial facet forms a convex on concave joint.

On eversion of the calcaneus on the talus, the posterior joint surface of the calcaneus must glide medially while the anterior and medial facets must glide laterally.

Close-Packed Position

Eversion.

Capsular Pattern

Inversion (varus) very restricted; eversion (valgus) is free.

FOREFOOT

Close-Packed Position

Supination of the forefoot relative to the calcaneus, such as decreasing the normal longitudinal arch, as happens when standing with feet wide apart.

Capsular Pattern

Pronation most limited.

ORIENTATION OF JOINT AXES

Remember that in the developing embryo the lower limb started out abducted and externally rotated so that the sole of the foot faced forward. During development, the leg must rotate medially and adduct. As a result, the femoral condyles are rotated inward (about 10° in the adult) in relation to the neck of the femur, and the shaft of the femur is adducted (forming an angle of about 125° in the adult) with respect to the femoral neck.

The shaft of the tibia is rotated about 25° outwardly so the axis of the ankle mortise is 25° outwardly rotated, relative to the knee.

The axis of the subtalar joint runs about 20° from back and out to front and in.

Index

Numbers followed by an f represent a figure; t following a page number indicates tabular material.